Psychiatry in Practice
Education, Experience, and Expertise

Edited by

Andrea Fiorillo
Department of Psychiatry,
University of Naples SUN, Naples, Italy

Umberto Volpe
Department of Psychiatry,
University of Naples SUN, Naples, Italy

Dinesh Bhugra
Institute of Psychiatry, King's College London, UK

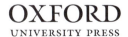
OXFORD
UNIVERSITY PRESS

OXFORD
UNIVERSITY PRESS

Great Clarendon Street, Oxford, OX2 6DP,
United Kingdom

Oxford University Press is a department of the University of Oxford.
It furthers the University's objective of excellence in research, scholarship,
and education by publishing worldwide. Oxford is a registered trade mark of
Oxford University Press in the UK and in certain other countries

Published in the United States of America by Oxford University Press
198 Madison Avenue, New York, NY 10016, United States of America

British Library Cataloguing in Publication Data

Data available

Library of Congress Control Number: 2015937789

ISBN 978-0-19-872364-6

Printed and bound by
CPI Group (UK) Ltd, Croydon, CR0 4YY

Foreword

Early career psychiatrists, as well as trainees in psychiatry, need a much broader exposure these days to a number of skills and competencies than ever before. These groups form the future of psychiatric practice. As there are variations in curricula and training patterns in Europe, often skills related to personal management and managing resources are not taught. This book fills that need. It has contributions by early career psychiatrists, with support from more senior colleagues, and that is what makes it unique. The European Psychiatric Association, being itself involved in education and training across Europe, is very pleased to support this exciting project.

This book successfully provides an overview of a range of skills and processes. The skills are needed in order to develop professionally, so that clinicians can provide services which will be efficient, efficacious, and engage patients and their families. The authors and editors have filled a major gap in the field and have done so very well. I hope that trainees and early career psychiatrists will benefit from this.

Professor Dr Wolfgang Gaebel
President, European Psychiatric Association

Preface

We are delighted to bring you this volume on psychiatry in practice. There are several novel things about this venture. First and foremost, this book combines the required clinical and non-clinical skills that psychiatrists of all ages need through their working careers. Secondly, the lead for each chapter has been taken by early career psychiatrists who are aware of what they require to function successfully. Thirdly, they have been ably supported by some of the senior and eminent figures in the field who have provided help, encouragement, and, most importantly, mentoring.

The book is aimed at all psychiatrists, but those in the early stages of training or who have just started to establish themselves will find it particularly useful on several key issues. We believe that there is much to be shared across Europe with varying training periods and programmes and healthcare systems. We expect that early career psychiatrists will continue to develop together, and plan and deliver services which will be culturally appropriate and sensitive for their patients.

We take this opportunity to thank the European Psychiatric Association for supporting this venture and Professor Wolfgang Gaebel for writing the Foreword. We are also thankful to our authors, both senior and less senior, for contributing effectively and delivering material on time in spite of their busy schedules. Finally, we would like to thank Pete Stevenson and Lauren Dunn and their team at Oxford University Press, who have been a total pleasure to work with.

Andrea Fiorillo
Umberto Volpe
Dinesh Bhugra

Contents

Contributors

Ahmed A. Abd Elgawad
Institute of Psychiatry,
Faculty of Medicine,
Ain Shams University, Egypt

Umut Altunoz
Centre for Transcultural Psychiatry
and Psychotherapy,
Wahrendorff Clinic,
Hannover, Germany

Olivier Andlauer
East London NHS Foundation Trust,
London, UK

Julian Beezhold
Norfolk & Suffolk NHS Foundation
Trust, Norwich, UK

Nagendra Bendi
Norfolk & Suffolk NHS Foundation
Trust, Norwich, UK

Sabyasachi Bhaumik
Learning Disability Service,
Leicester Frith Hospital, UK

Dinesh Bhugra
Institute of Psychiatry,
King's College London, UK

Giuseppe Carrà
Division of Psychiatry,
Faculty of Brain Sciences,
University College London, UK

Daniele Carretta
Department of Translational
Medicine and Surgery,
University of Milano Bicocca, Milan,
Italy

Marisa Casanova Dias
Camden and Islington NHS
Foundation Trust,
University College London Partners
training scheme,
London, UK

Francesco Cazzola
Bologna Transcultural
Psychosomatic Team,
Department of Medical and
Surgical Sciences,
Alma Mater Studiorum Bologna
University, Italy

Massimo Clerici
Department of Translational Medicine
and Surgery,
University of Milano Bicocca,
Milan, Italy

Patrick Corrigan
College of Psychology,
Illinois Institute of Technology,
Chicago, USA

Nicholas Deakin
Barts Health NHS Trust,
Queen Mary University,
London, UK

Giovanni de Girolamo
St John of God Clinical
Research Centre,
Brescia, Italy

Corrado De Rosa
Department of Psychiatry,
University of Naples SUN,
Naples, Italy

Valeria Del Vecchio
Department of Psychiatry,
University of Naples SUN,
Naples, Italy

Albert Diefenbacher
Department of Psychiatry and
Psychotherapy,
University Affiliated Hospital
of the Charité at Berlin,
Germany

Lisa Dixon
New York State Psychiatric Institute,
Columbia University Medical Center,
New York, USA

Annegret Dreher
Department of Psychiatry and
Psychotherapy,
University Affiliated Hospital
of the Charité at Berlin, Germany

Hussien Elkholy
Institute of Psychiatry,
Faculty of Medicine,
Ain Shams University, Egypt

Defne Eraslan
Department of Psychiatry,
Acibadem University, Istanbul, Turkey

Sara Evans-Lacko
Health Service and Population Research
Department,
Institute of Psychiatry, Psychology &
Neuroscience,
King's College London, UK

Silvia Ferrari
Department of Diagnostic-Clinical
Medicine and Public Health,
University of Modena and Reggio
Emilia; Department of Mental Health,
Modena, Italy

Clive Field
Surrey and Borders Partnership NHS
Foundation Trust,
Surrey, UK

Andrea Fiorillo
Department of Psychiatry,
University of Naples SUN,
Naples, Italy

Christian Foerster
Charité University, Berlin, Germany

Silvana Galderisi
Department of Psychiatry,
University of Naples SUN,
Naples, Italy

Shweta Gangavati
Leicestershire Partnership NHS Trust,
Leicester, UK

Domenico Giacco
Department of Psychiatry,
University of Naples SUN, Naples, Italy

Philip Gorwood
CMME-Sainte-Anne Hospital,
Paris, France

Iris Tatjana Graef-Calliess
Research group for Social and
Transcultural Psychiatry,
Hannover Medical School,
Centre for Transcultural Psychiatry
and Psychotherapy,
Wahrendorff Clinic, Hanover, Germany

Petra C. Gronholm
Health Service and Population Research
Department,
Institute of Psychiatry,
King's College London, UK

Sinan Guloksuz
Department of Psychiatry,
Institute of Psychiatry, Psychology &
Neuroscience,
Yale University School of Medicine,
New Haven, USA

Ahmed Hankir
Bedfordshire Centre for Mental Health
Research in Association
with Cambridge University,
The Royal Oldham Hospital,
Greater Manchester, UK

Cécile Hanon
Regional Ressource Center of Old Age
Psychiatry,
University Hospital of Paris Ouest, France

Andreas Heinz
Department of Psychiatry and
Psychotherapy,
Charité University Medical Centre,
Berlin, Germany

Marc H. M. Hermans
Child and Adolescent Psychiatry,
Mechelen, Belgium

Reinhard Heun
Department of Psychiatry and
Psychotherapy,
University of Bonn, Germany

Fritz Hohagen
Department of Psychiatry and
Psychotherapy,
University of Lübeck, Germany

Clare Holt
South London and Maudsley NHS
Foundation Trust,
London, UK

Muj Husain
Department of Experimental Psychology
and Nuffield Department of Clinical
Neurosciences,
University of Oxford, UK

Rutger Jan van der Gaag
Radboud University Medical Centre
Nijmegen, The Netherlands

Sarah B. Johnson
Department of Psychiatry and
Behavioral Sciences,
University of Louisville, USA

Vesna Jordanova
Institute of Psychiatry, Kings College,
London, United Kingdom

Nikolina Jovanovic
Unit for Social and Community
Psychiatry,
WHO Collaborating Centre
for Mental Health Services
Development,
Queen Mary University of London,
London, UK

Gurvinder Kalra
La Trobe Regional Hospital Mental
Health Services,
Traralgon, Victoria, Australia

Marianne Kastrup
Psychiatric Centre Copenhagen,
Centre for Transcultural Psychiatry,
Copenhagen, Denmark

Patrick Kelly
Child and Adolescent Psychiatry,
Bloomberg Children's Center,
The Johns Hopkins Hospital,
Baltimore, USA

Sayeed Khan
Learning Disability Service,
Leicester Frith Hospital, UK

Reza Kiani
Learning Disability Service,
Leicester Frith Hospital, UK

Tamas Kurimay
Department of Psychiatry and
Psychiatric Rehabilitation,
Saint John Hospital,
Budapest, Hungary

Linda Lam
Department of Psychiatry,
The Chinese University of Hong Kong,
Shatin,
Hong Kong

Zuzana Lattova
Max Planck Institute of Psychiatry,
Munich, Germany

Alexis Lepetit
Charpennes Geriatric Hospital,
University Hospital Lyon, France

Mario Luciano
Department of Psychiatry,
University of Naples SUN, Naples, Italy

Gregory Lydall
Department of Molecular Psychiatry,
Mental Health Sciences,
University College London, UK

Amit Malik
Formerly of Surrey and Borders
Partnership NHS Foundation Trust,
Surrey, UK

Giorgio Mattei
Department of Diagnostic-Clinical
Medicine and Public Health,
University of Modena and Reggio
Emilia, Modena, Italy

Adriana Mihai
Department of Psychiatry,
University of Medicine and Pharmacy,
Târgu-Mureş, Romania

Ana Moscoso
Department of Child and Adolescent
Psychiatry, Hospital D. Estefânia,
Lisbon, Portugal

Driss Moussaoui
Department of Psychiatry of Casablanca,
Ibn Rushd University Psychiatric Centre,
Casablanca, Morocco

Michael Musalek
Anton Proksch Institute, Vienna, Austria

Alexander Nawka
Institute of Neuropsychiatric Care,
Prague, Czech Republic

Carla Obradors-Tarragó
Centre for Biomedical Research
in Mental Health, CIBERSAM
Madrid, Spain

Maria Orlova
Moscow Research Institute of Psychiatry,
Moscow, Russia

Claudia Palumbo
Department of Medical Basic Sciences,
Neuroscience and Sense Organs,
University of Bari, Italy

Maja Pantovic Stefanovic
Clinic of Psychiatry,
Clinical Centre of Serbia,
Belgrade, Serbia

Olga Kazakova
Psychiatric Clinic of Minsk City,
Minsk, Republic of Belarus

Max Pemberton
St Ann's Hospital,
London, UK

Felipe Picon
Hospital de Clínicas de Porto Alegre,
Porto Alegre, Brazil

Luca Pingani
Human Resources Development,
Local Health Authority,
Reggio Emilia, Italy

Mariana Pinto da Costa
Hospital de Magalhães Lemos,
University of Porto,
Porto, Portugal

Anita Riecher-Rössler
Psychiatric University Clinic, Basel,
Switzerland

Florian Riese
Psychiatric University Hospital Zurich,
Division of Psychiatry Research and
Division of Psychogeriatric Medicine,
Zurich, Switzerland

Martina Rojnic Kuzman
Zagreb School of Medicine and
University Hospital Centre Zagreb,
Zagreb, Croatia

Wulf Rössler
Department of Psychiatry,
Psychotherapy and Psychosomatics,
Psychiatric Hospital,
University of Zurich, Switzerland

César Ruiz-Díaz
Psychiatry Department,
School of Medical Sciences,
National University of Asunción,
Paraguay

Jerzy Samochowiec
Department of Psychiatry,
Pomeranian Medical University,
Szczecin, Poland

Gaia Sampogna
Department of Psychiatry,
University of Naples SUN,
Naples, Italy

Norman Sartorius
Association for the Improvement of
Mental Health Programmes,
Geneva, Switzerland

Jordan Sibeoni
Department of Adolescent Psychiatry
Centre Hospitalier d'Argenteuil
Paris Diderot University, France

Giovanni Stanghellini
University of Chieti-Pescara,
Chieti, Italy

Philipp Sterzer
Department of Psychiatry and
Psychotherapy, Charité University
Medical Centre, Berlin, Germany

Ilaria Tarricone
Bologna Transcultural
Psychosomatic Team,
Department of Medical
and Surgical Sciences,
Alma Mater Studiorum Bologna
University,
Italy

Allan Tasman
Department of Psychiatry and
Behavioral Sciences,
University of Louisville, USA

Bino Thomas
Department of Social Work,
Christ University, Bangalore, India

Alex Till
Health Education North West,
Mersey,
UK

Julio Torales
School of Medical Sciences,
National University of Asunción,
Paraguay

Antonio Ventriglio
Department of Clinical and
Experimental Medicine,
University of Foggia, Italy

Umberto Volpe
Department of Psychiatry,
University of Naples SUN,
Naples, Italy

Michael J. Wise
Consultant Psychiatrist,
Wiser Minds, Manchester,
UK

Chapter 1

Role and responsibilities of psychiatrists

Andrea Fiorillo, Umberto Volpe, and Dinesh Bhugra

Introduction

In their classic volume, Hunter and MacAlpine[1] clearly highlighted, for the first time, the evolving role of psychiatry since 1535, although other accounts from earlier times in other healthcare systems also exist.[2,3] At that time, doctors dealing with mental illness were known as 'alienists'. The role and responsibilities of alienists were clear and well defined, as was their professional aim which was to protect society from madness and to place in custody those with mental illness. Asylums were established in different European countries throughout the seventeenth century and were usually located far away from urban areas. During the following decades, however, psychiatry emerged as a proper medical specialty and it still remains one, in spite of the many recent attempts to revert it to a social discipline only. The role of psychiatrists in society, their professional status, and their aims changed significantly in the twentieth century, in particular after the deinstitutionalization process at the end of the century. These changes significantly influence the current standards of clinical practice and the profession as a whole.

Various professional bodies have produced guidance papers on what it means to be a psychiatrist in these days, to further define the role and the responsibilities of psychiatrists in clinical and other settings. In this chapter, we will address the current role and main responsibilities for psychiatrists, reviewing the guidance provided by the Canadian Medical Education Directions for Specialists (CanMEDS) physician competency framework (adopted in 1996 by the Royal College of Physicians and Surgeons in Canada[4]), the Royal College of Psychiatrists,[5] and the Union Européene des Médecins Spécialistes (UEMS) in its charter on the training of medical specialists in the European Union (EU)[6,7].

Changes to society, changes to psychiatry

The last few decades have brought significantly rapid changes to many aspects of society, ranging from health to communication, from ethics to politics and economics. Such changes are in turn related to globalization, to economic and demographic drives on the one hand, and to the rapid spread of social media on the other. Psychiatry, as a significant component of the healthcare system, has also been profoundly affected by these changes. Some of these societal modifications are also reflected in the recent changes of psychiatric nomenclature—'doctors' are often called 'professionals', a 'psychiatrist' is now a 'mental health specialist', a 'patient' is known as a 'client', 'user', or in some circumstances even 'customer', while a 'psychiatric nurse' is called a 'care co-ordinator', 'case manager', or 'practitioner'. In this chapter, we will not adventure into detailing the pros and cons of such definitions; we want to highlight only that they reflect a change that is still happening. The role and responsibilities of psychiatrists may change under social pressures, but the core responsibilities of diagnosis and management remain in their hands.

The discipline and practice of present-day psychiatry deals not only with mental illness, but with behavioural and emotional disorders as well. Psychiatric practice often utilizes biopsychosocial approaches in understanding aetiological factors as well as management. Frequently, psychiatrists are accused of following the 'medical model' too closely,[8] and the critics ignore the fact that medicine itself is also a social discipline. Indeed, the term 'medical model' is used as a pejorative term to suggest that psychiatrists are not holistic in their approach, but only concerned with formal diagnosis and medication. Any social factor such as diet, religious views, and attitudes to alcohol and smoking, can affect how drugs are absorbed and act. Influences from society determine what is seen as deviant or sick and this may be more influential in psychiatry than in other medical disciplines. Social understanding of illness contributes to how symptoms are identified and what 'idioms of distress' are used.

Like all other doctors, psychiatrists deal with a wide range of conditions varying from childhood disorders (such as conduct disorders and nocturnal bedwetting) to dementia at the other end of the age spectrum, as well as co-morbidities such as addictions and severe mental illness, physical and mental illness, and personality disorders and mental illness. They also provide assessment and management of a number of conditions ranging from sexual problems to common mental disorders (such as depression and anxiety), from learning disability in children or adults to personality disorders. Depending upon the availability of resources, psychiatrists may themselves offer many interventions or supervise and support other professionals in the delivery of such interventions; these strategies include not only medical care, but also aspects of social care, psychological interventions (with or without medical treatments), and empowerment strategies for the most vulnerable and marginalized people in society.

Mental health and mental illness

Mental health was classically defined as the absence of mental disease[9] or, more recently, as a state of the organism which allows the full performance of all its functions or as a state of balance within oneself and between oneself and one's physical and social environment.[8,10] Mental well-being and mental illness can be seen as the opposite ends of a spectrum of conditions. In Maslow's hierarchy, mental and physical health are related to the satisfaction of basic needs such as food, shelter, and social functioning, but the so-called 'meta-needs'(such as beauty, goodness, justice, and wholeness) are also essential for satisfying personal needs.[11] Mental health is also an 'enabler' for the individual in forming and maintaining effective and intimate relationships. Mental health vulnerabilities can result from both internal and personal factors (such as low self-esteem, sense of entrapment, helplessness, and sadness) and from external or social and economic factors (such as poor housing, poverty, unemployment, discrimination or abuse, cultural conflicts, and stigma).[12]

Mental health also deals with how individuals think and feel about themselves, their life, and how they cope with adversities.[13] Mental health has been also defined as a state of equipoise and balance, in which individuals are at peace with themselves, able to function effectively socially, and to look after their own basic as well as higher needs.[9] Positive functioning usually includes managing changes, relationships, and emotions in a constructive manner. On the other hand, the expression 'mental illness' is used to describe a variety of behavioural patterns which disrupt a smooth functioning of life. It is arguably a catch-all definition for a largely medical model of pathology arising from biological vulnerabilities, social maladjustments, and psychological disturbances (within the framework of the classical biopsychosocial model of aetiology and management of psychiatric disorders[14]). These mental disturbances depend upon definitions of abnormality on the basis of statistical, physiological, psychological, behavioural, or humanistic paradigms.[15] Thus, what is 'abnormal', and how this is defined, lies at the very root of tensions between the professionals and society.

In the past two decades, concepts such as 'mental health issues' or 'mental health problems' have been used increasingly in Europe, giving the impression that these disorders carry with them a lower degree of distress, difficulty, and functional impairment. With these terms and approach, it seems that these conditions, although common, are not serious, or that they even lack any underlying pathophysiological cause. This devalues, minimizes, and underestimates the gravity and degree of disability caused by mental illness. It is therefore important to properly define the concepts of mental health and mental illness, so that the role and responsibilities of the psychiatrists will become clearer.

The role of stigma to access psychiatric interventions

The capacity of psychiatric interventions to improve mental state and even physical health is often underestimated by the general public and other professionals, although recent evidence shows that psychotropic drugs are among the most effective interventions available in the whole of medicine and that antipsychotic medication has comparative efficacy with medications used in general medicine.[16] Mental health services are an essential feature of any contemporary civilized society, but they are still too often stigmatized and neglected in terms of provision of resources and support. Internal stigma (from professionals) and external stigma (from society, policy makers, and others) have a major impact on patients, families, and carers.

Although research is progressing rapidly, specific biological markers that help with the diagnosing of psychiatric illnesses are still missing. The burden on society of neuropsychiatric conditions (a term used to include psychiatric conditions) is massive, but stigmatizing attitudes towards mental illness, mentally ill people, and psychiatrists makes it relatively difficult to obtain funding and treatments in many settings. Stigma towards the mentally ill and mental illness discourages those in need from seeking help. Psychiatrists may experience stigma from other mental health professionals and medical colleagues, contributing to a sense of rejection and isolation. Thus, a key challenge for society is to adequately deal with and significantly reduce stigma.

Historically, private 'madhouses' and 'public mental asylums' that looked after people with mental illness were often large austere institutions located beyond the limits of the cities and towns that they served. Although often set up with good intentions (and at times manifesting good standards of care), such institutions were among the first to suffer in economic crises in terms of resources and acquired terrible reputations, thus becoming further stigmatized. Although psychiatry should take responsibility for ill-conceived and sometimes harmful practices used in the past (just as in medicine and surgery), it is also important to acknowledge the huge strides that have been made by modern psychiatry towards delivering humane, evidence-based, and cost-effective treatments. Recognition of the damaging effects of social exclusion, stigma, and institutionalization on people with mental illness has led to policies of deinstitutionalization and of community care across the globe.

The laudable and welcome aim of deinstitutionalization is the empowerment of patients and their recovery. However, this has been implemented with variable enthusiasm, commitment, and success across the world, thereby sometimes resulting in new exclusion and stigma. The social and psychiatric authoritarianism, coercion, and abuse have, at times, been replaced by the all too frequent new reality of rejection and neglect. A study from six European countries[10] found that forensic beds had increased in all six countries and the number of general psychiatric beds had gone down in five countries; in only two of them, this reduction outweighed the number of forensic beds, thereby indicating an increase in containment. Such realities are a constant reminder that the practice of psychiatry requires clear moral and ethical frameworks based on preservations of human rights. Psychiatrists must have total commitment to the individual patient and his/her personal welfare. The patient is at the heart of the therapeutic interactions, being also surrounded by kinship, family, and society at large. Thus, it is critical to negotiate a clear 'contract' with society, which should be reviewed and updated regularly.

Mental disorders and their treatment

Psychiatric treatment requires commitment to work collaboratively with the mentally ill and their families as well as with other mental health professionals. Psychiatrists need to be clear about their responsibilities irrespective of resources. Psychiatrists as leaders need not only to engage with the public, but also to educate them. At the same time, psychiatrists have a key responsibility in providing clinical leadership in the development, quality assurance, efficiency, and protection of mental health services, which must be available to all citizens.

The challenges for psychiatry in the twenty-first century include the need to promote mental health and prevent mental illness. These notions need to be introduced into public health also through research, education, and teaching efforts. There is still a lot of debate about the concepts of mental disorder itself. Eisenberg[17] noted that the human brain is influenced by both biological and social factors and that nature and nurture stand in reciprocity; the fact that psychiatry is both biological and social often gets forgotten, as both sides of the argument may take on very reductionist views.

Role of the psychiatrist

There have been several debates on the role of psychiatrists worldwide, both in modern and ancient times. The Royal College of Psychiatrists[5] has recently proposed that the key aspects of the psychiatrist's role should be at least those listed in Table 1.1.

The CanMEDS[4] model puts the medical expertise at the core, along with the roles of communicator, collaborator, manager, advocate, scholar, and professional. Although the role of the psychiatrist as an 'enabler' and 'facilitator' is mentioned only in the section on communication, this can be considered as a significant aspect.

Table 1.1 Roles of the psychiatrist according to the Royal College of Psychiatrists

Patients' care	Patients need good doctors who make patients' care their main professional concern and who are competent, up to date, honest, and trustworthy. Doctors can and must deliver the best care patients need and deserve. Thus, like other physicians, the primary duty of any psychiatrist is the ability to diagnose and manage with the best evidence-based care for patients. Psychological and social factors contribute to understanding aetiology and management.
	A major responsibility for psychiatrists is to engage with patients and their families, keeping the individual at the core of the therapeutic interaction and alliance. They need to consider proximal factors which affect the patient, including employment, family, and peers, and also distal factors, such as society and culture. One of the major expectations of the psychiatrist is their ability to tolerate high levels of anxiety in situations of uncertainty, while controlling the team's anxiety and holding hope for the patient. A key skill of psychiatrists is to be empathic and engage patients in effective therapeutic relationships. For patients who are receiving treatments from primary care physicians and/or other mental health professionals, the psychiatrist must act as an advocate and set standards for high-quality care. Psychiatrists are uniquely trained and skilled in the application of the full biopsychosocial model, while other professions utilize a less holistic and more limited approach.
Management of complexity and severity	Medical expertise embedded in the psychiatrist's training and practice is the key to diagnosis and management, especially in complex situations. Co-morbidities, such as severe mental illness and addictions, or psychiatric disorders and underlying personality disorders, or a combination of physical and mental illness require complex and integrated interventions, and psychiatrists are best placed to deliver these. This ability to understand and manage the complexity of illnesses as well as complex healthcare systems is an important responsibility of psychiatrists.

(continued)

Table 1.1 (continued) Roles of the psychiatrist according to the Royal College of Psychiatrists

	With information overload and changing expectations from patients, the ability to sift through complex data and evidence and then apply this to the individual needs of the patient is a critical skill. Understanding the evidence and its application to clinical efficacy of medications or combined therapies is an important part of a clinician's role. Medication in mental disorders is one of many available strategies. Not surprisingly, it is the responsibility of psychiatrists to not only evaluate the patient, but also stop inappropriate treatments, whether they are medications or psychotherapies. This core expertise is the cornerstone of managing complexity in psychiatry. Patients should not be prescribed psychotropic medication unnecessarily, but neither should they be denied such medication out of ignorance or prejudice. Holding hope for the patient and managing patients' and their families' anxieties is part of the psychiatrist's clinical responsibility.
Risk assessment and management	Assessing and managing risks are important responsibilities of psychiatrists and must be agreed upon in an implicit contract between psychiatry and society. Local legal and statutory contexts should enable psychiatrists to determine and respond to risk. Managing risk in the context of stigma and discrimination is a particularly relevant skill that improves the therapeutic alliance and is a skill for which psychiatrists are well trained. In all cases, the least restrictive but appropriate approach should be used. Wherever possible, treatment must be carried out in explicit agreement and collaboration with the patient. Patient choice is extremely important. Sometimes, however, the patient's illness may cloud their judgement very severely. In such cases, the psychiatrist has to take on the responsibility for enacting compulsory detention and treatment under mental health law in order to protect the patient from harm.
Teaching and training	Psychiatrists, like all doctors, have a long-life commitment to reflective learning and also to teaching patients, families, and other health professionals. Key responsibilities of psychiatrists are the critical appraisal of available evidence, providing mentorship to junior colleagues or to other mental health professionals, and engaging in ethical research and training. Psychiatrists should be able to act as role models, educators, and mentors, and carry on the education of younger generations.
Research and innovation	Not everyone is interested in or able to carry out research, but all psychiatrists should be able to interpret new findings and their application to clinical settings. Psychiatrists, along with basic scientists, other mental health professionals, service users, and carers have key roles in researching the causes, the maintaining factors, and the appropriate treatments for mental disorders.

(continued)

Table 1.1 (continued) Roles of the psychiatrist according to the Royal College of Psychiatrists

	Innovation includes providing the right balance of efficacious and efficient mental health services. Community mental health services are necessary to support families and carers in shouldering the burden and providing effective treatments. However, these must be supplemented by hospital services, when needed. Psychiatric services within general hospitals are essential as poor physical health affects mentally ill people and as increasing longevity will lead to further medical co-morbidities in patients.
Advocate/facilitator/ enabler	Applying ethical principles and dealing with discrimination, prejudices, and stigma are important skills that psychiatrists must have. Stigma and discrimination against mental illness, mentally- ill individuals, and mental health professionals is a big challenge to overcome. Psychiatrists should advocate for their patients, their families, mental health services, and the profession as a whole. They must facilitate the patient's journey through the healthcare system, which can be a bewildering and complex process.
Clinical leadership	There is no doubt that multidisciplinary team work can help patients' recovery through a range of approaches in various settings (such as hospital, outpatients, and community mental health location). Psychiatrists must be able to provide leadership in planning and delivering services which are accessible and appropriate. Leadership skills include not only clinical decision making but also managing teams and their dynamics, and taking on ambassadorial roles while being aware of potential changes in policies and resource issues.

Source data from: Royal College of Psychiatrists, *Role of the consultant psychiatrist: Leadership and excellence in mental health services*. Occasional Paper OP74, Copyright (2010).

Physician's mission

The doctor's mission can no longer be considered as one of simply providing good clinical care to the patient. Other roles, such as management and leadership, are now necessary aspects of medical professionalism. Health policies are now strongly influenced by the often conflicting free market principles, such as value for money, competition, privatization, political agendas, and universal healthcare coverage. This implies that medicine has to face new economic and political pressures. To competently and successfully care for mentally ill patients, mental health professionals need to fulfil roles and bear responsibilities not only towards patients' care but also towards other team members, their institutions, and their wider academic and scientific community. The importance of psychiatrists participating or influencing administration structures and decisions must not be undervalued. If psychiatrists are not part of the decision-making process, the vacant space may be filled by other professionals, who will then shape the environment and conditions in which psychiatrists and patients interact, and in a way that may not always be beneficial to the patient.

Over the past years, several challenges—both 'internal' and 'external'—have emerged for the medical and psychiatric professions (Table 1.2).

Table 1.2 Internal and external challenges to the psychiatric profession

Internal factors	Decreasing confidence about diagnosis and classification
	Decreasing confidence about therapeutic interventions
	Lack of a coherent theoretical knowledge basis
External factors	Real or perceived discontent from patients and families
	Competition from other professions
	Negative image, stigma, and discrimination
	Repeated policy changes over which the profession may not have any control or input

Source data from: Hunter R, MacAlpine R. *Three hundred years of psychiatry, 1535–1860*, Copyright (1982); Carlisle Publishing; Royal College of Psychiatry. UEMS Section for Psychiatry. *Charter on training of medical specialists in the EU: requirements for the specialty of psychiatry*, Copyright (2000); *World Psychiatry*, 9, Katschnig H. Are psychiatrists an endangered species? Observations on internal and external challenges to the profession, p. 21–8, Copyright (2010); Royal College of Psychiatry. UEMS Section for Psychiatry—European Board of Psychiatry. *The profile of a psychiatrist*, Copyright (2005); *Int Rev Psychiatry*, 25, Fiorillo A, Malik A, Luciano M, Del Vecchio V, Sampogna G, Del Gaudio L, et al., Challenges for trainees in psychiatry and early career psychiatrists, p. 431–7, Copyright (2013), Informa.

Psychiatric competencies

Undergraduate (medical school) and postgraduate (residency programmes) training are crucial steps for the development of competent mental healthcare professionals. Traditionally, the core of postgraduate psychiatric training has consisted of a combination of clinical rotations in a variety of medical and psychiatric specialized services. This should ensure that experience is gained in treating patients in a wide range of settings (inpatient, outpatient, community, and emergency). However, there is still a huge variation in training between countries, and sometimes even within the same countries. Standards have been set by local, national, and international professional bodies, but often resources and the environment influence the levels and standards of training. Postgraduate psychiatric training schemes in the majority of European countries are developed and evaluated by national education policy makers. During the last decades, the emphasis has been on harmonization across different sites.[6] In Europe, the Section of Psychiatry of the UEMS was established to facilitate this process. In 2003, the UEMS made a number of recommendations for the effective implementation of training programmes in psychiatry, covering the structure of such programmes, competency-based training standards, standards for training institutions, trainers, and supervisors, and quality assurance mechanisms.[18] However, despite these directives, recent publications still show significant differences in content and quality of training curricula across Europe.[7,16,20,21]

Moreover, even with the promotion of these standards, important aspects of 'real-life' psychiatry are sometimes ignored in many educational and training programmes. This discrepancy has occasionally left trainees and young psychiatrists somewhere in the middle between traditional and contemporary psychiatrists, and unprepared to meet the needs of modern health services and society at large. With these dilemmas in mind, the definitions of core competencies (and of training) that a psychiatrist of the twenty-first century needs to acquire, are of outmost importance. Thus, the definition of the role of the psychiatrist implies the need for corresponding alignment of the education system.

Conclusions and the way forward

The challenges for psychiatrists in the twenty-first century will include the need to encourage the promotion of mental health and prevention of mental illness.[22] Similarly, research and teaching will need to become an essential responsibility for psychiatrists. Although the core underlying role of the psychiatrist will remain the same, responsibilities will change in relation to many factors including healthcare and social systems, as well as financial resources. However, it is essential that core competencies remain the same across countries so that competency-based training can be delivered. There is the need to agree on basic principles of psychiatric practice so that training curricula can be adapted accordingly. In any case, whatever competencies and roles will be considered, the main responsibility of psychiatrists worldwide will be to ensure that patients get the best possible consideration they need and deserve.

References

1 **Hunter R, MacAlpine R**. *Three hundred years of psychiatry, 1535–1860*. New York: Carlisle Publishing; 1982.

2 **Bhugra D**. Psychiatry in ancient Indian texts: a review. *Hist Psych* 1992; **10**:167–86.

3 **Caraka samhita,** *volumes I–VI*. Jamnagar, India: Shree Gulab Kunverba Ayurvedic Society; 1949.

4 **Frank JR**. (ed.) *The CanMEDS 2005 physician competency framework. Better standards; better physicians; better care*. Ottawa: The Royal College of Physicians and Surgeons of Canada; 2005.

5 Royal College of Psychiatrists (RCP). *Role of the consultant psychiatrist. Leadership and excellence in mental health services. Occasional paper 74*. London: RCP; 2010.

6 UEMS Section for Psychiatry. *Charter on training of medical specialists in the EU: requirements for the specialty of psychiatry*. Geneva: UEMS; 2003. Available at: http://uemspsychiatry.org/wp-content/uploads/2013/09/Chapter6–11.10.03.pdf.

7 UEMS Section for Psychiatry; participants of the fourth meeting of leaders of European psychiatry. *Consensus statement—Psychiatric services focused on a community: challenges for the training of future psychiatrists*. Geneva: UEMS; 2004.

8 **Szasz T**. Myth of mental illness. *Am Psychologist* 1960; **16**:113–8.

9 **Bhugra D, Till A, Sartorius N**. What is mental health? *Int J Soc Psych* 2013; **59**:3–4.

10 **Sartorius N**. *Fighting for mental health*. Cambridge: Cambridge University Press; 2002.

11 **Maslow AH**. *Toward a psychology of being*. New York: D. Van Nostrand Company; 1968.

12 Health Education Authority (HEA). *Mental health promotion: a quality framework*. London: HEA; 1997.

13 Mental Health Foundation (MHF). *What works for you?* London: MHF; 2008.

14 **Katschnig H**. Are psychiatrists an endangered species? Observations on internal and external challenges to the profession. *World Psych* 2010; **9**:21–8.

15 **Kristal L**. *ABC of psychology*. London: Michael Joseph; 1981.

16 **Leucht S, Hierl S, Kissling W, Dold M, Davis JM**. Putting the efficacy of psychiatric and general medicine medication into perspective: review of meta-analyses. *Br J Psychiatry* 2012; **200**:97–106.

17 **Eisenberg L**. The social construction of the human brain. *Am J Psych* 1995; **152**:1563–75.

18 UEMS Section for Psychiatry; European Board of Psychiatry. *The profile of a psychiatrist*. Geneva: UEMS; 2005. Available at: http://www.aen.es/web/docs/perfilpsiquiatraUEMS.pdf.

19 **Fiorillo A, Malik A, Luciano M, et al**. Challenges for trainees in psychiatry and early career psychiatrists. *Int Rev Psychiatry* 2013; **25**:431–7.

20 **Oakley C, Malik A**. Psychiatric training in Europe. *The Psychiatrist* 2010; **34**:447–50.

21 **Kuzman MR, Giacco D, Simmons M, et al**. Psychiatry training in Europe: view from the trenches. *Med Teach* 2012; **34**:e708–17.

22 **Bhugra D, Carlile A**. *Starting today—the future of mental health services*. London: Mental Health Foundation; 2013.

Chapter 2

How to develop leadership skills

Alex Till, Andrea Fiorillo, and Dinesh Bhugra

Introduction

Psychiatrists, as doctors, are legally and ethically bound to adhere to the standards outlined by their regulatory bodies. Although the priority for good doctors is to provide high-quality clinical care, they have wider responsibilities to their patients, colleagues, and the healthcare organizations in which they work. Leadership is one of these responsibilities and underpins all aspects of the medical care being delivered by the doctor, irrespective of their role within the hierarchy. It is vital not just for those responsible for creating and delivering the strategic vision for our mental health services, but also for those working on the front line of service delivery. Leadership must be held in high esteem, both by the individual developing their leadership skills and by the organization in which they work.

Aspiring to the highest standards of excellence and professionalism, with patients at the heart of care, is a common value throughout all healthcare organizations across the world. Unfortunately, however, the ability of healthcare professionals to deliver these high standards and provide the required quality of leadership within healthcare organizations has recently been questioned, particularly in the United Kingdom (UK).[1–3] While these incidents could be considered 'special cause variations', worryingly, anecdotal evidence suggests that the concerns highlighted in the UK are in fact present, to varying degrees, across numerous different healthcare organizations throughout the world.

As psychiatrists, we must learn from these incidents and review not just the extreme deviant behaviours but, more importantly, the common elements that underpin them; we must share the lessons learned and must prevent similar tragedies occurring within our own environment. Although the responsibility for this will not sit comfortably with all of us, naturally, as doctors, we assume this responsibility perhaps more so than our non-clinical executive counterparts, as we are often the front-line, visible face of healthcare teams. Furthermore, we are often effective at doing so; Goodall reviewed the top 100 hospitals in the United States and found a strong positive association between the quality of a hospital and whether the chief executive officer had a career background as a physician.[4]

The challenge faced, that will be integral to effective, safe, and cost-effective healthcare delivery, is how to develop strong and effective leadership within psychiatrists, how to drive an institutional culture where everyone, both directly and indirectly involved in care, puts patients first, and how patient safety is brought to the heart of mental healthcare delivery.[1,5] To secure this, and to do so sustainably, leadership development must not only be focused on those already high within organizational hierarchies but also towards those lower down, who are providing front-line care, around the clock, twenty-four hours, seven days a week.[1,2]

Harnessing these potentially powerful agents for change and cultivating their enthusiasm for excellence is complex and requires a multifaceted approach. It is clear, however, that disempowerment, alienation, and failure to engage doctors—some of the brightest people in any country—is a defining weakness in our healthcare organizations and that like all specialties, we within mental health must rapidly overcome them to harness this currently untapped resource of energy, creativity, and ideas.[6,7]

What is leadership?

In order to understand leadership, we must first ascertain a common definition, or at least a concept, of what leadership is and what modern-day mental healthcare requires from its leaders. Important in doing so is to distinguish between leadership and management. Often these terms are used interchangeably and while leaders at times can manage and, at other times, managers can lead, the two are separate entities and require two distinct skill sets.

Academics and leading think tanks have debated numerous varying definitions, models, and frameworks for both leadership and management over the years, and they often mean different things to different people in different contexts. Yet there are some definitions that are currently more popular and widely accepted than others. John Kotter, one of the world's best-known and highly regarded experts in the field of leadership and management, distinguishes between the two, stating that management regards coping with complexity, whereas leadership regards coping with change.[8] Loosely, this distinction is inherent among the majority of definitions which are summarized in Table 2.1.

While exact definitions vary, there are key attitudes and behaviours, considered essential for all healthcare leaders, that are common among the majority. Based on extensive research of the evidence base, the Institute for Healthcare Improvement in the United States and the National Health Service (NHS) Leadership Academy in the United Kingdom have developed such common frameworks based on dimensions that they consider to be interdependent and essential.[9,10] It is important to study and learn from these leadership models, outlined briefly in Boxes 2.1 and 2.2, in order to develop our skills and harness our leadership potential.

Table 2.1 Differences between leadership and management

Leadership	Management
Coping with change	Coping with complexity
Innovation	Administration
Long-term perspective	Short-term perspective
Challenging the status quo	Accepting the status quo
Originality	Imitation
Empowerment	Control

Adapted from Nanus B. *Visionary Leadership*, Copyright (1995), with permission from John Wiley & Sons Ltd.

Box 2.1 Institute for Healthcare Improvement—high-impact leadership

Mental models: *outline philosophies to adopt throughout the organization.*

1 Considering individuals and families as partners in their care.

2 Continually aiming to reduce operating costs in order to compete on value while improving outcomes, quality, and safety.

3 Reorganizing services to address new payment systems.

4 Valuing everyone within the healthcare organization as an 'improver'.

Behaviours: *outline behaviours to adopt and embed in the organization.*

1 Person-centred care.

2 Front-line engagement with both providers and recipients of care.

3 Relentless focus on the organization's vision and strategy.

4 Transparency of both positive and negative aspects of the organization and healthcare provided.

5 Unbounded thinking and collaboration across services involved in a patient's pathway of care.

Framework: *outline critical domains where leadership efforts should be targeted.*

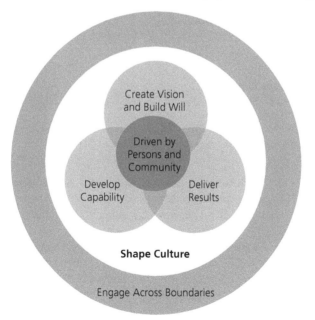

Reproduced from IHI White Papers, Swensen S, Pugh M, McMullan C, Kabcenell A, High-Impact Leadership: Improve Care, Improve the Health of Populations, and Reduce Costs, Copyright (2013), with permission from Institute for Healthcare Improvement.

Box 2.2 NHS Leadership Academy—the healthcare leadership model

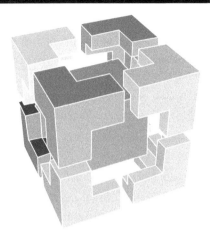

1 Inspiring a shared purpose

2 Leading with care

3 Evaluating information

4 Connecting our service

5 Sharing the vision

6 Engaging the team

7 Holding to account

8 Developing capability

9 Influencing results

Reproduced from NHS Leadership Academy, The Healthcare Leadership Model, version 1.0, Copyright (2013), with permission from NHS Leadership Academy

The strength of both these models and their advantage over set definitions is their dynamism and ability to guide individuals towards developing the behaviours required to lead, with attention focused on improvement rather than statements of simply what should be provided.

An additional vital aspect to leadership, that must not be forgotten, is followership. This is critical within psychiatry, particularly for psychiatrists who frequently act as heads of complex, multidisciplinary healthcare teams. As leaders, we must not view ourselves or be viewed by others as neither better, nor above, our followers; instead, we should be considered equals. In fact, some consider that rather than the leader, it is the early followers that are critical to any success.[11] As such, psychiatrists must ensure that, first, they are visible and easy to follow and, second, that they embrace, encourage, and support followers to attend to their developmental needs.

Leadership characteristics

Inspiring and enabling individuals to realize the collective vision they want to follow is the core essence of leadership. This, however, is not easily accomplished and requires multiple qualities and characteristics to be expressed by the psychiatrist, which we can consider at three distinct levels: personal, interpersonal, and organizational.[12] This should not be regarded as a complete, all-encompassing list; rather, these are some of the attributes widely considered to be core to successful leadership and aspects which all psychiatrists must look to develop.

Personal characteristics

This domain includes the qualities inherent within an individual that shape their own personality. Leaders must instinctively maintain a high level of passion and commitment in their work. In doing so, and with the imagination to create and communicate a clear sense of purpose, they rally and establish the same within their followers. Equally crucial is to show the courage and decisiveness that followers seek, particularly during times of uncertainty and change within the organization or team or, more specifically, within patient management. This often comes with the wisdom gained through practical experience and is especially effective and valued by followers if achieved through development and progression internally, within the organization.

Emotional intelligence underpins all this and is fundamentally about understanding yourself and others—a combination of self awareness, social awareness, self management, and relationship management.[13] Emotional intelligence is increasingly valued and recognized and, if not already, will become fundamental in recruitment.

Interpersonal characteristics

Interpersonal skills are essential to augment one's personal characteristics in order to achieve 'good leadership'. The ability to not just encourage and support followers but also to motivate and inspire them towards the collective vision is crucial, for both the organization as a whole and the individual patient. Truly effective leaders should be able to empower and develop their followers— at subordinate, peer, and senior levels—to higher levels of personal and professional development. In doing so, we increase our potential to deliver not only consistently high-quality care but also an effective and efficient service overall.

Organizational characteristics

Within healthcare organizations it is often easy to forget that we are not just responsible to the patient in front of us (although this must be the priority) but also, as employees, to our employer. Particularly as doctors, often highly regarded within healthcare organizations, we have a professional responsibility to act as role models in our behaviour and to show that we have the knowledge and ability to assess and analyse situations that do not just concern our immediate work environment but the organization as a whole. In order to do so sufficiently, we must maintain an awareness and understanding of healthcare policies, both nationally and locally, and include future policies that may directly or indirectly affect our patients. The truly proficient and successful leaders will then be able to articulate and convey their view and vision for the organization to their followers, in order to push for improved outcomes and high-quality care, turning challenges into opportunities.

While all psychiatrists should undoubtedly look to develop these characteristics, many within the profession may feel that they already possess a number of them and maintain them to a high standard. This is because, as psychiatrists, we embrace complexity and uncertainty with patients on a daily basis and are expected to overcome these challenges to produce management plans and diagnoses which predict potential problems and courses of illnesses. Using the biopsychosocial model to do so naturally provides psychiatrists with a greater insight and understanding of how to manage complexity and change. As leaders, psychiatrists should be able to transfer this into a leadership setting.[12]

Leadership styles

Encompassing the aforementioned qualities is vital, yet does not guarantee good leadership. To achieve this requires a consideration of not only one's own personal leadership style but also the leadership styles within the organization as a whole. Traditionally embedded within healthcare is a hierarchical, 'command and control', authoritarian, or 'autocratic' leadership style which stems from a culture whereby with rising seniority one gains 'legitimate' power. The danger of this is that autocratic leaders, due to their naturally controlling, close-minded, and power-orientated approach, often make independent decisions, resulting in demoralized staff and fear within the organization.[14] Led in this way, organizations as a whole, and specifically our most junior colleagues, become afraid of reporting errors and less inclined to admit mistakes.[15] This rhetoric of blame must be avoided; our existing leaders within psychiatry must welcome and respond to trainees directly, enabling them to speak up when they believe a lack of skills, knowledge, or resources is placing patients at risk of harm.[5]

Improving on this, a transformational leadership style or philosophy, comprising four key domains, commonly known as the 'four Is' (Table 2.2), is increasingly valued and considered to embody the essence of clinical leadership.[16] Transformational

Table 2.2 Transformational leadership—the four Is

Individualized consideration	Provision of personal attention, ideally through mentoring and coaching, to meet followers' needs.
Intellectual stimulation	Active encouragement of innovation and improvement from followers.
Inspirational motivation	Articulation of and motivation towards a clear vision which challenges and engages followers.
Idealized influence	Role modelled due to the trust and respect established from followers.

Source data from: Bass BM. *The Bass Handbook of Leadership: Theory, Research, and Managerial Applications*, Fourth edition, Copyright (2008), Free Press.

leaders, valuing that the development of 'followership' is both central and essential to achieve their vision, utilize the 'four Is' to broaden and satisfy the higher needs of followers. Effectively delivered, these domains help raise both the leader and their followers to higher levels, producing better outcomes and stimulating the intrinsic drive within followers to develop their own leadership skills and to provide the excellent care deserved and demanded by patients.[14,17]

To develop this further, while still maintaining a transformational style, at times leaders must consider, adjust, and adopt their approach, dependent on the composition of their followers and the task at hand. There are several different leadership styles and theories, none of which should be overvalued or discredited: they are merely different considerations of how leaders could, rather than should, act in different situations. Some of the most popular styles and approaches are outlined in Table 2.3.

Table 2.3 Leadership styles

Autocratic	Leaders are controlling and close-minded, unilaterally making decisions without consultation and expecting compliance. This is beneficial for quick decisive action during crisis periods but high risk, damaging morale and potentiating fear in followers who might otherwise challenge the leader's actions.
Democratic	Leaders encourage creativity, contribution, and collaboration from their followers to reach a consensus. While this generates engagement, democratic leaders are often uncomfortable making quick decisions when this process cannot be followed and this style can be ineffective.
Laissez-faire	Leaders oversee activity and provide support when required but otherwise let followers decide on their own course of action. Although followers value this autonomy, without the right skill set and knowledge base this can be highly inefficient and ineffective.
Visionary	Leaders strongly communicate with and mobilize followers towards a predetermined vision. While this maximizes commitment in followers, as they internally value the vision, often the guidance and understanding to achieve it is lacking.
Coaching	Leaders synchronize both personal and organizational goals, focusing on the follower's personal development. This, however, requires followers to be highly motivated; the danger is micromanagement and loss of the follower's sense of autonomy.
Pace setting	Leaders demand high standards and can produce timely results with a highly competent team. However, their targets are often hard to achieve and can damage followers' morale and confidence.

Leadership development and training

The ability of an individual to lead can be considered 'trait-based' (suggesting that certain individuals have an inherent leadership ability) or 'process-based' (suggesting that leadership is observable and can be learned).[18,19] While it is only natural that certain individuals will excel within leadership roles due to their inherent traits, it is undoubtable that all individuals can develop their leadership skills if given the right training, in the right environment, with the right opportunities.

Trainees are enthusiastic about this process of leadership development. They want to give more than is currently expected of them, contribute beyond basic service provision, and lead improvements that will positively impact on patient care and outcomes.[20] Significant consideration must therefore be paid towards harnessing this dedication and embedding strong, high-quality medical leadership at all levels of our mental healthcare organizations.

The ability of senior psychiatrists, and those established within formal leadership positions, to adopt the aforementioned transformational leadership style will be fundamental in driving leadership development among our early career psychiatrists, as will their mentoring and coaching skills. Leadership development should be a longitudinal key component of training and be integrated naturally within a trainee's clinical experience, rather than occurring in isolation.[21] We are fortunate that dedicated weekly supervision time is already embedded within our psychiatric training structure. Utilized effectively for leadership development, this available time presents the ideal opportunity for psychiatry to lead the way and show our colleagues from other specialties how to nurture trainees into strong clinical leaders.

'Quality improvement' is a vehicle through which existing leaders can cultivate and empower their trainees, and which trainees should utilize to achieve their leadership potential. Carefully implemented in the right way, this has the potential to encourage doctors to think of themselves as leaders not because they are personally exceptional, senior, or inspirational to others, but because they can see where improvements are needed and work with others to achieve these.[22] Fundamentally, quality improvement involves trainees influencing themselves and others to alter the behaviour of the healthcare provider (through systematic changes to methods and strategies), with the aim of improving patients' experiences and/or outcomes.[23,24]

There are numerous specific systematic changes to methods that can facilitate quality improvement; just to name a few, these include 'lean' methodology (focusing on waste reduction, flow, and value), 'six sigma' (focusing on product improvement and reducing 'defects'), and the 'model for improvement' (focusing on continuous 'Plan, Do, Study, Act' (PDSA) cycles). The 'model for improvement' is becoming increasingly popular, with its clear and simple formula, and particularly resonates with trainees testing out small-scale change within their workplace.[25]

Embedding leadership development through quality improvement into clinical practice and training creates an environment whereby trainees not only work but learn, and it is this that is likely to have the greatest impact, both on the individual and the organization.[26] From a developmental perspective, it is important to empower trainees and avoid merely using them as clerical assistants, engaged in laborious data collection and analysis for pre-existing quality assurance or improvement programmes. Utilizing the transformational leadership model, we must remember the intellectual stimulation required whereby leaders solicit their followers' ideas and solutions to problems, on a one-to-one basis, by establishing a relationship in which followers are openly encouraged to share their ideas and be creative, without fear of criticism following mistakes or failure.[14] Quality improvement tools, such as 'driver diagrams' (i.e., a type of structured logic chart with three or more levels), are ideal for this and their use, both by individuals on a personal level and by teams during improvement projects, should be strongly encouraged.

Facilitating quality improvement activity through this approach provides the ideal opportunity to engage trainees directly in open, constructive conversation, in which their opinions are respected and valued. This improves work's quality, patients' safety and helps to establish a culture which is firmly rooted in continual improvement.[5]

Without this guidance and support, there is a danger that the complexities and unanticipated challenges present in the healthcare system, which frequently form barriers to leadership, will leave trainees frustrated and feeling as though their skills and capabilities are undervalued. If a trainee is stifled in this way too early in their career, there is the risk that they will feel disillusioned and have potential doubts as to whether medicine can satisfy their ambitions and aspirations.[20]

External recognition can act as a powerful tool, helping to overcome this frustration and disillusionment. Within every individual there are both intrinsic and extrinsic motivators. Presentations, publications, and awards at national and international level act as a powerful extrinsic motivator to aid the development of trainees and to raise psychiatry's profile as a specialty which promotes trainees' leadership skills. Trainees must be encouraged and supported by their seniors in achieving this goal. In response, over time, inherent intrinsic motivators develop and drive our future leaders within mental health to seek not just external recognition but also internal satisfaction at improved outcomes and quality of care for patients, across a range of mental health settings. Additionally, these opportunities potentiate the development of networks external to their existing organization. Whether formally or informally, these networks can broaden trainees' exposure to leaders across a range of mental health services, further progressing their own personal development and the future of psychiatry through clinical and academic collaboration.

The future

The opportunity to create and develop a generation of engaged medical leaders is there to be seized and acted upon, particularly within the highly supportive training environment that we have within psychiatry. Leadership development must not remain a skill that is passively learned or considered to be an optional extra for trainees. We must not only identify potential leaders based on their inherent traits, but develop a process through which all trainees can develop their leadership skills. Without this, we risk creating a shortfall when existing leaders leave the profession which potentially could not only leave our specialty vulnerable, but our patients too.

Rather than continuing to allow traditional autocratic leadership styles to dominate, to the detriment of both medical staff and patients, we must learn to embrace, nurture, and support our trainees to acquire a transformational leadership style which develops the leadership behaviours outlined by the NHS Leadership Academy and the Institute for Healthcare Improvement and enhances their ability to act as powerful agents for change.

Focusing on integrating trainees into the wider quality improvement agenda through active opportunities to lead improvements to systems of care will help improve mental health outcomes and deliver high-quality healthcare for our patients.[5,27] Furthermore, through direct involvement and observation of the benefits derived from such improvements, trainees will enhance not only their leadership skills but also the care provided to patients.[27]

Supporting this development early in a trainee's career, with time allowed for its practical application, will harness their capacity to lead, utilize a large but undervalued part of the medical workforce, and avoid what is currently a wasteful oversight of 'not just the clinical leaders of tomorrow, but the clinical leaders of today' and a valuable resource lying dormant in our healthcare systems.[27]

References

1 **Francis R**. *Report of the Mid Staffordshire NHS Foundation Trust Public Inquiry: executive summary. House Paper 947*. London: The Stationery Office; 2013.

2 **Keogh B**. *Review into the quality of care and treatment provided by 14 hospital trusts in England: overview report*. London: Department of Health; 2013.

3 Department of Health. *Transforming care: a national response to Winterbourne View Hospital. Department of Health review final report*. London: Department of Health; 2012.

4 **Goodall A**. *Physician-leaders and hospital performance: is there an association? IZA (The Institute for the Study of Labor) Discussion Paper No. 5830*. Germany: IZA; 2011.

5 **Berwick D**. *A promise to learn—a commitment to act: improving the safety of patients in England. National Advisory Group report on the safety of patients in England*. 2013.

6 The King's Fund. *The future and leadership management in the NHS: no more heroes*. London: The King's Fund; 2011.

7 The King's Fund. *Leadership and engagement for improvement in the NHS: together we can*. London: The King's Fund; 2012.

8 **Kotter J**. *What leaders really do. Harvard business review on leadership*. Boston: Harvard Business School Press; 1998.

9 **Swensen S, Pugh M, McMullan C, Kabcenell A**. *High-impact leadership: improve care, improve the health of populations, and reduce costs. IHI White Paper*. Cambridge, Massachusetts: Institute for Healthcare Improvement; 2013.

10 NHS Leadership Academy. *The healthcare leadership model, version 1.0*. Leeds: NHS Leadership Academy; 2013.

11 **Sivers D**. *Leadership lessons from dancing guy*. Technology Entertainment Design (TED) Conference, 2010. Available at: http://sivers.org/ff.

12 **Bhugra D**. What makes a medical leader? *Adv Psych Treat* 2011; **17**:160–1.

13 **Goleman D**. *Emotional intelligence: why it can matter more than IQ*. New York: Bantam Books; 1995.

14 **Bass BM**. *The Bass handbook of leadership: theory, research, and managerial applications* (4th edn). New York, NY: Free Press; 2008.

15 **Edmondson AC**. Learning from mistakes is easier said than done: group and organizational influences on the detection and correction of human error. *J Appl Behav Sci* 1996; **32**:5–28.

16 NHS Confederation and The Nuffield Trust. *The modern values of leadership and management in the NHS*. London: NHS Confederation; 1999.

17 **Allio RJ**. Leaders and leadership—many theories, but what advice is reliable? *Strat Leader* 2013; **41**:4–14.

18 **Yukl G**. *Leadership in organizations* (6th edn). Upper Saddle River, NJ: Pearson-Prentice Hall; 2006.

19 **Daft RL**. *The leadership experience* (3rd edn). Mason, OH: Thomson, South-Western; 2005.

20 **Bagnall P**. *Facilitators and barriers to leadership and quality improvement. The King's Fund Junior Doctor Project*. London: The King's Fund; 2012.

21 The Royal College of Psychiatrists. *A college strategy for professional development in leadership and management*. London: RCP; 2012.

22 **Turnbull JK**. *Leadership in context: lessons from new leadership theory and current leadership development practice*. London: The King's Fund; 2011.

23 **Øvretveit J**. *Leading improvement effectively: a review of research*. London: The Health Foundation; 2009.

24 **Øvretveit J**. *Does improving quality save money? A review of the evidence of which improvements to quality reduce costs to health service providers*. London: The Health Foundation; 2009.

25 **Langley GL, Nolan KM, Nolan TW, Norman CL, Provost LP**. *The improvement guide: a practical approach to enhancing organizational performance* (2nd edn). San Francisco: Jossey-Bass Publishers; 2009.

26 **McKimm J, Swanwick T**. Leadership development for clinicians: what are we trying to achieve? *Clin Teach* 2011; **8**:181–5.

27 The Health Foundation. *What's leadership got to do with it? Exploring links between quality improvement and leadership in the NHS*. London: The Health Foundation; 2011.

Chapter 3

Evaluating mental healthcare systems by studying pathways to care

Adriana Mihai, Vesna Jordanova,
Umberto Volpe, and Norman Sartorius

Introduction

Despite the wide recognition of the importance of national mental health policies for the development of mental healthcare systems, more than 40% of the world's countries have no mental health policy and more than 30% have no national programme for mental health.[1,2] Political and economic problems, inefficient bureaucracy, and a lack of knowledge-based skills and resources are harsh realities for many countries, which may negatively affect the organization of mental healthcare systems.[3] European health systems face economic challenges that, among other effects, can lead governments to consider the reorganization of mental health services and savings that might be achieved by closing mental hospitals and other specialized services.

There are many ways to evaluate mental healthcare systems. There are several studies[4-8] which use descriptive methods to outline the structure of the mental health care system, legislation, and regulation. Policy makers and governments often evaluate the healthcare system using the number of psychiatrists, overall patient load, and other indicators of input and processing of mental healthcare. Another way to compare systems of mental healthcare is the evaluation of ease of access to services (and their quality) by the examination of patient pathways to care[9,10] and the assessment of barriers that prevent patients from asking or receiving help (e.g. mistrust, fear, stigma[11-15]). This chapter will focus on the evaluation of healthcare systems using information about the pathways that patients and their families took to reach the psychiatrists and to receive help. Pathways of care in 24 countries have been used in this analysis (see Table 3.1).

Pathways to care studies describe how people seek care for mental disorders and help to describe how mental health systems work. This is important because the accessibility of mental health services—which depends on the geographical position of the service, travel time from the patient's home to health service sites, and on other filters (such as stigma or being part of a population subgroup as an ethnic minority)—can be a decisive factor in the success of psychiatric treatment.[16] In our analysis, we will examine data that have been obtained through the pathways to care studies, which give an overall indication of the functioning of mental healthcare systems. This way of approaching

Table 3.1 List of countries included in the pathways to care analysis

No	Country evaluated	Reference
1.	Albania	[10]Gater R et al. 2005
2.	Bangladesh	[30]Hashimoto N et al. 2010
3.	Bulgaria	[10]Gater R et al. 2005
4.	Croatia	[10]Gater R et al. 2005
5.	Cuba	[19]Gater R et al. 1991
6.	Czech Republic	[19]Gater R et al. 1991
7.	India	[21]Lahariya C et al. 2010
		[30]Hashimoto N et al. 2010
		[25]Thomas B. 2012
8.	Indonesia	[19]Gater R et al. 1991
9.	Italy	[9]Volpe U et al. 2013
10.	Japan	[30]Hashimoto N et al. 2010
11.	Kenya	[19]Gater R et al. 1991
12.	Macedonia	[10]Gater R et al. 2005
13.	Mexico	[19]Gater R et al. 1991
14.	Mongolia	[30]Hashimoto N et al. 2010
15.	Nepal	[30]Hashimoto N et al. 2010
16.	Nigeria	[28]Adeosun II et al. 2013
17.	Pakistan	[19]Gater R et al. 1991
18.	Poland	[34]Pawłowski and Kiejna 2004
19.	Portugal	[19]Gater R et al. 1991
20.	Romania	[22]Mihai A et al. 2005
		[10]Gater R et al. 2005
21.	Serbia	[10]Gater R et al. 2005
22.	Spain	[19]Gater R et al. 1991
23.	UK	[19]Gater R et al. 1991
24.	Yemen	[19]Gater R et al. 1991

the evaluation of different systems of care not only gives a summary evaluation of the functioning of the care system but also presents a method that could be used by psychiatrists, at the beginning of their career, to examine their own service and to compare it to those in other countries.

The data offered by the pathways studies can make an important contribution to the formulation of mental health policies governing the organization of mental health services and psychiatry training provided to personnel in the primary care sector or in other sectors of social and general healthcare.[10,17] Pathway studies can also be used to generate health policies and to improve the quality of services. The encounter form (first used in World Health Organization (WHO) studies[18]), is a clear and concrete method of recording the elements of a pathway to care (see Appendix 3.1). Studies of pathways using this method are relatively simple and take little time. Data collection can be done as a part of routine assessment without the need of additional resources. These characteristics have allowed many to use the

Appendix 3.1 Pathways Questionnaire
(Slightly modified from Pathways Encounter Form[18])

INFORMATION ABOUT MENTAL HEALTH CENTRE	
1 Name of the institution	
2 Address of the institution	
3 Name of the interviewer	
4 Profession	
5 Date	
INFORMATION ABOUT THE PATIENT	
1 Coding number	
2 Age	
3 Gender	Male [ ] Female [ ]
4 Marital status	Single [ ] Married [ ] Widow [ ] Divorced [ ] Other [ ]
5 Economic status	High [ ] Average [ ] Poor [ ]
6 Personal mental health history	Yes [ ] No [ ]
7 Who suggested the consultation?	Patient [ ] Family [ ] Doctor [ ]
8 Patient lives in the area of research	Yes [ ] No [ ]
FIRST DECISION TO SEEK HELP	
1 Who was first seen?	GP [ ] Psychiatrist [ ] Social services [ ] Police [ ] Priest [ ] Native healer [ ] Other [specify] ....
2 How long ago?	Weeks [ ]
3 Who suggested the consultation?	Patient [ ] Family [ ] Neighbours [ ] Relatives [ ] Police [ ] Others [ ]
4 Reason (the most important symptom)	
5 How long ago did the problem begin?	
6 What treatment has been received?	
7 Duration of the delay	Hours [ ]

(continued)

THE SECOND CONSULTATION

1	Who carried out the consultation?	GP [ ] Psychiatrist [ ] Social services [ ]
		Police [ ] Priest [ ] Native healer [ ]
		Other [specify] … … … … … … … … …
2	How long ago?	Weeks [ ]
3	Who suggested the consultation?	Patient [ ] Family [ ] Neighbours [ ]
		Relatives [ ] Police [ ] Others [ ]
4	Reason (the most important symptom)	
5	How long ago did the problem begin?	
6	What treatment has been received?	
7	Duration of the delay	Hours [ ]

THE THIRD CONSULTATION (this and further consultations could be added, using the same questions)

DIAGNOSIS—ICD-10 AND DSM-V

1	First diagnosis
2	Second diagnosis
3	Third diagnosis

method, ensuring data are now available from a variety of regions, in developed and developing countries.

The pathways to care studies done in the same region, but at different times, can show the changes in mental health structure or changes in functioning in that region and the impact of legislation or mental health policy. Hence, they can be an important source of information for policy makers. In this chapter, we give examples of answers that pathway studies can give to some of the key questions related to mental healthcare systems.

Who asks for help, and for what?

Help could be sought by the patients, families, friends, police, state institutions, or third-party organizations. Help-seeking behaviour depends also on cultural and social factors, and not only on availability of mental healthcare provision.

The impact of different cultures on the recognition of mental health problems and the demand for help was presented by different authors.[19,20] In a study performed in India, 68.5% of patients first asked a faith healer for help.[21] In Europe, 10% of patients in Macedonia first seek help from traditional healers.[10] In Romania, 6% of patients repeatedly saw the priest before treatment in the mental health system was offered,[22] since they often considered the mental disorder as a 'possession' or a 'punishment' from a spiritual source.

In some countries, the police often ask for help in dealing with people who are mentally ill and this plays an important role in pathways to mental healthcare. In Romania, for example, 12% of patients admitted to psychiatric hospitals were brought in by the police.[22] Facts like these can help in the evaluation of the impact of laws enacted to protect the rights of patients with mental disorders and to avoid any kind of abuse or discrimination.[7,23]

In most of the countries studied, 'family members' and 'friends' were those who suggested seeking psychiatric care.[10,22] Referral delay was mainly caused by fear of stigma, lack of awareness about mental illness, and the insufficient availability of mental health services.[21]

In Eastern Europe, the behavioural disturbances associated with a risk to self or others where the main concern which led to seeking help from mental health services.[10] The differences between diagnoses of those seeking help from psychiatric services in different regions in the same country, and between different countries, are significant. We also found variations in the prevalence rates of mental disorders, as determined in longitudinal studies, within the same region,[24] which shows that the availability of community-based mental health services rather than the severity of symptoms determined help seeking.

Families often share the community's misconceptions about psychiatric disorders and have vague ideas about the care needs of the patient, complain about financial expenses, show inadequate coping skills, and feel helpless and burdened.[25] There are studies[26,27] which concluded that the variables associated with social support were more important than ethnicity in determining pathways to care. The positive role of families and friends in seeking care for mental illness were underlined by previous studies.[10,24]

Patients and their carers prefer to use general healthcare services because they are afraid of the stigmatization that can follow the diagnosis of mental illness or consultation of psychiatric services.[27] For example, Italian patients tend to refer to psychiatric services only in case of major mental disorders and when referral is highly needed.[9] In such situations, other professionals—such as psychologists, General Practitioners (GPs), and other physicians—play an important role in the treatment of mental disorders.

The needs of patients suffering with mental health problems differ from one region to another. While in developed countries, the primary needs for food and shelter are usually assured for all citizens, in low-income countries, these needs could become more important than the need for specialized healthcare services. Social networks and support from friends and families play a significant role in low-income countries. Poverty can also contribute to rates of somatic co-morbidity in people with mental illness.

In emergency situations, people usually seek help from GPs and/or local traditional healers. This is true for developed and developing countries. Native healers are popular in Macedonia, for example, and particularly among the rural population.[10] In Africa, traditional healers provide most of the treatment for the mentally ill.[28,29]

GPs play a limited role in the pathways to psychiatric care in many countries. Less than 20% of all referrals in Kenya, Albania, Mongolia, Japan, and Indonesia are to general healthcare services.[10,19,30] Pathways in Eastern Europe share many characteristics with countries of former Yugoslavia;[10] in these countries, the GPs have only a formal role—that of making the referral to secondary care—and are not involved in care planning and do not have a gate-keeping role. In Romania, the referral to psychiatric services is governed by regulations stating what has to be done by GPs and who can be referred to a specialist, which explains why the delay between primary care and the first contact with the psychiatric service is small (less than one week); similar situations were found in Albania and Cuba, and just a one-week delay in Serbia, Macedonia, the Czech Republic, and Spain. Primary care is not involved in care-seeking pathways in Tirana (Albania), and the mental health service itself manages a relatively high proportion of patients with mood and neurotic disorders (78%).[10]

The primary healthcare workers could act as gatekeepers toward the mental health system, being increasingly involved in diagnosis, referrals, and treatment of mental disorders.[16,31] The results of the available pathways to care studies, however, show that they do not play this role in most settings/countries.

The delay before seeking help

According to the 'critical period' hypothesis for schizophrenia,[32] a delay in mental health care may have serious consequences for the course and outcome of the illness. Several studies underline the impact of the duration of the untreated period on outcome in psychiatric disorder, and especially in psychosis.[33] In Europe, the delay before seeking help is less than 8 weeks in a majority of countries.[9,10] The interval before asking for help is much longer in Asia and South America, and could be almost 2 years (81 weeks) in India (Vellore) and several months in Mongolia (32 weeks) and Mexico (30 weeks). Religious beliefs could delay the access to professional help, with 68.5% of cases having first approached faith healers who then delayed contact with mental health services; magic and religious beliefs are among the most important social obstacles to seeking appropriate psychiatric treatment.[21]

The delay from first contact with healthcare agencies to reaching the psychiatric service

The mean time from first seeking care to the first psychiatric observation could vary from 0 weeks in Albania and Cuba[10,19] to 24 weeks in Mongolia and Bangladesh.[30] The total delay from the onset of the problem to the first psychiatric referral shows significant differences between different countries or even between different regions in the same country (for example, Vellore as opposed to Kathmandu). In 75% of evaluated countries, the delay before reaching psychiatric services is less than 12 weeks; in Europe, the exceptions are Portugal (20 weeks), Poland[34] (18 weeks), the United Kingdom (UK) (15 weeks), and Italy (13 weeks). In Asia, the differences in the delay are larger—India (Vellore, 100 weeks), Mongolia (56 weeks), Bangladesh (36 weeks), and Pakistan (16 weeks). In the majority of cases, the delays relate to the delay in first contacting healthcare services; except in Bangladesh, where the delay between the onset of illness and first contact with healthcare agents is 11 weeks, while access to psychiatric care is 25 weeks.

There are some medical systems where the patients, who want to contact a specialist, must first consult a primary care clinician. While these rules protect the hospital from overcrowding, they can also delay appropriate treatment of psychiatric disorders.[31] Countries such as Cuba, Yemen, the UK, Spain, Portugal, Bulgaria, and Czech Republic are characterized by this type of medical system and, as a consequence, more than 60% of referrals to psychiatric services are done by GPs. In other countries such as Albania, Kenya, Mongolia, and Japan, GPs play only a very small role as gate keepers; referrals to psychiatric services by GPs represent less than 15% of the total number of referrals. In these countries, direct access to psychiatric services is the principal way (40% of cases) to receive psychiatric care. In Kenya, the main route to psychiatric services is through hospital doctors (66%); while in the Yemen, Bangladesh, Indonesia, India, Mongolia, Romania, Macedonia, and Croatia, they make less than 10% of referrals.[10,19]

The delay between first care and psychiatric care varies between 6 months in Bangladesh and Mongolia, to 3 months in India and Poland, and a week or less in Cuba, Romania, the Yemen, Spain, Serbia, Macedonia, and the Czech Republic. (Such a small delay between the GP's consultation and referral to psychiatric services, as previously mentioned, shows that GPs in these countries play only a formal role, imposed by regulations, and do not really work as gatekeepers.) In India, Romania, Macedonia, Serbia, Croatia, Italy, and Pakistan direct access to psychiatric service remains important, occurring in more than 30% of total cases.

The impact of delay of access to appropriate care on people with severe mental illness can lead to a poor outcome.[35,36]

Conclusions

Pathway studies provide information about the functioning of healthcare systems and highlight those areas in which change is necessary. Such studies may also draw attention to significant delays in reaching care, which might help in the reorganization of referral systems and services. Data from pathway studies may serve people working within mental health facilities and policy makers, supporting them in their efforts to improve mental health provision within a certain country or across different countries. Using a standardized approach to these studies (such as that provided by the pathways questionnaire; see Appendix 3.1) may greatly help.

Pathway studies also show the role that stigma plays and the discrimination that patients with mental health problems experience while transiting through the mental health system of a certain country. They can also serve well as a method to evaluate the impact of changes to a healthcare system. Pathways to care studies are easy to carry out, do not require any substantial financial support, and may provide timely information about the way in which mental health services work and about interventions or changes that contribute to better use of resources and more effective care.

Psychiatrists at an early point in their career should be properly trained to evaluate pathways to care for their own patients. Systematic evaluations of the risk of delayed care or of peculiar routes to psychiatric care should be routinely performed in mental healthcare systems in order to ensure equal and high-quality provision of psychiatric care.

References

1 World Health Organization. *Mental health atlas 2011*. Geneva (Switzerland): WHO; 2011.
2 World Health Organization (European Regional Office). *Impact of economic crisis on mental health*. Copenhagen (Denmark): WHO; 2011.

3 White RG, Sashidharan SP. Towards a more nuanced global mental health. *Br J Psychiatry* 2014; **204**:415–7.

4 Epping-Jordan JE, Pruitt SD, Bengoa R, Wagner EH. Improving the quality of health care for chronic conditions. *Qual Saf Health Care* 2004; **13**:299–305.

5 Kohn LT, Corrigan JM, Donaldson MS. *To err is human: building a safer health system.* Washington, D.C.: National Academy Press; 2000.

6 Fistein EC, Holland AJ, Clare ICH, Gunn MJ. A comparison of mental health legislation from diverse Commonwealth jurisdictions. *Int J Law Psychiatry* 2009; **32**(3):147–55.

7 Mundt A, et al. Changes in the provision of institutionalized mental health care in post-communist countries. *PLoS One* 2012; **7**(6):e38490.

8 Xiang YT, Yu X, Sartorius N, et al. Mental health in China: challenges and progress. *Lancet* 2012; **380**:1715–6.

9 Volpe U, Fiorillo A, Luciano M, et al. Pathways to mental health care in Italy: results from a multicenter study. *Int J Soc Psychiatry* 2013; **60**(5):508–13.

10 Gater R, Jordanova V, Maric N, et al. Pathways to psychiatric care in Eastern Europe. *Br J Psychiatry* 2005; **186**:529–35.

11 Corrigan PW, Watson AC, Miller FE. Blame, shame, and contamination: the impact of mental illness and drug dependence stigma on family members. *J Fam Psychol* 2006; **20** (2):239–46.

12 Corrigan PW, Morris SB, Michaels PJ, Rafacz JD, Rusch N. Challenging the public stigma of mental illness: a meta-analysis of outcome studies. *Psych Serv* 2012; **63**:963–73.

13 Bijl RV, de Graaf R, Hiripi E, et al. The prevalence of treated and untreated mental disorders in five countries. *Health Aff (Millwood)* 2003; **22**(3):122–33.

14 Redaniel MA, Lebana Dalida NA, Gunell D. Suicide in the Philippines: time trend analysis (1974–2005) and literature review. *BMC Pub Health* 2011; **11**:536. Available at: http://www.biomedcentral.com/1471–2458/11/536

15 Damsa C, Andreoli A, Zullino D, et al. Quality of care in emergency psychiatry: developing an international network. *Eur Psychiatry* 2007; **22**(6):411–2.

16 Thornicroft G, Tansella M. *The mental health matrix. A manual to improve services.* Cambridge: Cambridge University Press; 1999.

17 Rogler LH, Cortes DE. Help-seeking pathways: a unifying concept in mental health care. *Am J Psychiatry* 1993; **150**(4):554–61.

18 World Health Organization. *Pathways of patients with mental disorders—a multicentre collaborative project.* WHO; 1987, pp.18–22. Available at : http://whqlibdoc.who.int/hq/1987/MNH_NAT_87.1.pdf. Accessed 20 February 2015.

19 Gater R, De Almeida E, Sousa B, et al. The pathways to psychiatric care: a cross-cultural study. *Psychol Med* 1991; **21**(3):761–74.

20 Sartorius N, Jablensky A, Korten A, et al. Early manifestations and first-contact incidence of schizophrenia in different cultures. A preliminary report on the initial evaluation phase of the WHO collaborative study on determinants of outcome of severe mental disorders. *Psychol Med* 1986; **16**(4):909–28.

21 Lahariya C, Singhal S, Gupta S, Mishra A. Pathway of care among psychiatric patients attending a mental health institution in central India. *Ind J Psychiatry* 2010; **52**(4):333–8.

22 Mihai A, Iosub D, Szalontay A. Pathway to psychiatric services in Romania. *Rom J Psychiatry* 2005; **8**(1–2):110–4.

23 **Bonnie RJ**. Political abuse of psychiatry in the Soviet Union and in China: complexities and controversies. *J Am Acad Psychiatry Law* 2002; **30**:136–44.

24 **Mihai A, Butiu O**. The family in Romania: cultural and economic context and implications for treatment. *Int Rev Psychiatry* 2012; **24**(2):139–43.

25 **Thomas B**. Treating troubled families: therapeutic scenario in India. *Int Rev Psychiatry* 2012; **24**(2):91–8.

26 **Cole E, Leavey G, King M, Johnson-Sabine E, Hoar A**. Pathways to care for patients with a first episode of psychosis. A comparison of ethnic groups. *Br J Psychiatry* 1995; **167**(6):770–6.

27 **Burnett R, Mallett R, Bhugra D, Hutchinson G, Der G, Leff J**. The first contact of patients with schizophrenia with psychiatric services: social factors and pathways to care in a multi-ethnic population. *Psychol Med* 1999; **29**(2):475–83.

28 **Adeosun II, Adegbohun AA, Adewumi TA, Jeje OO**. The pathways to the first contact with mental health services among patients with schizophrenia in Lagos, Nigeria. *Schizophr Res Treatment* 2013; 2013 769161.

29 **Patel V, Araya R, Chatterjee S, et al**. Treatment and prevention of mental disorders in low-income and middle-income countries. *Lancet* 2007; **370**:991–1005.

30 **Hashimoto N, Fujisawa D, Giasuddin NA, et al**. Pathways to mental health care in Bangladesh, India, Japan, Mongolia, and Nepal. *Asia Pac J Pub Health* 2010; **2**: 1847–57. DOI:10.1177/1010539510379395

31 **Jordanova V, Maric NP, Alikaj V, et al**. Prescribing practices in psychiatric hospitals in Eastern Europe. *Eur Psychiatry* 2011; **26**(7):414–8.

32 **Tait L, Birchwood M, Trower P**. Predicting engagement with services for psychosis: insight symptoms and recovery style. *Br J Psychiatry* 2003; **182**:123–8.

33 **Bhui K, Ullrich S, Coid JW**. Which pathways to psychiatric care lead to earlier treatment and a shorter duration of first-episode psychosis? *BMC Psychiatry* 2014; **14**:72. Available at: http://www.biomedcentral.com/1471-244X/14/72.

34 **Pawłowski T, Kiejna A**. Pathways to psychiatric care and reform of the public health care system in Poland. *Eur Psychiatry* 2004; **19**(3):168–71.

35 **Loebel AD, Lieberman JA, Alvir JMJ, Mayerhoff DI, Geisler SH, Szymanski SR**. Duration of psychosis and outcome in first-episode schizophrenia. *Am J Psychiatry* 1992; **149**:1183–8.

36 **Lieberman JA, Jody D, Geisler SH, et al**. Time course and biological correlates of treatment response in first-episode schizophrenia. *Arch Gen Psychiatry* 1993; **50**(5):369–76.

Chapter 4

Managing self: time, priorities, and well-being

Nikolina Jovanovic, Andrea Fiorillo, and Wulf Rössler

Case study

Theresa (28 years old) is in her second year of training in psychiatry. She has always wanted to become a psychiatrist and the day she got the post was one of the happiest days in her life. However, two years later, she feels she might be losing her enthusiasm. The head of the department demands extensive working hours from his team since there are not enough doctors to take care of the ever growing number of patients. What is also frustrating is that responsibilities and duties of the various team members are not clear, so everything needs to be negotiated day by day. This is not to mention the fact that keeping up with the administrative standards and paperwork, Theresa's least favourite bit, can take up to several hours per week. Theresa would rather spend that time with patients or catching up with the latest scientific publications. Altogether, quite often Theresa feels completely drained! Peter (34 years old), her partner, is also frustrated as he would like to spend more time with Theresa, and so would her parents and friends. In short—Theresa is quite desperate and questions if her position will ever improve and if there is another way of dealing with this situation.

If you were Theresa, what would you do? If you are not sure, or maybe share the same situation, keep on reading! We might have something that could help you.

Introduction

Would you not agree that being a medical resident is very stressful due to the long working hours, night shifts, inflexible schedules, and significant imbalance between professional experience and responsibility? This is not to forget that this period of life (usually one's late twenties or early thirties) is full of many life changes such as marriage, parenthood, shifts in the workplace, and estrangement from supportive networks.[1] Very few people would be able to claim the opposite. Furthermore, it has been identified that the field of psychiatry adds several very unique stressors to what has just been mentioned. These challenges range from the stigma of this profession, to particularly demanding relationships with patients and personal threats from violent patients, to difficult interactions with other mental health professionals within the multidisciplinary team. Other sources of stress are the lack of positive feedback, low pay, and a poor work environment. Finally, patient suicide is a major stressor, following which a majority of mental health workers report post-traumatic stress symptoms.[2] The co-occurrence of these stressors might induce mental health problems such as burnout syndrome, depression, substance abuse, and even suicide attempts.[3] Mental health problems could have devastating consequences on the careers of young doctors, eventually resulting in poor professional and academic achievements.[1]

At the same time, this period of life resembles the great excitement of student days. Immersing oneself into the new field, learning about different fascinating theories and achievements that moved the field forward over time, and discussing all that with peers and seniors is what makes this period so attractive and unique. It is probably one of the last formative periods in life and one should be able to make the most of it, while at the same time maintaining or even improving one's well-being. Therefore, the aim of this chapter is to move our energies into that direction. If you are a young doctor, this chapter might help you understand the importance of managing time and setting priorities in life. On the following pages you will be able to find some very useful techniques to help you with that task. If you are a senior working with young doctors, our aim is to increase your awareness of these problems in order that you can help young doctors in planning their careers and taking care of themselves.

Starting with the basic question—what do you want to do in your life?

The process of figuring out how best to spend one's own life is a demanding task. What this basically involves is getting to know yourself and who you are as a person, within the different aspects of your life. This includes setting short- and long-term goals in both your professional and private life, as well as defining your strengths and weaknesses that will help or prevent you from achieving your goals. In other words, it means that you should have a genuine interest in the things you want to do, you should be passionate about them, and they should make you feel good about yourself. Sometimes it is difficult to understand one's own genuine interests and not to incline towards other people's expectations (of parents, partners, seniors at work, etc.). However, the question should always be about what *you* want to do with your life. Others may have wishes and suggestions but, in the end, it is up to you to determine if what they want aligns with what you envision for yourself.[4]

Work life

Psychiatry as a medical discipline embraces many different and complex aspects such as neuroscience, public health, social medicine, internal medicine, psychology, psychoanalysis, and philosophy[5]. One can decide to work as a clinician or a researcher or as an academic. Curricular needs may be different if, for example, you want to work in an academic institution as opposed to a community service. For the former, publications in peer-reviewed and high-impact journals are strongly needed; also, it is important to attend national and international conferences, to develop teaching and presentation skills, and to be familiar with significant literature in your field of interest. Therefore, it is essential to choose your field of interest as soon as possible. One should bear in mind that this is one of the most difficult questions in life, as getting to know your true self is not easy, does not happen overnight, and can change over time. However, it is important to start thinking about it even today.

Box 4.1 brings together several questions that can be helpful in this task. Please note that there are no ideal careers, but in an attempt to have an enjoyable and successful career (and you can define success anyway you want for yourself), it is helpful to consider what you really want, what parts of your 'dislike' list you would tolerate, and which are absolute 'no goers'.

Box 4.1 Career management - questions to ask yourself when designing your professional life

- Why did I choose medicine?
- Why did I choose psychiatry?
- Do I feel adequate to treat persons with mental disorders? How much direct medical care do I want to provide? Research, writing, teaching, and administration are options that do not directly involve patient care. What option is best for me?
- How resilient am I? How do I deal with stress? How do I deal with negative experiences at work?
- Which parts of psychiatry are the most meaningful to me? Which parts of psychiatry do I like most?
- What type of patients and services fit best with my personality?
- If I pursue the clinical path, do I want to be a solo practitioner or part of a group practice? Do I want to work night shifts? Do I want to see lots of patients in short bursts or fewer patients in more depth and for longer?
- What subspecialty will suit me best?
- Would I like to pursue an academic career? Do I want to incorporate research into my career? Do I enjoy reading scientific papers? Am I good at teaching/ disseminating knowledge and skills in a meaningful manner?
- Which parts of psychiatry do I dislike most?
- What do I want to accomplish in my career? Am I an ambitious person? Am I a leader or do I prefer to be led by someone else? Do I need additional training regarding management skills? Would I like to have an international career?
- If I could pick and choose the most enjoyable and/or most meaningful parts of psychiatry to make the ideal career, what would I include? What would I exclude?

Source data from: *Practice Link*, 21, Harrison A, How to love your job, p. 69–71, Copyright (2011).

Private life

Medicine is a profession that requires significant time, effort, and personal sacrifice. However, our profession is just one of many ways to define ourselves. Knowing what you want, and your strengths and limitations, will allow you to set suitable priorities in life and to plan your career and private life in the best possible way. Please take a look at Box 4.2; these questions might help you in this process. The key thing is to find an appropriate life–work balance.

Box 4.2 Questions to ask yourself when setting priorities for your private life

- Ideally, what would I like to accomplish in my private life? (Consider your partner, family, hobbies, travel, other non-work interests, etc.)
- How big a role do these things play in my life at the moment? Is that enough? Is that by choice?
- Do I want to be in a relationship or single?
- Do I spend enough time with my partner? Is my partner satisfied with our relationship? Am I satisfied with it? If yes, what makes me happy? If not, what makes me dissatisfied?
- Do I (we) want children?
- Is the house/apartment where I/we live large enough?
- Is my salary sufficient for a whole family?
- Do I have enough time off work to spend with my children? What do we do in our time together? Am I happy with this? Do my kids complain? How do I feel about that?
- What about other family members, for example my parents? How often do I visit them? Is that enough? Do I invite them for dinner? What are we going to do once they will not be able to take care of themselves?
- Not to forget my friends—do I have time to meet them regularly? Do I plan joint activities? Do they complain that I do not spend enough time with them?
- Do I want to live in an urban/suburban/rural area? Does my ideal geographical location allow me to pursue my work goals and personal interests? Do I want to move closer to work to avoid long commuting? What is more important, work or home location?
- What are my hobbies and do I have enough time to practise them?

Source data from: *Practice Link*, 21, Harrison A, How to love your job, p. 69–71, Copyright (2011).

Personal time management and work–life balance

Being able to manage time allows us to find an adequate balance between work and leisure activities. However, 'balance' is a very individual thing and does not necessarily mean 50/50. It is you who determines what your 'balance' is.

Time itself is an interesting concept. There are 24 hours in a day, and 7 days in a week; that is a total of 168 hours per week. The European Work Time Directive (EWTD) limits the working time schedule to 48 hours per week[6].

According to 2000–2002 data from the American Medical Association (physician socioeconomic statistics), a general psychiatrist works on average 48 hours per week and the average for all specialties in the United States (US) is 53.9 hours[7]. So, in an average week, 120 hours are left for non-working activities (168 – 48 hours). How does that time get spent? The US Bureau of Labor Statistics states that an average US citizen spends 8.67 hours per day sleeping and 1.22 hours per day eating and drinking[8]. With a little rounding off, let us say that you spend 8.5 × 7 = 59.5 hours per week sleeping and 1.25 × 7 = 8.75 hours per week eating; that is 59.5 + 8.75 = 68.25 hours per week eating, drinking, and sleeping. This means that of the 120 hours per week that are not spent working, 51.75 hours are left over for activities like hobbies, personal care, family, socializing (120 – 68.25 hours). This leads to the question, how do *you* want to spend your 51.75 free hours?

Therefore, the next time you find yourself saying 'I don't have enough time', ask yourself what are you really saying? Sometimes people use that phrase to avoid doing things they dislike or are afraid of or simply think are unimportant. Please take a look at so-called 'time wasters' listed in Table 4.1. In the end, we all work within the confines of 24 hours per day. The key question is—are you happy with the way you use your time and could you use it more efficiently?

The Pareto principle

The Pareto principle, or the 80:20 rule, was first described by the Italian economist Vilfredo Pareto and states that 80% of the land in Italy is in the hands of 20% of the population. Since then, this rule has been applied to many areas in economics, business, and occupational health. In our context, this rule means that about 80% of our effective work is done in 20% of our working time. Thus, we spend 80% of our time perfecting

Table 4.1 Work-time wasters

Individual	Company
Lack of clear objectives, priorities, and daily/weekly/monthly plan	Unclear definition of professional duties and roles among co-workers
Lack of self-discipline	Lack of or unclear communication
Inability to say 'no'	Mixed messages from the management
Attempting too much at once	Telephone interruptions
Ineffective delegation	Drop-in visitors
Leaving tasks unfinished	Too many long meetings

things. This might be a good approach in our direct patient work but there are many areas of our daily business which do not require perfection (e.g. some administrative work). Therefore, we can save a lot of working time if we do not strive for perfection. To make the best of your time, make a list of your daily tasks and decide if a perfect result is required in each case. You will identify many work areas where such a perfect result is not necessary. After having identified these tasks, make a decision as to which other tasks then have priority. Be careful with your precious spare time.

The Eisenhower method

This method is assigned to the former US President Dwight D. Eisenhower. According to this method, there are tasks which are urgent and important. They should be handled immediately. Other tasks are important but not urgent. List these tasks according to importance. You can prioritize tasks on the list, but always keep this list in mind. Finally, there are tasks which are neither important nor urgent. Put these tasks in a waste-basket. Persons for whom these tasks might be important will get in touch with you again anyway. Again, try to identify in your life what is important/unimportant and urgent/not urgent. If you optimize your time management, you can gain time for 'more important' work. However, you also should be aware that optimal time management can be quite exhausting; therefore deliberately plan some recreational time within your working time.

Gender-related perspective on work-life balance

The balance between work and private life is challenging for both genders, although maybe due to slightly different reasons. Men are often focused exclusively on work and do not consider an alternative to their professional development, which can make them more vulnerable if they do not accomplish the expected career steps (especially in more traditional societies). Women often struggle to balance work and childcare responsibilities, and although several measures have been proposed to help families and women regarding this matter (e.g. career advice for female students and residents about the inherent characteristics of their chosen specialty, part-time working and flexible hours at certain points in a career, separate teaching and research career tracks to support clinical academics of the future), the implementation is still rather poor[9].

Be aware of mental health problems among psychiatrists

Physicians in general have high rates of mental health problems, including anxiety, depression, addiction, and increased suicide rates.[10] For example, approximately 10–15% of medical students and residents suffer from depression[11] and, on average, the US loses the equivalent of at least one entire medical school class each year due to suicide (approximately 400 physicians)[12]. The risk of completed suicide is up to 2.4 times higher in physicians than in the general population[13]. The reason for this might lie in the fact that very often, instead of asking for help, a depressed physician turns to social isolation and the use of alcohol, anxiolytics, and sedatives. Depression and alcoholism, together with knowledge of and easy access to lethal means, is what significantly increases the suicide risk. Results from the International Psychiatry Residents/Trainees Burnout Syndrome Study (BOSS) show that approximately 5% of studied European psychiatric residents meet the criteria for major depression and approximately 1% have attempted suicide, while the number of those with serious suicidal ideation goes up to 20% in some countries[3].

The specific role of burnout syndrome

Burnout syndrome stands for inadequate response to prolonged occupational stress, and conceptually is a triad of emotional overextension and exhaustion; negative, cynical, and detached responses to others; and feelings of inefficacy and reduced personal accomplishment[14]. Different studies report widely varying burnout rates among medical residents, ranging from 18% to 82% (up to 50% in psychiatry)[15]. According to the Maslach burnout inventory, burnout can be categorized into low, moderate, and severe level and, as discussed in the BOSS study, shows that European residents suffer from a moderate level of burnout[3]. The syndrome itself poses a significant challenge during early training years; its levels decrease in the second half of training, probably due to gained experience[16]. In general, the perception of losing control, time pressure, lack of respect and social support, as well as of a mismatch between the individual and the workplace, may be relevant factors for developing burnout syndrome.

The majority of studies in this field have focused on work-related risk factors (such as time demands, lack of control and work planning, poor work organization, and work–home interference), somewhat underestimating the contribution of individual (personal) variables (such as self-criticism, neuroticism, as well as a history of depression) to the onset of burnout. In their recent paper, Rossler and colleagues argue that this exclusive focus on the workplace environment, neglecting an individual's personality and/or predisposing mental disorder, leaves persons at risk, without appropriate treatment[17].Take care of your health!

As already mentioned, doctors make very bad patients and present late for treatment, often following a crisis at work or after a drink–driving offence[18]. Why is this? It seems that the list of barriers to seeking appropriate care seems to be significantly longer and more complex than for the general population. It includes inadequate education about causes and effective treatments of mental health problems; unwillingness to take time off from work and dedicate it to one's health; concerns over confidentiality, stigma, discrimination in medical licensing, hospital privileges, and career advancement[19]. Furthermore, physicians who decide to reach out for help may face limited understanding or sympathy demonstrated by their colleagues. Their problems may often not be taken seriously enough, which might lead to inadequate diagnosis and treatment. This highlights the need for specialist services, such as the Practitioner Health Programme (PHP), a confidential, London-based health service for doctors and dentists who have on average 5.5 new presentations each week, most of whom are doctors. Practitioners presenting to the service have considerable, often severe, mental health problems, similar to a cohort presenting to mental health services in the National Health Service (NHS).[20] Interestingly, follow-up data show that health practitioners treated at the PHP recover at a faster rate than patients who are not doctors or dentists and their recovery lasts longer.[21]

In general, treatment of depression and substance abuse in psychiatrists includes all validated procedures that are used in the general population. To our knowledge, there is no consensus on a biological approach to treat burnout. No clinical trials, including of pharmacotherapy, have been published. Hence, psychotropic drugs can only be used when a psychiatric disorder is clearly identified, as a co-morbidity of burnout. Most psychological interventions are group interventions and might include workshops on improving communication skills, on conflict resolution, and on stress management. Medical education can also be useful to reduce stress and improve self-efficiency and could include peer-support groups on difficult cases, attendance at lectures and conferences, or involvement in professional organizations. Supervision might be of great use in helping trainees; among other interventions, receiving positive feedback from supervisors is conducive to the development of positive self-efficacy beliefs[22].

Our aim is to increase awareness of this problem and motivate readers to seek help if they feel they need it and also to familiarize themselves with strategies that are helpful in preventing mental health problems.

Prevention strategies

Working as a physician inevitably includes high levels of stress, similar to those encountered by fire-fighters, policemen, managers, war reporters, or pilots. However, since it is impossible to completely eliminate stress from our everyday clinical work, the only way to increase resilience is to undertake whatever is known to preserve and improve physicians' well-being. Prevention strategies should focus on identified risk factors, both occupational and individual. This might lead to specific workplace interventions (primary prevention) and identification of at-risk trainees who might be offered psychiatric consultations or a more suitable workplace or specialty (secondary and tertiary prevention). An extremely powerful tool in prevention and/or early recognition of depression and other mental health problems is comprehensive education about risk factors and treatment options, starting with first-year medical students. For example, Japanese colleagues have developed a two-hour suicide intervention programme for medical residents, which consists of a one-hour lecture and a one-hour role-play session[23]. They have found that participants' confidence and attitudes significantly improve after the programme, but the effectiveness is limited after six months, which might indicate that education and intervention programmes should take place continuously.

Creating a defined boundary between work and home has also been strongly suggested. Maslach, cited by Ishak and colleagues, summarized effective working through burnout by stating: 'If all of the knowledge and advice about how to beat burnout could be summed up in one word, that word would be balance—balance between giving and getting, balance between stress and calm, balance between work and home.'[24]

Please take a look at Table 4.2 and the so-called biopsychosocial self-care formulation. As much as we may try, human beings do a very poor job of multitasking. That means

Table 4.2 Biopsychosocial self-care formulation

Bio	Psycho	Social
◆ Adequate:	◆ Exercise	◆ Family
• Sleep	◆ Relaxation	◆ Friends
• Rest	• Progressive muscle relaxation	◆ Significant others
• Food		◆ Children
• Exercise	• Guided imagery	◆ Pets
• Sex	• Deep breathing/ meditation	◆ Do you have a mentor?
◆ Addressing adequate preventive health measures:	• Supervision with peers or mentors	◆ Tending your personal comfort in places you inhabit most, e.g.:
• Going to primary care doctor, dentist, eye doctor, etc.	◆ Confiding in peers or friends	• Your home
	◆ Your own therapy	• Your work space
(a) Taking medications/ vitamins	◆ Sublimation (directing potentially negative emotions and energy into more positive experiences)	• Your mode of transport (car, bike, etc.)
(b) Proper nutrition		◆ Do you have control over finances?
◆ Making adjustments to lower work hours or stay home whenever needed	◆ Humour	◆ Making time for religion or spirituality
◆ Minimizing or controlling use of alcohol	• Reflecting on your own imperfect defences	◆ Do you have legal obligations that need to be filled?
		◆ Vacation
		◆ Hobbies

that when you make time for one aspect of your life, something else must get less. Therefore, the trick is not so much trying to cram in more but, again, trying to balance better.

Don't forget to exercise!

Does the thought of exercise seem more onerous than it is worth? Do you hate the idea of going to the gym? Certainly you are not alone. 'Exercise' should be part of everyone's day. Table 4.3 lists some exercise suggestions that involve minimal equipment and little, if any, money. Many of these exercises take up very little room and can easily be done inside, in your hotel, living room, kitchen, basement, or, if you are feeling particularly energetic, in a small hospital on-call room, which typically contains nothing more than a bed, a chair, and a desk. (In this case, we could call some of the exercises in Table 4.3 the 'call room workout'!) The exercises have been broken into two artificial categories. Of course, many of the exercises contain aspects of both, and almost anything can become a cardiovascular exercise if done long enough.

Table 4.3 The call-room workout

Body weight, strength, and flexibility	Cardiovascular
Upper body	◆ Walking laps around the hospital (can also be done in any indoor setting such as a shopping centre)
◆ Push-ups	
◆ Tricep dips	◆ Walking or jogging up and down the stairs
◆ Advanced: pull-ups	◆ Advanced: jumping rope
◆ Advanced: handstands against a wall (Handstand push-ups can also be done—prerequisite: the ability to support your bodyweight entirely on your hands; do not attempt unless you are comfortable standing on your hands already)	◆ Shadow boxing (prerequisite: knowledge of boxing, kick boxing, or other martial arts, as well as adequate flexibility to perform them safely)
	◆ Jogging on the spot
Lower body	
◆ Squats	
◆ Lunges	
◆ Calf raises (either on the ground or a raised platform, like the stairs)	
Core	
◆ Sit-ups/crunches (to the front to work the rectus abdominis, side to side for oblique muscles)	
◆ Advanced: leg lifts	
Flexibility	
◆ Stretching muscle groups and loosening up the joints	
◆ Yoga (consider doing it along with a video)	

Modified from Fiorillo A, Calliess IT, Sass H, How to succeed in psychiatry, in Blum J, Fiorillo A. *Choosing a career in psychiatry and setting priorities*, pp.197–210, Copyright (2012), with permission from John Wiley & Sons Ltd.

As always, the usual disclaimer: talk to your primary care physician before starting a new exercise programme, and start slow and with exercises you definitely know how to do, proceeding at your own pace. It is always helpful to loosen up the joints prior to doing any exercise. This is not meant to be a treatise on how to exercise. It is merely meant to provide interested parties with some ideas on how to do it cheaply using common household items.

Conclusions

Residency and the medical profession in general can be very stressful due to long working hours, night shifts, inflexible schedules, and a significant work–life imbalance. Therefore, in order to maintain a high level of service provision, while at the same time keeping or even improving mental health and well-being, one needs to learn a few 'tips and tricks'. The bottom line is to have a clear vision of professional and private life goals and some basic knowledge on managing time and priorities. It takes time and energy to achieve a desired life–work balance, but it is important to start thinking about these issues even today. Actions in that direction might include life changes such as moving home, reducing working hours, making time for personal psychotherapy, and changing jobs. Despite creating temporary discomfort, it might be worth the gamble because such changes can lead a person closer to their genuine interests. We hope some of the suggestions in this chapter might be useful for our readers. In the end, we would like to point out that everybody has teachers, mentors, and colleagues to ask for help and advice, and it is wise to use the experience and expertise of those who have gone before us.

References

1 **Tyssen R, Vlagum P**. Mental health problems among young doctors: an updated review of prospective studies. *Harvard Rev Psychiatry* 2002; **10**:154–65.

2 **Rössler W**. Stress, burnout, and job dissatisfaction in mental health workers. *Eur Arch Psychiatry Clin Neurosci* 2012; **262**(2):S65–659.

3 **Jovanović N, Beezhold J, Andlauer O, Mihai A, Johnson S**. Mental health problems of early career psychiatrists: from diagnosis to treatment strategies. In: *How to succeed in psychiatry: a guide to training and practice* (eds. Fiorillo A, Calliess IT, Sass H). Chichester: Wiley-Blackwell; 2012, pp. 283–95.

4 **Blum J, Fiorillo A**. Choosing a career in psychiatry and setting priorities. In: *How to succeed in psychiatry: a guide to training and practice* (eds. Fiorillo A, Calliess IT, Sass H). Chichester: Wiley-Blackwell; 2012, pp. 197–210.

5 **Kandel ER**. A new intellectual framework for psychiatry. *Am J Psychiatry* 1998; **155**:457–69.

6 Directive 2003/88/EC of the European Parliament and of the Council of 4 November 2003 concerning certain aspects of the organisation of working time. *Official Journal L 299*; 18/11/2003; pp. 9–19.

7 **Dorsey ER, Jarjoura D, Rutecki GW**. Influence of controllable lifestyle on recent trends in specialty choice by US medical students. *JAMA* 2003; **290**:1173–8.

8 US Bureau of Labor Statistics (Department of Labor). American time use statistics—2009 results. Bureau of Labor Statistics; 2013. Available at: http://www.bls.gov/news.release/pdf/atus.pdf.

9 **Dacre J, Shepherd S**. Women and medicine. *Clin Med* 2010; **10**:544–7.

10 **Brooks S, Gerada C, Chalder T**. Review of literature on the mental health of doctors: are specialist services needed? *J Mental Health* 2011; **I**:1–11.

11 **Goebert D, Thompson D, Takeshita J, et al**. Depressive symptoms in medical students and residents: a multischool study. *Acad Med* 2009; **84**(2):236–41.

12 **Andrew LB**. *Physician suicide*. Medscape; 2010. Available at: http://emedicine.medscape.com/article/806779-overview.

13 **Schernhammer ESI, Graham AC**. Suicide rates among physicians: a quantitative and gender assessment (meta-analysis). *Am J Psychiatry* 2004; **161**:2295–2302.

14 **Maslach C, Jackson SE, Leiter MP**. Maslach burnout inventory manual (3rd edn). Palo Alto, California: Consulting Psychologists Press Inc.; 1996.

15 **Prins JT, Gazendam-Donofrio SM, Tubben BJ, van der Heijden FM, van de Wiel HB, Hoekstra-Weebers JE**. Burnout in medical residents: a review. *Med Educ* 2007; **41**:788–800.

16 **Tzischinsky O**. Daily and yearly burnout symptoms in Israeli shift work residents. *J Hum Ergol* 2001; **30**:357–62.

17 **Rössler W, Hengartner MP, Ajdacic-Gross V, Angst J**. Predictors of burnout: results from a prospective community study. *Eur Arch Psychiatry Clin Neurosci* 2015; **265**:19–25.

18 **Strang J, Wilks M, Wells B, Marshall J**. Missed problems and missed opportunities for addicted doctors. *BMJ* 1998; **316**:405–6.

19 **Reynolds CF 3rd, Clayton PJ**. Commentary: Out of the silence: confronting depression in medical students and residents. Acad Med. 2009; **84**:159–60.

20 **Brooks S, Gerada C, Chalder T**. Doctors and dentists with mental ill health and addictions: outcomes of treatment from the Practitioner Health Programme. *J Mental Health* 2013; **22**:237–45.

21 National Health Service. *Practitioner Health Programme. Three-year report.* NHS; 2012. Available at: http://www.php.nhs.uk.

22 **Dory V, Beaulieu MD, Pestiaux D, et al**. The development of self-efficacy beliefs during general practice vocational training: an exploratory study. *Med Teach* 2009; **31**(1):39–44.

23 **Kato TA, Suzuki Y, Sato R, et al**. Development of 2-hour suicide intervention program among medical residents: first pilot trial. *Psychiatry Clin Neurosci* 2010; **64**:531–40.

24 **IsHak WW, Lederer S, Mandili C, et al**. Burnout during residency training: a literature review. *J Grad Med Educ* 2009; **1**(2):236–42.

Chapter 5

Managing financial resources in healthcare settings

Amit Malik, Clive Field, and Philip Gorwood

Introduction

While most doctors are reluctant to get involved in financial management of their hospitals/clinics/departments and so on (from here on, we will use the term *clinical services* or *services* to describe any of these healthcare settings), in a world where adequate financial health is often crucial for the long-term sustainability of services, it is essential that psychiatrists are aware of the broad concepts of how effective financial management can positively influence the delivery of services in which they work. Although healthcare financial management is a specialty in itself, this chapter covers some basic financial areas, knowledge of which psychiatrists might benefit from. As the world passes through challenging economic times and healthcare expenditure rises, year after year, the need to ably manage financial resources has never been greater. As the authors' extensive experience is that of working in state-funded services, this is reflected in a significant proportion of this chapter. However, the chapter also touches, more generally, on the psychiatrist's role in financial management, as this would be relevant to other models of healthcare funding.

In large healthcare organizations, formal corporate departments have responsibility for managing financial resources, and psychiatrists provide clinical input into this process, depending on either their formal roles (medical director, clinical director, etc.) or their informal leadership of the service they work in. Many of us who have eventually taken on formal medical leadership roles were at some point, usually early in our careers, involved in supporting our finance colleagues, in some informal capacity, with clinical input with respect to budgeting and service planning. In smaller organizations, and especially psychiatrist-run private set-ups, the medics are often a key part of the leadership team and play a more central role in the management of financial resources. Another aspect is the evolution of the relationship between the clinical services' administrative staff and the care professionals (such as psychiatrists). The role of financial and administrative staff in the organization and management of clinical activities is consistently increasing in many European countries. Being aware of the key priorities of the administrative staff, which are sometimes not concordant with the medical staff's point of view, might help clinical staff to better interact with them, therefore enabling them to be more efficient.

Box 5.1 Benefits of higher income

1 Further growth of the organization

2 Research and development to contribute to better outcomes for patients receiving these services

3 Bigger salary chest to recruit more staff and attract exceptional talent with higher renumeration

4 In a private organization, a key financial objective is to generate profits and distribute dividends among the shareholders.

This chapter briefly outlines why it is essential for organizations to have healthy finances and the role that a financial accountant plays in this process. It then looks at the two main drivers of financial health—cost and revenue. The area where psychiatrists could have greatest influence is in reducing the costs of providing clinical services or care while still maintaining quality and better outcomes, and a significant portion of the chapter focuses on this area. It then outlines how psychiatrists could support revenue enhancement for their organization. Finally, the chapter briefly looks at the finance-relevant steps that need to be undertaken to develop a new service either within an existing organization or independently.

Financial objectives of an organization

Robust management of financial resources provides a significant competitive advantage to services in a similar way that robust clinical and operational management does. Services that manage their finances efficiently can use the relatively greater financial resources available to enhance the overall value to patients and to people working in the services in a plethora of ways. In addition to creating a favourable revenue–cost balance, psychiatrists should support their organizations in making clinical and strategically sound financial investment decisions. All these efforts should lead to higher income that can then be re-invested (Box 5.1).

Working with financial accountants

The single most important message for psychiatrists, directly or indirectly responsible for managing financial resources, is the necessity to collaborate effectively with financial accountants/managers. Depending on their role and how much time they have allocated to a particular service, accountants/managers will usually be helpful to the growth of the organization (Box 5.2).

The crucial message is that accountants can give psychiatrists and managers financial figures relating to existing and new services, but it is the professionals (clinicians and managers) who need to use this information as a tool to make clinical and business decisions regarding their services.

Box 5.2 Roles of managers in healthcare organizations

1 Developing detailed cost accounts of their business

2 Giving cost estimates for new positions or services

3 Providing support for developing financial projections

4 Developing budgets for existing and new planned services

5 Preparing monthly/quarterly financial reports which highlight areas of underspend/overspend

6 Obtaining advice on tax and other regulatory implications of business actions

7 Assessing value for money by linking measures for effectiveness, efficiency, and economy.

Income, revenue, and costs

To start to fully understand the fundamental finance equation, *surplus (or deficit) = revenue – costs*, we should first explore costs and revenue separately.

Costs

Put simply, cost is the amount of money that is spent to deliver a service. Within health-care services, costs can largely be divided into pay and non-pay.

Pay costs

These include the salary and related costs for all the people working within or for a particular service. Within psychiatry, pay costs often constitute the most significant proportion (approximately 70–90%) of all expenditure within a large service. These costs include a number of components:

1 Salary

- Basic salary
- On-call supplements
- Any incentive payments or awards
- Any other benefits such as a rural service allowance or a recruitment/retention enhancement

2 Supplementary payments

- Any state dues, per employee (e.g. national insurance)
- Pension contributions

There are additional indirect costs of employing staff (including computers, phones, IT licences, office space, training costs, and travel allowances) but, depending on the organization, these either have a separate category of their own or are often added to corporate overheads. Regardless, these costs must be accounted for in planning for an increase in staff numbers.

Pay costs apply to medical staff, non-medical clinical staff, and to non-clinical personnel, although medical staff are by far the most substantial per capita expense in most countries. It is important to be cognisant of the cost breakdown, as doctors can often be guilty of thinking only of the first component (salary) when considering the cost of employing a new staff member, while the other costs can often add 20–25% to that figure, even before corporate overheads are included.

Non-pay costs

By definition, this includes all other costs of running a service, besides pay. Standard non-pay costs for a psychiatric service include drugs (medication), equipment, leasing costs, travel, training, consumables, investigation costs, and third-party costs such as cleaning and maintenance services and security services.

Drugs and investigations often form a large part of non-pay costs within psychiatric services and effective procurement of these can often lead to substantial cost savings.

Corporate overheads

Large organizations have corporate departments, whose functions are listed in Box 5.3.

The corporate entity usually does not generate any income itself and, therefore, the costs of the various crucial functions listed in Box 5.3 are charged to the clinical services that they serve. On the other hand, however, small independent clinical services lose any economies of scale that a well-functioning corporate entity would bring to bear when a number of such services are clubbed together within one organization. For instance, a psychiatric clinic with six psychiatrists, four psychologists, and twenty nurses requires some finance function but might not require a full-time finance manager. Therefore, if they were not part of a corporate entity, they might lose efficiency by having to employ a full-time person or by outsourcing this function to a local accounting firm, where the service would not have the same degree of interest, ownership, and customization. This function within a corporate entity could be served by a finance

---

Box 5.3 Functions of corporate departments in healthcare organizations

1 Finance

2 Human resources

3 Estates and facilities

4 Quality and risk management

5 Legal role

6 Information technology and management

7 Governance

manager who is also providing the same service to six other psychiatric clinics that are part of the same organization and can therefore share the cost of this individual. Obviously, this choice is not available to small stand-alone entities, like private clinics, that need to figure out customized and efficient solutions for each of the non-clinical support services.

Having understood the various aspects of costs, some broad principles for generating efficiencies within mental health services are explored (see Box 5.4). This is by no means an exhaustive list and is largely based on the authors' experience of financial management of psychiatric services.

Operational excellence The most significant valid means of reducing costs is by optimizing the operational capabilities of the service. Hopp and Lovejoy[1], in their 2013 treatise on hospital operations, have outlined a number of ways to achieve operational efficiency, and the authors of this chapter have referred extensively to this volume to enumerate numerous broad areas of achieving efficiency within a mental health setting:

1 *Reducing errors:* Errors contribute significantly to increased costs as time and resources then need to be expended in either rectifying them or, more significantly, indemnifying the patients or their relatives. So, developing a learning culture, implementing effective reporting systems for errors and near misses, using root-cause analysis methodology to investigate errors, and developing underlying remedial themes and disseminating them among the clinical and non-clinical workforce are all crucial elements of overall systemic enhancement that can help minimize errors in the long term and reduce operating costs of services.

2 *Simplification:* One way of improving efficiency and minimizing costs is to review each step of a treatment pathway and remove any steps that might not be necessary for improving overall patient care. In this instance, it is important to remember that seemingly redundant steps may act as a protective feature within care pathways, helping to mitigate the effects of errors when these occur. Therefore, unlike

Box 5.4 Principles for generating efficiencies within mental health services

1 Operational excellence

2 Use of technology

3 Early intervention and crisis support

4 Skill-mix reviews

5 Partnerships/outsourcing

6 Efficient procurement

7 Expense claim and approval guidelines

in the manufacturing industry, it might not be advisable to remove all these re-dundant steps from a care pathway in zeal to simplify things. For instance, in the case of in-patients, once a medication card is filled out by a ward doctor, it is often checked by the ward pharmacist and then again by the dispensing pharmacist. While a care process review might suggest removing the ward pharmacist's checks, this additional step often protects from medication errors, which can be costly for both providers and patients.

3 *Standardization:* While complex skills are required in diagnosing patients, most of the processes—from the point of receiving a patient referral to the point of dis-charge—can be standardized. All steps of care pathways should be reviewed, both in terms of the latest evidence base as well as for the process by which care is being delivered, to ensure that the service has a standardized care pathway, as far as is practicable, for most patients. Experienced senior clinicians can then use their judgement and experience to deviate from this pathway at certain points for a mi-nority of complex patients. For instance, the process for how a dementia patient is initially assessed, how collateral history is obtained, how they are examined, and what investigations are ordered, can all be standardized, or at least described ac-cording to precise guidelines that can be used in a majority of cases to facilitate the use of a relevant and efficient process. However, after these initial few steps, if further examinations or investigations are required because the presentation or assessment does not fit a particular diagnosis, then the care pathway should have enough flexibility to permit this. This will ensure that all patients are receiving the most efficient, evidence-based care, and deviations are only applied for the benefit of the few patients that cannot be managed through a standardized care pathway. Standardization will improve efficiency, reduce errors, and improve outcomes for all patients and, therefore, drive down costs.

4 *Measure variations in process (and outcomes):* Systems should be put in place to measure the process and outcome metrics of a standardized care pathway. In order to succeed, the metrics must be developed collaboratively with all stake-holders. Psychiatrists must involve their multiprofessional team at an early stage, to review care pathways as well as develop metrics. Unilaterally imposing metrics rarely gets the engagement necessary for performance improvement. Examples of metrics could include referral to assessment times, DNA (did not attend) rates for patient appointments, percentage of patients with completed diagnosis, percent-age of assessment reports sent to referrers within an agreed time frame, and per-centage of patients with completed risk assessments. Measurements can then be used to compare performance among teams (for larger organizations) and among professionals (for a team). The primary goal of performance measurements is not to create useless competition among teams or professionals, but to give bench-marks and raise awareness of the metrics and the rationale behind them. Psychi-atrists and managers should use any performance variations to address systemic problems that might be resulting in one team being an outlier. For instance, a high sickness rate within the administrative section in a team could be contributing to

referrers not getting assessment reports in time; and this backlog might not only be cost inefficient today but also might hurt revenues tomorrow. The discrepancy in waiting times for referrals can sometimes only become obvious when contrasted with other teams, and this then allows managers and clinicians to work together to resolve the problem and to communicate proactively with referrers to keep them engaged. However, not all performance variation results from systemic issues and, in some instances, issues with individual underperformance need to be addressed through both formal and informal mechanisms.

5 *Pooling*: Teams within organizations and professionals within teams often operate their patient pathways in silos that can lead to artificial queuing within a system that still has spare capacity. For instance, in the United Kingdom (UK), psychiatrists and nurses are often aligned to general practitioner (GP) practices and accept referrals only from specific GP practices. This can often result in a situation where one team has a waiting list, with the consequent stress and perceived need for more resources, due to a periodic spike in referrals, whereas another team has spare capacity. To circumvent such scenarios, three or four teams could come together to form a 'super team' so that the variability in demand could be distributed and collective resources could be utilized efficiently. This has the obvious moral hazard of 'free riding'; an inherently inefficient team will allow waiting lists to develop as they know that they will be rescued within the 'super team' structure. Intelligently designed metrics that collect data at the team and individual level will expose any such practices and allow colleagues to address these collectively or with support from their managers. Similar principles can also be applied to non-human resources, such as beds and investigations, where such carve-outs (dealing with only specific subsets of patients) can often result in queuing.

6 *Front-loading diagnosis and management (care) planning:* Many services have restructured themselves so that the most experienced and qualified professionals manage the most complex patients and other members of the teams manage patients presenting with a perceived lower level of complexity. This, in principle, is meant to prioritize more experienced professionals for relatively complex work. However, there have been recent suggestions that in chronic illnesses where there is no single, objective, gold standard diagnostic test (e.g. HbA1C for diabetes mellitus), the most experienced resources should collectively be deployed in diagnosing a condition and developing a management plan. This is because, if the condition is misdiagnosed, each stage of the resultant erroneous management plan will have a compounding effect on the overall error and the resultant patient care and cost implications.[2]

In addition to operational excellence, consideration should be given to the effectiveness of any clinical interventions, and practicable outcomes should be reviewed to ensure 'value for money' of costs incurred in delivering clinical services.

Use of technology There are multiple ways in which technology can be leveraged to create efficiencies. These could range from:

1 *Video conferencing:* Exploiting the potential of video conferencing could ensure that a psychiatrist can be present for the GP review in a remote nursing home, rather than having to drive him/herself all the way there, or that community nurses could attend care planning meetings for their patients via a video link.

2 *Digitization:* Using digital transcription technology to optimize the use of electronic health care records entry by healthcare professionals.

3 *E-prescribing:* Utilizing electronic prescribing programs to remotely prescribe medication for known patients.

4 *Tele-health:* Using tele-health devices to monitor and manage vulnerable patients at home rather than bringing them into hospital.

Bed-based versus community services (early intervention and crisis support) Intervening early, utilizing technology, and reconfiguring teams to provide intensive input might mean that some patients can be either managed at home during a relapse or crisis or could be discharged from hospital earlier, with the adequate support. Either way, this would imply that for patients, the trauma of a hospital stay could be minimized, while resources could be diverted from expensive bed-based services to community-based services.

Skill-mix reviews As technology and professional boundaries continually evolve, psychiatrists should always be asking if the right person is undertaking the right task within the care process. For instance, if senior experienced (and expensive) clinicians are spending a lot of their time entering clinical notes/data into a computer, it would be better to have more administrative staff so that clinicians' expertise can be utilized most efficiently. If senior nurses are visiting patients three times a week to monitor medication, it would be better to have support workers (health technicians) to undertake this task more cost effectively. Finally, if senior psychiatrists are spending a lot of time gathering background information rather than focusing on a therapeutic interaction, is it feasible, in some diagnostic groups, that nurse practitioners work alongside consultants in a clinic to gather this information and present the information to psychiatrists before the patient is seen by them—hence making the interaction more efficient and saving money in the process? These discussions need to take place collaboratively, among clinical teams and business and finance managers, to ensure that all stakeholders support the changes.

Partnerships/outsourcing Often, it is more effective and efficient to partner up with other organizations to deliver areas that are not one's core capability. For instance, a mental health organization might want to partner an acute hospital for a diabetes service for their schizophrenia patients, rather than employing staff directly to provide such a service. Similarly, a dementia memory service might want to outsource all their radiological investigations to a specialist provider so as to reduce the capital cost of buying a scanner and the revenue cost of its upkeep, of employing technicians, and of replacements when technology needs to be updated. This principle is equally applicable in non-clinical aspects of services as well; for example, patient notes could be dictated electronically and sent to a transcription company who can usually transcribe these and return them overnight for clinicians to review. Administrative staff can then be deployed in more patient-focused activities such as staffing clinics and entering patient-related data into computers. Similarly, in smaller organizations, it might be too expensive, per patient or per employee, to have an in-house pharmacy or payroll service, respectively, and these could be outsourced or provided through a service-level agreement with a third party.

Efficient procurement Getting the same materials/consumables from an alternative supplier might contribute to cost reductions. This is especially true where the cost of medication is borne by the healthcare service. Psychiatrists should work with their pharmacy colleagues to ensure that drugs are procured at the cheapest possible cost and, where available and when quality conditions are the same, generic formulations of medications are used. Similarly, procurement might also create efficiencies for other goods/services such as consumables used in inpatient units, electronic equipment, and training packages. However, psychiatrists are less likely to be involved in the procurement of these.

Expense claim and approval guidelines Most large organizations already have detailed guidance regarding who can claim and for which type of expenses. As a psychiatrist within a team, you might, as the senior professional, be asked to approve some of these expenses, especially for trainees working for you. In those instances, the role includes making oneself aware of the guidelines and ensuring that these are being followed robustly. In smaller organizations and private set-ups, guidelines will need to be established and should be flexible enough to not stifle the growth of a new venture but also should have adequate clarity to prevent any abuse. Audit systems should also be in place to review that expenses are being claimed and approved appropriately. Again, in small/private set-ups, some of this responsibility may fall upon the psychiatrist.

The list given here is by no means an exhaustive one, and not all areas will be applicable to all services. However, psychiatrists at an early stage in their career come into services with a fresh pair of eyes and should work with their senior colleagues, as well as with business and finance managers, to review the areas and assess if cost savings can be attained by making modifications. It is however crucial that new entrants, in their enthusiasm, do not jump in to make changes without fully evaluating the existing services and discussing the origins and history of the organization with more experienced colleagues who have been around for longer, as hasty changes could not only lead to more expenses but could also be expensive to reverse.

Revenue

Revenue is defined as 'the income generated from sale goods or services, or any other use of capital or assets, associated with the main operations of an organisation before any costs or expenses are deducted'.[3]

An organization may receive revenue from a wide range of sources (one or multiple institutional payers, private patients, insurance companies, etc.) and through different forms of payment systems. The most common ones include:

1 *Block contracts*: This is a fixed payment made to healthcare companies to provide care for a population regardless of the volume of services provided. This is usually the case with government contracts with a unitary healthcare provider for a geographical area.

2 *Fee per case*: Payment is made by the healthcare provider on the basis of diagnostic group/intervention undertaken. This payment could be through government contracts, health maintenance organizations (HMOs), insurance companies, or private payers.

3 *Capitated healthcare contracts*: This is a fixed payment, per patient, made to the healthcare company to provide all care to an individual patient. This method of payment has often been used by HMOs in the USA.

Astute readers would observe that both block and capitated healthcare contracts (fixed payments per population or patient, respectively) incentivize the healthcare providers to focus more on prevention and early intervention. This is because, for the same patient, the downstream costs of providing services in a crisis (either as an inpatient or in the community) are a lot higher than health promotion, prevention, and early intervention. Psychiatrists working in these services should therefore understand the additional financial imperative of collaborating extensively with their managers, public health officers, and primary care physicians to develop programmes and services that promote health and well-being and also to improve access to services. The authors are not suggesting that those working in private practices and other 'fee per case' services should not focus on health promotion and early intervention, but would like to highlight the clear financial incentives for doing so in the case of block and capitated contracts. The pros and cons of different types of contracts are beyond the scope of this chapter, but suffice it to say that none of the payment methods produce the perfectly desired incentives which would maximize both provider and payer interests.

Psychiatrists, where feasible, should also offer clinical input into contract negotiations with payers (commissioners) that might include government organizations, insurance companies, and HMOs. Clinical input can often make these negotiations more valid in terms of credibility, as well as provide a scientific basis for commissioning new services. Psychiatrists can also use a scientific evidence base, inculcate novel ideas, and break the deadlock in financially focused negotiations. To maintain long-term credibility, both internally and externally, it is crucial that psychiatrists who are given the opportunity to participate in these negotiations early in their career, aim to maximize the best interests of all patients that the negotiations relate to and not just the ones interfacing with their services.

Additionally, mental healthcare organizations might also receive funding through:

1 *Research and educational grants:* Psychiatrists who have interests, expertise, or qualifications in research or education, can apply, with the support of their managers, for research or educational grants that become available from either government bodies or private organizations. Such grants will help psychiatrists to pursue their interests in a funded manner, to provide their patients and colleagues with access to educational and research programmes, to raise the reputation of the organization, and to give the organization additional revenue. In undertaking such grant applications, psychiatrists should be cautious to run the finances of their applications past their finance colleagues to ensure that the grant would include

and cover the costs incurred by the organization (overheads) in achieving the objectives stipulated by the grant, as overheads can significantly reduce the grants finally available for research or education. Additionally, psychiatrists should ensure, through discussions with senior colleagues, that such activities are aligned to the strategic objectives of the organization. Finally, psychiatrists should guard against any conflict of interest both with regards to their duties towards their own organization and their duty of care towards their patients. When in doubt regarding a conflict of interest, one should always discuss grant applications with senior colleagues. Regardless, psychiatrists, when working for an organization, should never receive any funds directly and these should always be channelled through the appropriate organizational processes.

2 *Charitable contributions:* If psychiatrists come across an opportunity for the organization to obtain charitable funds, they should connect such charitable organizations to relevant business managers within their own organization. Psychiatrists might be approached initially, regarding such a contribution, following a presentation they may have made, externally, about the work that they or their organization is undertaking.

3 *Service-level agreement payments with other providers:* Occasionally, psychiatrists might be asked to provide services to other organizations, such as general hospitals or local businesses. This can potentially be revenue-generating work for the psychiatrist's employer organization. Should such an opportunity arise, psychiatrists should work with business and finance colleagues to develop a business plan and then negotiate a contract for such services. Psychiatrists can often initiate such opportunities through informal discussions with their primary care and hospital colleagues or through formal presentations regarding the importance of mental health input into general hospitals or local businesses. If psychiatrists choose to provide such a third-party service independent of their employer, they should follow organizational processes for declaring such alternative employment.

There are other ways in which psychiatrists can contribute to increased revenue for their organization. The most significant one is by utilizing skills/experiences gained during training to provide new services for which there is an unmet need. The authors' recent experience of these opportunities have included psychiatrists providing adult attention deficit hyperactivity disorder (ADHD) or fetal alcohol syndrome services. If psychiatrists are able to establish themselves as experts in novel therapeutic areas, this could increase the customer base of the organization and enhance its revenue.

Finally, psychiatrists—particularly those early in their career—can bring energy and enthusiasm to services and renew a focus on customer service; this can also help enhance the reputation of the organization and, indirectly, its revenue, by helping the service to win new contracts.

Finances and new services

Besides managing the costs and revenue of existing services, continual evidence-base and marketplace changes necessitate that new services are set up or existing services undergo a significant transformation. Either of the two scenarios requires an invest-ment decision. This could involve a small amount of finance (e.g. buying a new piece of software or hiring another member of staff) or a larger one (building a new unit). Psy-chiatrists should work closely with their finance and business colleagues in signposting potential technology shifts early, so that these can be included in the annual rounds of financial planning when organizational strategic plans are developed. Collaborative business cases should be developed for approval within the organization and should include:

1 Information on the demand for a new or modified service (market analysis and assessment of commissioners)

2 Details of the recommended service model

3 Findings of any pilots (proof of concept)

4 Cost analysis

5 Financial projections

6 Options analysis, with alternative models of providing the same or a similar service

7 Financial and non-financial support required within and outside the organization

8 Stages of approval

9 Implementation plan including set-up, recruitment, marketing, and launch

10 In-built success metrics and review processes.

The process is not that dissimilar for psychiatrists wanting to start their own private practice, except that the need for internal approvals would be redundant and one might have to hire a financial advisor and/or a business consultant to help with the financial modelling, cost analysis, and funding documents. Even if external funding is not re-quired, it is still important, in order to assess the viability of a new service, to go through the rigours of business planning, rather than relying on 'gut' instincts.

Conclusions

Effective management of financial resources is crucial for the success and long-term viability of all healthcare organizations. The extent to which psychiatrists, at an early stage in their career, get involved with finances of their service/organization will de-pend largely on the size and structure of the organization, as well as the additional management roles taken on by the psychiatrist. In fulfilling formal and informal fi-nancial responsibilities, the relationship between the psychiatrist and the finance and operational managers is crucial. Financial strength of a service/organization can be enhanced by efforts that impact on cost and/or revenue: psychiatrists can influence both of these. They should provide clinical input into initiating or planning for new ser-vices. Once again, the level of medical involvement in these decisions depends on the formal/informal management responsibilities of the individual and could range from peripheral (in a large organization) to integral (when psychiatrists are starting their own private service). Finally, while numbers can seem very daunting to many medics in general, modern-day physicians are unlikely to escape some involvement in the management of financial resources, and the best way to learn is to get involved, seek advice, and get one's hands 'dirty' by actually taking on responsibilities for such management.

References

1 **Hopp WJ, Lovejoy WS**. *Hospital operations: principles of high efficiency. Health care college.* New Jersey: FT Press; 2013.

2 **Christensen CM, Grossman, JH, Hwang J**. *The innovator's prescription: a disruptive solution for healthcare.* New York: McGraw-Hill; 2008.

3 Definition accessed from BusinessDictionary.com

Chapter 6

Managing difficult people in the workplace

Julian Beezhold, Nagendra Bendi, and Mariana Pinto da Costa

Introduction

Difficult people can be found in every workplace, and the difficulties can take different forms. Many different types of behaviour can be 'difficult', and dealing with these depends on experience, skills, and confidence. Examples of difficult behaviour may include bullying, undermining, unreliability, talking too much, not listening, failing to communicate or document, constant competition or criticism, making oneself very close to the boss, being rude and obnoxious, and forming exclusive cliques.

It is really important, even essential, that difficult behaviours are addressed and not ignored. The first response to difficult behaviour is often one of shock, particularly when there is a challenge to one's professional role. This can then change to anger and resentment, in turn potentially leading to harm to both oneself and the quality of work. That is why one must deal with difficult people from a position of objectivity and emotional control, early on, and not simply retreat or become a constant complainer oneself. Indeed, failing to address difficult behaviour can lead to being identified as both unable to cope and also as a difficult person yourself.

Sometimes dealing with this is more difficult, for example, when the behaviour is directed personally or undermines one professionally; at other times it can be easier to manage if it affects many others or if the person is generally unpleasant.

As psychiatrists, we usually work in multidisciplinary teams. In performing our role, we interact with various professionals (including senior and junior medical colleagues, nurses, psychologists, therapists, managers) in our day to day practice. Effective relationship with others in the team is a key factor in ensuring high quality and safe delivery of service. All too frequently, problems with care are exposed by 'whistle-blowers'. Yet if the workplace was run properly, there would be no need for whistle-blowing as the workplace culture itself would actively make it safe and routine for problems to be resolved within the organization. Of course, this cannot happen in a dysfunctional workplace struggling with 'difficult people'.

When working in a team, the primary task is to provide high-quality care for patients. However, there may be times when there are difficulties in getting along with senior and junior colleagues, or with other professionals. These days, there is an increasing awareness of the importance of problems in the doctor–manager relationship in the work environment. These problems can have a multitude of causes including, for example, interpersonal differences, working environment, or different styles of working arrangements. Fundamental to solving the problem is the understanding of how a conflict arises.

Understanding conflict between people

The Danish Centre for Conflict Resolution (DCCR) defines conflicts as: 'disagreements that lead to tensions within and between people'.[1]

The DCCR identifies three psychological areas forming part of the conflict process. First is the area with which we have no immediate interaction or influence over—the zone comprising the greater society, such as stakeholders. Indirectly, we may have some impact by electing those that participate in this zone. Second is the area of direct, interpersonal, face-to-face communication with others—the zone of relationships with co-workers. This is where our day-to-day conflicts most often take place, since we are in direct contact with people. In the third zone, we discover and learn how to improve our management of conflicts, including by sharing our daily situations while enjoying confidentiality and the benefit of support.

Almost all conflicts comprise a struggle over one or more of only a few dimensions, as listed in Table 6.1. Once there is conflict, then this can rapidly escalate (Table 6.2).

Table 6.1 Types of conflicts and proposed solutions

Dimension	Reasons for conflicts	Possible solution
Personal	It revolves around feelings and emotions such as one's identity (e.g. as a psychiatrist); loyalty to people, teams, and organizations; perception of acceptance or rejection by others; and the sense of one's own value.	Talking to each other, and understanding and finding solutions.
Value	Conflict arises around values that are important to the individual (e.g. ethical or cultural values).	Talking to each other, and understanding and finding solutions.
Instrumental	Reasons for conflicts include the aims, processes, and structures in the workplace. Disagreement could arise regarding what should be done and also how it should be done.	Problem-solving techniques.
Interest	The struggle for a variety of sometimes scarce resources such as funding, physical space, or even sufficient time is another potential source of conflict in the workplace.	Negotiation.

Source data from: Centre for Resolution of International Conflicts, University of Copenhagen, Øster Farimagsgade Copenhagen.

Table 6.2 Escalation of conflicts in the workplace

Disagreement	Not wanting the same thing
Personification	Feeling it is their fault
Problem expands	Believing there is always a problem with them
Dialogue stops	Gossip starts
Enemy images	Seeing them as bad
Open hostility	The idea that it is us or them
Polarization	Moving away from the opponent

Source data from: Centre for Resolution of International Conflicts, University of Copenhagen, Øster Farimagsgade Copenhagen

However, the good news is that with the right approach, the experience of working with many of the 'difficult' people that one encounters at work can be positively transformed. Indeed, resolving these issues can become richly rewarding. Practising successful techniques will result in greater skill, confidence, and, ultimately, a more productive and happy work environment. The rest of this chapter will look in more detail at specific types of 'difficult' people and methods of trying to address their behaviours.

How to be a good work colleague

One of the most important positive steps that one can take is to look at ways in which one can become a better work colleague. This is not done by educational attainment, number of publications, prizes and awards, or even patient feedback alone. Being a great work colleague is the most effective way of increasing personal job satisfaction, and will play a major part in gaining promotion and succeeding in one's career ambitions (see Box 6.1).

Box 6.1 The nine ways to become a better work colleague

1 Be as fair, open, and transparent as possible.

2 Always suggest solutions to any problems that you raise. This will make everyone else's life easier and create a very much more receptive environment to any concerns that you might need to raise. Simply reporting problems tends not to be a very welcome approach.

3 Avoid blaming others publicly, and as far as possible also privately, even when something is their fault. This simply creates enemies who will of course be keen to return the favour. It may be more helpful to focus instead on whether there were any system errors; in other words, could changing a system have prevented things going wrong?

Box 6.1 The nine ways to become a better work colleague (continued)

4 Treat all your colleagues professionally and with respect, and pay attention to language, tone, and volume. If you feel the need to shout or make hurtful comments, then it is better to remain silent.

5 Do not bypass colleagues or exclude them from lines of communication. Especially, do not raise issues forming part of a colleague's responsibility with their boss, without having first approached them. Instead, work on building a mutually trusting relationship.

6 Do what you say you are going to do, when you say you will do it, or let people know in good time (with a plan B) if you are unable to do so. This will ensure that your colleagues can trust and rely on you.

7 Give credit to others for their contributions towards your own success. Acknowledging, thanking, and valuing the efforts of your work colleagues is one of the most powerful positive actions that you can take to improving your own working life.

8 Aim to help your colleagues realize their maximum potential. It can be a source of great personal pleasure and satisfaction when you play a role in inspiring, facilitating, and supporting the achievements of others; and they will, in turn, be far more likely to help and support you, leading to a better and more productive workplace for all.

9 Above all, invest in valuing and appreciating your colleagues. Examples of how to do this include saying 'please' and thanking them for contributions; written and verbal compliments regarding their work (especially also copied to their boss); bringing in food (especially that you have made yourself); taking an interest in them as people by, for example, asking appropriately caring questions about personal matters and events; endeavouring to create and provide opportunities for them to achieve and advance including, for example, by supporting training; creating fun happenings such as a social/cultural activity or an inter-team sport event; and treating them with flexibility and humanity.

Types of difficult behaviour and specific strategies for dealing with them

Negativity

People can be negative either temporarily, in response to a specific trigger, or in a more persistent long-term manner. Such negativity should be dealt with differently in order to minimize the damage it causes.

Gossip can be considered as a special form of negativity and, in general, dealt with along the same lines. However, gossip is endemic, so it is important to be aware of features suggesting that it does need to be addressed. Gossip is out of hand and needs to be dealt with when it hurts colleagues' feelings, disrupts the working environment, harms morale and motivation, and starts to break down relationships. Where there is a culture of gossip, or when certain themes are prominent, it may be useful to reflect on whether

Box 6.2 How to deal with occasionally negative colleagues

- Listen fully to their issue and ensure that you properly understand the matter. You can do this by giving them enough time, asking questions, and clarifying any ambiguities or uncertainties.
- When they simply wish to let off steam and complain, then it is appropriate to listen, but with some clear boundaries attached. Simply listening, as they go on and on, will risk infecting you with negativity as well. When needed, change the conversation to a more positive subject.
- When there is a legitimate grievance, then consider offering your help in the form of advice and ideas for how they might resolve the issue. This should be short-term advice pointing them in the right direction to obtain further help. It is also important to be cognizant of your limitations and not become their therapist or career adviser.
- When you do not agree with your colleague's concerns, then you should let them know this in a sensitive and tactful manner, while emphasizing that you care about them and their feelings. You should gently, but firmly, then end the conversation and resist the temptation to prolong it or return to the same issues, under another guise, later on. This will then avoid encouraging further negativity in that colleague, and also discourage others from dumping their negativity onto you, and help prevent the creation of a culture of negativity.

there is anything that the organization should do differently. Remember too that with gossip, what goes around, comes around—if you gossip about others, then they will no doubt reciprocate.

Occasional negativity may be in response to a real or imaginary grievance but can often effectively be dealt with as detailed in Box 6.2.

Persistently negative colleagues require a decisive and different approach. Although there are almost always underlying reasons for their enduring negative outlook, as a work colleague, this should not be your concern. Their persistent negativity will, if allowed, risk infecting you. Essentially, persistent negativity is a choice, and the individual concerned really either needs a new job, treatment, or a different take on life (Box 6.3).

Ultimately, if there is no resolution, you have to put yourself first and consider whether it may be better to look, yourself, at moving. This is more likely to be the case where there is inadequate organizational support or will to address the negativity.

Bullying

Bullying is defined in many ways, but the essence is a subjective experience of being persistently treated unpleasantly by another person or people. It is a major source of work-related stress and ill health for individuals, and of loss of productivity for organizations.

Box 6.3 How to deal with persistently negative colleagues

- Spend your time with other, more positive, colleagues and actively avoid the negative persons.
- If you cannot avoid them, then set clear boundaries. Make it clear that you will not discuss or listen to negativity, but would rather focus on more positive matters.
- Try suggesting to them that they seek advice and help from their own boss, their union, or even the human resources or occupational health department.
- Draw the issue to the attention of your own boss, both for the purpose of sharing ideas for dealing with it and also because persistent negativity could potentially become a disciplinary matter.

Almost all employing bodies have policies that outlaw bullying; yet, despite this, bullying remains a common problem, with employees frequently reporting inadequate and ineffectual support from employers in dealing with it. Bullying must be dealt with as failure to do so will likely embolden and encourage the bully. Dealing with bullying requires courage and determination—but bear in mind that not dealing with it is likely to be even worse. There are five key steps that can and must, if needed, be taken to deal with bullying at work (see Box 6.4).

Box 6.4 The five steps to deal with bullying

1 Lay down clear boundaries for the bully regarding what is not acceptable behaviour. This involves deciding for yourself, in discussion with others if needed, what these boundaries are, and then telling the bully to stop the unwanted behaviour/s. This can be practised beforehand, but must be done. You will need to objectively, clearly, and unemotionally describe to the bully what unwanted behaviours you are experiencing, and also how this is impacting on your work. Then, go on to tell the bully exactly what behaviours you will no longer tolerate; be resolute in this. If the bully continues, then move onto the next step which involves confronting the bully with their own behaviour.

2 Confronting a bully is an action that you are in charge of, and that takes place on your own terms. You will need to verbalize the bully's actions (for example, by saying to them 'You are shouting at me' or 'You are behaving aggressively'). If he/she continues, then leave the room or terminate the call. Exactly the same approach can be used in meetings, including, if necessary, ending the meeting and reconvening later, and even excluding the bully if required.

> **Box 6.4 The five steps to deal with bullying (continued)**
>
> 3 Keep a detailed contemporaneous written diary of the bullying, with dates, times, and names of witnesses. This should also include information detailing how the bullying is negatively impacting on your work. Keep copies of any written evidence where this exists, including print-outs of any electronic items. Ensure that you keep this securely away from the workplace as this could be crucial evidence in the event that you become involved in formal processes or litigation.
>
> 4 Enlist the help of any other victims, especially encouraging them also to keep diaries detailing their own experiences of the bullying. Remember that this type of written evidence is what can make it possible for your employer to take formal action against the bully.
>
> 5 Finally, if the bullying continues, then you should formally complain to your employer, taking care to strictly comply with the organization's relevant policies and procedures. Your complaint should include the detailed written evidence collected as in these examples.

Unfortunately, sometimes there will not be a satisfactory outcome, and it may be that the best practical solution, even if it does not feel morally correct, is to look at other options for yourself, including different jobs.

What if the difficult person is your boss?

Difficult bosses are responsible for significant loss of productivity in the workplace. Staff are less likely to work at their best, more likely to lack motivation, less likely to contribute creatively and initiate problem solving, and more likely to make errors and lack pride in their work. Indeed, bad bosses are responsible for the majority of staff leaving their post due to work-related dissatisfaction. Whether a boss is bad or not depends on the interaction and balance between your needs, their skills, and the particular context in which you are working. Bosses can be just as difficult as other colleagues, but everything is made more challenging by the power relationship.

It may well be that the boss is blissfully unaware of their own failings. They may work to a whole different set of principles and values from those that drive you. They may believe that they are supporting you by their hands-on supervisory approach when you just want to be left to get on with the work independently. Alternatively, they may imagine that they are empowering you by leaving you to get on with the work when you actually want a more hands-on supervisory approach. Training for your boss is also important, and it can be that they are themselves poorly supported and out of their depth. It may sometimes be the case that your boss has decided to deliberately be difficult, perhaps because they learned from similar behaviour modelled by their boss (see Box 6.5).

Sometimes it may be that you have tried all these strategies but without success, in which case it may be necessary to consider a move to a different job or a different organization.

Box 6.5 What to do when the difficult person is your boss

- You need to keep your boss onside, and not accuse them of failings or make them feel that they are a bad boss.

- Enquiring about what they expect and want from you in order to reach targets and make their job easier can be a good starter. It may be that all that is required is a change of approach from yourself.

- It is really important to talk to your boss and make sure that they understand what you need from them in terms of feedback, support, and direction.

- Where the boss is aware of their behaviours, then it is important to inform them of the effect that this has on you and especially on your productivity. Occasionally, this may nudge the boss into trying to change. However, you will need to tactfully and privately keep them aware of the boundaries between acceptable and unacceptable behaviours.

- Ask for permission and get yourself a mentor who can act as a more experienced and supportive sounding board and adviser.

- If these steps fail, then consider going further up the organizational hierarchy, but strictly following any relevant policies. This is usually the point from which your relationship with your boss may never recover.

- If needed and relevant, you could ask other colleagues experiencing the same difficulties to join in this process. This is far more powerful than when a difficulty has been raised by one single individual. The risk with this, unless done with great care and thoughtful planning, is that you may yourself end up being perceived as the difficult person.

Holding difficult conversations

Difficult conversations can be about almost anything, but in this section we include topics such as annoying behaviours, habits, and even smells of employees that have an adverse effect on work or the workplace.

In many respects, this is similar to the skill of breaking bad news, in which most doctors are well versed. Nonetheless, we set out some basic principles here for guidance:

- Employers should not shirk or avoid their duty to have difficult conversations where required. Avoidance may lead to the individual suffering bullying and discrimination at the hands of their colleagues, personal harm, and ill health, and to even greater damage to productivity.

- There should always be a gentle lead-in to the topic, but after informing the person that this is a difficult conversation, it is best to then proceed directly to the subject of the conversation to avoid excessive anxiety.

- You should tell the person clearly and directly what the concern is, while avoiding judgemental or emotive language. It is imperative that they understand the issue, and do not get misled into thinking that it is not their concern.

- You should explain why this is a matter of concern for the organization including, if relevant, how it affects the organization.

- The person should be made aware, with an explanation of how, that the issue not only affects the organization and their colleagues, but also their own future career.

- Bear in mind that this is an individual problem that must be dealt with individually. Providing training to a group of staff to try and address the issue could result in the individual not realizing that they are the problem or, even worse, could end up as discrimination.

- Cultural sensitivity is important, and one should be cognizant of the individual's cultural background and norms, but at the same time, it should be made clear that what is important here is the culture and success of the workplace, especially when there is, in effect, a clash of cultural norms.

- It is appropriate and helpful to be open to ideas for possible remedial action or compromises that are in everyone's interest.

How to confront issues sensibly

Not many people look forward to confrontations. However, avoiding necessary confrontations in the workplace can come at a very high personal and organizational cost. In particular, there is a huge risk that people may simply continue, unaware of the concern caused by their conduct. We suggest some commonly acknowledged useful principles for successfully managing confrontations:

- Preparation is essential. This includes defining and describing the issue briefly, concisely, and clearly in an objective, factual, and non-emotive way. You will also need to decide what your desired outcome is before proceeding further.

- Tell the person, but avoid referring to your feelings as these are emotions rather than facts.

- After describing the issue, it is important to stop talking and allow the other person ample opportunity to respond, without interruption. Avoid defending your position, but do allow the other person to reply.

- Do not argue. You are there to state your position, not to defend it. It is important to listen properly to anything that the person says; you are not there to have an argument.

- Now, you should gently but firmly steer the conversation in the direction of your desired outcome, again stating this simply and clearly, and checking that it is understood.

- Remember that the issue is not about who is right or wrong, but rather, it is about achieving your desired outcome. Therefore you should not argue, no matter how great the temptation. However, you should negotiate, as required, in order to achieve the desired outcome.

General principles and techniques for resolving difficulties

Since difficult people at work can result in reduction of workplace productivity and cause increased stress levels, it is important to work towards the solution. As psychiatrists, we benefit from a wide array of skills, including:

◆ Communication skills in expressing views clearly and concisely

◆ Empathy in understanding others' viewpoints

◆ Skills in working towards resolution of the problems

◆ Ability to contact a senior colleague to discuss the problem.

Conflict resolution is about trying to find the common ground between both parties. It is from there that we can obtain solutions to our problems and renew our relations.

The language of solving conflicts is essential, with proper communication through verbal and non-verbal interaction. As there are ways of speaking and listening to others that block interactions, an open, facilitative communication style may need to be learned and practised (see Table 6.3).

In order to resolve a conflict, two aims should be fulfilled: first, to find sustainable and satisfying solutions to the matter; and second, to re-open the blocked relationship. To address the issues as well as the relationship, certain actions are needed. Both parties involved in the conflict should clearly speak out about their position; they should each disclose the facts, as they see them; they should speak about their feelings; they should clarify their underlying interests; they should express their deeper needs and try to understand each other's needs; they should offer various ideas for solutions, before agreeing on the best ones.

Table 6.3 Communication styles

Facilitative	Unhelpful
Calm and reassuring	Intimidating and aggressive
Describing one's needs/concerns	Blaming others
Listening	Interrupting
Explaining one's factual situation	Not listening or arguing with others
Sincere	Sarcastic
Real interest	Not interested in others
Candid	Rude and evasive
Genuine regret	Excuses
Focus on the problem	Focus on the person
Expressing one's views	Being defensive
Factual	Exaggerated and generalized

Source data from: Centre for Resolution of International Conflicts, University of Copenhagen, Øster Farimagsgade Copenhagen

The steps of basic conflict resolution reflect a certain way of thinking and they may be difficult to put into practice:[1]

- There should first be an opportunity that provides enough time and a suitable venue for both sides to explain their position and describe the effect on their work.

- There should be a direct conversation, and it should be acceptable that there may be legitimate and valid opposing views.

- These views need to be clearly communicated by both sides with each ensuring that they have properly understood the perspectives of the other.

- Next, participants should work towards agreeing on what the issues under dispute are.

- Creatively listing any feasible solutions follows, after which both sides should endeavour to negotiate and agree a practical, achievable outcome with which they are both satisfied.

Reference

1 Centre for Resolution of International Conflicts, University of Copenhagen, Øster Farimagsgade Copenhagen, http://cric.ku.dk/.

Chapter 7

Managing the media

Nicholas Deakin, Max Pemberton,
and Dinesh Bhugra

Case study: A scary prospect but one that can bring change

Ray is a new consultant psychiatrist. His hospital is experiencing a severe financial crisis as one of their main sources of income has been cut off, and a journalist from the local newspaper has called his office for a quote. The journalist starts asking about the scale of the cutbacks, then about the impact for patients, and then how the public could be endangered by people with mental illnesses 'roaming the streets' unable to access treatment. Ray starts to answer the questions but it becomes clear to him that the journalist has a very specific story in mind and keeps repeating herself until he agrees with her statements. A very negative story is printed, and he receives a call from the hospital management team asking why he made these statements and why he did not involve the hospital press office. He then receives numerous messages on his public Facebook profile from his current patients about the article and does not know whether he should respond.

Introduction

The media has tremendous power. It can be used to advance political points of view, to steer public opinion, to publicize advances in treatment, to highlight treatment or system failures, and to critically assess policy. Researchers who have analysed the treatment of psychiatry and mental illness in the media suggest that journalists have the ability to significantly distort public understanding of mental illness[1] and that while the profession generally gets 'a bad press', psychiatric patients in particular gain 'bad patient' status in the press.[2] The British psychiatrist Peter Byrne suggests that patients face their symptoms being used for 'infotainment' in the media, which also colours their expectations of management and offers an outlet for their opinions on their experience of the service.[2]

As well as seeking parity of mental health with physical health, using the media positively is one potential way to bring about more affirmative perceptions of psychiatry, psychiatrists, and mental illness among the general public and wider medical profession. This, however, requires psychiatrists to be 'media savvy' and to understand not only what the media and general public want to know but also how to present this in a safe, proficient, and succinct way. The media has many components—print media (such as newspapers, magazines, journals, free newspapers), electronic media (E-newspapers and online newspapers which may carry different content), social media (such as Facebook, YouTube, Twitter), and other instant media, films, and documentaries. There are

> ## Box 7.1 Criteria to be fulfilled for newsworthiness
>
> - ◆ Consistent with widely known facts
> - ◆ An interesting angle, altering what we know about the subject
> - ◆ Has 'human interest'
> - ◆ Seeks to educate and enlighten
> - ◆ Is informed—so delivered by an 'expert'
>
> Source: Reproduced from *Advances in Psychiatric Treatment*, 9(2), Byrne, P., Psychiatry and the media, p.135–143, Copyright (2003), with permission from the Royal College of Psychiatrists.

some general basic principles that need to be understood when dealing with the media. It is important to realise that if you feel uncomfortable dealing with or responding to the media, then you should not do it.

Newsworthiness

For a story, angle, or opinion to be considered worthy of broadcast, print, or discussion on social media, Bryne suggests analysis according to the following five points, all of which should be fulfilled (see Box 7.1). Issues that do not meet these criteria may well be of interest to more specialist media, such as medical or psychiatry related journals or comment pieces, or even social media, but will not generally be picked up by the national media.

Print media

Since the turn of the millennium and the technology revolution that this brought, there has been a steady decline in print media readership. Magazines and newspapers have suffered dropping circulation numbers as more and more people access their news on-line. However, despite this decline in readership, print media remain, for the time being at least, incredibly influential and important sources of information. They are trusted and respected by the general public. Mainstream print media still has considerable resources at their disposal and produce a significant output on a daily basis—the average broadsheet newspaper, for example, is the length of a novel. The content and opinion of newspapers is still considered incredibly important by politicians and policy makers and, of course, most newspapers and magazines now have an online presence, with many of them dominating the news agenda, blurring the line between old and new media.

In-depth studies conducted in Australia into the role that newspapers play in the formation of people's perceptions of mental illness have shown that people rank news and information media highly as an influential information source.[3] However, research has also shown that this can be trumped by direct contact with a mental health professional's or personal experience of mental illness. A sound understanding of the media and how it operates, therefore, means that there is a possibility for psychiatrists to use the media to communicate directly with readers and, in turn, that they can help offer a counterpoint to often biased and stigmatizing news coverage. This is not always easy to do, as editors will often chase the sensationalist headline and do not want this to be spoilt by a mental health professional attempting to redress the balance in the reporting. This said, news outlets have dramatically improved their coverage of mental health thanks to large-scale national campaigns, such as the 'Time To Change' campaign in the UK. Editors are gradually becoming more willing to print the views of professionals.

Mental health tends to be covered in four main areas in traditional print media and each of these has its own key considerations.

The news story

This is a report on a recent event and tends to appear towards the front of the newspaper. While it is intended to be entirely objective and a simple reporting of facts about a case, in truth, it is often biased in the way it is reported and the terminology used. Research conducted by the UK mental health charity Mind into reporting on mental health in newspapers has shown that a significant amount of news covered emphasizes negative aspects of mental illness, such as violence.[4] It is often these news stories that make the front page of newspapers due to the mixture of fear and fascination that such stories provoke in readers, making them appealing to editors. This can be seen at both a micro and macro level: incidents involving mental health patients; a notable individual such as a celebrity or someone in the public eye who makes a pronouncement about mental illness; hospital or health service issues relating to mental health; a charity or other non-governmental body that has issued a press release or report; and lastly, announcements by government or policy makers relating to mental health. While all of these news stories can have impacts on the psychiatric profession and patients, the most acute of these for the psychiatrist is when a patient under their care, or being cared for by the hospital where they work, is involved in an untoward incident which attracts the interest of newspapers. In these circumstances, reporters, from both newspapers and news agencies (organizations that gather news reports and then sell them on to media outlets) will often descend on the hospital hoping to speak to staff or patients. This can be very difficult and, unless informed otherwise by your hospital, it is also best to decline to comment. Remember that you are under no obligation to speak to the press or to provide them with your name or details. Many hospitals have a communications department which explicitly forbids staff from speaking to reporters. If approached, you should direct any journalists to this department. Remember that even a few sentences can easily be twisted or used to suggest something unintended, so it is better to be safe than sorry.

Excluding those that directly relate to you or your patients, news stories do provide the opportunity for psychiatrists to make statements or provide quotes to inform the reader of the key facts or considerations in the story. Often the media will have one or two key opinion leaders that they will turn to in times when such a quote is needed.

Unfortunately, they are not always the genuine experts and will often simply be people who are known to the media or who have some sort of media presence. In mental health in particular, this can often include unqualified individuals who opine on 'mental health'. There is an opportunity, therefore, for professional bodies representing psychiatrists to become organized so that they can provide experts to the media to give quotes relating to such news stories. This will ensure that the key messages are reported from the beginning, help balance reporting, and raise the public profile of psychiatry.

The human interest story

In newspapers, this type of story is usually featured towards the end of the paper and concerns a personal story that is in some way unique or interesting. These are usually longer pieces of journalism, written from a case study perspective, and will often be illustrated. In the case of mental illness, the theme of such stories is often one of resilience or overcoming adversity. The stories will often be tie-ins with books or films that are due to be released. Editors tend to be attracted to stories with a positive outcome, although occasionally a stark, shocking, or bleak narrative might be covered, providing it has some element of hope. For example, a story from a couple about how their daughter died from anorexia might end on how they set up a charity in her memory. Increasingly, television news and current affairs programmes will also feature 'human interest stories' and again, these are typically towards the end of the programme and will have the same appeal and serve the same function as human interest stories in print media.

The human interest story can be a great springboard to wider public debate and understanding of the affects of mental illness on people. It presents a 'just like you' view of people and promotes an empathic response to mental distress. Mental health campaigns will often get coverage by providing media outlets with access to individuals who have agreed to share their story with the media. Occasionally, psychiatrists will have patients that decide to do this and this can present a unique set of problems; while such coverage can have a tremendously positive impact on the public's perception of mental illness, it is not without risk for the individual and the psychiatrist may find him/herself offering advice and advocacy to the patient as they decide whether they should go ahead. It is important that the patient is aware of the possible ramifications to both their personal and professional life of speaking out about their problems and telling their story. They should be reminded that because of the internet, it is likely that they will be identifiable in one way or another. It should also be noted that the patient must have capacity, at that particular time, to make the decision to speak to the media. There are sometimes options such as using a false name, although increasingly newspapers and magazines feel this is inauthentic and limits the options for photography and therefore shy away from this unless there is a very good reason.

The opinion piece

This is an article in a newspaper or magazine that specifically reflects the author's personal view. Such articles tend to be placed after the news section, although this is variable depending on the publication. They are sometimes also called 'comment pieces'. They are not intended as an objective assessment of a situation and bias is implicitly assumed in the nature of this sort of writing. Opinion pieces are often intended to generate debate and controversy. They will often be in response to news stories that have been present in the media over the past few days, although not necessarily—sometimes opinion pieces themselves can shed light on a topic or event that is otherwise not receiving news attention, especially if the author has expert or personal knowledge of certain issues.

Editors will sometimes commission opinion pieces from external authors (not directly employed by the publication), especially if they are considered experts in the field or are known to hold particularly passionate, informed, or controversial opinions about a certain subject. Most newspapers will have a cohort of columnists. These journalists regularly contribute opinion pieces and will often write weekly on a specific day. Many develop loyal followings and their opinions tend to follow predictable patterns consistent with their political leanings. They are called upon to comment on current affairs and, within this remit, may cover mental health.

In addition to this, opinion pieces may also take the form of a 'leader'. This is a series of short comments (typically three) published in the newspaper that are not attributed to an individual writer but which represent the official stance or view of the paper. They are usually guided or written by the senior editorial team and will often have political undertones.

The opinion piece offers psychiatrists a platform to write detailed accounts, to lay out arguments point by point, and to give a passionate, informed, and intelligent defence of key areas affecting mental health. If you are approached to write an opinion piece, think carefully about what you want to say and also, if it is controversial in nature, the impact this may have on career prospects. Authors of pieces that are highly critical of government policy, for example, will often opt for the use of a pseudonym. Many opinion pieces open with some 'colour'—a description of a scene to draw the reader in—but be mindful of patient confidentiality at all times.

If you have an idea for an opinion piece, then many publications welcome unsolicited contact. Make sure you approach the commissioning editor for the relevant section and outline your article briefly in no more than one paragraph. Email is usually best and can be followed up by a telephone call if appropriate. If you are unsure of who to approach initially, contact the publication switchboard and ask for the name of the person who commissions for either the comment section or health section. Remember that newspapers and magazines are not there to tell a 'worthy' story; they are there to sell a product, and if the story you want to promote is not deemed to be commercial (i.e. of suitable interest to the general public), they are unlikely to print it. Unfortunately, not all stories—while fascinating to the author and often very important to the people they affect—are of interest or relevance to the general public. However, that does not mean you should not persevere and keep approaching different news outlets with your ideas. Likewise, when inaccurate, harmful, biased, or dangerous reporting on mental health topics is noted, it is important that all those with training and expert knowledge in the subject challenge the media on this. Reporting offensive or stigmatizing reporting to relevant media regulators is easy and quick to do, will mean that the media are further encouraged to improve their reporting, and is strongly encouraged by advocates of fair treatment of psychiatric illness in the media.

The consumer health article

This provides information about a certain topic and is intended to be educational. Depending on the publication, it may be relatively simple and cover the basics of a condition (such as an article explaining what depression is) or more in depth and technical (such as an article covering recent advances in treating depression). Unlike the opinion piece, this form of coverage aims to report only the established facts about a topic, presenting any controversy about it in an even-handed way with opposing views acknowledged. These articles will sometimes be prompted by recent news stories, which might see a particular condition receive press coverage, and so a consumer health article is published to educate readers about this subject in more depth, using the news story as the 'peg'. This might happen, for example, after news reports of a famous person who has committed suicide; this might trigger consumer health articles on suicide or depression. However, consumer health articles can also be unrelated to any current affairs and instead might be prompted by the personal interest of the commissioning editor, press releases from industry or charities, or by the idea of the journalist.

These articles are usually written by professional journalists, but they will often rely on specialists, professionals, or experts in the field to provide quotes or to confirm accuracy. There is also the opportunity for professionals to approach commissioning editors directly with ideas for consumer health articles, and again, this opens up the possibility for psychiatrists to educate the general public.

Social media

Recent years have seen new types of media flourish. The UK General Medical Council defines social media as 'web-based applications that allow people to create and exchange content.'[5] These include networks focused on social interaction, professional communication, and career progression, as detailed in Table 7.1. Psychiatrists and doctors, along with the general public, use all these.

Social media have bought tremendous opportunities for clinicians to socialize, discuss work, discuss their home lives, and update others on what they are up to. They can be used for professional advancement, through national and international networks.[3] Some use them to engage patients and fellow health professionals in discussions around health, health policy, and public health, and to disperse relevant information about health or service provision. The British Medical Association states that most doctors use these networks appropriately, without experiencing any danger, but warns that some just do not realize the risks that they are exposing themselves to. [6] Box 7.2

Table 7.1 Types of social media with examples

Social networks	Facebook, Twitter
Content communities	Youtube, Flickr, Instagram
Professional forums	Doctors.net, sermo.com, and doc2doc
Career-focused networks	LinkedIn

Box 7.2 Notable cases where social media has led to professional repercussions

- In June 2009, nurses and doctors faced disciplinary action for posting pictures on Facebook of themselves lying down in locations around the hospital as part of the international 'lying down game'.[4]
- Medical boards in Australia have investigated doctors for revealing information on social networking sites which could be used to identify individual patients.[7]
- A civil servant in the UK government revealed on her personal Twitter account that she was 'struggling with a wine-induced hangover' at work. The tweets, intended for friends, were reported in the national press.[4]
- A junior doctor in the UK was suspended for six months after using inflammatory language about a senior leader in the health service.[5]

describes some cases where there have been significant repercussions for doctors and health professionals based on their social conduct.

To avoid such occurrences affecting your practice, organizations such as the British Medical Association, a committee led by the Australian Medical Association, the Canadian Medical Association, and the General Medical Council (UK) have produced guidance to follow.[5-7] Such guidance rests on the premise that the professional–personal boundary is blurring and any inappropriate activity online is rapidly dispersed and may be difficult to withdraw. It is particularly important for psychiatrists, given the vulnerability of patients with mental illnesses and the power balance than can exist between the clinician and patient. Of course, the guidance does not seek to curtail the use of social media among doctors, as it has the potential to bring many professional and personal benefits to the user. Instead, it is about being sensible online and seeking to maintain the status of the profession in the public eye, so we can continue to enjoy patient trust long into the future. The following pointers form the basis of this guidance, which applies to all doctors:

- You have a duty to maintain patient confidentiality. This is an ethical and a legal duty in many countries, and applies not just to the statement of facts but also the sum of related facts, which observers could put together.[5-7]
- You should maintain high privacy settings and politely refrain from accepting Facebook friend requests from patients.[5-7]
- Think about the potential impact on professional relationships, especially with multidisciplinary team members, before allowing others to access your personal information.[6]
- You should refrain from publishing informal, personal, or derogatory comments about patients or colleagues on the internet.[5,6] In particular, there are strict rules in place in many countries against bringing the medical profession into disrepute.[6]

- ◆ You should be conscious of what image you project online and how this could affect your career—including progression and potential disciplinary action.[6] This includes sharing information about activities that may seem unprofessional or joining groups which may be seen as inflammatory or prejudiced.[4]
- ◆ You should declare any conflicts of interest if these apply[6]—these include pharmaceutical companies, healthcare organizations, and biomedical companies.[5]
- ◆ You should be familiar with local guidance on social media.[5]

Blogs

Blogs are discussions published online which appear in reverse chronological order on a designed website. They were initially written by individuals, either under their own name or a name chosen by them, but have increasingly been adopted by companies, organizations, politicians, print media, and even medical journals. Blogs relating to medicine exist to dispense health advice, advice to colleagues, act as diaries, share commentary on health politics, and share health news. Medical issues are also covered by doctors writing blogs for the general press, including in newspapers such as *The Guardian* (which has 'Guardian Healthcare' and 'ABC News'). They are a fantastic way to engage the public and other professionals in debate, with the comment function being enabled on many blogs. However, much as with social media, there is also the potential for psychiatrists and doctors to face consequences if they publish material that is deemed to be offensive, insensitive, or against professional guidelines. The authors would recommend that you use the bullet points from the 'social media' section of this chapter to govern your use of blogs, and always remember that once information is published on a blog, it can be considered public information that is impossible to retract.

Broadcast media - radio and television

Broadcast media gives you unrivalled access to many viewers at the same time, the presentation of which is often embedded in relevant, factual news broadcasts and can be either live (broadcast as you are talking) or recorded (where you have an interview and certain extracts are broadcast).

Before you agree to any broadcast, you should be aware of the news story, the programme, the likely audience, when it will be broadcast, what aspects the interviewer wants to cover, whether you will be 'debating' with someone (and if so, what their position might be), how long it will be, whether it will be live or recorded, and what timescale you would have to work to. If the interview relates to your work organization, professional association, or could be very controversial, then you should seek advice from colleagues and, where applicable, the relevant press office. You will also need to ensure that you have knowledge of the law and professional guidelines in the relevant area, and facts should be to hand. Statistics are a great way of making your point succinctly, and national information databases, professional associations, research, and charities are useful resources for obtaining these.[2]

Writing three key points, for any broadcast interview, and then working out how to say these as succinctly as possible, is probably the best way to approach this. You also need to remember some basic principles:

- The general public do not have medical degrees or significant knowledge about mental illness, so do not use terms or abbreviations which they will not be familiar with. If you do use specialist vocabulary, explain this. Never use acronyms without first giving a very clear explanation of what each letter stands for.

- Use statistics in an easy to understand way—so, half is easier to understand than 1 in 2, which is simpler than saying 50%.

- Speak slowly.

- When asked a question, it is fine to take a moment to think about the answer before speaking.

- Do not feel under pressure to keep talking to avoid silence; it is the job of the interviewer to keep the conversation moving, not yours.

- Use natural breaks to allow people to digest your comments.

- Do not ramble.

- Stay calm.

Appearing on television can be daunting, not just because it could be live but also because so much depends on your appearance. Indeed, Byrne suggests that viewers will 'remember what you were wearing'.[2] Here are some top tips (see Box 7.3 and 7.4).

In contrast to television, where your appearance is of upmost importance, listeners on the radio depend on your voice to convey emotion and enthusiasm for the subject. Some people find that smiling can help elicit this. Answers should be succinct enough to offer short 'sound bites' which can be aired and which contain the main point or points you wish to put across. Some tips when participating in broadcasts are reported in Box 7.5

Box 7.3 Guidance for television interviews

- You should avoid busy clothes, bright colours, and striped or patterned fabrics. Striped clothes, in particular, will often appear distorted when viewed on a screen and most television programmes will insist you do not wear them anyway.

- Look at the interviewer, not the camera, so your piece will look like a conversation rather than attempt to take over the screen.

- Practise to make sure you do not do anything which could distract viewers from your message - such as moving your hands excessively or saying the word 'erm' repeatedly.

- Try to smile, regardless of how unnatural it feels.

- Ask the interviewer what question they will start with.

Box 7.4 Guidance on how to respond to media requests

1 Only agree if it is your area

2 Check who the programme is aimed at

3 Have key messages and stick to them

4 Sound bites are good - but be careful

5 Consider appearance and body language

6 Appear interested and interesting

7 Remember speech volume, tone, and pacing

8 Include analogies and anecdotes

Box 7.5 Golden tips for when participating in broadcasts

1 What is the journalist's motive? Can you clarify the agenda? Is it education? Is it sensational story?

2 Think of your message and stick to it.

3 Do *not* let the journalist lead; avoid answering leading questions.

4 Give short, sharp, and interesting responses.

5 If you use a good phrase, feel free to use it again.

6 Avoid jargon and acronyms—viewers/readers may not be aware what they mean.

7 Enjoy the experience - and look/sound as though you are enjoying it.

8 Be up to date.

Byrne suggests listening to broadcasts, considering how points are argued, and then contacting the programmes or news desks to suggest angles and offer yourself for interview. He feels this will make presenting to your consultant colleagues much less daunting![2]

Media training

Organizations for doctors and psychiatrists, such as the British Medical Association and the Royal College of Psychiatrists, offer media training to either members or committee members that is tailored to fulfilling the needs of inexperienced doctors and those looking to improve their performance in the media. Such training helps to build theoretical knowledge of how the media works but often combines this with the development of practical skills—for example, recording yourself performing sample television interviews and watching them back critically. If you are unable to find a course within your professional association, then your hospital trust, local health provider, or commercial companies sometimes offer similar courses. They will usually count towards hours of continuing professional development (CPD).

Conclusion

The media offers the young and established psychiatrist alike, a unique way to interact with the general public to raise awareness and dispel myths about mental illness. Particularly if you develop specialist expertise, you have an exclusive ability to inform debate and policy through the media. There are numerous ways to do this, with both new and traditional media offering routes towards exposure. However, this does not come without risks and you should always be aware of your professional obligations and etiquette. This includes not only print and new media around mental health but also your personal social media activity.

References

1 **Salter M**. Psychiatry and the media: from pitfalls to possibilities. *Psychiatric Bulletin* 2003; **27**:123–5.

2 **Byrne P**. Psychiatry and the media. *Advances in Psychiatric Treatment* 2003; **9**:135–43.

3 **Pirkis J, Francis C**. *Mental illness in the news and information media: a critical review*. Mindframe National Media Initiative, Commonwealth of Australia; 2012.

4 British Broadcasting Corporation (BBC) Health. *Media 'unfairly stigmatises mental illness'*. BBC; 2000. Available at: http://news.bbc.co.uk/1/hi/health/635415.stm [accessed July 2014].

5 General Medical Council (GMC). *Doctors' use of social media (2013)*. Available at: http://www.gmc-uk.org/guidance/ethical_guidance/21186.asp.

6 British Medical Association (BMA) Medical Ethics Department. *Using social media: practical and ethical guidance for doctors and medical students*; 2012. Available at: http://bma.org.uk/-/media/Files/PDFs/Practical%20advice%20at%20work/Ethics/socialmediaguidance.pdf.

7 Australian Medical Association Council of Doctors in Training, the New Zealand Medical Association Doctors-in-Training Council, the New Zealand Medical Students' Association, and the Australian Medical Students' Association. *Social media and the medical profession: a guide to online professionalism for medical practitioners and medical students*; 2010. Available at: https://ama.com.au/sites/default/files/documents/Social_Media_and_the_Medical_Profession_FINAL_with_links_0.pdf.

Chapter 8

Mentoring and career coaching

Umberto Volpe, Andrea Fiorillo, Nikolina Jovanovic, and Dinesh Bhugra

Case study: 'What apples can do for you!'

Apples changed John's life for good. John was a trainee in psychiatry, in his fourth year of training. He was a brilliant physician and an avid learner. He used to succeed in almost every aspect of clinical and research training. However, the institution in which he worked was strongly entrenched in a psychoanalytical milieu and John was not exactly a fan of Freud's approach to psychiatry. While attending a conference, John was fascinated by a lecture on research in psychiatric neuroscience. However, since he did not feel confident enough on that topic and knew that he could not ask his tutors to start an experiment in that field, he suppressed his enthusiasm. During a coffee break after the lecture, John found that apples were available to eat. Coincidentally, the neuroscientist who had delivered the lecture also had a passion for apples; and thus the two met. They started talking about neuroscience and the conversation ended with an e-mail address exchange. Following that, John decided to write to the neuroscientist, who provided him with suggested readings on neuroscience. During his final year of training, John visited him for short periods, and he eventually became involved in an experiment and even more enthusiastic about neuroscience. Right after graduation, John applied for a PhD position in the neuroscience laboratory of his mentor. John has run his own laboratory for three years now.

Introduction

The term 'mentor' comes from Greek mythology: in the ancient epic Greek poem 'The Iliad', Mentor was an old and trusted friend of Odysseus, who placed him in charge of his son Telemachus when he had to leave for the Trojan War. According to Homer, the goddess Athena often visited Telemachus, disguised as Mentor, to offer advice, protection, and guidance in his time of difficulty. The first modern usage of the term, however, can probably be traced back to a seventeenth-century French book that relates the adventures of Telemachus; however, in the book (*Les aventures de Télémaque* by François Fénelon), Mentor became the leading character of the story.[1] The book had a great impact on many people at the time and, since then, the definition of 'mentor' has come closer to the modern sense of a special learning relationship between a senior teacher and a less experienced 'mentee'. In its 1750 edition, the *Oxford English Dictionary* already included the word 'mentor', reported as a commonly used term. In the 1970s, use of the concept spread worldwide, mainly in business training contexts, later expanding into the healthcare sector.

Definitions

Mentorship might be broadly defined as a personal relationship in which a more experienced and/or knowledgeable person (the 'mentor') helps to guide a less experienced and/or knowledgeable person (the 'mentee'), with the aim of developing the skills and competences of the person in receipt of mentorship.

Different from other forms of teaching and/or tutoring, the focus of mentoring programmes is totally determined by the goals, ambitions, and skills of the mentee. Usually, it is for the mentee to identify the issues about which he/she wants to be mentored, and the mentor is supposed to provide the most adequate solutions to such issues. Several forms of mentoring and tutoring exist and these are summarized in Table 8.1 to show the similarities and differences.

Table 8.1 Mentoring and related tutoring processes

Type	Core characteristics	Similarities	Differences
Training	◆ Acquiring new job functions	◆ Transfer of knowledge and skills	◆ Programmes are *not* tailored to individual skills or needs ◆ Not always sufficient to ensure effective skills transfer
Coaching	◆ Make lasting changes in one's life ◆ Development of activities ◆ Finding the right attunement ◆ Developing skills ◆ Performance improvement	◆ Oriented towards full- potential achievement ◆ Focus on interpersonal skills ◆ Designed to suit one's personal needs ◆ Assistance with further career • 'Live' environment	◆ Not directly focused on pursuing significant transitions in work career ◆ Not all coaches work within the area of their own personal competence ◆ The coach may work outside the organization (consultant approach)
Counselling	◆ Exploring personal issues and professional problems through discussion ◆ Promotion of self-awareness and goal achievement	◆ Leading the client towards self-directed actions	◆ More 'in-depth' relationship, with special focus on personal issues
Consultancy	◆ Development of practices, processes, and structures	◆ Experts' advice on specific issues	◆ More strategic role ◆ Less 'live' training ◆ Individual up-skilling is not the primary goal

Box 8.1 The six steps of the mentoring process

◆ Finding the focus of mentoring
◆ Mentor–mentee match
◆ Defining the shared goals of mentoring
◆ Planning schedule/meetings
◆ Training (discussing issues and finding solutions)
◆ Review over time

Box 8.2 Crucial elements of the mentoring process

◆ Relationship
◆ Development
◆ Communication
◆ Transfer of knowledge
◆ Sharing experiences
◆ Coaching approach
◆ Constant support
◆ Evaluation over time

Many similarities exist, particularly between mentoring and coaching, but mentoring frequently involves a younger colleague following the path of a more senior and wiser colleague, with the opportunity of sharing experience and knowledge (allowing the mentee to open the door to otherwise out of reach opportunities). On the other hand, coaching is usually less focused on professional or specific skills.

Typically, a mentoring activity involves many different goals, practices, and skills; however, some steps are common to many mentoring programmes (Box 8.1).

The mentorship process is far from being a simple one, as at the core of the activity lies the special relationship between the mentor and the mentee, with a specific focus on the personal and professional development of the mentee. Thus, mentoring may require a broad range of different techniques, and it often involves several domains, abilities, and processes, Consequently, it may take different forms, with varying degrees of formality. Although a precise and unequivocal definition of mentoring is probably not achievable, a tentative list of the main elements underpinning the concept is provided in Box 8.2.

What are the advantages of mentoring?

The advantages of mentoring are multiple, both for the mentor and the mentee. A tentative list of the most significant positive changes that mentoring may induce is provided in Table 8.2.

Table 8.2 Advantages of mentoring for mentor and mentee

Mentor	Mentee
◆ Increase in professional and personal networks	◆ Increase professional skills
◆ Develop from others' experience	◆ Training to adapt to changes
◆ Provision of new job dimensions; feeling 'refreshed' about own work	◆ Knowledge about one's own organization
◆ Chance to broaden skills/knowledge	◆ Positive impact on future career

When mentoring programmes are set up to help newcomers acclimatize more quickly and effectively to their new organization, the organization can usually offer some clear advantages in terms of easier integration, stronger shaping of professional culture, and operational style. It has been claimed that newcomers who are paired with a mentor are twice as likely to remain in their job as those who do not receive mentorship.[2] Potentially, the person being mentored networks better, becomes more easily integrated in an organization, and obtains more experience and advice along the way. Pompper and Adams recently affirmed that 'joining a mentor's network and developing one's own is central to advancement'.[3]

The process of mentoring

The process of mentoring usually starts with the exploration of the mentee's needs, skills, self-reflections, and motivations for professional change, which culminates in the definition of his/her new professional goals.

The second crucial step for mentoring is the 'matching' of mentor and mentee. In our opening case study, the mentor search happened by chance; and informal mentoring takes places in organizations that are developing a culture of mentoring but do not have formal mentoring in place yet. The match is most often achieved by a 'mentoring co-ordinator' who chooses from a database registry the right mentor for the right mentee. In order to build a proper 'mentoring database', both mentors and mentees are usually asked to complete a 'mentoring profile'. This usually consists of a written and/or online form, in which they specify their areas of interest, time available, recent achievements, future projects, etc. Mentees are matched with mentors by a designated mentoring committee (usually consisting of senior members of the training organization) or the mentoring co-ordinator. The matching committee often reviews the mentoring profiles and makes matches based on areas for development, mentor strengths, overall experience, skill set, location, and objectives for the mentorship. In some organizations, depending on the programme format, mentees may self-select their mentors. This form of mentoring choice may enhance the quality of matches because the greater the involvement of the mentee in the selection of their mentor, the better the outcome of the mentorship.

One successful example of a mentoring programme is the one developed and carried out by the European Psychiatric Association.[4] This programme is based on an informal meeting, which usually occurs during the annual European Congress of Psychiatry, between several mentors (chosen from among the officers of the Association) and several mentees (selected from among the most promising European early-career psychiatrists). After this first initial and relaxed meeting, the mentor–mentee pair are free to interact as long as they want in order to improve career opportunities for the mentee.

> "I am inspired every day by having the picture of my mentor on my desk, close to my PC".
>
> Silvia Ferrari (European Psychiatric Association mentee, 2011)

In these days, technology can be used to facilitate matches and to maintain the mentoring relationship. For example, the use of an online mentors' database may allow the mentees to search and select a mentor based on their own needs and interests. This mentee-driven methodology increases the speed at which matches are created and reduces the amount of administrative time required to manage the mentoring programme.[5]

The definition of goals within the mentoring process is usually achieved through the match between the mentee's ambitions and new ideas and the mentor's experience and real-world evidence (in terms of available resources and evaluation of feasibility). One approach to goal setting is the 'SMART' one:[6] this is an acronym to guide in the setting of objectives, the letters of which broadly conform to the words Specific, Measurable, Attainable, Relevant, and Time-bound, which should define the basic characteristics of an individual's goals (Table 8.3).

Once broad goals and specific objectives are defined, mentor and mentee should meet to discuss issues and find proper solutions to the problems posed by the mentee. Meetings are vital for communication. Properly run meetings save time, increase motivation, and solve problems. Meetings often create new ideas and initiatives. The choice of structure and style of the meeting depends on several factors such as the situation (circumstances, mood, atmosphere, background, etc.), the organizational context (the implications and needs of the project or of the organization), the mentor's and mentee's needs and interests, the specific aims of the meeting, and the time schedule of both mentor and mentee. Usually an 'agenda' of the meeting should be circulated in advance

Table 8.3 The SMART technique to define goals

Letter	Word	Meaning
S	Specific	Significant, stretching, simple, sustainable
M	Measurable	Motivational, manageable, meaningful
A	Achievable	Appropriate, agreed, assignable, attainable, actionable, action-oriented, adjustable, ambitious, aligned with corporate goals, aspirational, acceptable
R	Relevant	Result-based, results-oriented, resourced, resonant, realistic, reasonable
T	Time-bound	Time-oriented, time-framed, timed, time-based, time-specific, timetabled, time-limited, trackable, tangible, timely, time-sensitive

in order to better define goals and roles of the meeting. During the meeting, both mentor and mentee should agree upon outcomes, actions, and responsibilities. The mentee should take notes, to be sent after the meeting to the mentor, to define and follow up agreed actions and responsibilities.

When setting the time and date of the meeting with the mentor, the mentee should ensure the chosen date causes minimum disruption for all concerned. For meetings that repeat on a regular basis, the easiest way to set dates is to agree them in advance, at the first meeting, when everyone can commit there and then. Better still is to schedule a year's worth of meetings if possible, so that dates can be circulated well in advance, which helps greatly to ensure people keep to them and that no other priorities encroach. Conversely, leaving it late to agree dates for meetings will almost certainly inconvenience people, which is a major source of upset. Times to start and finish depend on the type and duration of the meeting and the attendees' availability but, generally, it is worth trying to start early and plan to finish by the end of the working day. Breakfast meetings are a good idea in certain cultures, but can be too demanding in more relaxed environments. If attendees have long distances to travel (i.e. more than a couple of hours), overnight accommodation on the night before should be considered (this usually also allows for a much earlier start). As for the meeting venue, many mentoring meetings are relatively informal and are often held in meeting rooms 'on site' or at national/international congresses (thus eliminating the need for extensive planning). In order to properly plan meetings, Table 8.4 can be used as a general scheme.

Along with the scheduled meetings, the mentor and mentee should review, over time, the results obtained by the mentee, paying special attention to unveiling possible problems and obstacles to the fulfilment of the mentee's professional achievements. Accurate and thorough evaluation of a mentoring programme represents the best practice for determining the effectiveness of the programme itself, and it may help in reshaping mentoring objectives and outcomes, when necessary. The evaluation of the mentee's

Table 8.4 Checklist for mentoring meetings

	Done	**Additional comments**	**Date**
Agenda			
Date			
Time			
Venue			
Notification			
Notes of last meeting			
Directions/map			
Materials (as required by agenda items)			
Reference material for ad hoc queries			
Priorities			
Outcomes			

outcomes should be done by using objective measures wherever possible, to ensure that the relationship is successful and that the mentee is achieving his/her personal goals.

Mentoring programmes should be neither too short, nor too long. No rule is available in this respect and mentoring relationships may last a few months or several years, depending on the goals and on the relationship of the mentoring pair. However, it is also a specific duty of the mentor to ensure that mentees develop personal competencies, do not develop unhealthy dependencies on the mentoring relationship (as possible in those cases when the mentoring programme lasts longer than necessary), and receive the just appropriate level of expertise.

Characteristics and typology of mentoring

Basically, there are two broad types of mentoring relationships: formal and informal. Informal relationships develop on their own, while formal mentoring usually refers to a structured process, supported by an organization and addressed to specific target populations. In some organizations, mentoring is provided by employers and is of professional nature; more often, mentorship is an unpaid activity with philanthropic goals. The mentoring process can be short term (usually when it develops around a particular issue) or long term (when it focuses on a range of issues and often lasting for years).

Mentoring techniques

An effective mentoring practice usually moves through three main stages. Each stage builds on the learning from the previous and within each stage, there are responsibilities for both the mentor and the mentee. A graphical representation of the basic stages of mentoring is provided in Fig. 8.1.

During the first stage of the process (exploration), the role of a mentor is to provide information (when requested by the mentee), to ask probing questions to help the mentee make initial judgements, to reflect back to the mentee what he/she has learned, and to guide the mentee through thinking about the implications of potential conclusions. The second stage is to agree what actions should be taken (understanding) and how to make them happen (action), just by guiding the mentee towards identifying actions that he/she can implement. After actions are agreed, the third stage is for the mentor to ensure that these are recorded and then monitored through regular review and feedback (evaluation).

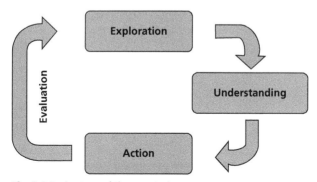

Fig. 8.1 Basic steps of the mentoring process.

There are many kinds of mentoring relationships, from school or community-based relationships to e-mentoring relationships. These mentoring relationships vary and can be influenced according to which type is in effect. Recently, several models have been used to describe and examine the mentoring relationships that can emerge (see Table 8.5).

Many different techniques may be used by mentors according to the situation and the mindset of the mentee; although the most commonly used techniques are summarized in Table 8.6.[7] Of course, no single technique is pre-eminent; mentors should, rather, look for 'teachable moments' in order to 'expand or realize the potentialities of the people in the organizations they lead'[8] and underlining that personal credibility is as essential to quality mentoring as is skill.

Table 8.5 Mentoring models

Cloning	The mentor tries to produce a duplicate copy of him/herself
Nurturing	Parent-like relationship; usually in a safe and open environment
Friendship	Less hierarchical relationship; usually works with peer mentor
Apprenticeship	Less on personal or social aspects; professional relationship is the sole focus; the apprentice will learn by working on the job with the mentor

Buell C. Models of Mentoring in Communication. Comm Rev, 2004; 53: 56–73.

Table 8.6 Mentoring techniques

Questioning	Observe, listen, and ask questions; this facilitates the mentee's own thoughts, in order to let him/her find solutions and set actions, without assuming a directive approach
Facilitating	Setting appropriate goals and providing help for finding methods and solutions, with a one-to-one approach
Networking	Developing new alliances to let the mentee achieve his/her own goals
Accompanying	Taking part in the learning process, side by side with the learner
Sowing	Preparing the learner before he/she is ready to change—what you say will make sense and have value to the mentee when the situation requires it
Catalysing	Plunging the learner straight into change, provoking a different way of thinking, a change in identity, or a re-ordering of values
Showing	Using examples to demonstrate a skill or activity; presenting own behaviour
Harvesting	Usually used to create awareness of what was learned by experience, and to draw conclusions; frequent use of such questions as 'What have you learned?' or 'How useful is it?'

Source data from: Aubrey B & Cohen P. *Working Wisdom: Timeless Skills and Vanguard Strategies for Learning Organizations*. Wiley, London, 1995: pp. 23, 44–47, 96–97.

Table 8.7 Qualities of mentor and mentee

Mentor	Mentee
◆ Knowledge and skills in the field of interest	◆ Intention to broaden skills
◆ Interest in being a mentor	◆ Personal and professional growth
◆ Available time	◆ Learn from experience
◆ Listening skills	◆ Ready to change
◆ Patience	◆ Humble
◆ Supportive attitude	
◆ Non-judgemental attitude	

Mentoring figures

The most usual form of mentoring is 'one-to-one' mentoring, which involves face-to-face interaction between two persons—the mentor and the mentee—whose profiles are depicted in Table 8.7.

Besides the classical 'one-to-one' mentorship, multiple mentoring practices are applied in specific contexts. These practices have been given the name of 'mosaic mentoring', and are based on the concept that almost everyone can perform one or other function for someone else. The model is seen as useful for people who are 'non-traditional' in a traditional setting. A related concept is the mentoring 'phase model',[5] in which, initially, the mentee proves him or herself worthy of the mentor's efforts; then, coaching and a strong interpersonal bond between mentor and mentee develops; and finally, during a phase of separation, the mentee experiences more 'autonomy'. After mentoring is completed, there is more equality in the relationship (a phase of role redefinition). The idea has been well received in medical education literature.[9]

High-potential mentorship

High-potential mentoring programmes are used to mentor the mentees deemed to have the potential to move up into leadership roles. Here, the mentee (or 'protégé') is paired with a senior-level leader (or leaders) for a series of career-coaching interactions. These programmes tend to be smaller in scale than more general mentoring programmes and mentees must be selected to participate. Within high-potential mentoring, the mentee often carries out a series of short-term jobs in different areas of an organization, in anticipation of learning the organization's structure, culture, and methods.

E-mentoring

E-mentoring is a means of providing a guided mentoring relationship using online software or email that began to gain popularity around the 1990s. Telephone communication has also been occasionally used and is known as 'telementoring'. Nowadays, there are a variety of online mentoring technology programmes available that can be utilized to facilitate this mentee-driven matching process. E-mail communication and Skype calling are now a standard part of job activities and have been revealed as particularly useful in maintaining the relationship between mentors and mentees, especially if the mentor does not belong to the same training institution or not even to the same country. Newer options are the use of FaceTime, Google Hangouts, and video chat through Facebook or other professional social networks.

Professional e-mentoring programmes have been officially launched in the USA and in the UK and other European countries. Some controversies have recently emerged on the use of e-mentoring programmes, as they have been unfavourably compared to 'face mentoring', due to their lack of visual and/or social cues, making the mentoring relationship less personal (with the risk of providing less feedback to the mentee). On the other hand, e-mentoring is less time-consuming and tends to promote more honest feedbacks.

Facilitated mentoring

Classical mentoring is characterized as an informal, often spontaneous enabling relationship between an older mentor and a younger mentee; this relationship is based on a shared wish to work together, usually for a long period, without financial compensation for the mentor. On the contrary, 'facilitated' mentoring tends to privilege a professional setting, with a paid mentor focused on the specific training needs of the mentee.[10] Mentors may also receive other benefits such as prioritized registration, course credit, and references.

Peer mentoring

In some training institutions, mentorship programmes are offered by senior students/trainees to support younger students and trainees in programme completion and transitioning to further education or the workplace. A typical peer mentoring relationship is that of alumni with mentees. Peer mentoring can be defined as a relationship between a person who has lived through a specific experience (peer mentor) and a person who is new to that same experience (the peer mentee). Peer mentoring programmes are often implemented to promote health and lifestyle changes (e.g. patients' self-help groups).

The peer mentor is supposed to challenge the mentee mind with new ideas, but should also ensure sensibility, confidence, and reliability. The peer mentor should be selected also on the basis of good social skills. Peer mentoring provides individuals with education and support, but it differs from classical mentoring in two main aspects.[11] First, in peer mentoring, mentors and mentees are close in age, experience, and educational level (which usually also constitute the criteria for matching), and they may also overlap in their personal identities. Second, peer mentoring programmes are more structured and planned in advance, with specific guidelines and a set of activities to be achieved within a predetermined amount of time.

Peer mentoring programmes have many advantages. Because junior mentors are closer in age, knowledge, and authority to their mentees, they may more easily feel free to express ideas, ask questions, and eventually take risks, with lower risks of any sense of inferiority for the mentee. Furthermore, peer mentors can probably better manage both the personal and academic problems of their protégées, which may increase mentor–mentee compatibility. Both participants usually report that peer mentoring allows them to easily establish the right pace of the programme, to develop more effective interpersonal and communication skills, and increase self-esteem, patience, and empathy.[12] On the other hand, peer mentoring detractors tend to note that it may leave junior students without reliable guidance and vulnerable to peer pressure and unsupervised rivalry.

Conclusions

Mentoring programmes offer both advantages and disadvantages, as summarized in Table 8.8.

The concept of mentoring has become increasingly popular over the past few decades, both in education and management. Mentoring has been advertised as necessary in order for students and trainees to flourish in their environment. However, one of the main criticisms of peer mentoring is the lack of research to show how peer mentoring relationships work, how they develop, and what their outcomes are. The lack of research and of solid knowledge concerning mentoring programmes leaves the field open to improvisation, which might be detrimental to mentees.[13] While there is an abundance of articles on the topic of mentoring in the educational setting, more stringent research standards and more definitional consistency is still desperately needed. Another major criticism of mentoring is that the programmes often target students in need of help, who are frequently perceived as unlikely to succeed unless successful adults help them (the so-called 'deficiency model' of mentoring);[14] although mentoring may extend well beyond this model, clarification in this area is still required. Finally, a more subtle criticism of mentoring refers to the relative lack of supervision and structure, as most programmes rarely have direct supervision of full-time university staff.

On the other hand, as Plutarch once said, 'the mind is not a vessel to be filled, but a fire to be kindled': professional development does not consist of mere academic achievements, and transmission of information and mentoring programmes usually support the entire learning process of the mentee. Furthermore, it also has positives for the mentor. Mentees may benefit from increased personalized attention in a one-on-one setting and being able to work at their own pace. Sessions are customized according to the mentee's individual questions, needs, and learning styles, and they gain a greater mastery of the material and concepts while developing creativity and critical thinking skills. The mentor may also gain a deeper understanding of the material or subject

Table 8.8 Advantages and criticisms of mentoring programmes

Advantages	Criticisms
◆ Help in adapting faster to a new academic environment	◆ Based on a 'deficiency model' (mentees are perceived as in need of help and unlikely to succeed unless successful mentors help them out)
◆ Give the sense of being connected to a community (where one may otherwise feel lost)	◆ Unreliable assessment of outcomes
◆ Identify mentors as positive 'role models' (academic success and good communication and social skills)	◆ Insufficient literature coverage

Box 8.3 Practical hints to get your mentoring programme started

◆ Identify your possible mentor

◆ Find or meet your mentor

◆ Communicate with him/her outside of meetings (confidentiality issues)

◆ Define the goals

◆ Select areas of interest

◆ Schedule meetings (frequency, length, location, goals/outcomes/plans)

◆ Evaluate over time

that they are teaching, as this relationship often encourages greater dedication to their own studies so that they may more effectively communicate what they have learned. The mentor gains a deeper sense of responsibility and dedication. Additionally, both mentors and mentees tend to develop more effective interpersonal communication skills; mentees learn how to effectively form and pose questions and seek advice; and, furthermore, their self-esteem, empathy, and patience increase as they practise active listening and concentration. Mentors gain valuable practice in effective teaching strategies. Often, the mentor also serves as an important role model which, in turn, can shape academic skills and work habits as well as personal values (e.g. dedication to service, empathy, and internal motivation).

Although mentoring programmes are appealing to most people and seem easy to implement and develop, there is little research to offer evidence for their positive role. Future studies should fill this gap, particularly in the medical field, in order to ensure the delivery of effective mentoring programmes (see Box 8.3).

References

1 **Roberts A**. The origins of the term mentor. *Hist Educ Soc Bull* 1999; **64**:313–29.

2 **Kaye B, Jordan-Evans G**. *Love 'em or lose 'em: getting good people to stay*. San Francisco: Berrett-Koehler Publishers Inc.; 2005.

3 **Pompper D, Adams J**. Under the microscope: gender and mentor–protege relationships. *Pub Relat Rev* 2006; **32**:309–15.

4 **Fiorillo A, Calliess IT, Giacco D**. Why should I pay for it? The importance of being members of psychiatric associations. In: *How to succeed in psychiatry—a guide to training and practice* (eds. Fiorillo A, Calliess IT, Sass H). Chichester: Wiley-Blackwell; 2012.

5 **Bullis C, Bach WB**. Are mentor relationships helping organizations? An exploration of developing mentee–mentor–organizational identification using turning point analysis. *Comm Quart* 1989; **37**:199–213.

6 **Doran GT**. There's a S.M.A.R.T. way to write management's goals and objectives. *Manag Rev* 1981; **70**:35–6.

7 **Aubrey B, Cohen P**. *Working wisdom: timeless skills and vanguard strategies for learning organizations*. San Francisco: Jossey Bass; 1995, pp. 23, 44–7, 96–7.

8 **Posner B, Kouzes J**. *Credibility*. San Francisco: Jossey Bass; 1993.

9 **Parsloe E, Wray MJ**. *Coaching and mentoring: practical methods to improve learning*. London, UK: Kogan Page; 2000.

10 **Morton-Cooper A, Palmer A**. *Mentoring, preceptorship and clinical supervision: a guide to professional roles in clinical practice*. Oxford, UK; Wiley-Blackwell; 2000.

11 **Holbeche L**. Peer mentoring: the challenges and opportunities. *Career Dev Int* 1996; **1**:24–7.

12 **Karcher M**. *Cross-age peer mentoring*. Alexandria, VA: Research in Action; 2007.

13 **Tyler JL**. The death of mentoring. *Hosp Health Netw* 1994; 68: 84.

14 **Fields CD**. Black peer mentors, cooperative advocacy beneficial to morale. *Black Issues High Educ* 1996; 19, 84: 68.

Chapter 9

How to organize and manage scientific meetings

Olivier Andlauer, Carla Obradors-Tarragó, Clare Holt, and Driss Moussaoui

Introduction

Scientific meetings are a vital part of the academic and clinical life of any psychiatrist. They offer a unique chance to hear from experts about the latest developments in the specialty, to fulfil every doctor's duty of continuing professional development (CPD), and to network with colleagues. Admittedly, the internet and online journals provide the modern psychiatrist with more information than he or she will ever be able to read but they will never replace the real-life experience of attending a scientific meeting, as testified by the success of local, national, and international conferences.

Organizing a scientific meeting is a unique experience that requires excellent scientific, organizational, and also human skills. Even though nothing can ever guarantee that a meeting will be successful, there are mistakes that can be avoided, and steps that are inescapable. To our knowledge, the most up-to-date peer-reviewed article that deals with this subject dates back to 1990.[1] The World Psychiatric Association has published a detailed booklet on this topic, the scope of which covers mainly the organization of big international conferences.[2] Of course, on the internet, numerous websites give advice on how to organize a conference, some of them being very insightful, while some others miss very crucial points.

Our aim in this chapter is to provide psychiatrists with practical information to make sure their meeting, whatever its size, will be a success. We will start by defining the different types of scientific meetings. We will then detail the two main parts that have to be taken care of when organizing a meeting: the scientific content (dealt with by the scientific committee) and the practical organization (dealt with by the local/organizing committee).

Definitions

There are a variety of scientific meetings, which differ in aim, size, and duration (see Table 9.1). The main aim of congresses, conferences, and lectures is to develop and share knowledge. They give the opportunity for speakers to present their experiences or

Table 9.1 Different types of scientific meetings, with indicative size and duration

	Type of scientific meeting	Aim	Description	Number of participants	Duration (days)
Develop/share knowledge	Congress	Exchanging ideas	Large meeting	200+	4–7
		Sharing new data	Wide variety of lectures, symposia, and workshops		
		Networking			
		A general theme, but broad range of different topics	National or international level		
	Conference	Same as above	Smaller scale than a conference	50–200	2–4
		More focused on one topic of interest	Regional or national level		
	Lecture/ grand rounds	One specified topic	Lecture from an expert, usually visiting from another institution	10–200	½
Develop skills/pragmatic approach	Seminar/ school	Networking	Small groups	10–50	1–5
		One specified topic	Interactive		
	Workshop	Networking	Small groups	10–50	1–3
		One specified technique	Interactive		
	Research team meeting	Getting to know each other	Meeting of different research teams that work on the same subject	3–15	1–2
		Exchanging ideas			
		Discussing one research protocol/results			

Source data from: *How to organize a conference: step by step manual.* Copyright (2003), IAPSS.

research results, and for all participants to learn from each other. For seminars, workshops, and team meetings, the emphasis is more on developing skills, like learning a new technique. They are therefore of a smaller size, because they have a more personalized and interactive approach.

The content (sessions) of each type of meeting can also vary, depending on the main expected outcome (see Table 9.2). Some use a top–down approach, with one teacher and many learners, whereas others apply a more transversal approach, based on interactivity and exchanges between peers.

Sessions can be combined together in a variety of different ways. The right type of sessions for a scientific meeting must be decided based on the aim(s) that the organizers want to achieve and the resources that they can access. It is therefore very important to start by defining the core of the meeting—its scientific content.

Table 9.2 Different types of sessions in a scientific meeting, with indicative sizes and durations

	Type of session	Aim	Description	Number of participants	Duration (hours)
Top-down approach	Plenary lecture	Teach Present new data	An expert presents a comprehensive overview on a specific topic	15+	½ –1½
	Symposium	Teach Present new data Compare ideas	A series of 2–4 experts present, one after each other, complementary information on a specific topic	15–100	1–2
	Round table	Exchange ideas Reach a consensus	2–5 experts present complementary and diverging points of views on a specific topic Talk one after another or open discussion between the experts	10–200	1–3
Transversal approach	Meet the expert	Teach Inspire Exchange ideas	An expert presents a short overview of his work, and then answers questions from the audience	10–50	½ –1½
	Workshop	Teach Improve skills	1–3 experts Small groups work under supervision to gain experience in a specific skill	5–30	2–6
	Poster session	Present new data	A researcher presents preliminary work	3–30	½–1

Scientific content

Theme of the meeting

Every scientific meeting has a theme. Even the biggest psychiatric congresses (like the congresses of the European Psychiatric Association, the World Psychiatric Association, or the American Psychiatric Association), who gather a wide range of speakers and cover hundreds of different topics, have a general theme.[1] Usually, the theme of the meeting is obvious to the organizers, because that is this theme that originally led them to organize the meeting. For large international events, it is usually the president of the association that chooses the theme.

Except for very large congresses, it is advised to choose a theme that is clear and precise, relevant to a certain audience, and original. Ideally, it should be appealing, or even a little bit provocative, to catch the attention and interest of potential participants.

Scientific committee

The scientific committee has the responsibility of deciding on the theme of the meeting, its programme and sessions, and the relevant speakers and chairs of these sessions. One of its duties is also to organize the review process of submitted abstracts.

The scientific committee should consist of knowledgeable experts in the scientific field of the meeting, as they are responsible for the scientific programme.[3] It is also important to make sure that the scientific committee represents different types of expertise: biologists and doctors; young and senior psychiatrists; public and private practitioners; clinicians, academics, and researchers; and carers or service users, when relevant. It is also very helpful to include in the scientific committee, members who have a good professional network. They can then invite speakers who they know are good presenters and who are more likely to accept the invitation. Committee members with a large professional network will also advertise the meeting widely.

Scientific programme

Constructing the scientific programme is the main task of the scientific committee. There are four main issues that need to be defined: topics, types, scheduling, and speakers for the sessions. All of these are of capital importance for the success of the meeting, and imply making some difficult judgement calls. If the meeting is organized by a psychiatric association, a general assembly should be scheduled into the programme.

Topics of the sessions

The topics of the sessions have to be carefully considered. They should obviously relate, directly or indirectly, to the theme of the meeting. When choosing the different topics for the sessions, it is important to consider the whole coherence of the meeting. Multiple sessions on the same topic should be avoided, even if all the sessions proposed by the committee or submitted via abstracts are of high scientific quality. It is possible to offer to merge two sessions into one if they appear to be both interesting and of good scientific quality, but overlapping. A balance between the different fields and scientific points of view should be considered, as well as between clinical and theoretical sessions. Added value is frequently provided by original or more 'general public' lectures (e.g. from a famous personality), but this should remain as a minor part of the programme. It is necessary to provide the participants with what will be relevant to them, but also to surprise them by choosing some unexpected topics.

Types of sessions

The type of session will be based on its topic and aim. Table 9.2 outlines the different types that can be considered, according to the aim of the scientific committee for the session. A balance between the different types of sessions should be attained.

Scheduling of the sessions

Defining the scheduling of the sessions can become a very tricky exercise, and a general rule in this area is that 'less is more'. Indeed, people have a tendency to build very ambitious programmes, with a very tight schedule from early in the morning until late in the afternoon, and with very short or no breaks. This is a mistake, as time needs to be given to participants to 'breath' between the sessions. Moreover, it must be considered that some sessions might run 5–10 minutes late, and therefore some extra time between the sessions should be allowed to avoid all of the following sessions running late too. No matter how enthusiastic and motivated the participants will be, they will need time to eat lunch, go to the bathroom, walk from one room to another, or simply have a coffee and a quick chat between two sessions. A scientific meeting with a very dense programme will make the participants tired, and sessions in the afternoon will not have the attention they deserve. People will also be more likely to 'miss' the afternoon sessions if they have been overwhelmed by a very busy programme in the morning.

Speakers and chairs of the sessions

Finding a good speaker is a difficult task. The very first quality for a speaker is to be an expert in his or her field. Unfortunately, in most of cases, this is not enough to ensure that a high-quality presentation will be delivered. It is also important for a speaker to communicate his or her message as clearly as possible (see Box 9.1). Having seen the speaker in a meeting beforehand is helpful to make sure that the presentation will achieve its goal of passing the information onto the audience. When inviting the speakers, it is essential to make sure that they are aware of what is expected from them. They should be contacted early enough to increase their likelihood to be available and to therefore agree to participate. It is important to invite the most renowned experts in the field, but also to avoid inviting speakers that everyone has already seen. Less well-known speakers might not attract as many participants but they might have the advantage of being more dedicated and of trying harder to make their presentation as best as possible. They are also more likely to surprise the audience with an original point of view.

Box 9.1 What makes a good speaker?

- Being knowledgeable
- Being clear
- Have a defined message
- Making a structured presentation
- Speaking slowly rather than quickly
- Having good adaptive skills
- Using as few slides as possible
- Inviting questions
- Inspiring

Box 9.2 What makes a good chairperson?

◆ Being knowledgeable

◆ Keeping the schedule on time

◆ Being discrete

◆ Having good adaptive skills

◆ Inviting questions

◆ Having good diplomatic skills

◆ Gently but firmly interrupting irrelevant or long questions

A good session chairperson is also crucial (see Box 9.2). Tasks of a chairperson include introducing the speakers and putting them in context and making sure the session is running on time (which involves timely management of the speakers and of questions from the audience). The chairperson therefore needs to be knowledgeable about the topic of the session, but also have good organizational and diplomatic skills. Indeed, it is not easy to interrupt a lengthy question or a speaker who has only reached his second slide after 20 minutes.

Submission and review of abstracts

Congresses and conferences usually rely, at least partly, on submissions from the psychiatric community. Once the theme of the meeting and the scheduling of the sessions have been established, a call for abstracts should be sent, which would usually also appear on the website and first flyers for the meeting. The call for abstracts should clearly state a deadline for submission, the topics and types of sessions that can be submitted, and the format of the submission.[4] An online submission, via email or an online form, is always the easiest way.

Once all the abstracts have been received, the scientific committee will review them according to predefined rules. The best submissions will therefore be selected; but the scientific committee should also be allowed to reject or select some submissions based on other criteria than purely scientific content. Such criteria might include the need to balance the types and topics of the sessions, or the wish of organizers to put forward a topic that is less attractive but needs support (e.g. a new topic or field, a very interesting and innovative approach). Otherwise, there is a risk that only the 'big names' and already well-established speakers/teams will be selected.

Continuous medical education/continuous professional development courses and credits

Continuous medical education (CME) or continuous professional development (CPD) has become an important issue in a number of countries. Participants attending the meeting might therefore expect to receive CME/CPD credits. It reinforces the positive, high-profile, and high-quality image of the meeting, and rewards participants for their attendance. For national or smaller-scale meetings, the local authority should be contacted to enquire about the procedure for applying for CME/CPD credits. This usually involves a fair amount of paperwork, including the need to detail the scientific content of the meeting, its relevance, and the quality assurance process that is in place (satisfaction survey among participants, pre- and post-tests, etc.).

Networking opportunities

Networking opportunities are also an important part of a scientific meeting. They are relevant to the scientific content, especially of workshops or seminars, because these types of meetings usually gather clinicians or researchers from the same field of interest. Providing them with opportunities to network is therefore one of the scientific roles that the meeting can achieve. These opportunities can be created during the meeting (by allowing long enough breaks between sessions or by using interactive sessions such as workshops), and also by exchanging participants' emails or creating an online community through social networks.

Practical organization of a scientific meeting

Shortly after having defined a theme and the scientific outline of the meeting, it is time to start planning its practical organization. Regardless of the particular type of meeting, the organizational process can be consistently divided into three key phases: preparation, execution, and evaluation.[5] Execution and evaluation constitute the tip of the iceberg: it is actually the first phase (preparation) that will take most of the workload and time. The complexity of each of these phases, and thus the time, money, and manpower necessary to devote to them, will depend on the particular meeting being organized.

The following three subsections deal in more detail with the three organizational phases. It is important to remember that this is a general guide which should be used flexibly and modified according to the particular requirements of the meeting.

The preparation phase

Where and when?

When deciding on the venue for the meeting, the first question to answer is which country or city the meeting can or should take place in. While this is clearly an issue for international meetings, and even for meetings at a national level, there may be several cities that are potential contenders. As a general rule, it is sensible to select a place that is local to at least some of the committee members, as this will make certain aspects of organization, such as booking the venue and selecting caterers, much more straightforward. In addition, it is important to consider where the majority of participants are likely to be travelling from, as this will suggest the selection of a place that is easily accessible. Fig. 9.1 provides a guide to some possible venue options, including the advantages and drawbacks of each.

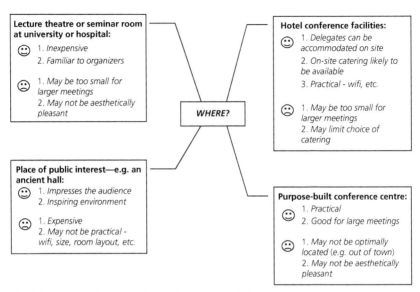

Fig. 9.1 Venue options, and their advantages and drawbacks.

Before confirming the venue, it is important for a committee member to make a visit to it. This final check should be done with a critical eye and with the following questions in mind:

◆ Is the venue sufficiently accessible by public transportation?

◆ Does the venue meet the necessary technological requirements (e.g. computers connected to overhead projectors, wireless internet access)?

◆ Do the meeting rooms have any negative features (e.g. inadequate visibility of the 'stage area' or poor acoustics)?

◆ Will the meeting rooms cater for the style of sessions planned (see Table 9.3 for some ideas for different types of room set-up)?

◆ Are there suitable areas in which to conduct the registration of participants or to serve food?

Setting the date and booking the venue go hand in hand, and it is useful to come up with several potential dates for the meeting in order to allow more flexibility when booking the venue. Indeed, the chosen venue might not be available at the date of the meeting. Therefore, the earlier the date and venue are set, the better. Box 9.3 provides some additional tips to bear in mind when setting the date for the meeting.

Planning and organization

The next steps in the preparation phase require the organizers not only to consider exactly what needs to be achieved, but also the rate at which progresses should be made. Essentially, the organizers need first to develop a checklist of all the tasks necessary to make the meeting possible, and then create a timeline for completion of each task,

Table 9.3 Different types of room set-up

Setting	Pros	Cons
Theatre Style	Accommodates large groups	Often no writing surface Allows for minimal group interaction
Hollow Design	Promotes group interaction Writing surface available Accommodates quite large groups (25–30 people)	No focus point if there is a speaker or chair of meeting Speaker or chair of meeting aren't easily distinguished from other participants
'U' Shape	Allows group interaction Can accommodate a speaker	Eventually (for groups over about 25 people) the sides of the 'U' become too long, hindering group interaction
Classroom Style	Allows note taking Speaker can see all participants Accommodates large groups in limited space Allows discussion among smaller groups after a large group activity	Interaction only possible between subgroups of participants
'V' Shape	Allows discussion among small groups after a large group activity Creates a more enclosed and interactive feel	Limits the interaction between attendees of different tables

Box 9.3 Tips for setting the DATE of the meeting

Days off: avoid public holidays

Advance planning: ensure the date gives enough time to organize the meeting

Topic overlap: ensure date does not clash with other similar meetings

Eminent speakers: check availability of key speakers before finalizing the date

bearing in mind the proposed date of the meeting. By setting clear targets early on in the preparation phase, organizers really could save themselves time (and stress!) in the long run.

Table 9.4 gives an overview of the stages involved in each of the organizational phases of a scientific meeting; it also provides a suggested timeline for the preparation phase according to the size of the meeting. This suggested schedule provides a useful starting point, which can then be adapted to the specific needs of the meeting.

In addition, it is important to be clear about who has responsibility for doing what; otherwise work may be duplicated or, even worse, not done at all. For a small-sized meeting, this may involve simply dividing tasks between existing committee members. However, for larger meetings, it may be sensible to have several subcommittees, that are each in charge of a different aspect of the organizational process, and a professional congress organizer to deal with the main practicalities involved in the organization.[6] Examples of areas that may be usefully covered by subcommittees include:

- ◆ Scientific programme (e.g. to finalize the sessions and secure speakers)
- ◆ Finances (e.g. to finalize the budget and secure sponsorship)
- ◆ Publicity (e.g. to handle advertising and produce printed programmes)
- ◆ Entertainment (e.g. to plan social events)[7]; opening and closing ceremonies are important moments, as well as cultural activities
- ◆ Technical support (e.g. to maintain the website and source audio-visual equipment).

Creating subcommittees may require recruitment of new members into the organizational committee. Clearly, while it is important to select people with the relevant expertise, it is also necessary to consider whether or not members will be able to devote sufficient time to the planning process, including being able to attend committee meetings. One way to make this easier for everyone is to schedule some meetings as video conferences (e.g. via online conference services) rather than expecting people to always meet face to face. It is also extremely useful to ensure that the chairperson of the organizing committee has an overview of each subcommittee's progress, for example via regular progress reports.

Budgeting

Another essential practicality of the organization of a meeting is to plan and handle finances. It is vital to accurately construct the budget from the very beginning (i.e.

Table 9.4 Proposed timeline for preparation phases according to the size of the meeting

	Before the meeting								During the meeting		After the meeting
Congresses	24 months	18 months	12 months	9 months	6 months	3–4 months	1 month	2 weeks	Registration day	Meeting days	Post meeting
Small events	6 or more months	4–5 months	3–4 months	2 months	4–6 weeks	3 weeks	2 weeks	1 week			
Course	12 weeks	8 weeks	6 weeks	4 weeks	2 weeks	1 week	3 days	1 day			
	Define the theme(s) and the aim	Book catering services or restaurants	Advertise the event	Send the letters of confirmation of attendance	Check availability of participants	Close applications	Prepare the material	Prepare the meeting room(s) and the registration desk	Check that registration is set up	Check equipment (especially audio-visual) an hour before	Prepare the minutes of the meeting
	Decide type, size, and scope	Book other social activities and entertainment (if applies)	Reach the targeted audience	Arrange trips and accommodation of speakers and/or other participants	Close abstract submission	Send the participants information about the hotel	Confirm with speakers again and check whether their needs have changed	Put up signs	Welcome attendees	Check the catering each day	Evaluate development of the meeting
	Decide the location (city, country)	Preliminary agenda	Launch the call for papers	Contracts with restaurants, catering, transportation, and hotels	Finalize agenda and session schedule	Confirm guest/meeting room arrangements			Distribute registration packets	Monitor expenses	Reimburse the costs or pay the honorary fees to speakers and/or participants (if applies)
	Set the date	Send official invitations	Open the registration	Determine transportation needs of attendees		Confirm menus			Make sure refreshments are available	Check if hotel is sold out	TAKE YOUR DESERVED REST!
	Book the venue	Confirm sponsorship and arrange layout of stands, etc.				Confirm special dietary needs			Be ready to sort out any problems that occur		
	Contact important speakers and check availability					Send the final documentation			Confirm meal timing		

(continued)

Table 9.4 (continued) Proposed timeline for preparation phases according to the size of the meeting

	Before the meeting								During the meeting		After the meeting
									Registration day	Meeting days	Post meeting
Congresses	24 months	18 months	12 months	9 months	6 months	3–4 months	1 month	2 weeks			
Small events	6 or more months	4–5 months	3–4 months	2 months	4–6 weeks	3 weeks	2 weeks	1 week			
Course	12 weeks	8 weeks	6 weeks	4 weeks	2 weeks	1 week	3 days	1 day			
	Prepare a checklist and a tentative timeline			Decide on materials needed in registration packet		Printing company (if needed)					
	Appoint committees (if applies)			Define and design signs, banners, room signage		Update website or intranet site					
	Prepare the budget					Submit daily schedule to hotel					
	Contact sponsors (if needed)					Assemble registration packets					
						Cut-off date to join special events					

Source data from: *BMJ*, 300(6727), Wright DJ. How to organise a medical symposium for general practitioners, pp. 799–801, Copyright (1990), BMJ Publishing; IAPSS. How to organize a conference. Step by step manual, Copyright (2003); *BMJ*, 2(6137), Capperauld I, Macpherson AI. Organise an international medical meeting. II: Scientific programme, pp. 616–7, Copyright (1978), BMJ Publishing; *BMJ*, 2(6140), Capperauld I, Macpherson AI. How to do it. Organise an international medical meeting. V: The final programme, pp. 805–7, Copyright (1978), BMJ Publishing; *Archives of disease in childhood*, 80(6), Wacogne ID, Diwakar V, Anderson JM. How to organise a paediatric MRCP (UK) part II training course, pp. 570–2, Copyright (1999), BMJ Publishing.

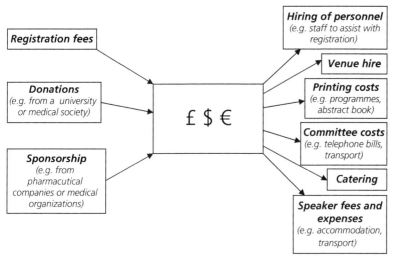

Fig. 9.2 Budget planning for a meeting.

expected income and expenditure) and monitor it continuously. Essentially, the final budget report should confirm forecasts without any surprises! The main ingoings and outgoings involved in organizing scientific meetings are shown in Fig. 9.2.

There is no general rule, but some guidance can be found that registration fees should cover at least about 60% of the total cost of the meeting:[6]

$$\text{Registration fee} = 60\% \times \frac{\text{Total estimated cost} + 10\%}{\text{Number of attendees}}$$

If the fee is exaggeratedly high, the budget should be revised and/or the feasibility of organizing this meeting should be reconsidered. If many donations or sponsorships are received, then the registration fees can be lowered.

In short, before spending any money, a predicted budget (based on research into likely outgoings such as catering, accommodation, and venue fees) should be formulated. This in turn will allow the registration fees to be set at an appropriate level. In addition to the registration fees, some income for the meeting may come from donations or sponsorships. One way to secure sponsorship, for instance from pharmaceutical companies, is to offer sponsors the opportunity of a trade exhibition (a stall where they can display information about their services or products). In other words, sponsorship may be easier to come by if the sponsor feels that there is a tangible benefit to be gained.

A further consideration relating to registration fees is in what form they should be collected. The most straightforward method for collecting registration fees is to have a designated bank account (for example, an account which is registered in the name of the educational organization to which the scientific meeting is affiliated). Using the personal account of one of the committee members should not be considered as an option. It is important to produce regular budget reports and to ensure that the accuracy of these reports is verified. All invoices must be carefully collected and recorded.

Who is coming?

Given that a large proportion of the budget is made up of the registration fees, it is important to advertise the meeting appropriately widely and sufficiently far in advance. Some ideas about different potential modes of advertising are as follows:

- E-mails (personal invitations or group e-mails sent to the target audience)
- Flyers/leaflets (distributed to professional or academic associations, postgraduate centres, research centres, universities, or hospitals)
- Press releases, short notices, or advertisements placed in related web page(s), peer-reviewed journal(s), or newspapers (this latter option is extremely expensive)
- Website devoted to the meeting (probably most relevant to large conferences)
- Social media (e.g. a Facebook page or Twitter profile).

Whatever modes of advertising are used, it is necessary to be consistent in including key pieces of information such as:

- Meeting date and venue
- Costs and logistics of registration—including early bird fees and fees for different types of participants (e.g. concessions for students or allied health professionals)
- Overview of the scientific programme
- Important deadlines (e.g. for registration, for abstract submission, or for signing up to events like the conference dinner).

Execution of the meeting

After all the hard work of planning the meeting, there should not be much to do except to make sure everything is running smoothly and according to the programme. On the day of the meeting, committee members should arrive well in advance to make sure that everything is in order at the venue, such as meeting rooms and registration desk, and audio-visual equipment. In addition, it is sensible for at least some of the committee members not to be involved in mandatory planned activities, so that they can oversee the overall running of the meeting and can troubleshoot any unexpected complication. In large meetings, it is likely that staff will be hired to help participants with the registration process, provide general information and directions, and serve food and drinks during breaks.[8]

Particular attention should be given to time management; for example, ensuring that chairpersons and speakers are fully aware of both the length of their sessions and the timings of coffee and lunch breaks. A copy of the agenda can be placed in each meeting room to provide a gentle reminder of the importance of timekeeping. If a session is running behind schedule, a subtle wave at the speaker and chairperson might help to remind them that it is important to keep the meeting on time.

Evaluation of the meeting

During the meeting, participants should be asked to provide feedback about the meeting in general and about each specific session. In order for a course to be recognized as part of a CME/CPD programme, gathering feedback on the course is a mandatory requirement. An effective way to ensure a high response rate is to issue certificates of attendance to participants only once they have returned their evaluation forms. These should be carefully designed such that they are as short as possible while still covering enough ground in order to provide constructive feedback. After the scientific meeting, the organizing committee should discuss the feedback collected and analyse any areas that were less well received and thus could be improved in the future.

Conclusions

Organizing a scientific meeting is a very demanding but also immensely rewarding task. No matter whether the meeting is a gathering of a few enthusiasts, or a major international event, defining a scientific programme and dealing with the practicalities of the organization are challenges that will require cohesion and constant work of the members of the committees. From the scheduling of the sessions to the choice of the venue, nothing should be left to chance. Box 9.4 summarizes some important tips to keep in mind when organizing a scientific meeting.

With the development of information technology, recent years have brought tremendous changes in the way teaching can be delivered. It is now possible to hear the most renowned experts and the best lecturers in any field without the need to leave one's

---

Box 9.4 Ten commandments of a good congress organizer

1 Choose the best possible team (and professional congress organizer, if relevant) and work hard together.
2 Be optimistic—but beware of your optimism.
3 Always have one or more alternative scenarios ready.
4 Decrease your expected figure of attendees and income (by about 25%).
5 Increase your expected figure of expenses (by about 25%).
6 Beware of the time left before the beginning of the congress—advance your deadlines instead of postponing them.
7 Make the people around you happy, and do not expect thanks from them.
8 Delegate to the right people whenever possible, and motivate them.
9 Be attentive to details (the devil is in there) but keep in mind the whole picture.
10 Do not exhaust all your energy before the opening of the congress, and *when nothing goes wrong, start to worry*!

Source data from: Moussaoui D. How to organize a psychiatric congress. Copyright (2002), World Psychiatric Association.

chair at home, and sometimes even for free. Moreover, raising issues ranging from energy wasted in transport, to political games of influence, to the blurred relationship with the pharmaceutical industry, some authors have questioned the need to continue organizing scientific meetings.[9-11] However, we believe that scientific meetings represent an integral part of a psychiatrist's professional life. They still provide important opportunities to learn, teach, and stay up to date, while also being inspired, exchanging knowledge, and networking with peers.[12] There is no doubt that a successful scientific meeting, no matter its size or budget, contributes to creating a sense of pride in belonging to a fascinating specialty.

References

1 **Wright DJ**. How to organise a medical symposium for general practitioners. *BMJ* 1990; **300**(6727):799–801.

2 **Moussaoui D**. *How to organize a psychiatric congress*. World Psychiatric Association; 2002, http://www.psychiatry.sk/cms/File/how_to_organize_a_psychiatric_congress_2002.doc.

3 **Zhao B**. *The soul of the conference: effective technical program development*. 2011, IEEE Panel of Conference Organizers (POCO), Beijing, China, https://www.ieee.org/documents/2011_07_22_confcom_panel_zhao.pdf.

4 **Capperauld I, Macpherson AI**. How to do it. Organise an international medical meeting. II: scientific programme. *BMJ* 1978; **2**(6137):616–7.

5 **Chang RY, Kehoe KR**. *Meetings that work: a practical guide to shorter and more productive meetings*. San Francisco: Jossey-Bass/Pfeiffer; 1994.

6 **Capperauld I, Macpherson AI**. How to do it. Organise an international medical meeting. I: committees and budgets. *BMJ* 1978; **2**(6136):541–4.

7 **Capperauld I, Macpherson AI**. How to organise an international medical meeting. VI: the social programme. *BMJ* 1978; **2**(6141):875–7.

8 **Capperauld I, Macpherson AI**. How to do it. Organise an international medical meeting. V: the final programme. *BMJ* 1978; **2**(6140):805–7.

9 **Green M**. Are international medical conferences an outdated luxury the planet can't afford? Yes. *BMJ* 2008; **336**(7659):1466.

10 **Ioannidis JP**. Are medical conferences useful? And for whom? *JAMA* 2012; **307**(12):1257–8.

11 **Dobbing J**. How to organise an international medical meeting. *BMJ* 1978; **2**(6140):827.

12 **Drife JO**. Are international medical conferences an outdated luxury the planet can't afford? No. *BMJ* 2008; **336**(7659):1467.

Chapter 10

Raising funds for research and educational activities

Martina Rojnic Kuzman, Umberto Volpe, and Dinesh Bhugra

Case study

Robert was a trainee in psychiatry, very much interested in neurofeedback. He went abroad to learn this technique and apply it to psychiatric patients. Since none of his supervisors were skilled in this technique, Robert had to himself pay for this training. When he came back to his department, he wanted to use neurofeedback with his own patients. However, his supervisor was not convinced by this approach and refused to fund this activity because of budget limitations. Of course, if Robert had himself been able to raise funds for this activity, his supervisor would have had no objection to starting to use neurofeedback. Regretfully however, Robert had no knowledge of how to obtain such funds. After a few years, he was still looking for funds and his efforts resulted in nothing.

Introduction

Fundraising may be defined as the process of soliciting and gathering voluntary contributions of money or other resources, by requesting donations from individuals, businesses, charitable foundations, or governmental agencies.[1]

Traditionally, fundraising consisted mostly of face-to-face interaction (e.g. asking for donations on the street or at people's doors), but this process has significantly expanded and, nowadays, fundraising may represent a quite complex procedure that requires great experience, a strong research background, and even specific administrative training (especially when submitting large fund requests, granted by national or international governmental agencies). However, especially during the earliest stages of a psychiatric career, smaller funds can be obtained for low-budget and/or local projects, from different sources. Here, we describe, in brief, the latter crowdsourcing type of fundraising, applied to the field of mental health.

While fundraising has a long history, it was not treated with a scientific/research-based approach until the early 1990s. Since then, mainly following the work of Henry A. Rosso in the United States,[2] lots of fundraising principles and hypotheses have been researched and tested in practice, and it has become a specific subject taught in many universities.

Why is fundraising necessary?

The last few decades have brought tremendous rapid changes in society worldwide, greatly influencing its various aspects including health, communication, ethics, politics, and economics. After the 1990s, those changes consequently affected nearly all areas of the health and educational systems, as well as care and research in psychiatry.

Over the last few years, additional factors have affected the redistribution of funds into the mental health sector including the more rational distribution of welfare funds, the international economic crisis (and the consequent shortage of research funding), new rules for funding activities, the emergence of new financing bodies (mainly, a more prominent role for the private sector), and competition among research and health organizations. These days, clinical, educational, and research policies are strongly influenced by the principles of cost effectiveness, commodification, and competition.[3] Such a sudden shift has greatly influenced both the health sector and the health political agendas, inducing significant modifications in the way medical research is produced and funded; a brief account of the major changes that characterized research in mental health over the past decades is provided in Table 10.1.

Table 10.1 Recent shifts in mental health research policies and funding opportunities

Requirement	Before 1990s	After 1990s
Technology	Not necessarily demanding	Very demanding
People	Psychiatrists, psychologists, neuroscientists, other medical specialists	As before, but also other mental health professionals, molecular biologists, mathematicians, statisticians, information technicians
Collaboration	Closed, local	Open, global, multidisciplinary
Topics	Basic, clinical, social, epidemiological issues	Higher degree of interdisciplinary co-operation and stronger emphasis on translational research
Finance	Research activities could have been run with modest amounts of money	Need for larger funding, even for small projects (mainly to cover the costs of personnel and technology)
Dissemination of results	Slow and via traditional means (e.g. congresses, local publications)	Faster and global process; policy for results' dissemination has to be declared within the research project
Applicability	Not always applicable	Increasing demands for accessibility, immediate applicability, and translational impact
Ethical issues	Less strictly regulated	High demands on ethical issues; necessary part of any fund request

(continued)

Table 10.1 (continued) Recent shifts in mental health research policies and funding opportunities

Requirement	Before 1990s	After 1990s
Motivation	Intrinsic and from local environment	Intrinsic, plus larger scope encompassing national/ international environments
Location	Small and top research centres	Mostly top research centres; often collaboration between top centres is necessary

Furthermore, the role of psychiatrists is no longer seen as just providing good clinical care as their responsibilities towards team members and their institutions have grown. Now, clinical psychiatrists are expected to ensure state of the art clinical care and, preferably, to participate in research projects.[4] This process of evolution of the psychiatrist's role started decades ago in North America.[5,6] In other countries, and especially in Europe, the process has more recently become apparent: research work is strongly encouraged within psychiatric training in many European countries, in accordance with existing guidelines on mental health training.[7] This has led to a greater pressure on early-career psychiatrists to be involved in research activities, although official European training curricula rarely provide structured rules for such activities.[8] Consequently, research is usually regarded as extracurricular and requires external funding. For motivated trainees, it might be problematic accessing significant funding opportunities.

How to raise funds?

Over the last decades, besides traditional governmental bodies and official organizations, many non-governmental and professional organizations have expanded their funding opportunities and promotional activities. Thus, the landscape of funding has become significantly more complex and the lack of knowledge of the 'funding market' may represent the first obstacle to accessing funds. An account of currently available funding sources is provided in Table 10.2.

When searching for funding, forward planning is necessary and usually entails the development of a proper 'strategic plan'. In order to develop a well-structured action plan, many issues have to be taken into account. A tentative general scheme of the whole process of fundraising is summarized in Fig. 10.1 and practical 'step-by-step' guidelines for early-career psychiatrists are included to assist them in obtaining their own funding for educational and research activities.

Step 1: Develop a good idea

Usually, the first step is to develop the initial idea which lies at the core of the research/ educational project. If one is applying for a research project, the idea usually comes from reviewing previous work on the topic and identifying the research gaps. If the

Table 10.2 Who provides funds?

Public funding sources	Private funding sources
◆ International and supranational governmental agencies (e.g. EU)	◆ Pharmaceutical companies
	◆ Non-profit associations
◆ National governmental agencies (e.g. Ministry of Health)	◆ Professional associations
	◆ Families' associations
◆ Local institutions (e.g. universities, local health units, hospitals)	◆ Patients' associations
◆ Institutional student scholarships	◆ Religious groups
	◆ Charities
	◆ Private foundations
	◆ Philanthropic organizations
	◆ Public broadcasters
	◆ Political bodies
	◆ Individuals

aim of fundraising is to run a new clinical or rehabilitation activity, the idea could be more general and the definition of the core idea less specific. However, it still usually requires definition of the mission (e.g. the main purpose of the activity, what the project or the organization does, who is involved, and how the goal is to be achieved) and of the vision (e.g. the future achievement aims of the organization/project, the

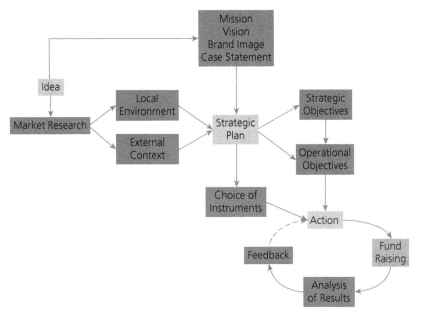

Fig. 10.1 The fundraising process.

guidance and inspiration needed for the organization to focus on achieving its aims) of the fundraising project. It might also be advantageous to summarize the mission and the vision of a fundraising activity in the form of a logo and/or a specific mission statement. An example of a successful fundraising logo and statement is provided in Fig. 10.2.

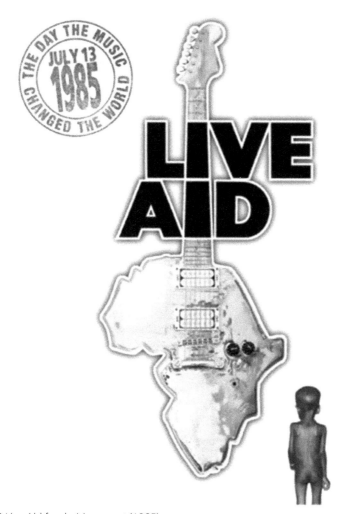

Fig. 10.2 Live Aid fundraising event (1985).
Live Aid was a dual-venue concert, held in London (UK) and Philadelphia (USA) on 13 July 1985. The event was organized by Bob Geldof and Midge Ure to raise funds for relief of the ongoing Ethiopian famine. It was one of the largest-scale television broadcasts of all time, with an estimated global audience of 1.9 billion, across 150 nations, and around £150 million was raised for famine relief as a direct result of the concerts.

Original and innovative ideas are always a good start. However, less innovative ideas are also worthy of funding if one can demonstrate that they will contribute something that is lacking. For example, although a course of treatment in depression may not be innovative enough for psychiatrists, it may fit very well as an innovative course for neurologists working in a setting where it was proved that post-stroke depression is not properly recognized and consequently undertreated.

Step 2: Search the 'market'

Before further steps are taken, it is advisable to develop the idea as an initial project and research the available funding options. If the initial idea does not comply with currently available grant options, one may choose to wait for a further grant opportunity to become available, adapt the project in order to fit current funding requirements, or expand the search for funding options.

There are a number of grants aimed at specific career stages, including some especially devoted to young psychiatrists and/or early-career psychiatrists.[9] In general, there are two main types of fundraising possibilities. The first includes the search for funds available through official programmes and issued by usually large governmental and international organizations. Such funding opportunities are rarely available to early-career psychiatrists; high-profile research proposals put forward by experienced researchers generally have a higher chance of getting these funds. The second opportunity is for raising funds from donors who are non-governmental bodies, such as local interest groups or local health agencies. Early-career psychiatrists should give these funding opportunities considerable attention since not only is there a greater chance of being funded but also, these days, they provide significant donations at both national and international level. (For example, according to the National Survey of Giving, Volunteering, and Participating (NSGVP) in Canada, healthcare donations account for up to 20% of education and research fundraising and about 5% of all donations.)[10] Actually, there is a third opportunity to raise funds for initiatives in the mental health sector, which is to approach pharmaceutical companies: especially when a new drug is going to be launched, local representatives may be more amenable to be involved in projects.

Step 3: Explore the local/external contexts

When developing the core project idea, it should be always evaluated within the local context (i.e. taking account of all the figures to be involved in the future project, such as the mental health professionals, the patients, and their families) and the impact it may have on the external and more general environment. While an internal audit may be easy to conduct and can strongly influence the definition of the vision and mission of the activity, often proper market research is necessary to test the impact of the activity on the target audience, trying to reach the highest possible number of users.

Step 4: Develop a strategic plan

Having defined the main topic of the project and having learned about realistic funding opportunities, the development of the final strategic plan is mandatory in order to properly present your ideas to a potential donor. This step includes defining the strategic objectives of the plan (which should comply with the mission of the funding donor) and the operative objectives, as well as choosing the main instruments to use in the application for fund raising.

Often, funding bodies provide detailed instructions as to their requirements (sometimes, especially for larger grant applications, a proper instruction manual is provided). Careful reading of such instructions may avoid your funding proposal being rejected for not complying with the donor's requirements. However, some general hints concerning how to structure your fundraising project draft are provided in Table 10.3.

Table 10.3 What a fundraising plan should include

Core idea, mission, vision	This lies at the very heart of the application and should be scientifically sound but also clear (always ask yourself: 'Is the project understandable to a layperson?') and appealing to the donor (mostly in terms of clinical impact). Clearly express what is the main and secondary aims of your project.
Background information	A potentially fundable mental health project should always start from the evidence base already available, and it should clarify what the present project will obtain as a potentially innovative outcome (with respect to what is known about your topic).
Skills and knowledge required	With rapidly developing knowledge, teamwork becomes a precondition for every project. For example, a collaboration between young psychiatrists with a special interest in clinical work with patients with depression and a basic scientist with a specialism in the same topic may present a project team capable of a more complex, interdisciplinary approach to the same subject, thus potentially increasing the applicability of the project's products.
People involved	The successful accomplishment of a project requires a successful team of collaborators. The team should comprise a leader who is eager to take responsibility and enough manpower to perform the field work. It is always of added value to have renowned experts in the topic of the project ('big names')—in at least a mentoring capacity. International collaboration may further contribute to the strength of the project team as it offers ways to share experience and to increase the flow of knowledge and the dissemination of results. There are a number of associations and networks of peer groups consisting of psychiatric trainees and early-career psychiatrists which are effectively performing numerous researches and educational and clinical projects. This presents an enormous opportunity for getting involved in all kinds of international projects and of meeting and connecting with distinguished researchers working at research institutions, opening up the possibility of future collaboration.
Timing and financial administration	This is essential to provide the donor with a clear idea about when and how funds will be spent. The application should contain detailed descriptions of the project and of its financial structure.
Ethical aspects	Ethical aspects that should be respected include the protection of privacy, confidentiality, accuracy, relevance, accountability, and honesty. There are a number of documents issued by philanthropic organizations and associations defining the ethical aspect of fundraising (e.g. see[11]).

Table 10.4 lists the mandatory documents and the most commonly required other items for the majority of official fundraising calls. Some funders actively welcome a preliminary approach by the applicant and may even advise on how to pitch the application. Some also hold seminars for teaching and explaining their funding calls so that applicants can learn about the required focus and strategy for their applications.

Table 10.4 Usual documentation for a fundraising call

◆ Covering letter	It can be used to give a more personal note to the application itself. It summarizes the intent, aims, and outcomes of the project and presents the team. This is the place to outline the most important past successful projects of the team.
◆ Title page	Provide a focused, clear, catchy title which reflects the mission and vision of your project.
◆ Executive summary	The abstract of the project is a very important part of the proposal, as it gives a quick overview of the project and directs the reviewers further. Thus, it is advisable to write it last.
◆ Introduction	The project background should focus on the most important and recent knowledge on the topic, and provide a link to the goals and objectives of the project.
◆ Core proposal	The idea that lies at the heart of the project should be clearly stated here.
◆ Goals and objectives	This should include a hypothesis which is clear and straightforward. Using numbers/bullets may help better organize this section.
◆ Methodology	The methods section should contain the description of the subjects or participants of the project, the research methods (e.g. description of genotyping techniques, assessment scales, statistical tests), and the protocol of the project in sufficient detail to make the reader understand who (of the team members) is going to do what (project activity) at any given point.
	Pay special attention to providing references for the instruments to be used in the project, to reassure the donor that the methodology is robust and scientifically sound.
◆ Results and outcomes	Project outcomes and results should be very straightforward and clearly stated, and correspond to the hypothesis and aims of the project. Also, clear identification of the target population is necessary (who will benefit from the project and to whom are the project results directed?).
◆ Evaluation	This implies the description of internal and external methods of evaluating project performance throughout its duration (e.g. the congruence of the project proposal with the practical performance at any given time; the evaluation of the project outcome and results; the evaluation of the level of participants' involvement). Internal evaluation may include personal evaluation of the team leader(s) by other team members, evaluation questionnaires, and meeting of the project participants; while external evaluation is conducted by independent specialized organizations. A careful evaluation of obstacles and unexpected situations is advised. Also, it is advisable to identify methods to counteract such obstacles and to develop a back-up plan for unexpected situations.

(continued)

Table 10.4 (continued) Usual documentation for a fundraising call

◆ Budget (summary and/ or detailed)	A well-defined financial plan is of great importance. The calculation of the costs should be transferred into a carefully developed financial plan. A realistic approach to the calculation of costs is strongly advised. Overestimation of costs (as in 'ask for more to get less') or underestimation of costs may both send a message that financial aspects have not been carefully enough considered. Preliminary applications may need only limited detail, whereas a full application will require all financial details.
◆ Manpower	The description of the team of collaborators should give enough information on the manpower of the project, the leadership and organizational structure of the project team, the involvement of the new learners, and of communication among the team members. The curricula vitae of the team members should serve as complementary proof (e.g. in addition to the usual CV format, there should be details of professional experience in the area of the project, leadership skills, networking, management skills, past projects successfully fulfilled by the team of collaborators).
◆ Dissemination of results	Dissemination of the results is frequently overlooked by the applicants; however, this is of great importance to the reviewers and especially to the potential funders of the project. A well-defined dissemination plan includes project promotion from the very beginning. Usual dissemination media include both professional/scientific media and general media (e.g. popular websites). It is advisable to include cost-effective dissemination strategies.
◆ Ethical issues	Ethical aspects of the proposal and of the research should always be included in the proposal. In large application calls, there are usually standardized documents detailing all the ethical issues that have to be mentioned.
◆ Future plans/ sustainability/ applicability	A future plan relies on the products and outcomes of the project and on the benefits for the participants and for the target groups. A description of the potential benefits for the applicant (e.g. field specialization, finished PhD), applicant organization (e.g. acquisition of a new treatment method, organization of a new service), and wider scientific and general community (e.g. international publication, future international collaboration) is strongly advisable. Strategies that will ensure the impact and the sustainability of the project outcomes and results, after the project is finished (or the funding period is over), should be defined and outlined in the proposal.
◆ Appendix	If needed or explicitly required. It may include administrative details, graphs, diagrams, organigrams, Gant charts, etc.

It is self-evident that projects with a higher probability of success have better chances of being funded. Thus, every strategy that could increase the applicability of the project should be mentioned (e.g. use of interdisciplinary approach, specific technological advancements, good dissemination plan).

Finally, formal accuracy is always welcomed by project reviewers, so it would be wise to double-check that all necessary documents are submitted and written in a clear

Table 10.5 Linguistic style of a project/fundraising proposal

- ◆ Always prioritize conceptual clarity and a concise and consistent style: sentences should be short, clear, and grammatically correct.
- ◆ Jargon and non-standard abbreviations should be avoided.
- ◆ It is advisable to adapt the language style to the profile of the reviewers: use medical and scientific language in scientific project proposals; avoid too specialized and medical language for educational projects.
- ◆ Numbered lists, bullet points, and other such features may help to organize the text.
- ◆ Graphs and tables may be good visual tools where appropriate (e.g. to summarize your previous work, a previous hypothesis or idea, work plan).
- ◆ Adapting old proposals or collapsing different projects into a new one should be avoided to prevent the risk of fragmentation.
- ◆ The project should be understandable to a layperson (one could ask a colleague or friend who has not been involved in the project to read the proposal before submission).

and concise style, without typographical errors. Sometimes, it might particularly be advisable to adapt the style of writing according to the project reviewers/readers who will decide upon the allocation of funds. For example, when asking for funding from donors pertaining to some specific interest group outside psychiatry or when applying for official calls for general educational projects, the reviewers may not necessarily be experts in the field of psychiatry; in such cases, the content of the proposal and the writing style should be clear to an 'average layman'. In the case of scientific foundations or large grant applications, the reviewers may more often be experts in the field of the project proposal; for such proposals, the use of medical, technical, and scientific language is not only appropriate but necessary. Also, the style and tone of the proposal is equally as important as the content and should follow at least the general principles shown in Table 10.5.

When asking for money from private donors or companies, or when an institution refers to a specific person as being in charge of the project, it is customary to send, along with the project proposal, an accompanying application letter, the content and structure of which is illustrated in Box 10.1.

Often, trivial errors may jeopardize the obtaining of funds, even if the main idea is worth funding. Box 10.2 summarizes the most common mistakes made when writing a grant application and can be used as a checklist before sending out the fundraising proposal.

Step 5: Get into action

Once the funding proposal has been prepared and after the review process is completed, you will be notified about the outcome of your proposal. If the funding has been granted, the project is on its way to achieving the planned goals. Sometimes, the funders may ask for certain changes to the protocol before agreeing on funding, and the project leader has to judge whether these changes will significantly alter the project and if it is worth making them.

Box 10.1 How to approach a potential donor with a letter

An 'application letter' should always contain:

- The name and address of the recipient
- Date and place
- An introduction of the applicant and a description of the group/organization that the applicant represents (possibly with reference to previous projects successfully performed by the organization)
- A short background note explaining the core of the problem leading to the purpose of the project
- Description of the 'target' group
- Description of the main activities of the project
- Description of the project outcomes, including a well-defined dissemination plan
- Financial plan of the project
- Conclusive remarks
- A kind salutation
- The applicant's signature
- The applicant's contact details

Box 10.2 Common mistakes when applying for funding

- The grant call is too competitive for the career stage of the applicant and the project plan is too ambitious or just not achievable.
- The project idea or the main hypothesis is not clearly defined.
- The background of the project does not outline the 'need' for the project.
- The content of the proposal is written in a language not understandable by the reviewers.
- The team of collaborators does not have a large enough workforce to execute the planned activities.
- The financial plan and requirements are not adequately addressed and/or explained.
- There are no plans for the dissemination of results.
- International or interdisciplinary collaboration is not stressed enough.
- There is no evidence of similar projects/research on the applicants' and collaborators' curricula vitae (CV).

Box 10.3 A start-up meeting is needed to . . .

◆ Introduce all team members to each other

◆ Set the basis for good communication and collaboration among all members

◆ Reiterate the aims and activities of the project (and eventually plan the needed changes)

◆ Review the anticipated main outcome and secondary results of the project

◆ Establish tasks and individual responsibility for the tasks

◆ Make sure that all members are aware of their specific tasks

◆ Define a plan which everybody agrees on (in case of unplanned hurdles)

◆ Plan promotional activities

◆ Agree on further action points (usually circulated within the minutes of the meeting)

Once the funds have been received, an initial or 'start-up' meeting with co-workers is necessary before actually commencing a project or an activity, in order to co-ordinate all the necessary group work and ensure the most efficient allocation of tasks (see Box 10.3).

While the project is ongoing, it is advisable to evaluate regularly both the performance of project tasks and the finances. It is necessary to stick to the project proposal plan and act whenever the tasks are not fulfilled as planned, reporting this to the funder.

While it is correct to assume that the funder is interested in the results, one should not disregard other aspects that may be important for the specific funder (e.g. keeping track of administration, other contractual obligations with the funder such as the use of their logo in all promotional activities).

Step 6: Keep track of the project administration and verify the outcomes

Although probably the most annoying aspect of any research or educational project, keeping records of project progress is a very important task. For governmental or large funded programmes, a substantial amount of administrative information will be required by the funding organization and stated in the official calls and the contracts. However, even the donations received from non-governmental organizations or official calls should be carefully administrated, as the records serve as proof of the activities performed. Minutes of any meeting should be prepared and approved by all team members, as they will help the project to progress to the agreed plan. Further documents which may be useful as administrative records of fund management may include personal testimony (possibly in a written form), participation records (e.g. attendance forms), public information (available, for example, through leaflets, the internet, newspapers, journals), or scientific publications related to the project.

Besides the eventual specific requirements of the donor, feedback is an essential part of a project in itself; it allows the project leader or any team member to verify that all procedures have been run correctly, that the quality of the results is acceptable, and that the funds are being spent in a correct way.

Follow-up meetings should be scheduled in advance and minutes from such meetings should be prepared. If negative outcomes are reported, it is a responsibility of the project leader to verify the achievability of the objectives and the correct use of means, as well as to change the objectives and instruments if necessary.

Conclusions

To raise funds for clinical and/or research activities is one of the most challenging tasks for early-career psychiatrists nowadays, but it represents also a strongly encouraged activity for those who want to make a real impact in their community. Furthermore, in times of economic crisis and consequent shortage of funds for such activities, there is greater competition for these funds and fundraising becomes a necessary skill for most early-career psychiatrists.

As pointed out in this chapter, it is also true that many funding opportunities are simply not known or properly explored by early-career psychiatrists. Increasing the chances of obtaining funding may be achieved just by widening the search of the funding market. Learning how to search and find funding opportunities is also a matter of experience: we have tried, within this chapter, to define a practical approach to fundraising, to provide the most useful hints, and to advise about the most common mistakes. However, writing successful grant applications or even smaller fund requests from private donors is an ability that grows with experience. Probably the best way to learn how to write funding proposals, is to do it—even if making errors in the beginning. Within this field, we learn much by seeking and blundering, and often do not appreciate good advice. The successful applicant will profit from his mistakes and try again, in a different way, since the only way to really fail to learn is probably by not learning from the failures.

Finally, the reader should bear in mind that most of the fundraising applications are aimed at promoting local or large activities with a clear humanitarian scope that is intended to positively affect the community. Thus, the best reason to try fundraising within the mental health field is the one long advised by the Greek philosopher Plato: 'good actions give strength to ourselves and inspire good actions in others'.

References

1 **Tempel ER, Seiler TL, Aldrich EE**. *Achieving excellence in fundraising*. Hoboken (USA): Wiley; 2011.
2 **Rosso HA, Tempel ER**. *Achieving excellence in fundraising*. London: Josey Bass/Wiley; 2003.
3 **Radder H**. *The commodification of academic research*. Pittsburgh: University of Pittsburgh Press; 2010.
4 Royal College of Psychiatrists (RCPsych). *Role of the consultant psychiatrist. Occasional paper 74*. London: RCPsych; 2010.
5 **Burke JD Jr, Pincus HA, Pardes H**. The clinician-researcher in psychiatry. *Am J Psychiatry* 1986; **143**(8):968–75.

6 **Honer WG, Linseman MA**. The physician-scientist in Canadian psychiatry. *J Psychiatry Neurosci* 2004; **29**(1):49–56.

7 UEMS (Union Européenne des Médecins Spécialistes) Section for Psychiatry. Charter on training of medical specialists in the EU: requirements for the specialty of psychiatry. *Eur Arch Psychiatry Clin Neurosci* 1997; **247**(Suppl 6):S45–457. (Revised 2003; available at: http://uemspsychiatry.org/wp-content/uploads/2013/09/Chapter6–11.10.03.pdf)

8 **Kuzman MR, Giacco D, Simmons M, et al**. Psychiatry training in Europe: views from the trenches. *Med Teach* 2012; **34**(10):e708–7017.

9 **Fiorillo A, Malik A, Luciano M, et al**. Challenges for trainees in psychiatry and early career psychiatrists. *Int Rev Psychiatry* 2013; **25**(4):431–7.

10 **McClintoch N**. *Understanding Canadian donors. National Survey of Giving, Volunteering and Participating (NSGVP)*. Canadian Centre for Philanthropy; 2004.

11 The Association of Fundraising Professionals (AFP). *AFP code of ethical principles and standards*. Adopted 1964; amended September 2007. Available at: http://www.afpnet.org/files/ContentDocuments/CodeOfEthicsLong.pdf.

Chapter 11

Medical mobility: how to gain further skills

Maria Orlova, Marisa Casanova Dias, Domenico Giacco, and Marc H.M. Hermans

Case study

John was browsing emails when his attention was caught by a message from his national association, inviting applications for an exchange programme to several European countries. He looked through the offerings, chose two programmes and applied. In a couple of weeks John received two invitations and accepted the offer from the eating disorders programme, which was an area he had a special interest in. He successfully negotiated the process of attaining study leave with his supervisor and got in touch with the future host. As accommodation was not provided, he arranged to stay with friends he had in the city.

After arriving, he was introduced to the staff and made a presentation about best practices in his home institution. Together with his supervisor they planned the activities for the following weeks. These varied from taking part in the ward rounds and community based clinics to engaging with the trainees in the eating disorders unit and in their teaching programme. He was also invited to take part in the teaching of medical students where he presented a lecture on anxiety disorders, their diagnosis and treatment. The supervisor offered him the opportunity to write a paper on different aspects of John's scientific interest. In addition to the observership placement, he had the opportunity to attend a conference on eating disorders.

As he returned to his daily practice, he felt refreshed, full of enthusiasm and shared his experience with his colleagues. The exchange created a new understanding of psychiatry in his home country. And his knowledge and skills on the topic of eating disorders improved. John is continuing his training and currently hosting an exchange trainee from Portugal. He aims to subspecialise in eating disorders.

Source data from: EFPT Exchange Programme, http://www.efpt.eu/page.php/exchange, reproduced under the Creative Commons Attribution License (4.0)

Introduction

'Medical mobility' is defined as the ability of doctors to move to a different country for professional reasons. Over the past few decades, mobility of citizens in general has increased due to improvements in transport, the economy, and the changing political landscape.

Enlargement of the European Union (EU) created more possibilities for travelling and working in different countries within Europe. As a legal framework for professional mobility, the European Parliament and the European Council adopted Directive 2005/36/EC on the recognition of professional qualifications, which affects hundreds of professions regulated by member states across the EU, including medical doctors, nurses, midwives, and dentists.[1] According to this directive, 'Freedom of movement and the mutual recognition of the evidence of formal qualifications of doctors . . . should be based on the fundamental principle of automatic recognition of the evidence of formal qualifications on the basis of coordinated minimum conditions for training'.[2]

Learning mobility (transnational mobility for the purpose of acquiring new knowledge, skills, and competences) is seen by the EU as 'one of the fundamental ways in which young people can strengthen their future employability, as well as their intercultural awareness, personal development, creativity and active citizenship'.[3]

Outside Europe, there is not yet a legal framework for the recognition of professional qualifications (e.g. a doctor from UK wishing to work in Brazil), but many regions are moving in that direction. The Association of South East Asian Nations (ASEAN) Economic Community (AEC) will be implemented in 2015, and Latin America is taking the first steps towards harmonisation of medical training. In addition, bilateral agreements exist between some countries for the purpose of recognizing professional qualifications and facilitating the movement of medical doctors.

Increased mobility of patients and doctors is changing clinical practice. This emphasizes the need for cultural awareness and cultural competence of medical professionals. Culture shapes the clinical presentation of mental disorders as well as interactions between doctor and patient within mental health services.[4] Doctors now need different skills than the ones traditionally taught at undergraduate and postgraduate level (Fig. 11.1).

At an undergraduate level, elective rotations abroad are very attractive. Participating in an international rotation is reported to 'provide educational benefits in knowledge (e.g., tropical diseases, cross-cultural issues, public health, alternative concepts of health and disease, and health care delivery), enhanced skills (e.g., problem solving, clinical examination, laboratory expertise, and language), and fostering attitudes and values (e.g., idealism, community service, humanism, and interest in serving underserved populations)'.[5] The World Federation for Medical Education (WFME) has recently recognized electives organized by the International Federation of Medical

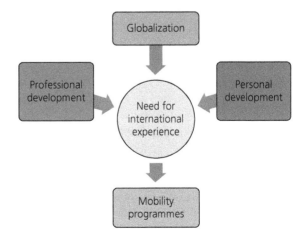

Fig. 11.1 Need for international experience.

Table 11.1 Types of medical mobility

Length
Short-term: 1–3 months
Medium-term: from 3 months up to 1 year
Long-term: more than 1 year

Modality
Observership
Clinical placement
Research placement

Students' Associations (IFMSA) since 1951. In its global standards for postgraduate medical education,[6] the WFME states that there must be a policy on accessibility of individualized training opportunities at other sites within or outside the country and for the transfer of training credits, and the exchange of academic staff and trainees should be facilitated by the provision of appropriate resources and mutual recognition of training elements. However currently, at postgraduate level, being able to spend time abroad is still mainly dependent on bilateral agreements.

In psychiatry, the European Federation of Psychiatric Trainees (EFPT) has been organizing an exchange programme for psychiatric trainees since 2011.[7] In 2014, the European Psychiatric Association launched the 'Gaining Experience Programme' for early-career psychiatrists (up to five years after completion of specialist training).

Medical mobility can take several forms (Table 11.1). Migration can be considered a form of mobility, with a permanent or semi-permanent character, but we will not cover it in this chapter. Instead, we will focus on temporary, short-, or medium-term medical mobility, as that is the modality most relevant for early-career psychiatrists (ECPs) as a means of gaining further skills to improve clinical practice.

In the following sections, we will take a practical approach to guide readers who want to gain additional skills abroad. We will cover the benefits and challenges of mobility programmes and illustrate this with real-life examples of trainees who participated in short-term mobility programmes for psychiatric trainees—the EFPT exchange programme.[8]

The reasons for taking part in a mobility programme

A review of the literature[9] identified several areas most frequently reported to benefit from medical mobility:

a) *Professional development*: 'increased cultural competence, deeper understanding of professional practice issues through comparative experience, increased compassion toward patients, increased communication skills, increased appreciation for and/or knowledge of public health, increased appreciation for and confidence in clinical skills, effect on public service career orientation, and increased awareness of resource use'.

b) *Personal development*: 'value of experiential learning, increased sense of independence and confidence, general personal growth, development of a broadened perspective on patient care and cross-cultural communication'.

c) *Advantages for medical institutions*: 'increased attractiveness for students, the overall value of an international program, development of new curricular materials' and, for the host society, gains such as the creation of libraries in one case and developing evidence-based medical educational seminars in another.

Mobility programmes can have an impact at several levels, both directly and indirectly. The most obvious benefit of going abroad is to learn about a specific area of psychiatry and to explore similarities and differences in the manifestations of psychiatric disorders and their treatments. It makes it possible to enhance existing skills and to gain new skills in areas which are not available, or only scarcely available, in one's home institution or country, including subspecialties (for instance, child and adolescent psychiatry, forensics, old age psychiatry) and particular domains of expertise (for instance, eating disorders, programmes for homeless people, day hospital care, electroconvulsive therapy, or psychotherapy). Another benefit is to be temporarily involved in a different healthcare organizational model (Box 11.1).

At the same time, exploring a foreign training scheme gives the possibility to experience psychiatric training programmes that differ in duration, quality assurance systems, curricula, competencies, didactic structure, level of supervision, and methods of evaluation.[10] Evidence shows similarities and differences among training schemes throughout Europe, despite efforts for uniformity.[11]

Another area which can be developed through a temporary foreign placement is that of cultural sensitivity (Box 11.2).

While experiencing a different treatment model or a different tradition of psychiatric care, one is not only learning but also critically reflecting and comparing. It brings new perspectives to routine practice (Box 11.3).

Box 11.1 Feedback from a trainee

'... there is a difference in the organisation of care. There is a private and a public system; the public system works strictly with "catchment areas". In these areas the consultant psychiatrist is responsible for all patients, be it out-patient clinics or patients admitted under the mental health act. This provides patients with continuity of care; their consultant is responsible for their care at home as well as in the clinic. I feel that specialized supraregional facilities sometimes suffer from the strict financial boundaries of the catchment areas, but in general, patients are better taken care of and followed through the various stages of their illness, by the same healthcare providers. I considered this as a great strength of the system.'

Source data from: EFPT Exchange Programme, http://www.efpt.eu/page.php/exchange, reproduced under the Creative Commons Attribution License (4.0)

Box 11.2 Feedback from a trainee

'The biggest difference I noticed is the more paternalistic approach . . . I also noticed that the workers use less physical distance [between the doctor and the patient] than in my country.'

Source data from: EFPT Exchange Programme, http://www.efpt.eu/page.php/exchange, reproduced under the Creative Commons Attribution License (4.0)

Box 11.3 Feedback from a trainee

'The approach of the patient has a strong non-medicalising aspect, with less focus on "danger" and giving the disease as a concept a much smaller place in relation to the life of that person. I will probably try to experiment with using less quickly the diagnosis in my communication but to use more the perspective of that person's life.'

Source data from: EFPT Exchange Programme, http://www.efpt.eu/page.php/exchange, reproduced under the Creative Commons Attribution License (4.0)

Box 11.4 Adapted from a trainee's feedback

Peter wanted to subspecialize in child and adolescent psychiatry. However, competition is very high in London and, unfortunately, he did not succeed in obtaining a higher training post. Then he decided to apply for the EFPT Exchange Programme, and he spent two weeks in a child and adolescent department in Denmark. He thoroughly enjoyed the experience, which made him sure that it was what he wanted for his career, and he applied again for a training post in child and adolescent psychiatry. When he attended the selection interview, he was very surprised at how interested the panel were in his exchange experience and spent the majority of the interview discussing it. In the end, he was offered a training job in his area of interest. Peter is soon due to become a consultant child and adolescent psychiatrist.

Another advantage of mobility programmes is the possibility to continue communication with colleagues met, through future joint projects based on common clinical, research, or academic interests. Online collaboration is now feasible and effective. Finally, a few lines on a curriculum vitae outlining international experience make it more attractive when applying for jobs (Box 11.4).

Challenges of medical mobility: funding, time off, and accreditation

The most obvious but manageable challenge is to find funding for a mobility stay. There are usually local, national, or international grants you can apply for. However, it is better to be prepared for the fact that no grants may be available. Most expenses will go on travelling and accommodation. Since the latter requires the biggest budget, it is wise to explore, in advance, the possibility of free accommodation (for example, in the hospital) or some that is as cheap as possible (for example, in a student dormitory). Your local co-ordinator might suggest an affordable hostel. Perhaps you can arrange your exchange visit in a city where you have friends to stay with, or choose a time when flight tickets are available at a lower rate. The internet makes these arrangements quite easy.

The most frequently reported barrier for trainees, however, is finding the time off from work and family responsibilities. If one's training scheme does not allow for taking time abroad, the trainee has to organize it to fit in with the training requirements and work responsibilities, which will limit the flexibility. The timing and the length of the mobility programme can be negotiated with supervisors both at home and in the host institution. For short periods of time, using annual leave allowance, study leave, or unpaid leave might be the best solution.

In undergraduate training, accreditation for mobility programmes of 6–12 months' duration is common. The most popular programme in Europe is the Erasmus.[12] However, at postgraduate level, there is no international accreditation system yet. It is left to individual institutions or training programme directors to decide, case by case. If you want your international experience to be counted as part of your training, please check with your supervisor and institution. The possibility of accreditation differs between countries and institutions. In order to maximize the chances of it being counted towards your training, you can discuss with your supervisors in the home and host countries, the possibility of some kind of assessments: for example, you could do a 'Case based Discussion' or give a presentation at a seminar or conference.

Medical mobility in practice

Once you have chosen your programme, applied, and received an invitation, you have finished the application process. However, be prepared for more paperwork since the receiving institution may ask for additional documentation. Usually, you will be informed by local co-ordinators about all the details. So, stay in touch and check your emails regularly.

Following your arrival into the new setting and the introduction to the local staff, these colleagues might expect you to present on best practices in the home setting—the so-called 'exchange in action'. According to one's preferences, slides or video may be used.

If your mobility programme is an observership, you will shadow a clinician. You will not evaluate patients nor issue prescriptions, but you will observe the day-to-day practice of your colleagues. You will see how psychiatrists and other professionals provide care to patients in a different clinical setting. Through observing, you will see what the usual working day looks like and what the responsibilities are of a given doctor within a given healthcare setting (Box 11.5). Depending on the setting, you will be attending morning meetings, case discussions, ward rounds, and journal clubs, or you may be involved in teaching or research activities. Do contact your hosts in advance to clarify

Box 11.5 Feedback from a trainee

'From the outset, I was made to feel a part of the team; observing clinicians on the ward and in the outpatient clinic, shadowing those on call in the assessment unit and contributing to diagnostic and treatment discussions'

Source data from: EFPT Exchange Programme, http://www.efpt.eu/page.php/exchange, reproduced under the Creative Commons Attribution License (4.0)

Box 11.6 Feedback from a trainee

'The team was open to my visit, collaborative and interested in my opinions and experience. During the weeks I built a good relationship with my fellow interns that allowed us to extensive reflections on professional and personal issues.'

Source data from: EFPT Exchange Programme, http://www.efpt.eu/page.php/exchange, reproduced under the Creative Commons Attribution License (4.0)

these possibilities! Be engaged during your stay, participate actively by paying close attention, ask questions, and take notes.

It may be recommended to keep a journal[13] in which you can record the amount of time spent in different clinical settings and leave notes regarding perceptions, reflections, new ideas, and gaps in knowledge that you would like to fill. Wearing a name badge mentioning your observership status will probably facilitate communication with doctors and patients (Box 11.6).

How to prepare

For a successful observership, it is necessary to be well prepared. The first and most important factor for success is language proficiency. The better your knowledge of the local language, the more you will benefit from the experience. There will be some differences in the level of language proficiency needed depending on the clinical setting. If you are going to observe activities in the electroconvulsive therapy (ECT) department or another instrumental and laboratory setting, you have to be confident in your ability to understand and to ask questions. However, if you are attending a psychotherapeutic setting, it is essential to communicate fluently in the host language. Not being proficient in the local language should not prevent you from gaining experience but, to get the most from your observership, choose a setting where you will feel comfortable with your level of knowledge of the language. Usually, you can expect local trainees and staff to communicate with you in English. If you are not proficient enough in the local language, you may choose to stay for a shorter period, just to 'experience the spirit' of that setting and healthcare system (Box 11.7).

Box 11.7 Feedback from a trainee

'During meetings, those present would attempt to speak in English, but during lapses my neighbour would often translate. When seeing a patient with another doctor, they would discuss the case with me both before and after; when the patient felt comfortable, assessments were carried out in English but even when this was not possible, I discovered the opportunity to test my powers of observation of non-verbal communication'.

Source data from: EFPT Exchange Programme, http://www.efpt.eu/page.php/exchange, reproduced under the Creative Commons Attribution License (4.0)

Box 11.8 Feedback from a trainee

'The presentation I gave about my own training and the mental health care system in which I work allowed me to take a step back and think about these aspects from a wider perspective. From the questions and feedback I received, it was a real pleasure to be able to give this talk'.

Source data from: EFPT Exchange Programme, http://www.efpt.eu/page.php/exchange, reproduced under the Creative Commons Attribution License (4.0)

Settings of interest could be those not available in your training scheme, or possible or attractive avenues for your future career. Leisure and social activities are usually not part of the exchange programme. Your hosts might be able to spend some time with you, but expect you to be able to take care of yourself. Ask your co-ordinator about this in advance and consult about suggestions for leisure time. It may sound obvious, but sometimes trainees mark, as a disadvantage, that there were not enough social activities provided by the host. Preparing for your stay by reading about the country's culture and its traditions will probably make you feel more comfortable while visiting.

Do not forget to prepare your own contribution. Whether your hosts will ask you to present or not, it will be appreciated if you have information to share (Box 11.8).

What is next?

When you are back at your ordinary workplace, you will usually (although this varies between programmes) be expected to make a presentation about your experience. Make it your moment of glory! It is time to offer your feedback and to discuss your reflections. You can share what you have learned, compare treatment settings, and illustrate best practices. You can cover cultural differences and describe the patient–clinician model as you have experienced it in the host country. You will be in a good position to comment from a different angle on current local practices, and you can encourage and suggest colleagues to gain such an experience.

> ## Box 11.9 10 steps for a successful international experience
>
> 1 Assess opportunities for mobility.
> 2 Choose the institution for your placement and gather information about it.
> 3 Prepare the documents for the application in advance.
> 4 Make arrangements with your supervisor for the leave period.
> 5 Apply and check your emails regularly until you receive the confirmation.
> 6 Be prepared for a considerable amount of paperwork as a part of your acceptance process.
> 7 Be open to share information and good practices from your country/home institution.
> 8 Use the exchange period to build enduring links with new colleagues, juniors, and seniors.
> 9 When you are back, report to your colleagues and provide feedback to host institutions and exchange programme providers.
> 10 Maintain your links and use them to shape your career.

It is likely that you will be asked to fill out feedback forms about organizational aspects of a programme. In most cases, you will receive a certificate or another document stating that you have completed an exchange programme.

The ways you will continue your new friendships and collaborations may vary. You may keep in touch by email or social networks. You may invite your new friends/colleagues to your workplace to give a presentation or to an exchange programme in your institution, or you may start a joint research project or write a paper together.

Consider the opportunity to contribute, yourself, to exchange activities in your local setting: you know from your personal experience how important this is. Consider giving support to the newcomer; this may be language support, accommodation support, or even organizing social activities.

Finally, do not forget that despite the fact that your international experience has finished, you are only at the beginning of your professional career, with more opportunities to come! In Box 11.9 some tips for your successful international experience are reported.

Conclusions

In the current globalized world, medical mobility provides opportunities to gain international experience and to enhance psychiatric skills. Be aware that challenges are manageable and the experience is unique. Consider this way of learning, since it is not only beneficial for yourself as a professional and as a person, but also for other parties, such as the receiving and home institution.

References

1 **Costigliola V.** Mobility of medical doctors in cross-border healthcare. *EPMA J* 2011; **2**:333–9.

2 Directive 2005/36/EC of the European Parliament and of the Council of 7 September 2005, on the recognition of professional qualifications, March 2011. Available at: http://eur-lex. europa.eu/LexUriServ/LexUriServ.do?uri=OJ:L:2005:255:0022:0142:en:PDF

3 EUR-Lex (Access to European Union Law). Council Recommendation of 28 June 2011—'Youth on the move'—promoting the learning mobility of young people. (2011/C 199/01). Available at: http://eur-lex.europa.eu/legal-content/EN/NOT/?uri=CELEX:320 11H0707(01).

4 **Kirmayer LJ.** Rethinking cultural competence. *Transcult Psychiatry* 2012; **49**:149–64.

5 **Thompson MJ, Huntington MK, Hunt DD, Pinsky LE, Brodie JJ.** Educational effects of international health electives on U.S. and Canadian medical students and residents: a literature review. *Acad Med* 2003; **78**:342–7.

6 World Federation for Medical Education (WFME). WFME global standards for quality improvement in postgraduate medical education (PGME). Available at: http://www.wfme.org/ standards/pgme.

7 **Casanova Dias M, Orlova M, Pinto da Costa M.** Training abroad? Not so difficult. *Lancet Glob Health* 2013; **1**:e136.

8 EFPT exchange programme website: http://www.efpt.eu/page.php/exchange

9 **Mutchnick IS, Moyer CA, Stern DT.** Expanding the boundaries of medical education: evidence for cross-cultural exchanges. *Acad Med* 2003; **78**:S1–5.

10 **Zisook S, Balon R, Björkstén KS, et al.** Psychiatry residency training around the world. *Acad Psychiatry* 2007; **31**:309–25.

11 **Kuzman MR, Giacco D, Simmons M, et al.** Psychiatry training in Europe: views from the trenches. *Med Teach* 2012; **34**:e708–17.

12 Erasmus programme website: http://www.erasmusprogramme.com

13 **Dye D.** Enhancing critical reflection of students during a clinical internship using the self-S.O.A.P. *Internet J Allied Health Sci Prac* 2005; **3**.

Chapter 12

Building an academic career in psychiatry

Florian Riese, Maja Pantovic Stefanovic, Andrea Fiorillo, Allan Tasman, and Norman Sartorius

Introduction

An academic career can be one of the most appealing professional pathways for early career psychiatrists (ECPs). You might become the first person on this planet who has understood a certain biological mechanism or else, you might become a world-renowned expert for a psychiatric disease. This chapter is intended as a practical guide for ECPs who wish to pursue that difficult path and contribute to our field by high-quality research and teaching—often alongside an equally successful clinical career. However, such a career is not easy to achieve: even if you and your environment combine all the elements to build an academic career, you may not be successful. Being in the right place at the right time can often be the missing ingredient for advancement in an academic career. This chapter therefore mainly aims to encourage you to seize your opportunities. The future of psychiatric care depends on whether the brightest and most motivated ECPs continue to enter an academic career—which cannot be taken for granted.[1] Throughout this chapter, we will highlight the most important factors and pitfalls in building such a career. You will find case examples and 'quick tips', that we believe offer useful advice. We do so on the basis of the literature and mainly from our personal experiences at different stages of our own academic careers.

The first steps into academia: seize your opportunities

Case study 1: Maria is currently on a six months' rotation in a substance abuse outpatient clinic. She has not participated in any research so far, but she would love to do so. The consultant psychiatrist who runs the service invites Maria to contribute to the writing of a protocol for a small non-pharmacological intervention study to improve sleep in opioid addiction. Maria declines since the project does not match her primary interest in psychiatry, which is psychosis.

The very first steps into academic psychiatry can be highly diverse. Many ECPs enter academia through formalized PhD programmes that are offered in major teaching hospitals and associated universities around the world. In some places, dedicated research or leadership tracks during residency training facilitate academic careers.[2] Especially in the USA, significant efforts have been made to teach psychiatric residents the basics of research methodology and thus create a better foundation for entering academic medicine.[3] Beyond such facilitated entry points, the opportunity to start academic activities may sometimes present itself unexpectedly. Especially in the beginning of your academic career, we advise you to seize such opportunities. Even if a proposed research project does not completely match your personal interests (as in Case 1), it can be extremely valuable for learning research skills, finding a mentor, and building a network. Over time, you will develop your own academic profile and can become independent.

If you do not have any research opportunity, try to create your own ones. Often, senior academics are extremely welcoming towards enthusiastic younger colleagues: you may well be the only ECP in your hospital who is seriously interested in an academic career. Most established researchers have unanalysed data that they are happy to make available on the basis of scientific co-operation and shared authorship. Analysing such datasets can lead to high-impact publications without the need to collect your own data in a time-consuming process.[4] Another way to start your academic career is to engage in trainee-led research activities. In Europe, there are several successful examples, including those supported by the European Psychiatric Association (EPA), the European Federation of Psychiatric Trainees (EFPT), and the World Psychiatric Association (WPA).[5–8] Finally, contributing to your field through academic activities other than research may also set you on the path to an academic career.

Academia is much more than research

Research is an important building block for most academic careers—but it is clearly not the only one (see Table 12.1). Many academicians, even some well-known leaders, gained their prominent positions primarily through academic activities other than

Table 12.1 Academic activities beyond research

Academic activity	Example
Publication of clinical or educational texts	This book chapter
Technology transfer	Implementation of a new clinical method or electronic tool
Improvement of clinical practice	Development of evidence-based treatment algorithms or clinical pathways
Teaching	Courses for medical students; bedside teaching of residents
Scholarly presentations	Grand rounds; invited lectures in other institutions
Policy development	Contribution to local or national guidelines
Contribution to conferences	Organization of workshops
Participation in relevant boards and committees	Institutional review board; national committee on postgraduate psychiatric education
Consulting	Contributing to planning of new psychiatric outpatient clinic; advising the regional government on resource allocation in mental health

research. We emphasize this point because we would like to encourage you to follow your interest in an academic career—even if you are working in an environment with limited research opportunities or you lack the desire to do research. Even in the leading academic medical centres around the world, only very few scholars lead research. Instead, most (if not all) perform other academic activities on the basis of their clinical work assignments, or have leadership responsibilities for either clinical or educational programmes (see Case 2; see also the section 'Becoming a leader in the field').

Case study 2: During her postgraduate psychiatric training, Emilia became more and more interested in personality disorders, especially in the treatment of borderline personality disorder. In order to be able to help her patients better, Emilia attended a course on dialectical behavioural therapy (DBT) in a different city. After becoming a consultant, she managed to convince the head of the psychiatric department to create a specialized DBT service, which until then had not been available. In the following years, Emilia acquired extensive clinical expertise in DBT and also went to several international courses and conferences on the topic. Over time, she found herself to be a respected expert on DBT: psychiatrists from other hospitals often consulted with her and she participated in an effort to develop national clinical practice guidelines for treatment of personality disorders. She inspired several younger colleagues to focus their careers on DBT and other forms of psychotherapy. A few years later, Emilia was asked to participate in an international multicentre study on DBT, which was later published in an international medical journal.

As illustrated by Case 2, not all successful academic careers require research, but all do require participation in academic activities. Depending on the stage of your career and which academic career track you are following (research, education, clinical), career advancement will require varying amounts of the different 'academic ingredients'. If you are aiming for a tenure-track professorship in psychiatric genetics, your research output will be critical, maybe even the only measure of your academic success. If you are pursuing an academic career in psychiatric education, it may be more important to contribute to a new curriculum for medical students or to publish a textbook. We advise research-oriented academicians to become competent in other areas of academic activity. Similarly, clinicians and medical educators may considerably enhance their profile by seizing the opportunity for participation in research. Like other competencies, academic competencies are acquired through observation (e.g. seeing how a senior colleague delivers a lecture), training (e.g. attending courses on medical education), and practice (e.g. delivering lectures and scholarly presentations yourself).

Making yourself essential: mastering a crucial technique

Case study 3: Senol is a late-stage trainee in psychiatry and has collaborated on several research projects that use magnetic resonance (MR) spectroscopy in neuropsychiatric disorders. Over the course of these projects, he has learned to perform MR scans and to use the MR data processing software. He has also acquired a good knowledge of the necessary statistical analyses. The postdoctoral fellow from the neuroradiology department who taught him these skills has moved on to an assistant professorship in another city. Senol is now the most experienced researcher in MR spectroscopy in the hospital and is therefore asked to participate in a new study on brain tumour metabolism.

The initial phase of an academic career is usually a period of intensive learning and offers the greatest opportunity to acquire highly specialized technical knowledge and skills. As in Case 3, such knowledge and skills can make you essential for the realization of a whole set of research projects which may even extend beyond your own department. In this way, you may produce a disproportionately high number of publications in a limited time.

> **Quick tip 1: Develop your technical knowledge and skills!** Then, let others know that you have this expertise.

> **Words of wisdom:** An investment in knowledge pays the best interest. (Benjamin Franklin)

Examples of methodological skills that are currently extremely valuable in psychiatry research are analysis of imaging data, behavioural testing in animals, and statistical analyses of longitudinal data. A lack of technical skills can, on the other hand, severely restrict your academic potential.[9] Later in your academic career you will often have to draw from your hands-on technical expertise when you teach and supervise more junior colleagues. In later career stages, skills like leading a team, initiating academic collaborations, and acquiring research funding will also become more important.

Mastering a specific clinical skill (e.g. skills in the application of standardized methods of assessment) can also be the foundation of a non-research academic career (see Case 2). Alternatively, clinical psychiatric skills such as mental status assessment or delivering psychotherapy may become research skills in the context of clinical trials. This is of particular interest since, in clinical trials, psychiatrists cannot be replaced with researchers from other professions, such as biologists or psychologists.

> **Quick tip 2: Be sure about your goals!** Identify what you want to achieve in your academic career and what you need to get there. An academic career is more like a marathon than a sprint: from your first steps in academia to becoming a postdoctoral fellow, assistant professor, associate professor, and full professor, you will be journeying for a long time. It will help you to keep going if you know what your goals are and what motivates you. Depending on how far you want to go, you will need to plan your career differently.

> **Words of wisdom:** The three great essentials to achieve anything worthwhile are first, hard work; second, stick-to-itiveness; third, common sense. (Thomas Edison)

Factors influencing academic progress

A number of internal and external factors influence an academic career. Internal factors include your ability to generate new, creative ideas; your working habits; the image you have of yourself and of academia; and also your tolerance of frustrating experiences (since progress may be slow, your results may be negative, and your papers may be rejected). Important external factors are the quality of the academic environment, availability of time and money for academic activities, mentorship, and professional networks. Having a social network and a supportive partner will also help a lot. Unfortunately, the key factors in an academic career—ideas, time, and money—seem to behave like the electrons described by Heisenberg's uncertainty principle: you will never be able to pin down all three of them at the same time. Sometimes you will have ideas and money but no time; sometimes, time and money and no ideas; and sometimes, ideas and time but no money. You will need to work with what you have got.

Time

External factors that influence your academic career may include the local clinical and educational system, the available research facilities, and the local academic culture. However, most of these environmental factors boil down to how much support you receive from senior colleagues, especially how much time you can dedicate to academic activities. For certain aspects of academic career development, time can replace other resources. For example, many types of research projects can be performed practically without funding but may require investment of substantial amounts of time (e.g. secondary analysis of existing datasets, survey studies).[7,8,10–12] Time is also required to put together applications for research grants, so that your time and creativity may convert to money later on.

Since time is such a precious asset, you should become an expert in managing it. If you find it difficult to balance clinical and academic activities, you are not alone—almost everybody has to undergo that struggle.[13] Research time competes with your other important aims (e.g. gaining clinical expertise or spending time with friends and family) and your institution (e.g. taking care of more patients or backing up senior colleagues so that they can perform academic activities themselves). Hence, if you are interested in an academic career, you should ideally be working in an institution that can offer you the necessary freedom from other duties. On the other hand, engaging in academic activities is particularly challenging for ECPs who work outside the major university centres. International mentorship programmes or collaborative initiatives between university centres and peripheral psychiatric teaching institutions may help to reduce that bias.

Money

A second obstacle for building an academic career is lack of funding, particularly research funding. Research is expensive and it will likely become even more expensive in the future, since most insights from small, low-budget projects have already been made. Most low-hanging fruits have been harvested. Not only is money required to free your own time from other duties such as the regular clinical workloads, but in many kinds of research, money is needed also for equipment, consumables, or outsourcing services. Funds allocated to research are most frequently directed to researchers who have already achieved preliminary results in a project or who have a track record of successful research. From the perspective of the funding agencies, this decreases the chances of funding projects that are likely to fail. From the perspective of an ECP, this makes establishing yourself as a researcher very hard, since only by using your own money will you become a fully independent researcher. Therefore, becoming knowledgeable about the available funding opportunities is essential for academic progress.

A number of national science funding agencies, and also some international organizations such as the European Commission, offer grants targeted particularly at young researchers. These grants often aim at 'capacity building' (i.e. allowing junior researchers to acquire critical research skills that make them valuable contributors to their local research environments). Some of these grants also require the junior researcher to spend some time abroad. Do it! Working in different academic environments can greatly improve your scientific network. Still, the first phase of almost all research careers is spent using money that senior colleagues have acquired for their projects.

As we have pointed out before, there are other ways to an academic career than research. Likewise, there is funding for non-research academic activities (e.g. for continuing medical education activities or technology transfer). These funds are often smaller than research grants but tend to be less competitive, so they are often good entry points for a line of work.

> **Quick tip 3: Go to where the money and success are!** Even if an academic project from an established and productive group does not completely match your own interests, it will get you published and within a network. This will make it much easier to acquire your own funding later.

Mentors

Another external factor that can impact on the development of an academic career is the presence of a suitable mentor. High-quality mentoring may not only accelerate the process of academic education but also opens the way into various academic fields for young researchers.[14,15] Mentors may help by guiding career decisions, giving input to your particular research project, facilitating access to funding, and making their own professional network available to you. Ideally, you should look out for a local mentor that can support you throughout everyday academic activities, on a regular basis. In addition, you should try to find a second, international mentor who you can refer to for the wider perspective. Recently, several scientific organizations have established programmes to promote such international mentorship (e.g. the EPA Mentorship Programme and the European College of Neuropsychopharmacology (ECNP) Certificate Programme). Another excellent way to find an international mentor is to participate in scientific conferences. Especially during the social programme of conferences, there is usually an opportunity to meet potential mentors in a more casual way.

Quick tip 4: Find a mentor and network! Start when you are young. Your network is your strength; you will grow together.

Words of wisdom: Coming together is a beginning; keeping together is progress; working together is success. (Henry Ford)

Professional networks

Today, practically all research projects and many other academic activities require intensive collaboration between different sites, different medical specialties, or different professions. Being open to such collaborations and extending your network can greatly advance your career. Building networks requires social skills: some people have them, others have to learn them. They can be learned but this will take time—which will be wisely invested! You will find opportunities to network and build academic collaboration primarily during scientific congresses and meetings. Do not be frustrated by your first international congress though—you will know many more people and have a much better experience during the next one.

The first steps to building your own network may be difficult; later on, it will rapidly grow on its own. An excellent way to speed up this networking process is participation in summer schools and other national or international short-term programmes. There are many examples of such activities—often organized by the major psychiatric associations, but also by local universities or hospitals. Such programmes usually offer educational activities on research and leadership skills,[16] but (equally important) they also let you meet your peers.

Publish or perish

Case study 4: About six months ago, Lisa finished her part of a research project that makes use of a national health insurance database. For the preparation of the publication, she relies on the technical contribution of several other researchers. Lisa has now moved on to a consultant position on a busy psychiatric inpatient ward and has no further time to dedicate to research. Since Lisa previously was the person who motivated the other contributors and co-ordinated their efforts, she is now afraid that the paper will never be published.

If a research project is not published (Case 4), it might as well never have been done, because nobody will know about its results. Not to publish is a waste of resources and can be considered unethical. Therefore, no research project is finished before it has been published. A sufficient number of good-quality publications is also evidence of a researcher's credibility and will open the way to research funding and, later, to academic advancement. Ideally, you should produce a constant stream of publications, some of them in high-impact journals. Keep in mind, however, that advancement in your academic career is not based merely on the number of your publications, but even more so on the impact of your research on the practice of medicine. We therefore encourage you to aim for quality and relevance in your research and work actively towards the dissemination of your results (e.g. through scholarly presentations; see Table 12.1).

Getting published is not easy, especially when you have never done it before. When you prepare for publication, check which journal is most suitable for your manuscript. Also think about the time a journal usually takes before it rejects a paper. You do not want to have your manuscript lying around on an editor's desk for several months before it is rejected without a proper peer review. Refer to the author guidelines for how to shape your manuscript. Most journals have word limits and tell you what figures should look like and which citation style to use. Submit the best manuscript you are capable of producing: if it is sloppily written, who will believe in the quality of your research? Invest time in the covering letter, using it to explain why your research is interesting for the readership of that particular journal and why it will make a citation impact (since editors want their journals to have increased reference in citation indexes). Properly and respectfully address all comments from the reviewers: they are colleagues that donate their time to improving the scientific quality of other people's work. If your manuscript is rejected, do not despair—it frequently happens to Nobel Prize winners as well. Publishing always means exposing yourself and your work to public scrutiny.

> **Quick tip 5: Do not take reviewers' comments as personal!** They are only meant to improve your work.

> **Words of wisdom:** Success is not final, failure is not fatal: it is the courage to continue that counts. (Winston Churchill)

Fear of rejection is considered an important reason that prevents researchers from publishing,[17] and this may be even more pronounced in young researchers who are often insecure and doubtful about their work.[18] Incorporate what you have learned from the peer review and send a better version of the manuscript to another journal. Ultimately, your article will be published if you are persistent enough.

The ethics of an academic career: personal integrity and professionalism

---

Case study 5: Marc is an ECP who is also pursuing a PhD degree in psychiatric epidemiology. His main research project deals with the prevalence of post-traumatic stress disorder (PTSD) in his country. His first paper on the project is currently under review. Now, his boss has been invited by a journal editor to contribute a paper for a special journal issue on PTSD. Marc does not have new data, but his boss tells him to 'use a subset of the old data', 'make some new tables', and 'get the draft of the new article done by next week'. Regarding Marc's concerns about double publication of data, his boss responds: 'We don't know if the first article will be accepted anyway.'

Table 12.2 Examples of scientific misconduct

Scientific misconduct	Description
Fabrication of the data	Publication of fabricated or intentionally misleading research data (e.g. invented data, manipulation/omitting of the data for the purpose of scientific/economic profit)
Plagiarism	Taking credit for research that the scientist has not participated in (e.g. lacking citations, ungrounded co-authorship)
Unethical research	Violations of ethical principles for research using human subjects (e.g. lack of informed consent, motivational bias) or animals (e.g. violation of animals' rights)

Source data from: Principles for good scientific and ethical conduct, http://www.dtu.dk/english/Research/Research-at-DTU/Principles_for_good_scientific_and_ethical_conduct, [retrieved on May 2014]

Since the outcome of a research project is unknown at its beginning, success cannot be guaranteed—failure is a possibility. Personal ambition may then send a researcher down the slippery slope of scientific misconduct, the intentional or negligent violation of the norms of scientific conduct, or unethical behaviour (see Table 12.2 for examples). Even in successful projects such as the one described in Case 5, situations may arise where a researcher's integrity is being tested. Often a sense of urgency creates such situations: grant application deadlines, the approaching end of a clinical trial recruitment period, or the need to beef up your curriculum vitae in order to apply for the next position.

Table 12.3 The principles of good scientific practice

Principle	Description
Scrupulousness	Research is carried out scrupulously and free from expectation of results and pressure to publish
Reliability	Research conduct and data reporting are reliable; knowledge transfer (teaching, lay publications, etc.) is granted
Verifiability	The data are verifiable at all times
Impartiality	Scientific judgement and behaviour are unaffected by other interests (prejudice, personal affections, economic interests, etc.)
Independence	Independent and free scientific judgement and behaviour

Source data from: Barry MJ, Cherkin DC, YuChiao C, Fowler FJ, Skates S. A Randomized Trial of a Multimedia Shared Decision-Making Program for Men Facing a Treatment Decision for Benign Prostatic Hyperplasia. Disease Management and Clinical Outcomes, 1(5), Copyright (1997), Elsevier.

Scientific misconduct undermines the public trust in research and poisons the evidence base of medicine. If it is discovered, it will also destroy your academic career. Adherence to the principles of good scientific practice (Table 12.3) is therefore strictly required. Likewise, adherence to the standards of professional conduct is important in other areas of academia. For example, failure to disclose conflicts of interest (e.g. ties to the pharmaceutical industry) may harm your doctor–patient relationships or make you unacceptable to serve on guideline committees. Asking yourself 'Would my patients approve if they knew about this?' and 'Would my colleagues approve if they knew about this?' will often help you discern acceptable from unacceptable behaviour. Written guidelines for professional conduct have been issued by many medical organizations. Since academicians (especially educators) serve as role models for other professionals, they should be knowledgeable about these guidelines and should hold themselves to the highest professional standards.

Becoming a leader in the field

Building your career in academic psychiatry does not stop at the production of publications—it requires you to establish yourself as a leader in the field. The concept of leadership is complex and you will find a more detailed discussion in another chapter of this book (Chapter 2). In the context of an academic career, think of leadership as 'stepping out of the ivory tower'. Leadership means communicating not only with your direct peers but also with all other parties that are interested in your work (e.g. other medical specialties, patient organizations, scientific organizations, the general public). Leadership means setting scientific, clinical, and political goals and inspiring other people to work towards them.

As mentioned, it is important that you seize your opportunities to practise your leadership skills. When invited to hold a seminar in your hospital or to give a presentation at a conference, do it! It may require some (unpaid) extra work, but you will benefit in multiple ways. First, it will help you to focus and improve your knowledge of the topic. Secondly, the audience will perceive you as an expert on what you are presenting. Maybe someone in the audience is planning a similar event in the future and is still looking for a speaker: a single presentation may thus trigger a whole set of invitations. Thirdly, you will train your presentation skills. Since speaking in public is of such fundamental importance, you should train your ability as much as possible. Media training will help you to prepare for communication with the wider public.

Another important element of becoming a leader in your field is participation in professional associations (e.g. the national psychiatric associations, the EPA, the WPA). In these associations, decisions are made that shape how psychiatry is practiced (e.g. through the formulation of guidelines). Participation in this process lets you influence the outcome but also gives you exposure to other experts in the field—an excellent networking opportunity. It also provides you with advance knowledge about ongoing developments in the field. In this way, you may become the one in your hospital who is introducing a novel technique or leading the efforts to adapt to a new set of rules. For similar reasons, participation in the governing bodies of your hospital or university is very important.

Where to go? Finding and establishing your own niche

The landscape of psychiatry is extremely broad and while some areas are more competitive and crowded (such as neuroimaging in depression and schizophrenia), others are neglected (delirium, catatonia, or palliative care psychiatry). In our experience, most successful academic psychiatrists have not initiated their careers thinking 'I want to find a new treatment for depression' and then really discovered one later on. Rather, their academic focus has evolved over time and been shaped by the internal and external factors described in this chapter. Sometimes, developing your academic career calls for strategic thinking similar to that engaged in competitive sports. Once you and your coach (mentor) have identified what your preferences, predispositions, and obstacles are, and once you have learned the rules of the game, the time has come to decide in what league you are going to play.

The good thing about academia is that whatever league you choose to play in, you can always mix and match between them—choose one field, but also co-operate with other colleagues and conduct multidisciplinary research. Indeed, transferring your expertise from one academic area into another can be extremely fruitful. The transfer of preclinical basic research results into early clinical trials ('translational medicine') is even considered the high point of academic achievement in medicine. However, very few researchers have such an opportunity during their careers. Finally, having established your niche, it is important not to forget that you may outgrow it: be prepared to find, or create, a new one.

Remain open to constant change

Today's ECPs are training for a future that is impossible to predict. This has always been a problem, but has become even more prominent because of the fast pace at which the world is changing.[19] These rapid changes are maybe even more pronounced in the academic setting. In an instant, a scientific breakthrough can make much of your expertise obsolete: once Alzheimer's disease can be prevented, there will be a lot less demand for treatment of its behavioural and psychological symptoms. Therefore, ECPs in academia need to remain open to adjusting their career if personal beliefs or external demands change. In order to prepare, we advise you to diversify your capital. Capital diversification is a concept long known in the business world. It implies actions to diminish the overall risk so that the positive performance of some investments will neutralize the negative performance of others. In building your academic career, your intelligence, hard work, preferences, creativity, and goals are your most valuable assets. Diversify your investment into more than one area: do research if you can, but also build clinical expertise, contribute to psychiatric associations, engage in teaching, etc. Putting all your eggs into one basket may not take you very far in your academic career. In the end, be prepared to walk away: if you do not succeed in academic psychiatry, there are many other things in life. On the other hand, it may well be you who advances psychiatry through a major research finding or another eminent academic contribution.

References

1 Fiorillo A, Malik A, Luciano M, et al. Challenges for trainees in psychiatry and early career psychiatrists. *Int Rev Psychiatry* 2013; **25**(4):431–7.

2 Arbuckle MR, Gordon JA, Pincus HA, Oquendo MA. Bridging the gap: supporting translational research careers through an integrated research track within residency training. *Acad Med* 2013; **88**(6):759–65.

3 Fitz-Gerald DMJ, Kablinger A, Manno B, Carter OS, Caldito G, Smith S. Psychiatry residents' participation in research. *Acad Psychiatry* 2001; **25**(1):42–7.

4 Blazer D. Independent research by early investigators: an underutilized option. *JAMA Psychiatry* 2014; **71**(4):357–8.

5 Kuzman MR, Giacco D, Simmons M, et al. Psychiatry training in Europe: views from the trenches. *Med Teach* 2012; **34**(10):e708–17.

6 Jauhar S, Guloksuz S, Andlauer O, et al. Choice of antipsychotic treatment by European psychiatry trainees: are decisions based on evidence? *BMC Psychiatry* 2012; **12**(1):27.

7 Fiorillo A, Luciano M, Giacco D, et al. Training and practice of psychotherapy in Europe: results of a survey. *World Psychiatry* 2011; **10**(3):238.

8 Riese F, Oakley C, Bendix M, Piir P, Fiorillo A. Transition from psychiatric training to independent practice: a survey on the situation of early career psychiatrists in 35 countries. *World Psychiatry* 2013; **12**(1):82–3.

9 Goldstein JL. On the origin and prevention of PAIDS (paralyzed academic investigator's disease syndrome). *J Clin Invest* 1986; **78**: 848–854.

10 Jovanovic N, Beezhold J, Andlauer O, et al. Burnout among psychiatry residents. *Die Psychiatrie* 2009; (**6**):75–9.

11 Volpe U, Fiorillo A, Luciano M, et al. Pathways to mental health care in Italy: results from a multicenter study. *Int J Soc Psychiatry* 2014; **60**:508–13.

12 Farooq K, Lydall GJ, Malik A, Ndetei DM, ISOSCCIP Group, Bhugra D. Why medical students choose psychiatry—a 20 country cross-sectional survey. *BMC Med Educ* 2014; **14**(1):12.

13 Ahn J, Watt CD, Man L-X, Greeley SAW, Shea JA. Educating future leaders of medical research: analysis of student opinions and goals from the MD-PhD SAGE (students' attitudes, goals, and education) survey. *Acad Med* 2007; **82**(7):633–45.

14 Rieder RO. The recruitment and training of psychiatric residents for research. *Psychopharmacol Bull* 1988; **24**(2):288–90.

15 Pincus HA, Haviland MG, Dial TH, Hendryx MS. The relationship of postdoctoral research training to current research activities of faculty in academic departments of psychiatry. *Am J Psychiatry* 1995; **152**(4):596–601.

16 Mihai A, Ströhle A, Maric N, Heinz A, Helmchen H, Sartorius N. Postgraduate training for young psychiatrists—experience of the Berlin Summer School. *Eur Psychiatry* 2006; **21**(8):509–15.

17 Scherer RW, Langenberg P, Elm von E. Full publication of results initially presented in abstracts. *Cochrane Data Syst Rev* 2007; (**2**):MR000005.

18 Gillin JC. Postresidency research training of psychiatrists. *Psychopharmacol Bull* 1988; **24**(2):291–2.

19 Sartorius N. Training psychiatrists for the future. *Asia-Pacific Psychiatry* 2009; **1**(3):111–5.

Chapter 13

Curriculum development for psychiatric training

Marisa Casanova Dias, Florian Riese, and Allan Tasman

What is a curriculum?

The term *curriculum* is derived from Latin and refers to 'a running, course, career'. In education, a curriculum is the course of educational activities that you have to go through (and master) before you reach a certain formal qualification. In most places, curricula are nowadays available in written form and normally comprise lists of learning objectives, minimum levels of required knowledge and skills, suggested teaching methods, and methods for evaluation of educational progress. In other words, a curriculum is a set of educational rules and provides a framework to enable learning to take place. Similar to a contract, this set of rules has to be respected by all involved parties, both educators and learners. A curriculum (especially in written form) provides learners with the security that if they manage to become proficient in the delineated areas and pass the required assessments, they will obtain the desired formal qualification (e.g. they will be allowed to hold the title of 'psychiatrist'). For educators and the general public, a curriculum enforces minimum standards for what a 'psychiatrist' should know and be able to do.

While educational curricula exist in many contexts, this chapter focuses on psychiatric training at postgraduate level—from the moment doctors choose psychiatry as their medical specialty after graduating from medical school until the moment they become ready for independent practice as qualified psychiatric specialists. The 'race track' (Fig. 13.1) in this case is the career of physicians specializing in psychiatry. Although this chapter gives examples for early career psychiatrists, the suggestions are applicable to other career stages.

The content and methods of the postgraduate psychiatric training profoundly shape future psychiatrists. If they are more likely to work in community-based settings or hospitals, in one subspecialty or another (see Case 1), if they are more medication-oriented or put a stronger emphasis on psychotherapy, how they interact with other medical specialties, and so on, all depend—at least partly—on their psychiatric training curriculum.

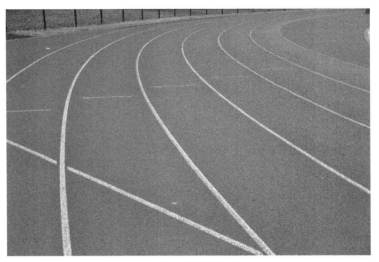

Fig. 13.1 Running/race track: representation of career progression.

Case study 1: Sam has just completed his postgraduate psychiatric training and is looking for his first position as a consultant. Unfortunately, the job market in the city where he lives is tight. There are two job offers for consultant positions but in old-age psychiatry. Since old-age psychiatry was not part of the mandatory curriculum, Sam so far has had very little exposure to it and he is unsure if he would be up to the task. Instead of applying for one of the two positions in old-age psychiatry, he therefore decides to apply for a position in a mood disorders clinic in a different city.

For the field of psychiatry in general, other curricula (such as for undergraduate medical education, nursing, or for mental healthcare workers' education) are also of fundamental importance: they determine to a large extent how non-psychiatrists perceive and interact with our profession and, subsequently, with our patients. Case 2 exemplifies the importance of the psychiatric curriculum in nursing training. When psychiatric nursing was included in their training, nurses felt more confident with psychiatric patients, which has led to better care. However, the same case illustrates that incomplete training can lead to false beliefs (e.g. danger)—hence the importance of a balanced curriculum content. The guiding question behind the development of a psychiatric curriculum therefore is 'What kind of psychiatrists will patients need in the future?', which should never be forgotten during the development process.

Case study 2: In a three-year nursing course, psychiatric nursing is taught during a four-week module. One week of the module is dedicated to dealing with patients' violent behaviours. After the course, the evaluation form reveals that nursing students feel substantially safer and less uncomfortable when having to deal with violent patients. However, nurses were also much more likely to endorse statements such as 'psychiatric patients are dangerous'.

The importance of taking part in curricular development

For early career psychiatrists (ECPs), there are few similarly rewarding experiences as being able to directly influence the knowledge, skills, and behaviours at stake in their own professional career. Who we become depends on what we learn. Where we 'run' is laid out by the design of the 'race track' (i.e. the curriculum). Educational curricula therefore profoundly shape the image and practice of psychiatry as well as the profile of individual psychiatrists, as illustrated in Cases 1 and 2. Consequently, involvement in curricular development has the potential to make a lasting impact on the practice of psychiatry. Table 13.1 summarizes the advantages of ECP involvement in curriculum development. As with research, there will be a delay until the effect of curricular modifications finds its way into clinical practice. However, ECPs have almost their entire career in psychiatry still ahead, so they are uniquely suited to adopt a long-term perspective. Maybe in ten years from now, all recently graduated colleagues will have trained in old-age psychiatry and the demand for such specialists will finally be met. We need the best professionals in order to improve patient care and clinical outcomes. That can only be achieved through a training curriculum that reflects healthcare needs and is effective in practice.

Another reason for involvement of ECPs in curricular development is that trainees or recently qualified specialists often know best what should be included in the curriculum and how it should be delivered. As the target audience and the ones who will experience the curriculum first-hand, they are important stakeholders in its development and can influence its quality. Traditionally, medical training curricula have been developed via an exclusive top–down approach: a regulatory body (e.g. a national psychiatric association) develops a curriculum, without trainee involvement, and enforces its implementation. Recently, however, a bottom–up approach to training has become more popular: trainees themselves have taken the initiative to survey different aspects of training across a variety of countries to understand the status quo and areas for development.[1,2]

Table 13.1 Advantages of ECPs involvement in curriculum development

For ECPs	For organizations that develop training curricula
Contributing to shaping own profession	Stakeholder input on educational aims
Taking an expert role	Stakeholder input on educational methods, resources, and pace
Reflecting on education may lead to more sustained motivation to learn	Decreasing resistance to implementation
Networking opportunities	Capacity building: the enthusiastic trainees of today will be the programme directors of tomorrow
Rewarding experience	Cost efficient
Preparing for future leadership functions	Social responsibility

The European Federation of Psychiatric Trainees (EFPT) went further by suggesting standards of psychiatric training that were agreed by consensus of its 35 member countries.[3]

Curriculum development—a process within a national and international context

As we have pointed out before, who we are as psychiatrists is fundamentally shaped by the psychiatric curriculum that we undergo. However, the development or reform of a psychiatric curriculum is exposed to conflicting interests. It occurs in the context of local educational traditions, political interest groups, professional and social context, and is limited by the available resources (see Case 3).

Case study 3: Although the training curriculum states that trainees should have an active role in teaching medical students and other health professionals, John is having difficulties in gaining these competencies. He is training in the countryside, where there are no teaching hospitals and therefore no medical students, and there is no tradition that junior doctors can teach other professionals.

Political and economic influences may also lead to shortening of the length of the curriculum in order to produce the medical workforce faster (see Case 4).

Case study 4: Mary will now finish her specialty training at the same time as her friend Joana (who started a year earlier) because the government decided that five years was too long to train in psychiatry when there was a shortage of psychiatrists in her country. This means that she will get less exposure in substance misuse disorders and child and adolescent psychiatry than Joana, and is worried that she will not be able to gain the necessary skills.

It is also worth noting that mobility of health professionals, like citizens in general, is increasing (see Chapter 11). This means that psychiatrists will have to acquire the knowledge and skills to deal with patients from different cultural backgrounds in a professional manner. This is something that ECPs might not have learned during their training, as teaching of global health competencies is not widely disseminated (see Case 5). A commission on medical education for the twenty-first century noted that there is currently a 'mismatch between present professional competencies and the requirements of an increasingly interdependent world'.[4] Therefore, curricula need to take into account cultural variations that emerge from patients' and healthcare professionals' mobility.

Case study 5: Peter failed to diagnose depression in a patient that attended his clinic because she denied feeling low in mood. Instead, she only referred to feeling 'weak', 'imbalanced', and 'tired', which are the expressions of depressive symptoms in her Chinese culture, where depression is expressed somatically.

While at undergraduate level, the curriculum can be defined with a degree of precision, at postgraduate level, learning occurs alongside clinical work, which limits the time and resources available. Therefore, the curriculum needs to be more flexible. Clinical commitments vary widely, so the challenge is ensuring that all psychiatrists achieve the intended learning outcomes despite the variability (nationally and internationally) of the clinical experiences and the resources (length of training, working hours, population demographics, variability of clinics, faculty expertise, etc.). After obtaining the title of 'specialists', ECPs are even more limited in the time that they can dedicate to learning: thus the concept of curriculum loses its meaning. At that stage, learning will be guided by individual needs and the framework of revalidation or recertification requirements.

The curriculum as a means to harmonisation of training

A psychiatric curriculum should be primarily based on knowledge and skills required for future psychiatrists. One of its functions is to provide a template or framework to enable learning to take place in a standardized way.

While local organizations can create curricula adjusted to their own resources and particularities, national and international bodies have provided curriculum frameworks in an attempt to standardize curricula—and with it, educational standards—across regions. These efforts are driven by the increase in number and mobility of today's trainees. Fifty years ago, it might have been possible to personally know the handful of psychiatric trainees in your region and judge their fitness to practice based on your own experience. Today, there might be dozens of trainees in your hospital, many of them having studied medicine in another country or at least in another university.

In Europe, the international frameworks for training standards are issued by the Union Européenne des Médecins Spécialistes (UEMS), which is the representative organization of the national associations of medical specialists in the European Union and its associated countries. It is the European body responsible for setting standards for high- quality healthcare practice that are transmitted to the authorities and institutions of the EU and the national medical associations, stimulating and encouraging them to implement its recommendations. For psychiatry, the Charter on Training[5] and the European Framework for Competencies in Psychiatry,[6] both issued by the UEMS Section of Psychiatry, are of fundamental importance, and many national psychiatric curricula have been developed based on these models.

In the United States, the Accreditation Council for Graduate Medical Education (ACGME) and the American Board of Psychiatry and Neurology have recently developed the Psychiatry Milestone Project.[7] Milestones are the necessary knowledge, skills, attitudes, and other attributes, organized in a framework that allows for the assessment of the development of the trainee in key dimensions of the competencies in a specialty.

The Royal Australian and New Zealand College of Psychiatrists (RANZCP) oversees the training and qualification of psychiatrists in Australia and New Zealand. By the end of 2015, its new competency-based Fellowship Program for psychiatry training will have been rolled out, replacing the previous training programme.

In other parts of the world, there have been attempts to create international frameworks of competencies, but none is currently established yet. The Association of South-East Asian Nations (ASEAN) Economic Community (AEC) will be implemented in 2015. Doctors in South-East Asian countries (ten nations and East Timor) are one of the professions which will be allowed to move and work in other countries (similar to the current situation in the European Union). In Latin America, the first steps are being taken to devise an integrated international curriculum framework. The Education Committee of the Asociación de Psiquiatría de América Latina (APAL) collected and examined the psychiatric training programmes available throughout Latin America in order to standardize them and allow for homologation of certification. The ultimate aim is to allow psychiatrists from the Latin American countries to move and work in other neighbouring countries.

Learning objectives and models of teaching

Medical education looks quite different today from what it did in the past (see Table 13.2). Traditionally, medical education followed an 'apprenticeship model'. A future psychiatrist would work alongside one or more senior colleagues and learn through observation of their behaviour. He would also read textbooks to gain knowledge about the theoretical background of his work. After a certain period as an 'apprentice', an assessment of the candidate's fitness for independent practice would (or would not) have followed, usually testing knowledge of psychiatric theory. Subsequently, the right to practice independently as a psychiatrist was awarded. The limitations of such a model are obvious: what you learn mainly depends on the qualities of your direct teacher, the setting in which you work, and on your intrinsic motivation to learn.

Over time, many curricula developed that followed a more 'time-based' model. These would require learners to rotate through different wards or hospitals for predefined periods of time, thereby increasing their exposure to different patients and different educators. However, that puts too much emphasis on the duration of a rotation, rather than the abilities acquired. Trainees learn at a different pace and this model does not allow for flexibility.

Table 13.2 Changes in medical education approaches

Traditional model[10]	The SPICES model[11]	The PRISMS model[12]
Teacher-centred	Student-centred	Practice-based, linked with professional development
Knowledge-giving	Problem-based	Relevant to students and communities
Discipline-led	Integrated	Inter-professional and interdisciplinary
Hospital-oriented	Community-oriented	Shorter courses taught in smaller units
Standard programme	Electives (+ core)	Multi-site locations
Opportunistic (apprenticeship)	Systematic	Symbiotic (organic whole)

Source data from: Flexner A. *Medical education in the United States and Canada: a report to the Carnegie foundation for the advancement of teaching*, Copyright (1910), The Carnegie Foundation for the Advancement of Teaching; *Med Edu.*, 18 (4), Harden RM, Sowden S, Dunn WR. Educational strategies in curriculum development: the SPICES model, pp. 284–297. Copyright (1984), John Wiley & Sons Ltd.; *Med Educ.*, 35 (6), Bligh J, Prideaux D, Parsell G. PRISMS: new educational strategies for medical education, pp. 520–521, Copyright (2001), John Wiley & Sons Ltd.

Currently, the most common model is a 'competency-based' one. In this approach, trainees are assessed against predefined competencies. It promotes learner centredness, and focuses on outcomes and abilities. In this model, time is not a marker of learning but, rather, another resource for learning.[8] Society today demands accountability and transparency from medical education, which has led to the move to outcomes-based or objectives-based curricula.[9]

The curriculum development process

There are no evidence-based approaches to optimal curriculum design, which tends to be rather ideology-based,[13] so it changes in response to the dominant political, societal, and professional concerns—and so do the teaching, learning, and assessment methods. To develop a curriculum that is adapted to the patients', educators', and trainees' needs requires an iterative and ongoing process. In other words, it is never 'finished'. The process can be summarized as a cycle (see Fig. 13.2) although the phases of curricular development are often not as clearly defined as the cycle indicates. However, all phases need to be taken into consideration for the development process to succeed. Usually, the process is directed by a core group of people, designated by the organization that issues the curriculum. As described, stakeholder involvement (e.g. trainees) helps to increase the fit to real-world needs.

Phase 1: Plan

Study the past if you would define the future.

Confucius

In the majority of cases, a curriculum is not developed from scratch. It usually already exists in some form, either locally, nationally, or internationally, which is then adapted to the intended purpose. Most likely, there is also a governing body responsible for the

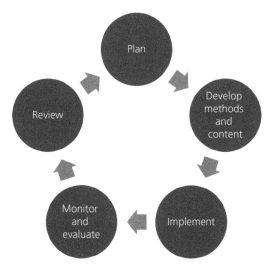

Fig. 13.2 Phases of curricular development.

Box 13.1 Curriculum development team

◆ Teachers (including tutors and supervisors)
◆ Educationalists
◆ Managers
◆ Patients
◆ Carers
◆ ECPs

oversight of the psychiatric training. The starting point for developing a curriculum is then to do an assessment and analysis of needs. The best way to identify the weaknesses of the old curriculum is by collecting feedback both from trainees and trainers. Lay members and patient and carer representatives are also important in this process. Areas in need of change may be related to content (e.g. add or delete topics) or means of delivering (e.g. lectures, seminars, clinical placements, e-learning). Resources also need to be considered (e.g. faculty expertise, variety of training sites, diversity of patient population, time allocated, educational equipment and materials, technological support). After the main issues are identified, it is time to form a team for curriculum development (Box 13.1). This is the chance for ECPs, as the main stakeholders, to influence the future of the profession.

ECPs can get involved in the needs' assessment and analysis (e.g. running a focus group or survey to identify the areas for improvement). They can also get involved through national trainees' associations or international associations, which may already have statements on what trainees deem as important topics for the curriculum and that can be used as lobbying documents (e.g. EFPT statements[3]). The World Psychiatric Association[14] and the World Federation for Medical Education[15] have produced standards that can be used as a framework and against which to benchmark postgraduate psychiatric training.

Phase 2: Develop the content and methods

> Learning without thought is labour lost; thought without learning is perilous.
>
> *Confucius*

Firstly, *aims and intended learning outcomes* have to be established. These should cover knowledge, skills, and values and be linked to appropriate assessment methods (see Fig. 13.3). In medical education, it is common to use the structure of the CanMEDS framework[16] to organize the intended learning outcomes (see Fig. 13.4). The CanMEDS Physician Competency Framework describes the knowledge, skills, and abilities that specialist physicians need to demonstrate for better patient outcomes. It is based on the seven roles that all physicians need to have to be better doctors: medical expert, communicator, collaborator, manager, health advocate, scholar, and professional.

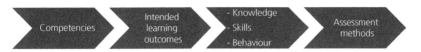

Fig. 13.3 Curriculum organization.

Although broad curriculum objectives can be established, it is better to devolve the detailed planning and design to those who will be delivering the course, so that they have ownership of their programme. To ensure standardization, robust quality assurance mechanisms will be required. At European level, the European Framework for Competencies in Psychiatry (see Fig. 13.5) serves as a benchmark[6] which is then used by the different national psychiatric associations to guide the development process of their national curricula.

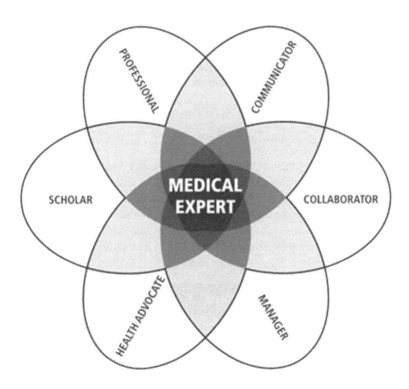

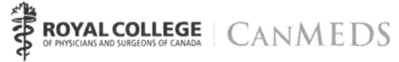

Fig. 13.4 CanMEDS definition of the roles of a physician.
Reproduced from Royal College of Physicians and Surgeons of Canada, Copyright (2005), with permission.

UEMS Section and Board of Psychiatry – COMPETENCY FRAMEWORK FOR PSYCHIATRY

2 Communicator

Definition

To provide humane, high-quality care, psychiatrists establish effective and empathic relationships with patients and their carers, other physicians, and other health professionals. Communication skills are essential for the functioning of a psychiatrist and are necessary for obtaining information from, and conveying information, to patients and their families. Furthermore, these abilities are critical in eliciting patients' beliefs, concerns and expectations about their illnesses and for assessing key factors impacting on patients' health.

Competencies

The psychiatrist is able to:

2.1 establish a therapeutic relationship with patients

	Knowledge	Competence	Performance
	Knowledge tests WE OE	Clinical examinations ASCE CE	In-training assessment DBD DOP MSAP
2.1.1 be aware of factors influencing the patients' reactions to the physician and others, and one's own reactions when dealing with patients.			DBD MSAP
2.1.2 communicate effectively and empathically, both verbally and non-verbally		ASCE	DOP MSAP
2.1.3 establish, maintain and conclude appropriate therapeutic relationships with patients and carers			DBD MSAP
2.1.4 facilitate a structured clinical encounter		ASCE	DOP

Fig. 13.5 Example section of the UEMS European Framework for Competencies in Psychiatry.

Reproduced from European Union of Medical Specialists, *European Framework for Competencies in Psychiatry*, Copyright (2009), UEMS.

Secondly, the curriculum *content* has to be selected. Box 13.2 summarizes potential sources of content which needs to reflect the knowledge, skills, and values expected of fully trained psychiatrists, to meet the day-to-day demands of clinical practice. The content has to be in line with the current expectations of professional bodies and societies. It needs to fit with the local cultural environment. For instance, if there is a move from hospital-based to community-based treatment in psychiatry, the curriculum will need

Box 13.2 Sources of content

- Previous curriculum
- National professional associations
- International professional associations
- Trainee/junior doctors' associations
- Allied health professionals
- Patient groups
- Carer and family groups
- Scientific literature
- Healthcare policies

to reflect that (e.g. by increasing the number of training rotations in the community). The curriculum should also provide a graduated sequence to the content: from simple to complex, from general to specific (e.g. in the UK, the Royal College of Psychiatrists established a core curriculum for the initial three years of postgraduate training and a subspecialty curriculum for the final three years).

Thirdly, the *teaching and learning methods* need to be delineated. These are shaped by the governing trends in healthcare and education (e.g. evidence-based medicine, cost effectiveness, the use of different teaching means—formal vs. informal, computer-based, etc.). The methods also depend on the resources available:

a) *Staff* (faculty and administrative): There should be an appropriate number of faculty members (the number will determine whether small-group or larger-group teaching can take place); the faculty should have the appropriate knowledge and skills (in general and in subspecialty topics); 'train the trainer' courses may be helpful to build capacity within the faculty; a large training scheme will require administrative personnel to organize and run it.

b) *Equipment and facilities*: Equipment should be adequate for the chosen teaching and learning methods (e.g. technological support for an online lecture); facilities and clinical services to teach the various components of the curriculum should be available (e.g. teaching how to assess suicidality might require experience in an emergency setting or simulation facilities in addition to a didactic seminar).

c) *Material*: There should access to medical library facilities, the internet, and electronic journals (e.g. for finding current, accurate, relevant learning materials).

Finally, the *assessment methods* need to reflect the intended learning outcomes and be in line with the teaching and learning methods used. One of the fundamental discussions in curriculum development relates to if and how to assess learning outcomes. Society today demands accountability and transparency from medical education; therefore, learning outcomes and their assessment take a prominent role. This stage of development presents another excellent opportunity for ECPs to become involved (e.g. by writing multiple-choice questions (MCQs), making suggestions for Objective Structured Clinical Examination (OSCE) stations, designing a logbook, participating in review panels, removal of trainees from training and appeals procedure).

Phase 3: Implementation

You can't cross a sea by merely staring into the water.

Rabindranath Tagore

In order for a curriculum to be effective, we need to make sure that there is no mismatch between the formal curriculum that is published and what happens in practice. Stakeholder involvement is vital in this process. While some stakeholders may work with the curriculum development team and have a more hands-on approach, others can be involved through consultation (e.g. with health jurisdictions and health services).

Regardless of the scope of the curriculum (international, national, or local), it is important to have an implementation strategy. The strategy needs to include clear communication of the content and use of the curriculum, and to be cascaded to the relevant people (e.g. university departments responsible for training, training programme directors, tutors and supervisors, assessors and trainees). The use of resources needs to be realistic for the context in which the curriculum is to be implemented (see the section 'Phase 2: Develop the content and methods').

Oversight of the curriculum is determined by national or local requirements. The most common scenario is that there is a training programme director who oversees the implementation of the curriculum locally and is responsible for the allocation of resources. ECPs can aid implementation by disseminating information on the curriculum to those on the ground, more directly involved with training activities—training programme directors, and educational and clinical supervisors and trainees.

Phase 4: Monitoring and evaluation of curriculum success

> Everything that can be counted does not necessarily count; everything that counts cannot necessarily be counted.
>
> *Albert Einstein*

Monitoring refers to a continuous check to detect problems at any level of implementation. Trainees and ECPs are likely to be the first ones to notice such problems, so they are well placed to become actively involved at this stage (see Case 6).

Case study 6: A group of trainees from the EFPT is collaborating with UEMS on a research study to look at how the European Framework of Competencies is translated at national level, by surveying the experiences and opinions of trainees regarding their national curricula competencies.

Evaluation should be done throughout the curriculum development process. For effective evaluation, a strategy needs to be developed which can include different phases: design, collecting data, evaluation report, communicating results. Well-planned, periodically scheduled evaluations give timely, accurate information about the effectiveness of the process and feed into the development cycle. According to the World Psychiatric Association template for psychiatric education,[14] the most effective approach for evaluating the curriculum is to create a permanent education committee in which both trainees and the faculty are represented, who can bring forward concerns and proposed changes for discussion by the committee on an ongoing basis. Table 13.3 suggests markers of curriculum success and how they relate to the curriculum development cycle.

Phase 5: Revision

> Change is the end result of all true learning.
>
> *Leo Buscaglia*

The development of the curriculum is a continuous process that involves a wide community including laypeople, trainees, medical managers, psychiatry experts, and trainers.

In the initial phase of curriculum development, an assessment of needs was performed (see the section 'Phase 1: Plan'). The curriculum should be revised against this

Table 13.3 How to assess curriculum success

◆ Recruitment and retention	Is the purpose of the curriculum right? Are we attracting the right people? Once in training, do they continue in psychiatry or change specialty?
◆ The syllabus can be covered in the time allocated for it	Is there adequate planning?
◆ Transparency in outcomes	Does it address the views and experiences of the various stakeholders?
◆ Graduation rates	Does it help learners to attain the intended learning outcomes?
◆ Trainee assessment results (e.g. exams, formative assessments)	Are there trends of shortcomings in trainees' outcomes/assessments of knowledge and skills?
◆ Aggregated performance results	How do trainees rate the teaching they receive (e.g. lectures, clinical rotations)?
◆ Visitation schemes	Are teaching staff and resources appropriate?

original needs' assessment. However, we should be aware that needs change and they are perceived differently by the different groups involved. Trainees have the right and the duty to report when needs have changed and it is time to revise the curriculum (see Box 13.3).

There are no strict guidelines on how often a revision should occur, but it is widely accepted that an extensive formal revision should occur at least every five years, and a less formal revision every year. It does not mean that a curriculum must be reformed so often, but it is useful to go through the revision process to elicit areas that need to be addressed.

Box 13.3 Warning signs that it is time to revise the curriculum

- ◆ Lack of time to cover the curriculum
- ◆ Lack of training resources
- ◆ Use of obsolete material
- ◆ New treatments not being taught/out-of-date treatments still being taught
- ◆ Learning activities not directly related to meaningful clinical tasks and to career development
- ◆ Work beyond level of competency
- ◆ Low or very high examination pass rates

Box 13.4 Examples of how ECPs can get involved in the curriculum development process

♦ Run a focus group or survey to understand the needs

♦ Present the results at key meetings to raise awareness

♦ Get involved through national trainees' associations or international associations, which may already have statements on what trainees deem as important topics which can be used for lobbying at stakeholder meetings

♦ Join curriculum development teams

♦ Meet the training programme director and suggest methods of teaching relevant to the training setting (e.g. small group, problem-based learning, distance learning)

♦ Aid implementation of the curriculum by liaising with programme directors and training supervisors

♦ Participate in assessments: write multiple-choice questions (MCQs) or Objective Structured Clinical Examinations (OSCE) stations

♦ Participate in visitation schemes

♦ Participate in review panels, appeals procedures, etc.

♦ Report to the training director or to the national association when the curriculum is no longer fit for purpose

Conclusions

The purpose of a psychiatric curriculum is to produce competent and capable psychiatrists to enhance the standards of patient care. It outlines the breadth and depth necessary to become a specialist able to work in a variety of settings.

To develop a curriculum is a complex task, with many challenges.[17] The needs are diverse and so are training resources (e.g. faculty to provide adequate supervision, range of clinical settings available locally). The curriculum design is a reflection of the current educational, professional, political, social, and economic situation. A curriculum should only be reformed or created if there is a need. ECPs have to be at the heart of its development. Box 13.4 gives examples of how ECPs can get involved in the process. The curriculum should be practical, valid, and applicable to the desired context. ECPs, through their involvement in curricular development, have the potential to make a lasting impact on the practice of psychiatry, both for themselves and for the lives of patients that are affected.

References

1 Oakley C, Malik A. Psychiatric training in Europe. *Psychiatrist* 2010; **34**:447–50. DOI: 10.1192/pb.bp.109.026062

2 Kuzman MR, Giacco D, Simmons M, et al. Psychiatry training in Europe: views from the trenches. *Med Teach* 2012; **34**(10):e708–17. DOI: 10.3109/0142159X.2012.687481

3 European Federation of Psychiatric Trainees. *EFPT recommendations on standards of psychiatric training*; 2013. Available at: http://www.efpt.eu/images/library/File/EFPT%20 STATEMENTS%202013%20revision_2.pdf.

4 **Frenk J, Chen L, Bhutta ZA, et al**. Health professionals for a new century: transforming education to strengthen health systems in an interdependent world. *Lancet* 2010; **376**:1923–58. DOI: 10.1016/S0140–6736(10)61854–5

5 European Union of Medical Specialists / Union Européenne des Médecins Spécialistes (UEMS). *Charter on training of medical specialists in the EU*; 2003. Available at: http:// uemspsychiatry.org/wp-content/uploads/2013/09/Chapter6–11.10.03.pdf.

6 European Union of Medical Specialists / Union Européenne des Médecins Spécialistes (UEMS). *European framework for competencies in psychiatry*; 2009. Available at: http:// uemspsychiatry.org/wp-content/uploads/2013/09/2009-Oct-EFCP.pdf.

7 Accreditation Council for Graduate Medical Education (ACGME) and the American Board of Psychiatry and Neurology. The psychiatry milestone project. *J Grad Med Educ* 2014; **6**(1):284–304. DOI: http://dx.doi.org/10.4300/JGME-06–01s1–11

8 **Frank JR, Snell LS, Cate O, et al**. Competency-based medical education: theory to practice. *Med Teach* 2010; **32**(8):638–45. DOI: 10.3109/0142159X.2010.501190

9 **Rees CE**. The problem with outcomes-based curricula in medical education: insights from educational theory. *Med Educ* 2004; **38**(6):593–8. DOI: 10.1046/j.1365–2923.2004.01793

10 **Flexner A**. *Medical education in the United States and Canada: a report to the Carnegie Foundation for the Advancement of Teaching*. New York City: The Carnegie Foundation for the Advancement of Teaching; 1910.

11 **Harden RM, Sowden S, Dunn WR**. Educational strategies in curriculum development: the SPICES model. *Med Educ* 1984; **18**(4):284–97.

12 **Bligh J, Prideaux D, Parsell G**. PRISMS: new educational strategies for medical education. *Med Educ* 2001; **35**(6):520–1. DOI: 10.1046/j.1365–2923.2001.00984.x

13 **Swanwick T**. *Understanding medical education: evidence, theory and practice* (2nd edn). Chichester, UK: John Wiley and Sons; 2013.

14 **Tasman A, Kay J, Pichet U, et al**. *WPA template for undergraduate and graduate psychiatric education*; 2011. Available at: http://www.wpanet.org/uploads/Education/Template_for_Undergraduate_and_Graduate/WPA-Template-rev.pdf.

15 World Federation for Medical Education. *WFME global standards for quality improvement*; 2003. Available at: http://www.wfme.org/standards/pgme.

16 **Frank JR**. (ed.) *The CanMEDS 2005 physician competency framework: better standards, better physicians, better care*. Ottawa: Royal College of Physicians and Surgeons of Canada; 2005.

17 **Mackey AB, Tasman A**. Psychiatric residency curriculum: development and evaluation. In: *Teaching psychiatry: putting theory into practice* (eds. Gask L, Coskun B, Baron D). Chichester, UK: John Wiley & Sons; 2010.

Chapter 14

Social media and e-learning for professional development in psychiatry

Olivier Andlauer, Alexander Nawka, Gregory Lydall, Sinan Guloksuz, and Silvana Galderisi

Introduction

Today's generation relies on the internet as their main source of information and uses it for a variety of purposes, including establishing and maintaining professional connections.[1] We could paraphrase René Descartes's famous quote as 'I share, ergo, I am', capturing how important sharing ideas and new thoughts has become in the modern world.

The internet is a place where everybody can express their thoughts or knowledge, thus creating more information than anyone will ever be able to read, available at any time, from everywhere. In the field of medical education, including in mental health, social media and e-learning have attracted a lot of attention from the media, the general public, and also regulators and institutions. From unrealistic hopes of a way to deliver optimal education, to fear and rejection of these unknown technologies, clarification is needed on what to expect from information technology in medical education for psychiatrists.

In this chapter, we will describe how social media and e-learning can help improve professional development in psychiatry. We will also discuss the limitations and potential pitfalls for the mental health professional of engaging with information technology.

Social media and professional development

Access to reliable and high-quality information and research data, as well as membership of different professional associations, are important for professional development.[2] This trend is supported by the development of the internet which now allows publishing of user-generated content, including by professional groups.[3] Psychiatrists today may post their contributions online, Tweet, write blogs, and share pictures and videos. All of these may erode the boundaries between the social and professional spheres, which are particularly important in psychiatry.[3]

Social media enables people with similar interests to form groups, allowing them to share resources with friends and colleagues. Such resources may include educational materials, research data collection, and important health information.[3] Other benefits include engaging people in public health and policy discussions; establishing national and international professional networks; and facilitating patients' access to information about health and services.[4]

One purpose of all this connecting is to establish a network of contacts. Thanks to shared contents, doctors 'meet' others in social networks, and can get their feedback, share their experience, discuss issues of interest, and thus develop professionally. If a doctor can create a network of contacts, and gain certain influence, then he/she becomes one of its network nodes, meaning that he/she is becoming a person via which information is efficiently spread through the network.[2]

A key way to use social media for professional growth is in participation in online discussions on interesting and relevant topics with partners who can increase psychiatrists' knowledge. It is important to realise that the contacts established on this occasion do not have to be maintained forever. Once an online contact or network is not useful anymore, involvement can be stopped at any time. Connections can be chosen according to one's own rules, interests, and timetables.[2]

With the transformation of Facebook from a popular internet website to a mobile-based platform, social media have taken root among people, up to the point of becoming one of the most widely-used online tools.[1] In certain cases, however, the use of social media can lead to a breakdown of boundaries in the physician–patient relationship.[3]

Facebook

With over a billion active users, Facebook is the world's largest online social networking service.[5] After registration, users can create their own personal profile, add other users as friends, exchange messages, share relevant information, or join various common-interest user groups.[5] This is why many physicians, including psychiatrists, have created their own Facebook pages. Doctors are advised to maintain separate pages for private and professional purposes.[4] Typically, the information published on such professional pages includes recent medical news, self-promotional materials such as television or radio appearances, and advertisements promoting other professional institutions, usually from the realm of healthcare or related areas. Facebook should very rarely be used as a tool for direct communication with patients. However, this does not stop anyone, including patients, employers, and appraisers from looking up a psychiatrist's online profile.

With regard to the nature of a therapeutic relationship, it is necessary to establish certain professional boundaries between a psychiatrist and their patients.[1] If the patient's request for online 'friendship' is accepted, this boundary between the professional and private sphere gets diluted.[6] The terminology itself implies that a transition in the relationship has occurred.

Even though it is, in the end, a physician's choice, it is advisable to decline such invitations. The UK guidance on this issue recommends that 'if a patient contacts you about their care or other professional matters through your private profile, you should indicate that you cannot mix social and professional relationships and, where appropriate, direct them to your professional profile.'[4]

Limits can be set up via 'privacy settings' options, so that patients on Facebook, whether they are part of the physician's network or not, have only limited or no access to his/her private content. Another option is to switch off the public search function, which makes a profile invisible to public search engines and therefore impossible for a patient to find a physician's profile.[1] It is worth noting that Facebook changes their privacy settings and related policies from time to time, and psychiatrists are advised to keep up to date with these.

However, it seems that the professional potential of Facebook has not yet been fully appreciated, and its use for the practice of psychiatry has been rather limited so far because of the aforementioned interferences of the social, family, and professional spheres, as well as local regulations.[1]

For the benefit of professional development, as with any other online network, groups can be created where people who share the same interests can exchange information. Such information could be research updates in a specific field, as well as digests of important psychiatric news and articles.

Twitter

Twitter is an online social networking and microblogging service that enables users to send and read short (up to 140 characters) text messages, called 'tweets'.[7] You gain access to these tweets once you become a follower of another user. Twitter users may be any person, company, or cause, including psychiatrists and mental health institutions.

Registered users can both read and post tweets; non-registered users can only read them. With Twitter, a doctor can reach the general public and colleagues. Through tweets, followers can quickly learn about interesting events, research news, presentations, lectures, job opportunities, or any kind of statement,[1] and it can therefore be used for professional development. In this regard, it is advisable to create a group of approximately 100 users whose tweets you are following and then decide whether you find this network useful or not.

LinkedIn

LinkedIn is a business-oriented social network used for professional networking. With more than 250 million members in over 200 countries, it is today, the world's largest networking service of its kind.[8] A LinkedIn profile is, in essence, an online curriculum vitae, displaying information on the user's job experience, education, references, and skills.[1]

LinkedIn is an excellent tool for recruiters who are looking for new employees, as well as for job seekers who can search among job offers published directly on LinkedIn pages or get information about vacancies via their network.[1] This makes LinkedIn a useful recruitment, networking, and self-promotion tool, but it is not suitable for acquiring new patients.

Groups of interest can be created on LinkedIn to start and share discussions. Educational material, as well as links to interesting websites and news, can be shared between professionals.

Generally, one needs to keep in mind that many patients have profiles on the same networks as physicians do. If a professional receives a request for friendship or sharing, he/she risks stepping over the boundaries of a professional relationship. Such requests, therefore, should be politely declined, preferably in person and with the justification that it may harm the professional relationship and lead to issues around privacy protection.[1]

ResearchGate

ResearchGate is a social network for scientists and researchers to share papers, ask and answer questions, and find collaborators.[9] The site includes profile pages, comments, groups, and job listings. Members are encouraged to share raw data and negative experiment results (as well as successes), so that their peers can avoid repeating the failed scientific experiment. ResearchGate reports to have over 4 million members[9] and can be useful if a doctor is pursuing an academic career.

Social networks and dilemmas

Information shared on the internet by psychiatrists can be a minefield of potential dangers. Disclosure of patient-identifiable information can undermine the assurance of doctor–patient confidentiality, an issue of particular importance in psychiatry. This may affect a client's willingness to talk to a psychiatrist openly about his/her problems.[3] Studies analysing Facebook profiles of medical school students carried out in 2013 found that 16% of these profiles contained professional-related content, violating the accreditation guidelines for a healthcare professional.[10]

Another potential issue is the excessive and careless disclosure of private information by the psychiatrist. In a therapeutic relationship, self-disclosures should be presented only rarely, for a limited time, and only when they are likely to have a positive therapeutic impact for the patient.[11] The majority of published private information on social networks does not meet these criteria.[3]

Due to these negative aspects, many psychiatrists simply ignore social media. However, this attitude misses the potential advantages. Like so often, it is the dose that makes the poison. When used in an appropriate way and with a sound guiding framework, there is no reason to avoid social media.[12] This framework includes not publishing private content where it may be accessed by patients; to protect the physician's private life and their therapeutic relationship with patients; and to avoid liability.[3] In making decisions, the psychiatrist should remember that most of the internet is a public place, and information is nearly impossible to remove, and therefore a good knowledge of who can access the information is required. If in doubt, it would be advisable not to publish private information online.

In one survey, 58% of psychiatrists reported that they never or rarely evaluated the way they present online.[13] The ever more frequent use of social media in medicine brings up a plethora of ethical, legal, and therapeutic questions which have to do with guarding boundaries in professional life. Psychiatrists should, however, pay attention not only to the content published by themselves directly, and to their potential recipients, but also regularly check what kind of information is published about them online by others, as this information can be incorrect or intentionally harmful.[3] Koh et al.[13] conclude that discipline-specific guidelines for psychiatrists' interactions with social media and electronic communications are needed.

Another challenge is the huge amount of information coming from social networks. To avoid being overwhelmed by this mass of incoming data, one needs to keep contacts well organized within the network. Practically, this means sometimes deleting non-active network members or setting up rules about communication requirements for group membership.[2]

These precautions should be inculcated as part of psychiatric training[14] so that psychiatrists in the twenty-first century will be able to navigate themselves through the dramatically developing social media arena as cautious yet active members.[3] On some social networks, it is possible to create a specific profile for professional purposes only. This makes it feasible to share useful information about mental health with the public, patients, and colleagues, and at the same time to keep a professional distance from patients. Clear rules should be set, from the beginning, on how the network will be used, and the boundaries between private and public life defined.

If psychiatrists decide to become active contributors and recipients of information in the framework of social media, they have to pay attention not to leave negative 'digital footprints' behind, because these can easily be found by patients.[3] Social media can enhance professional development in many ways. The choice of the most suitable social media, and to what degree one is prepared to be involved, are entirely up to ourselves.

Another dilemma that modern psychiatrists have to face is the therapeutic implication of the use of social media. Of course, the same limitations and dangers exist in the use of social media to interact with patients as in their use for professional development, especially regarding the need to maintain boundaries and confidentiality. However, the existence of social media cannot be ignored because patients use them to communicate with peers and other patients, and they can benefit from the doctor's use of social media.[4] This question is beyond the scope of this chapter, which is why we will not develop it further.

Newsletters and digests and professional development

Online newsletters and digests are valuable for keeping up to date with recent advances in psychiatry. They are particularly helpful when time is limited, as they review, summarize, and concisely report current research.

Some online newsletters and digests require paid subscription, whereas others are completely free. Although they provide a great amount of valuable information, some of them, particularly free alternatives, are funded by the pharmaceutical industry, and thereby contain advertisements or agendas that might be unappealing to some. Moreover, readers should be aware of industry ties that could create conflicts of interest. Fortunately, authors are generally required to disclose such conflicts, consistent with the policy of scientific journals.

Besides these commercial newsletters and digests, it is also possible to create a personalized digest that is customized according to one's interests and sent via e-mail, periodically (e.g. daily, weekly) and in a specified format (e.g. summary, abstract), by using the free search engine PubMed (https://www.nlm.nih.gov/bsd/disted/pubmed-tutorial/040_015.html). Another free search engine, Google Scholar, which provides a similar service, also allows users to build their own personal reference collection (http://scholar.google.com/intl/en-US/scholar/help.html#alerts),

Online open access journals and professional development

A recent study examining the availability and the use of relevant medical information sources in psychiatric training among 32 European countries showed that access to online medical information was 'sufficient or above needs' in the majority of countries.[15] However, this study also demonstrated that there were obstacles that prevented adequate access to medical information, and mainly to scientific journals, which were chosen as the most preferred source of information.

In an era of rapidly evolving scientific knowledge, immediate access to the most recent information, through online scientific journals, is not only required for research activities but also necessary for providing high-quality clinical care to patients. The excessive cost of journal subscriptions, that was once deemed to be an obstacle preventing access to information in primarily low-income countries, has recently arisen as a problem in developed countries.[16]

In this regard, an open access publishing system might be beneficial in providing free and equal access to current scientific literature. The era of open online access journals (OAJ) began in the late 1990s, concurrent with the growth of the internet, and there are now more than 10,000 OAJs.[17]

The key advantage of OAJs is their free access to articles, without the requirement of a journal subscription; therefore, OAJs can provide access to scientific literature for psychiatric trainees without institutional journal subscriptions, and for early career psychiatrists working in private practice with no institutional resources. Moreover, OAJs give young investigators an opportunity to share their work with a wider audience, thereby increasing the chance of their work being known and cited.

Notwithstanding its advantages, OAJs have been criticized for the requirement to pay for publication costs, which might be unaffordable for young investigators. Moreover, it has been argued that the 'pay to publish' system creates a conflict of interest for editors of OAJs arising from the financial gain per article which, in turn, might lead to a decline in overall quality through a lax peer-review process.[18] Indeed, a spoof study submitted to 304 OAJs was accepted for publication by 157 of them, even though the study had serious methodological and ethical flaws.[19] This experiment showed considerable diversity in the quality of open access journals. However, it might be argued that traditional peer-review journals, and particularly less prestigious ones, suffer from the same problem. In addition, even high-profile journals can have their own editorial biases by, for example, selecting articles not only on their methodology but also on their foreseen citation impact.

Recently, the USA and the UK have undertaken an initiative to make taxpayer-funded research articles freely available to readers.[20,21] Together with the rise of open access publishing, this initiative has made traditional peer-review journals revise their publishing policy by providing open access options for authors. In addition, the World Health Organization (WHO), together with the major publishers, initiated the Health InterNetwork Access to Research Initiative (HINARI programme) to help low- and middle-income countries to gain free or low-cost access to one of the largest collections of medical literature.[22]

Overall, online access to medical journals is one of the most important necessities for continuing medical education and professional development; however, it appears that trainees in low-income countries and early career psychiatrists with no affiliation to wealthy institutions struggle to access medical journals. Given current conditions, on-line OAJs offer a unique and practical opportunity to follow recent advances in psychiatry, albeit with some concerns over the quality of the peer-review process.

E-learning and professional development

Definitions and brief history

The term 'e-learning' refers to the use of internet technologies to enhance knowledge and performance (Box 14.1). E-learning is considered a useful tool in medical education at both undergraduate and postgraduate levels because it can help with the achievement of those learning objectives required to reach competency[23] and with maintaining competencies during postgraduate professional development. Evidence of e-learning application to postgraduate training and professional development is currently limited, but growing. The authors have therefore, where necessary, focused on and extrapolated from the medical undergraduate literature and from other fields.

Box 14.1 Definitions

E-learning: refers to the use of internet technologies to deliver knowledge. E-learning is also called web-based learning, online learning, distributed learning, computer-assisted instruction, or internet-based learning.[23]

Learning object: any grouping of materials that is structured in a meaningful way and is tied to an educational objective.[39]

MOOC: massive open online course offering a collection of online resources—typically, a series of video or multimedia lectures following a predefined schedule of weekly topics, and associated work. Classified into cMOOCs and xMOOCs.[24]

cMOOCs: connectivist MOOCs, emphasizing 'creation, creativity, autonomy, and social networked learning'. cMOOCs focus on knowledge creation and generation.

xMOOCs: a more traditional, teacher-centred learning approach, with content presented through short video lectures and learning tested through quizzes. xMOOCs focus on knowledge duplication.

Podcast: a multimedia file, mainly audio or video, distributed over the internet. These can be downloaded to a personal computer or a mobile device.

Historically, there have been two common e-learning types: distance learning and computer-assisted instruction. Distance learning uses information technologies to deliver instruction to learners at remote locations from a central site. Computer-assisted instruction (also called computer-based learning and computer-based training) uses computers to aid in the delivery of stand-alone multimedia packages for learning and teaching. These two modes have been subsumed under the term 'e-learning' by the integrating technology of the internet. More recently, with the advent of massive open online courses (MOOCs; Box 14.2), the potential for collectivism, feedback, assessment, and other interactions has opened up new ways of learning.[24]

Box 14.2 MOOC resources

◆ https://www.futurelearn.com/—brings together content from 12 different institutions. The involved universities are Birmingham, Bristol, Cardiff, East Anglia, Exeter, King's College London, Lancaster, Leeds, Southampton, St Andrews, Warwick, as well as the Open University.

◆ http://www.coursetalk.com—a search, discovery, rating, and sharing site for learners to explore a broad array of online courses.

◆ https://www.edx.org/—edX offers interactive online classes and MOOCs from the world's best universities including the Massachusetts Institute of Technology, Harvard, Berkeley, University of Texas, and the Karolinska Institutet (https://www.edx.org/school/kix).

◆ https://www.coursera.org/—an education platform that partners with top universities and organizations worldwide, to offer courses online for anyone to take, for free.

◆ http://www.france-universite-numerique.fr/moocs.html—French MOOC collection.

◆ https://iversity.org/—German MOOC collection.

◆ http://www.jhsph.edu/departments/mental-health/prospective-students-and-fellows/online-and-continuing-education/moocs.html—Johns Hopkins School of Public Health.

◆ http://online.stanford.edu/courses/topic/9—Stanford University's online medicine courses.

◆ http://in2mentalhealth.com/2013/06/12/trainings-and-short-courses-in-global-mental-health-and-mhpss/—training and short courses in global mental health and mental health and psychosocial support (MHPSS).

◆ http://www.moocsuniversity.org/academic-mooc-pathways.html—MOOCs University partners with accredited higher education institutions worldwide to create 'MOOCs to academic certification and degree' pathways for the serious MOOC learner.

◆ http://www.mooc-list.com/—MOOC List is an aggregator (directory) of MOOCs from different providers.

Advantages of e-learning

The role of e-learning in postgraduate professional development is evolving as the role of educators and the expectations of learners changes. An emphasis in medical and postgraduate education on lifelong learning and competency-based education has encouraged educators to move away from merely delivering knowledge to becoming 'facilitators of learning and assessors of competency'.[25]

E-learning offers a solution to the challenges of increasing medical knowledge, decreasing time available, and decentralization of medical care. It does so by providing an efficient way of delivering both continuing medical education and postgraduate training to many geographically dispersed users. It is also considered relatively easy to update and standardize content, improve learning delivery, measure outcomes, and enhance accountability.[23]

E-learning enables learners to use the tool at a convenient time and place and to control the learning sequence. It can therefore be personalized according to an individual's learning style and working life commitments. There is also evidence that internet-based learning is cost effective and achieves higher learner satisfaction scores than more traditional learning methods.[23,26]

Automated tracking and reporting of learners' e-learning activity and assessment of outcomes may reduce the administrative burden on educators.[27] Cost savings related to e-learning may include travel, accommodation, lecture rooms, and time away from the workplace.

E-learning technologies offer educators new opportunities to use adult learning theory in their teaching. This theory states that adults learn by relating new learning to past experiences, by linking learning to specific needs, and by the practical application of learning.[27]

By personalizing learning, allowing flexibility and opportunistic learning, enhancing learner participation, and offering interaction and feedback, a well-designed e-learning system can enhance engagement and interest, improve knowledge acquisition and retention, and improve attitudes in learners. Interactivity offers a stronger learning stimulus by focusing on active learner-centred teaching rather than a passive teacher-centred model. E-learning has demonstrated evidence of improved content utilization, knowledge retention, motivation, and engagement.[28]

Limitations of e-learning

E-learning is still currently closer to a traditional lecture than a clinical setting. However, with its development, the use of patients (or actors) in simulated clinical scenarios, followed by robust assessment of outcomes, may improve learning. It may be that knowledge, skills, and attitudes develop using e-learning, but the importance of 'real-life' clinical interaction should not be forgotten.

Where e-learning is the simple transfer of a traditional lecture into streaming video or audio, careful consideration will need to be given to improving engagement to enhance learning and encourage bidirectional learning and interaction. Principles of good lecturing (e.g. timing, pace, voice, volume, lighting, use of visual aids, opportunities for questions and answers) still apply; however, new teaching and technology skills may be needed in the e-learning arena.

Another disadvantage is dishonesty. Several studies have shown that medical students may report reduced attendance at online lectures, supported by studies which measured timing and interaction and showed significant levels of 'irregular activity'.[29,30] E-learning management systems should be robust so as to detect unusual behaviour, but also encourage real-time interaction because this enhances learning and is likely to reduce 'gaming' and dishonesty.

When using e-learning technologies in 'high-stake' examinations to obtain specific qualifications, security is a key issue, with programs to detect plagiarism becoming standard and rigorous efforts made to verify the identity of the candidate.[31]

Hare[31] notes that:

> attempting to deliver the whole [specialist examination] curriculum in this way might be a good starting point to convey factual information in a structured manner. However, the trainee would again lose the chance to hear local specialists' lectures on their personal areas of expertise . . . In any case, actually acquiring the necessary skills for psychiatric practice (eliciting symptoms, considering the differential diagnosis, formulating treatment plans and explaining them to patients in a variety of contexts) will always require considerable experience with real patients.

The author also notes that getting informed consent to use online video clips of patients demonstrating psychiatric signs and symptoms would be problematic.

Another major disadvantage of not being in the same room is the loss of human interaction with the lecturer or patient. Eye contact, body language, gut feeling, awareness of feelings brought out by the patient (countertransference), and the potential for positive role modelling are all factors considered important in adult learning, and even more so in psychiatry which already has a recruitment and image problem.[32]

Finally, potential cost savings will need to be offset against the costs of technology and expertise needed in developing robust e-learning systems, and against the risks of learners 'gaming' e-learning systems to achieve results without actually learning.

MOOCs

MOOCs have revolutionized access to learning. They are typically associated with high-quality institutions, and offer free or low-cost courses in a wide variety of subjects (see Box 14.2). The current emphasis is on undergraduate subjects, with the enrolment sometimes of tens of thousands of students from around the world.

Once the technology costs come down, MOOCs may be used for more specialist postgraduate training. Young psychiatrists will need to search for an appropriate course and may wish to get advice from their supervisors as to the appropriateness of the course and the value of investing the time.

Distance tutoring

Improved transport, as well as the decrease in its cost, has made it easier for students and teachers to cross borders and travel abroad. In addition to email communications, online conference tools like Skype allow easy and free contact between two people based anywhere in the world, and online storage services give the opportunity to work on shared documents. It is therefore now possible for students to receive online tutoring. This phenomenon expands the range of possibilities for students and teachers, and develops links between institutions, while keeping continuity in professional development and medical education.

Continuing professional development—what to expect from e-learning

Notwithstanding the advantages and limitations discussed, e-learning is growing. Continuing professional development (CPD) through e-learning is available in many countries. The main advantages are the lower cost compared to traditional CPD; high-quality, easy online access; assessments; and provision of evidence (e.g. a printed certificate).

A meta-analysis focusing on e-learning in the health professions has been conducted by Cook et al.[33] From the 201 eligible studies, effect sizes of knowledge and skills were large for e-learning, when compared with no intervention, but were small when compared to traditional teaching, suggesting a similar effectiveness. A more recent review showed that in comparison with other instruction, technology-enhanced simulation was associated with small to moderate positive effects.[34]

E-learning for CPD or continuing medical education (CME) has been more specifically reviewed by Wutoh et al.[35] They found, from 16 eligible studies, that internet-based CME programmes were just as effective in imparting knowledge as traditional formats of CME. However, the authors commented that, as most traditional CME courses fail to change physician practices, little is known as to whether the positive changes in knowledge shown with e-learning are translated into changes in practice.

An example of streaming lectures and slide shows is available through the European Psychiatric Association (EPA) website. The EPA has developed an online offering of lectures delivered by senior psychiatrists at recent EPA conferences, along with access to their PowerPoint slides. They are published on the European Psychiatric Network (http://europsychiatric.com/; Fig. 14.1). Similarly, the World Psychiatric Association offers online videos of lectures from some of the most prominent psychiatrists in the world (http://www.wpanet.org/videoIndex.php). The Royal College of Psychiatrists in the UK chose to set up its own independent CPD website in 2007 to provide learning materials designed for trained psychiatrists (http://www.rcpsych.ac.uk/workinpsychiatry/cpd.aspx). It now offers podcasts and interactive multimedia modules, for an annual subscription well below the cost of a day's attendance at a conference.[31] The American Psychiatric Association has also developed a comprehensive website providing CME courses for psychiatrists (http://www.apaeducation.org/).

When considering which e-learning CPD provider to access, readers may wish to compare the offerings against the following criteria:

- Ease of access and use
- Languages
- Automated record of learning
- Quality of associated institution
- Acceptability by national psychiatric or medical regulator (accreditation)
- Cost
- Time commitment

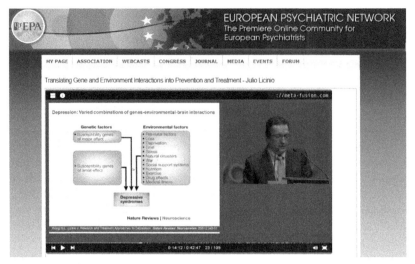

Fig. 14.1 EPA conference lectures online.
Reproduced from the European Psychiatric Association, with permission from the European Psychiatric Network.

Being an e-teacher

Developing an e-learning module combines traditional knowledge transfer, adult learning theory, and modern technology. Teachers can no longer rely merely on having good knowledge of the area of learning and an engaging smile. A successful e-teacher will consider how to use e-learning technology to enhance attention, learning, retention, interactivity, and then assess learner understanding and outcomes—all with learners whom they may never meet.

Content comprises all instructional material. The content in a 'learning object' can comprise documents, pictures, simulations, movies, sounds, etc. (For a more complete set of definitions, see Box 14.1).

Structuring learning objects in a meaningful way implies that the materials are arranged in a logical order, are related, and have a clear and measurable educational objective. E-teachers should consider best practice guidelines in developing learning objects (Box 14.3). A systematic review showed that interactivity, practice exercises, repetition, and feedback were associated with improved e-learning outcomes.[36]

Content must then be managed, delivered, and standardized. Use of a learning management system to facilitate storage, delivery, and tracking of e-learning, to automate administration and supervision, and to measure outcomes across the institution is recommended. There are numerous commercially available learning management systems available, each with their particular strengths, and this number is growing.

Standardization is needed when creating new e-learning material to promote usability and compatibility and to facilitate widespread use. An example from the USA is the Sharable Content Object Reference Model (SCORM). SCORM specifications prescribe the manner in which a learning management system handles e-learning.[37]

Box 14.3 Summary of design guidelines for authors of learning objects

Designing to enable learning

- Keep your educational goal in focus.
- Choose meaningful content that directly supports your educational goal.
- Present content in appropriate ways.
- Select appropriate activity structures.
- Consider assessment issues.

Designing the learner's experience: graphic design guidelines

- Each page or screen should be visually balanced.
- Use physical placement on the screen or page to establish and strengthen visual relationships between items.
- Select one or two visual elements and use them throughout the piece to create a sense of rhythm.
- If elements in your design are not the same, make them very different (not just slightly different) to create contrast.
- All elements should work together to create a harmonious whole.

Designing the learner's experience: usability guidelines

- Be consistent in the use of design elements, language, formatting, appearance, and functionality.
- Allow learners to control their interactions; give them the freedom to choose how to complete tasks.
- Follow established standards of design and use conventions that are familiar to learners.
- Simplify the design wherever possible, and stick to basic principles of aesthetics.

Designing for accessibility

- Design for device independence.
- Provide alternative formats for visual and auditory content.
- Allow learners to control moving content.

> ### Box 14.3 Summary of design guidelines for authors of learning objects (continued)
>
> ## Designing for reusability
>
> - Solve the copyright problem for others who want to reuse your materials.
> - Make sure your learning object is self-contained and can stand on its own.
> - Design your learning object so it may be used by a diverse audience.
>
> ## Designing for inter-operability: adding metadata
>
> - Include appropriate metadata in learning objects you author.
> - When you add learning objects to a collection or library, provide requested metadata information.
>
> ## Choosing a technology and development tools
>
> - Choose a technology and a tool your primary developer is comfortable using (or learning).
> - Choose a technology that supports the features you want to include in your learning object.
> - Choose a tool that is supported by your institution's instructional technology staff, if applicable.
> - Choose a tool you can afford.
>
> ## Care and feeding of your learning objects
>
> - House your learning objects on a secure, stable computer with permanent internet access.
> - Provide contact information, copyright and use licences, technical requirements, and version information. Keep these current.
> - Provide sample assignments, usage tips, links to related resources, and other support material.
>
> Source data from: Smith Rachel S., *Guidelines for authors of learning objects*. Copyright (2004), NMC: The New Media Consortium.

The future of e-learning

Technology will continue to advance, and access to available information will grow exponentially. Adaptive and collaborative learning are likely to be areas of growth in e-learning. Adaptive learning uses technology to assess skills, knowledge, and attitudes at the beginning of e-learning in order to deliver personalized and appropriate levels of teaching.[27]

In order to reduce the isolation of learners sitting before a screen, e-learning may help by developing collaborative learning technologies. These may allow for interaction (by blogs, forums, instant messaging, voice, or video). Interaction may be between learners across the globe, or with the teaching team, depending on whether the e-learning is 'live' or pre-recorded. Studies of collaborative learning in medicine have shown improved learner satisfaction, knowledge, self-awareness, changes in practice, and achievement of course directives.[38]

With the internet making knowledge available to all, the reputation of educational institutions increasingly rests with the quality of their assessments. Using electronic methods to assess students is in itself an evolving discipline. E-learning systems can incorporate diagnostic tests to pitch the content to the correct level, formative assessments to help the student check their understanding as they progress through an activity, and summative assessments to gain a credit and/or grade.[31]

Numerous research opportunities exist within the e-learning field including translation of e-learning to postgraduate (speciality) training; assessing effectiveness and cost effectiveness of different e-learning methods compared with traditional teaching; measuring and improving retention, outcomes, and quality; and incorporating e-learning into a 'blended-learning' strategy.[23]

Conclusions

In these days, social media are omnipresent in our lives, and offer a unique opportunity to share medical knowledge. Some of these tools have been available for years now, and there has therefore been time to find ways to share ideas and knowledge in the most efficient way.

E-learning developments, combined with the rapid pace of technological advancement, have the potential to revolutionize medical and postgraduate education.[23] E-learning can be increasingly individualized (adaptive learning), it can enhance interactions (collaborative learning), and it can alter the role of the teacher (from disseminator to facilitator and assessor).

It is hard to imagine a world without the internet and social media. The easy and free availability of so much information of variable quality offers both challenges and opportunities. As professionals, our role can be to engage with this process, focus on quality and evidence, and ensure learners achieve the most effective learning possible, to the ultimate benefit of our patients.

However, it is also difficult to imagine a world, especially for psychiatrists, without intense and prolonged face-to face encounters between professionals and patients, and between trainees and teachers. The type and degree of emotional involvement/reaction, with its positive and negative effects, cannot be provided by any computer-based interaction, the goal of which should be to complement interpersonal interactions.

References

1 **Luo J**. How to use social media—and when. *Psychiatric News* 2013; **48**(10):22–25. Available at: http://psychnews.psychiatryonline.org/newsarticle.aspx?articleid=1688791.

2 *Claireot's blog Using social media for professional development at the Leeds #SMSm-health. Claireot's blog.* 20 September 2012. Available at: http://engagecomms.co.uk/communications-tools/the-art-of-blogging-in-the-mental-health-sector-smsmhealth

3 **Appelbaum PS, Kopelman A**. Social media's challenges for psychiatry *World Psychiatr.* 2014; **13**(1):21–3.

4 General Medical Council. Doctors' use of social media. London, UK: General Medical Council; 2013.

5 Wikipedia; Facebook; 22 June 2014; http://en.wikipedia.org/wiki/Facebook.

6 **Devi S**. Facebook friend request from a patient? *Lancet* 2011; **377**(9772):1141–2.

7 Wikipedia; Twitter; 22 June 2014; http://en.wikipedia.org/wiki/Twitter.

8 Wikipedia; LinkedIn; 22 June 2014; http://en.wikipedia.org/wiki/Linkedin.

9 Wikipedia; ResearchGate; 22 June 2014; http://en.wikipedia.org/wiki/Researchgate.

10 **Ponce BA, Determann JR, Boohaker HA, Sheppard E, McGwin G Jr.**, Theiss S. Social networking profiles and professionalism issues in residency applicants: an original study-cohort study *Journal of Surgical Education* 2013; **70**(4):502–7.

11 **Henretty JR, Levitt HM**. The role of therapist self-disclosure in psychotherapy: a qualitative review *Clinical Psychology Review* 2010; **30**(1):63–77.

12 **McCartney M**. How much of a social media profile can doctors have? *British Medical Journal* 2012; **344**:e440.

13 **Koh S, Cattell GM, Cochran DM, Krasner A, Langheim FJ, Sasso DA**. Psychiatrists' use of electronic communication and social media and a proposed framework for future guidelines *Journal of Psychiatric Practice* 2013; **19**(3):254–63.

14 **DeJong SM, Benjamin S, Anzia JM, et al.** Professionalism and the internet in psychiatry: what to teach and how to teach it *Academic Psychiatry* 2012; **36**(5):356–62.

15 **Gama Marques J, Andlauer O, Banjac V, et al.** P-852—access to information in psychiatric training (ATIIPT) among the delegates to the European Federation of Psychiatric Trainees (EFPT) 2011 forum. *European Psychiatry* 2012; **27**(S1):1.

16 **Sample I**. Harvard University says it can't afford journal publishers' prices. *The Guardian*; April 2012. http://www.theguardian.com/science/2012/apr/24/harvard-university-journal-publishers-prices

17 **Lebert M**. DOAJ offers 10,000 open access journals from 124 countries in 51 languages; 11 December 2013; http://marielebert.wordpress.com/2013/12/11/doaj/.

18 **Balon R**. Perilous terra incognita—open-access journals *Academic Psychiatry* 2014; **38**(2):221–3.

19 **Bohannon J**. Who's afraid of peer review? *Science* 2013; **342**(6154):60–5.

20 **Butler D**. US seeks to make science free for all. *Nature* 2010; **464**(7290):822–3.

21 **Corbyn Z**. White House petitioned to make research free to access; 25 May 2012; http://www.nature.com/news/white-house-petitioned-to-make-research-free-to-access-1.10723.

22 WHO; HINARI Access to Research in Health Programme; 22 June 2014; http://www.who.int/hinari/en/.

23 **Ruiz JG, Mintzer MJ, Leipzig RM**. The impact of E-learning in medical education. *Academic Medicine* 2006; **81**(3):207–12.

24 **Siemens G**. MOOCs are really a platform; 25 July 2012; http://www.elearnspace.org/blog/2012/07/25/moocs-are-really-a-platform/.

25 **Chodorow S**. Educators must take the electronic revolution seriously *Academic Medicine* 1996; **71**(3):221–6.

26 **Bandla H, Franco RA, Simpson D, Brennan K, McKanry J, Bragg D**. Assessing learning outcomes and cost effectiveness of an online sleep curriculum for medical students *Journal of Clinical Sleep Medicine* 2012; **8**(4):439–43.

27 Gibbons A., Fairweather P., Gibbons A., Fairweather P. Computer-based instruction. In: *Training and retraining: a handbook for business, industry, government, and the military* (eds. Tobias S, Fletcher JD, American Psychological Association's Division of Educational Psychology). USA: Macmillan Reference; 2000; pp. 410–42.

28 Clark D. Psychological myths in e-learning. *Medical Teacher* 2002; **24**(6):598–604.

29 Lanier M. Academic integrity and distance learning. *Journal of Criminal Justice Education* 2006; **17**:244–61.

30 Bigeni J, Bigeni S, Balzan M. E-learning: are all users in front of the computer all the time? *Journal of European CME* 2013; **2**(22826).

31 Hare E. E-learning for psychiatrists. *Psychiatric Bulletin* 2009; **33**:81–3.

32 Farooq K, Lydall GJ, Bhugra D. What attracts medical students towards psychiatry? A review of factors before and during medical school. *International Review of Psychiatry* 2013; **25**(4):371–7.

33 Cook DA, Levinson AJ, Garside S, Dupras DM, Erwin PJ, Montori VM. Internet-based learning in the health professions: a meta-analysis. *Journal of the American Medical Association* 2008; **300**(10):1181–96.

34 Cook DA, Brydges R, Hamstra SJ, et al. Comparative effectiveness of technology-enhanced simulation versus other instructional methods: a systematic review and meta-analysis. *Simulation in Healthcare* 2012; **7**(5):308–20.

35 Wutoh R, Boren SA, Balas EA. E-learning: a review of internet-based continuing medical education. *Journal of Continuing Education in the Health Professions* 2004; **24**(1):20–30.

36 Cook DA, Levinson AJ, Garside S, Dupras DM, Erwin PJ, Montori VM. Instructional design variations in internet-based learning for health professions education: a systematic review and meta-analysis. *Academic Medicine* 2010; **85**(5):909–22.

37 Fallon C, Brown S. *e-Learning Standards: A Guide to Purchasing, Developing, and Deploying Standards-Conformant E-Learning Boca Raton; St. Lucie press*; 2002.

38 Wiecha JM, Gramling R, Joachim P, Vanderschmidt H. Collaborative e-learning using streaming video and asynchronous discussion boards to teach the cognitive foundation of medical interviewing: a case study *Journal of Medical Internet Research* 2003; **5**(2):e13.

39 *Elusive vision: challenges impeding the learning object economy (a white paper).* San Francisco: Macromedia Inc; 2003.

Chapter 15

The philosophical basis of psychiatry

Nicholas Deakin, Dinesh Bhugra, and Giovanni Stanghellini

Case study: applying some structure

Stephanie was reflecting on her years as a trainee psychiatrist, and the most challenging patient experiences she had encountered. She thought about how much she had appreciated having a senior consultant with whom she could discuss patients' treatment plans or to whom she could refer with ease for a senior opinion when she had a dilemma deciding on the best way forward. Now she had recently started working as a consultant psychiatrist, she was increasingly being telephoned by her juniors when they faced ethical dilemmas. In the past month, she had had one trainee traumatized by unwanted advances from a manic patient, a new trainee who was added on Facebook by her patient, and a colleague who wanted advice when detaining a patient with a severe eating disorder. It was not until she read up about different ethical theories and ways of tackling dilemmas in practice that she could offer structured, logical advice to her colleagues, which she herself could find invaluable when faced with ethical challenges at work.

Introduction

In basic terms, ethics concerns 'several different ways of examining and understanding the moral life.'[1] Philosophically speaking, living a moral life involves following norms about what is right and wrong, which are so commonly upheld by society that 'they form a stable (although incomplete) social agreement.'[1] Robertson contends that when a professional group, who practice a set of 'virtues' to promote public good, asserts these norms, then they are accredited with the professional autonomy and ability to self-regulate.[2]

The moral deliberations in psychiatry require an awareness of ethical theories, professional guidelines, and relevant legislation. We will aim to give an overview of these in this chapter, but readers should familiarize themselves with their own local statutory law and professional guidelines. Also, they must be aware that conflict between different values is indigenous to human affairs, and this includes within psychiatry. Referral to a given ethical theory cannot be used as a way to escape personal moral responsibility.

Mason and Laurie argue that while decisions regarding healthcare for physical conditions often depend largely on patient consent, for the psychiatrist, they often have to 'treat the unwilling.'[3] The importance of mental health treatment to wider society is also integral to this thinking, so scholars such as Bartlett argue that such treatment involves social control, and the duty of the law is to determine when this can be justified.[4]

This chapter seeks to explain key ethical theories and their philosophical basis, professional guidelines, and mental health law principles, to help aid decision making during the inevitable ethical dilemmas we may face as part of our work. It is in this way that we can look after the most vulnerable members of society in a manner that is right, proper, and justifies the trust that the public put in psychiatrists.

Ethics in psychiatry: guidelines for doctors and psychiatrists

A major aspect of professionalism is about self-regulation, which has a moral and ethical aspect. This has been the case in medicine for millennia. Since the time of Hippocrates in the fifth century BC, doctors have been expected to comply with codes of practice that seek to build public trust through commitment to patient care and professionalism. In the words of the original Hippocratic Oath, used for centuries, doctors pledged that they would 'follow that system of regimen which, according to my ability and judgement, I consider for the benefit of my patients, and abstain from whatever is deleterious and mischievous.'[5] Beauchamp and Childress comment that this approach does not offer help in contemporary ethical dilemmas such as truthfulness, confidentiality, research ethics, and the distribution of limited resources.[1] This prompted them to propose a new theory of morality, now commonly known as the 'four principles approach', that will be discussed in this chapter. The World Medical Association (WMA) attempted to update the Hippocratic Oath for modern medical practice in the Declaration of Geneva (2004), with a focus on changing patient expectations away from paternalism and towards a shared decision-making approach.[6]

Psychiatry is one of the medical specialties where the clinician has the legal authority to detain and treat patients who may be seen as at risk to themselves and to others. This special context and treatments used by psychiatrists have led scholars to propose that ethical practice as a psychiatrist commands special principles and practice. The American founders of bioethics, Beauchamp and Childress, note that the need for patient autonomy to be curtailed by other ethical principles or for the protection of others gives rise to unique challenges.[3] Radden highlights the vulnerability of patients with mental health issues, the special contribution of the therapeutic relationship towards treatment outcome, and the need to bring about change to character and behaviour.[7,8]

The code of ethics of the professional body for psychiatrists in the UK (the Royal College of Psychiatrists) draws on guidance from the WMA, the American Academy for Psychiatry and the Law, and the Royal Australian and New Zealand College of Psychiatrists (Box 15.1). This code comprises 12 key duties ascribed to psychiatrists to safeguard good ethical practice and the respect that society has for psychiatrists.

Box 15.1 The Royal College of Psychiatrists' (UK) code of ethics

1 Psychiatrists shall respect the essential humanity and dignity of every patient.

2 Psychiatrists shall not exploit patients' vulnerability.

3 Psychiatrists shall provide the best attainable psychiatric care for their patients.

4 Psychiatrists shall maintain the confidentiality of patients and their families.

5 Psychiatrists shall seek valid consent from their patients before undertaking any procedure or treatment.

6 Psychiatrists shall ensure patients and their carers can make the best available choice about treatment.

7 Psychiatrists shall not misuse their professional knowledge and skills, whether for personal gain or to cause harm to others.

8 Psychiatrists shall comply with ethical principles embodied in national and international guidelines governing research.

9 Psychiatrists shall continue to develop, maintain, and share their professional knowledge and skills with medical colleagues, trainees, and students, as well as with other relevant health professionals and patients and their families.

10 Psychiatrists have a duty to attend to the mental health and well-being of their colleagues, including trainees and students.

11 Psychiatrists shall maintain the integrity of the medical profession.

12 Psychiatrists shall work to improve mental health services and promote community awareness of mental illness and its treatment and prevention, and reduce the effects of stigma and discrimination.

Source data from: Royal College of Psychiatrists, Good Psychiatric Practice: Code of Ethics. College Report CR186 Copyright (2014).

The ethical theory underpinning psychiatric practice

In the next sections, we summarize the major ethical theories that should be considered in ethical decision making, together with the philosophical basis for these. We have also attempted to highlight the key benefits and limitations of each group of theories when applied to psychiatric ethics. For a full critique of theories, we recommend readers to refer to ethics textbooks, journal articles, or specific books on mental health ethics.

Principlism

The work of Beauchamp and Childress has been most influential in developing ethical reasoning for clinicians in the twenty-first century. They propose that the most ethically correct discourse is determined by the relative contributions of the principles of respect for patient autonomy, beneficence, non-maleficence, and justice—as defined in Box 15.2.

Box 15.2 The four principles according to Beauchamp and Childress

- **Respect for autonomy**: to value the decision-making capability of autonomous persons to facilitate reasoned, informed choices
- **Beneficence**: to provide overall benefit when balancing benefits, risks, and burdens
- **Non-maleficence**: to avoid causing harm
- **Justice**: fairness in the distribution of risks and benefits

Source data from Beauchamp T, Childress J, Principles of Biomedical Ethics, p. 1, 2, 15, 6, Copyright (2009), Oxford University Press

This seeks to create a general moral framework to guide all ethical thinking. The four principles are each 'prima facie', which means that they must be maximized in every situation, unless there is conflict between the principles, at which point this should be specified and a balance achieved. The principle(s) with the most weight would have supremacy when making a decision.[1] The British Medical Association (BMA) suggests that when these principles are in conflict with each other, then 'beneficience comes more to the fore if the patient has impaired mental capacity.'[5]

Those who support these theories consider that the four principles approach allows justification and explanation of all universalizable norms of medical ethics—some go as far as saying that they 'constitute moral DNA.'[9] At the very least, the approach constitutes a useful instrument for psychiatrists to articulate the core clinical aspects of ethical dilemmas.[10] It has become the cornerstone of ethical teaching for students and young clinicians around the world.[11] However, even Beauchamp and Childress admit that the framework is 'sparse'[1] and, therefore, could lead different clinicians to different answers, even when they are equipped with an identical scenario. Also important is the relative size of the population who holds a view on the common morality, and their respective influence, with Lee maintaining that, in practical terms, the majority view always predominates.[12] Forensic psychiatrists in particular have argued that they often find themselves with conflicting professional duties—to the patient for their treatment, to staff in the forensic setting, and to reduce the risk to wider society.[13] The challenge of applying this theory to psychiatric practice has been emphasized by Beauchamp and Childress themselves, who noted that the treatment of 'the unwilling'[3] makes psychiatry unique.

The four principles approach can be used 'with astounding ineptitude or dazzling virtuosity'[14] but does offer a really useful checklist for clinicians—especially in their early years of practice—to ensure that they consider the key concepts that are central to medical ethics. Ideally though, the four principles will be used in conjunction with established professional judgement, an assessment of the social context,[11] and wider frameworks to reach moral conclusions in medical ethics.

Virtue ethics

Grounded in Aristotle's work, virtue ethics originally concerned the four cardinal virtues of courage, temperance, justice, and prudence.[2] He claimed true happiness was found with rational reasoning and that this should involve finding a medium between contrasting or alternative views.[15] In modern medicine, virtue ethics is more concerned with the virtuous characters of doctors rather than their actions or the outcomes of these. The BMA holds that these are self evidently 'an important part of what it means to be a good doctor' and that they highlight what society expects from doctors.[5] The professional codes of ethics that psychiatrists abide by have some basis in virtue ethics.

Virtue ethics is arguably impractical to apply in specific situations, particularly given the lack of guidance on moral norms.[5] It leaves doctors in a potentially frustrating position of seeking to act as idealized, ethical supermen,[16] with the pressure of contrasting expectations and conflict within ethical dilemmas. Principles, and rules, help foster collective decision making and ensure the public trust in mental health professionals is maintained. For these reasons, it is difficult for psychiatrists to act based on virtues alone, and scholars have concluded that other theories should be considered along with virtues when making ethical decisions.[17] Thus, it is crucial that training in psychiatry incorporates some of these other theories.

Deontology

In contrast to utilitarian approaches to ethics, which consider consequences, deontological theories focus on what duty purports what ought to be done. The theory was born out of the European Enlightenment, by Immanual Kant, who held that people should be free to make rational, moral choices that are right in themselves and based on 'good will'. A moral deed is one motivated exclusively by pure reason, free of any influence of natural inclinations. Kant defined the 'categorical imperative' as the necessary factor for universal moral law. These categorical imperatives demonstrate the need for universality and the importance of the action, not intentions or intended consequences. Box 15.3 contains formulations of Kant's categorical imperatives.

Box 15.3 Formulations of Kant's categorical imperatives

- Act only according to that maxim whereby you can at the same time will it should become a universal law

- Act as if the maxim of your action were to become through your will a universal law of nature

- Act in such a way that you treat humanity, whether in your own person or in the person of another, always at the same time as an end and never simply as a means

- The idea of the will of every rational being as a will that legislates universal law

Source data from Kant I, Groundwork for the Metaphysics of Morals. p. 421–431, Copyright (1785/1997), Cambridge University Press

Modern approaches, such as those by the Royal College of Psychiatrists, to produce codes of ethics, are grounded in deontological reasoning.[18] In theory, following the 12 ethical guidelines quoted earlier in this chapter will help psychiatrists negate challenging decisions. They stand, no matter what the context, though they still leave some room for individual interpretation. The idea that 'reason' is the marker of human function is integral to psychiatry, and central to psychiatric ethics.[20] This is a key strength of using the theory in mental health ethics. Indeed, scholars such as Warren have argued that one of the main issues facing psychiatrists (in comparison with doctors more generally) is that capacity to reason may be harmfully impaired for psychiatric patients.[19,20] At this point, a psychiatrist must aim to restore this capacity to reason and may only intervene with forced or involuntary treatment while it is impaired.[2]

Despite this, many others claim that deontology is fatally flawed as a theory. O'Neil lists several key problems.[21] Firstly, categorical imperatives are too abstract to facilitate action and are 'empty'. Secondly, the strict universal goals of deontology have been criticized as forming rigid and insensitive rules, which neglect human impulses and can be difficult to apply. Some claim this can reduce psychiatrists' actions to merely fulfilling their professional duties rather than acting out of any compassion or desire to relieve suffering.[2] Finally, like principlism, the theory can be criticized for offering little or no guidance on how to balance conflicting duties or in the case of when a wrong action is pursued.

Utilitarianism

Jeremy Bentham, the British Victorian social reformer, is known for articulating a consequentialist theory of ethics which determined that we should judge each action by how much utility results. He held that this was determined by maximizing the amount of pleasure within society, according to his 'hedonic calculus'. Thus, an action was deemed good if it maximized pleasure and minimized pain for the greatest number. Mill later iterated this theory to give relatively greater weight to higher-order pleasures (such as cultural or intellectual pleasures) than to lower-order or more primitive pleasures (such as satiety).[22]

On the one hand, utilitarianism appeals to the scientific mind. It fits well with approaches to public policy,[23] where it is politically advantageous to maximize benefits to the majority. It has an 'instrumental value' in psychiatric decision making.[20] However, it is difficult to ascribe weight to, and balance, preferences. The focus on outcomes may lead to disregard for common morality and professional guidelines if greater overall benefits may result from ignoring these.[5] Furthermore, there are problems around unexpressed preferences (which clinicians may be unaware of) and granting harmful preferences.[24] It also commands that physicians function entirely rationally, forgetting any human connection with the patients, and may involve actually harming a disadvantaged group, such as those with mental illnesses, for the sake of the majority. These criticisms are well summarized by Kymlicka:[27] 'When the question is whether to defend an oppressed majority against a small privileged elite, utilitarianism gives us a clear, progressive answer. But when the question is whether to defend an oppressed minority against a large, privileged majority, utilitarianism gives us vague and confusing answers.'

The consequences of moral decisions in psychiatry should not be forgotten but, as with principlism, the strong criticisms of taking a purely utilitarian approach mean that it should not alone form the de facto ethical reasoning methodology for psychiatrists or doctors generally.

Communitarian ethics

Communitarian approaches to ethics deflect many ethical decisions away from the individual towards consideration of what would be appropriate in the community generally. When applying this to psychiatric ethics, the British psychiatrists Fulford and Hughes suggest that a psychiatrist must tackle issues of personhood based on the social and cultural context of the encounter.[25] Robertson and Walter suggest that communitarianism requires consideration of 'the values constricted by psychiatrists, the factors that determine these values, as well as the multiple relationships the profession has in different contexts within its community . . . [accounting for] the influence of history, societal values, the law and culture.'[26] This presents problems when practices, such as the ostracizing of individuals with mania or female genital mutilation, are accepted by particular communities[5] even when they seem contrary to professional obligations and a wider sense of the common morality. The BMA also highlights concerns about conflict and discrimination within the group. On the other hand, the approach may be particularly helpful when considering public health, genetic disorders, and areas of community conflict.[5]

Narrative ethics

Narrative ethics holds that to solve any ethical dilemma, it is necessary to explore the story and individual context. It involves a holistic assessment of the patient's situation, including their life, social context, values, and medical experience.[5] Ideally, this would include the triangulation of views of family members and the multidisciplinary team. Its ideal aim is to become an exchange of views that admits no external referee, but only the responsibility shared by the partners to define the terms of one's own discourse. This reciprocal explication of one's own discourse, the exposition of the values at play in it, and the elucidation of the words through which one's position is expressed, paves the way to an exercise of cooperation during which no one view prevails over others. Its final aim is not validation or invalidation aimed at some form of consensus; rather, clarification aimed at coexistence. As Ricoeur states, it is 'a confrontation of opinions refereed by the effort of definition.'[27]

This approach will offer excellent clarification of the ethical issues, but lacks both structure to ensure all relevant factors are taken into account and any ethical framework for analysis or application. It should therefore be used in conjunction with other approaches to ethics in psychiatry.

The psychiatrist as a moral agent: reaching conclusions in ethical dilemmas

There is no consensus as to the exact approach that psychiatrists should take when approaching an ethical dilemma.[28,29] In reality, whether they do so consciously or not, most psychiatrists use approaches from all the theories discussed here when tackling everyday dilemmas. Attempting to tackle ethical problems using different philosophical approaches leads to consideration and balancing of all the relevant issues, and allows justification of actions and decisions to colleagues and patients. Given the profound ethical difficulties that psychiatrists will experience, Bloch and Green suggest that psychiatrists 'have no choice . . . but to respond as moral agents.'[31]

In the age of increased scrutiny of practice, acting as an independent moral agent does not, in itself, protect psychiatrists from litigation and damage to reputations. Using context-specific advice for psychiatrists (such as in the codes from the American Psychiatric Association, the Royal College of Psychiatrists, or the Royal Australian and New Zealand College of Psychiatrists) or international codes of ethics (such as guidance from the World Psychiatry Association), together with advice from your regulator and medical protection society, will ensure safe, effective, and acceptable practice.

Mental health law and psychiatry

The World Health Organization (WHO) states that mental health law can protect human rights, improve the provision of psychiatric services, and promote the integration of those with mental illness into communities.[29] Law is a lever for ensuring that the public can accept decisions which limit the autonomy of patients with mental health disorders.[30] Many argue that mental health law is created to minimize the tension between legalism—the need to put limits on the power of mental health professionals—and patient autonomy.[31] Despite this, 25% of countries lack mental health law. The other 75% have either distinct mental health law acts or sections of law with provisions for those with mental health needs.[32] The WHO has produced ten basic principles of mental health law that are essentially based on analysis of relevant law around the world. They are reproduced here, with suggestions for implementation, and offer a useful framework for practice (Table 15.1).

There is not the space here to cover the mental health law of each jurisdiction, although psychiatrists need to be familiar with this. Instead, as an example of one approach, we will briefly summarize how involuntary treatment and informed consent are dealt with in the England and Wales Mental Health Act and Mental Capacity Act. (These two topics are covered in detail in Chapters 32 and 21, respectively.)

Involuntary treatment

The Mental Health Act 1983 (amended in 2007) defines when involuntary treatment may be permissible. Obviously, most patients' interactions are purely voluntary—with a patient agreeing to trial a medication or talking therapy, or to be admitted to an inpatient unit. Where involuntary assessment is required, the Act sets out what is permissible to compulsorily admit someone for assessment or treatment. The provisions are designed to permit safeguards for patients and ensure their liberty is not unnecessarily curtailed. For example, for many of the longer detainment periods, review panels and second opinions from specially approved doctors are required. These safeguard provisions are even more stringent for procedures like electroconvulsive therapy, brain surgery, and hormone implantation.

Table 15.1 The WHO ten basic principles of mental health law

WHO principle	Proposed ways for clinicians to achieve this
Everyone should benefit from measures to promote their mental well-being and to prevent mental disorders	◆ Promote behaviours which contribute to enhancing mental well-being ◆ Identify and act on the causes of mental illness
Everyone in need should have access to basic mental healthcare	◆ Use evidence-based practice ◆ Offer culturally appropriate care ◆ Ensure primary care provision includes basic mental healthcare ◆ Ensure care is geographically accessible, including psychotropic medications and talking therapy
Mental health assessments should be made in accordance with international best practice	◆ Promote quality training ◆ Refrain from using non-clinical criteria to assess risk ◆ Use holistic assessment
Persons with mental health disorders should be provided with healthcare which is the least restrictive	◆ Use community resources where appropriate ◆ Train for crisis management
Consent is required before any type of interference with a person can occur	◆ Always presume patients have capacity ◆ Make context-dependent capacity assessments ◆ Given patient's verbal and written information regarding treatment options ◆ Take advance, personal, and family wishes into account
When a patient finds it difficult to understand the implications of treatment, they should be able to seek advice from others	◆ Ensure patients are aware of the role of health advocates, family members, social workers, or lawyers
Decisions made by officials (e.g. judges) or surrogate (representative) decision makers, and by healthcare providers, should be open to appeal	◆ Ensure you understand the legal system in your country, and the room for appeal ◆ Involve professional bodies where necessary

Source based on: Reproduced from Mental Health Law: Ten Basic Principles, Copyright (1996) with permission from the World Health Organization.

Informed consent

In the UK, as in most countries, informed consent is a requirement before assessment or treatment. The only exception is when a person lacks capacity to make a decision that might have legal consequences, such as agreeing to treatment, when the Mental Capacity Act (2005) applies. For this to be the case, the patient must be 'unable to make a decision for himself' regarding a specific issue, at a specific time 'because of an impairment of, or a disturbance in the functioning of, the mind or the brain'.[32] A study by Owen et al. in 2008 found that 60% of all patients admitted to psychiatric hospitals lacked capacity, as did over 85% of compulsorily detained hospital patients.[33] As clinicians, we must be aware of this, and also able to accurately assess a patient's capacity. The BMA has summarized the statute law and case law, and recommends that a formal assessment of capacity relies on a clinician being able to establish that a person:

1 Understands what the treatment is, its purpose and nature, and why it is being proposed

2 Understands its principal risks, benefits, and alternatives

3 Understands, in broad terms, what will be the consequences of not receiving the proposed treatment

4 Retains the information for long enough to make an effective decision

5 Weighs up and balances the information

6 Makes a free choice (being free from undue pressure or coercion).[5]

Case study: Law in action - Re. C (adult refusal of treatment), Court of Appeal 1994

68-year-old C suffered from paranoid schizophrenia, having both grandiose and persecutory delusions. He believed that he was a highly successful, internationally renowned physician. He was transferred to a general hospital during a period of imprisonment in a secure hospital after he developed severe gangrene in his foot. The surgeon believed that C had an 85% imminent chance of dying if the leg was not removed, but the patient was adamant that he did not want his foot amputating and would rather die with two legs than live with one. He maintained this, even though he knew he may die if he kept his leg, and was content to follow all other medical advice and treatments as long as his rejection of amputation was respected. The Court ruled that even though his schizophrenia did impact on his general capacity, he could understand the risks and benefits of keeping his leg, and had come to a decision. The hospital was therefore unable to remove his leg unless he changed his mind, now or in the future; and his conservative treatment was progressing well at the time of his hearing.

Conclusions

Successful psychiatrists are able to interweave their clinical acumen with awareness of the social, cultural, ethical, and legal considerations that affect patients. It is easy to focus on building clinical knowledge as a training psychiatrist, but these other factors are as important for successful, safe practice in union with patient preferences and the trust placed in the profession by society. In particular, as there is no dominant, universally agreed way to analyse ethical dilemmas, it is imperative that all psychiatrists have an awareness of the major ethical frameworks and are able to use these. National ethical guidance and the law as applied to mental health are important points of reference to ensure safe, defensible practice, as where patient autonomy is limited, the potential for claims of abuse is very high. More emphasis on this and case-based small group or individual study should be incorporated into psychiatric training to ensure that the profession continues to command respect from society at large and that trainees feel equipped for the challenges they will face in practice.

References

1 **Beauchamp T, Childress J**. *Principles of biomedical ethics*. New York: Oxford University Press; 2009, pp. 1, 2, 6, 15.

2 **Robertson M**. *An overview of psychiatric ethics*. New South Wales: Health Education and Training Institute; 2009, pp. 6, 14.

3 **Mason J, Laurie G**. *Mason and McCall Smith's law and medical ethics* (8th edn). Oxford: Oxford University Press; 2010.

4 **Bartlett P**. The test of compulsion in mental health law: capacity, therapeutic benefit and dangerousness as possible criteria. *Med Law Rev* **11**; 2003:326–52.

5 British Medical Association (BMA) Medical Ethics Department. *Medical ethics today*. London: Wiley-Blackwell; 2012, pp. 10–12, 136, 887.

6 World Medical Association (WMA). *Declaration of Geneva*. Geneva: WMA; 2006.

7 **Radden J**. Notes towards a professional ethics for psychiatry. *Austral New Zeal J Psychiat* 2002; **36**:52–9.

8 **Radden J**. Psychiatric ethics. *Bioethics* 2002; **16**:397–411.

9 **Gillon R**. Ethics needs principles—four can encompass the rest—and respect for autonomy should be 'first among equals'. *J Med Ethics* 2003; **29**:307–12.

10 **Robertson M, Ryan C, Walter G**. Overview of psychiatric ethics III: principles-based ethics. *Australas Psychiat* 2007; **15**(4):281–6.

11 **Ebbesen M, Anderson S, Pederson B**. Further development of Beauchamp and Childress' theory based on empirical ethics. *J Clinic Res Bioeth* 2012; S6:e001.

12 **Lee M**. The problem of 'thick in status, thin in content' in Beauchamp and Childress' principlism. *J Med Ethics* 2010; **36**:527.

13 **Sen P, Gordon H, Adshead G, Irons A**. Ethical dilemmas in forensic psychiatry: two illustrative cases. *J Med Ethics* 2007; **33**(6):337–41.

14 **Sokol D**. Sweetening the scent: commentary on 'What principlism misses'. *J Med Ethics* 2009; **35**:233.

15 Aristotle. *The nicomachean ethics*. Oxford: Oxford University Press; 1998.

16 **Dyer A**. *Ethics and psychiatry: toward a professional definition*. New York: American Psychiatric Press; 1988.

17 **Robertson M, Walter G**. Overview of psychiatric ethics II: virtue ethics and the ethics of care. *Australas Psychiat* 2007; **15**(3):207–11.

18 **Robertson M, Morris K, Walter G**. Overview of psychiatric ethics V: utilitarianism and the ethics of duty. *Australas Psychiat* 2007; **15**(5):402–10.

19 **Wakefield J**. The concept of mental disorder: on the boundary between biological facts and social values. *Am Psychol* 1992; **47**:373–88.

20 **Wakefield J**. Disorder as harmful dysfunction: a conceptual critique of DSM-III-R's definition of mental disorder. *Psychol Rev* 1992; **99**:23–39.

21 **O'Neil O**. Kantian ethics. In: *A Companion to ethics* (ed. Singer P). Oxford: Blackwell; 1991, pp. 175–85.

22 **Bentham J**. *An introduction to the principles of morals and legislation*. London: Althone Press; 1970/1823.

23 **Robertson M, Walter G**. A critical reflection of utilitarianism as the basis for psychiatric ethics. *J Ethics Ment Heal* 2007; **2**(1):1–4.

24 **Kymlicka W**. *Contemporary political philosophy*. New York: Oxford University Press; 2001.

25 **Hughes J, Fulford K**. Hurly-burly of psychiatric ethics. *Austral New Zeal J Psychiat* 2005; **39**(11–12):1001–7.

26 **Robertson M, Walter G**. *Ethics and mental health: the patient, profession and community*. Florida: CRC Press; 2014, p. **64**.

27 **Ricoeur P**. *Anthropologie Philosophique*. Paris: Seuil; 2013, p. 124.

28 **Bloch S, Green S**. An ethical framework for psychiatry. *Br J Psychiat* 2006; **188**:7–12.

29 World Health Organization (WHO). *Mental health legislation and human rights: mental health policy and service guidance package. Geneva*: WHO; 2003.

30 **Golver-Thomas N**. *Reconstructing mental health law and policy*. London: Butterworths; 2002.

31 **Fennell P**. Inscribing paternalism in the law: consent to treatment and mental disorder. *J Law Soc* 1990; **17**:29–51.

32 Mental Capacity Act 2005: S2(1). London: Her Majesty's Stationery Office (HMSO).

33 **Owen G, Richardson G, David A, Szmukler G, Hayward P, Hotopf M**. Mental capacity to make decisions on treatment in people admitted to psychiatric hospitals: cross sectional study. *BMJ* 2008; **337**:448.

Chapter 16

How to build a strong therapeutic alliance in mental healthcare: things to do, things to avoid

Muj Husain, Claudia Palumbo, and Dinesh Bhugra

Case study: a case of different agendas

Farah is a psychiatrist in her second year of training. She had been seeing a patient, Samuel, who was suffering from depression, and as part of a holistic plan, medication was prescribed, alongside cognitive behavioural therapy (CBT). Farah suspected that Sam was not taking his medication and wondered whether he was experiencing side-effects. When reviewing Sam in clinic, Farah asked specifically about side-effects but he told her there were no problems at all. Farah felt Sam seemed distant. However, there were no immediate concerns, so Farah increased the dose of medication and arranged to review him again in a few weeks.

At the follow-up appointment, Farah asked if a senior colleague, Dr Ediae, could sit in to observe her and to offer feedback. Dr Ediae agreed and, after the encounter, discussed how things went. They both noticed Sam had seemed reticent but, again, he reported no problems with his treatment plan. One of Dr Ediae's suggestions for Farah was that the relationship between her and her patient seemed a bit strained and that she could try booking a longer appointment next time, with a view to exploring this further. Farah did this and started by asking Sam how he had been, as she usually did. Sam replied 'fine, I'm doing OK'. Farah then decided to explore more and asked him how he was finding their sessions. He said he had been finding them helpful and appreciated being able to talk about his problems. Farah then went on to what he thought about his illness.

Listening to Sam, it became apparent that he did not understand why he was having separate CBT sessions and had missed appointments. He wanted to see just one health professional, as he found building up trust difficult. It turned out that medication was not the issue after all. Farah realized that when she first saw Sam, she had made an assumption about what his concerns might be. She reflected on this and changed the way she approached her first encounters with patients, to focus more on their concerns and building up a shared understanding and agreement about the treatment plan.

In Sam's case, Farah was able to talk to Sam about the CBT and explain why he needed to see someone else. She also spoke to the CBT therapist afterwards; together, they were able to address Sam's concerns and help him re-engage with therapy. Farah was pleased to see that the next time she saw Sam, his symptoms had started to improve.

Introduction

The therapeutic relationship between the clinician and the patient is at the heart of engagement and treatment. Psychiatrists in particular use a number of strategies when offering treatment, with medication combined with talking therapies and social interventions. It is inevitable that in long- term chronic conditions, patients need supportive therapy as well. In addition, engaging carers and families is important. This engagement is strongly influenced by the patient's and the carers' explanatory models of what the patient is experiencing and from where else they may have sought help. In this chapter, we describe the concept of the therapeutic alliance, what it means, and factors which may be influencing this core activity of healthcare.

What is the therapeutic alliance?

The term 'therapeutic alliance' has often been used interchangeably with terms such as 'working relationship' or 'therapeutic relationship'. At its simplest, it is defined as a rational agreement or contract which supports a patient's treatment.[1] It has been described as the 'cornerstone of treatment in medicine' and is an essential part of the relationship between a patient or carer and their health professional (such as a doctor, care co-ordinator, or psychotherapist). The therapeutic alliance matters because the quality of the relationship we form with our patients is an important predictor of how our patients do. So, a better therapeutic alliance means that we are offering better care and better outcomes for patients.

Freud was the first to propose the concept of the therapeutic alliance as distinct from transference and counter-transference in a relationship.[2] He felt that there was an aspect of the relationship between the therapist and patient which was conscious, positive, and reality-based. This has since been recognized as an important part of the therapeutic relationship and is referred to as the 'therapeutic alliance'.

The key elements defining the therapeutic alliance are those aspects of the patient–health professional relationship which are collaborative, reality-based, non-transferential, and rooted in empathy. It may be explicit, but there are usually unspoken elements to the mutual understanding shared by a patient and health professional.

Bordin (1979) has usefully described the therapeutic alliance as having three components:[3]

1 **Bonds:** the reciprocal positive feelings the patient and health professional share with each other. These include mutual trust, regard, and confidence.

2 **Goals:** a set of targets or outcomes for the interaction endorsed, shared, and valued by the patient and health professional.

3 **Tasks:** both the health professional and patient must share beliefs and a commitment to undertake the tasks required of them as part of the therapeutic journey.

Although the concept has its theoretical roots in psychotherapy, the relationship we build with our patients, based on shared goals and mutual trust, is the key to all interactions between health professionals and their patients—from the inpatient psychiatric

Box 16.1 Where does the therapeutic alliance happen?

The setting in which we speak to patients has an impact on the relationship. It encompasses both external factors which influence the consultation and a set of expectations about what the consultation may involve. External factors include noise or distractions (e.g. in a busy emergency department), the degree of privacy and comfort, and even staffing levels on a ward. The expectations that come with a particular setting are likely to be different for healthcare professionals and patients, and may not always be immediately obvious. Many patients would feel more comfortable seeing a doctor in their own home but, for some, the home may be a place of current or past distress. It is important to be aware that the setting can influence the therapeutic relationship you are building. Here are a few tips:

◆ Take steps to minimize factors such as noise and other distractions.

◆ Ensure privacy and comfort wherever you can.

◆ Ask your patients what they expect and explain the purpose of the consultation and environment, particularly in relation to the setting, to the patient.

ward to psychodynamic therapy; from psychiatric assessments in an emergency department to the management of chronic mental illness over the course of months or years. Indeed, the concept is just as applicable outside of psychiatry and is relevant to all healthcare professionals—particularly as so much of medicine has a mental health component, but also because medicine is increasingly about the long-term management of chronic disease and lifestyle (Box 16.1).

Does the therapeutic alliance make a difference?

There is a considerable and growing body of evidence that the quality of the therapeutic alliance between patients and health professionals is a key predictor of clinical outcomes and the success of an intervention. Many psychotherapeutic modalities show similar rates of success: it has been proposed that the key 'ingredient' of psychotherapy (i.e. the factor that makes the difference) is not the type of therapy but the relationship and alliance between the patient and health professional.[4] This has been described as the 'pan-theoretical approach' to understanding the therapeutic alliance.

Research in this area is complicated because there are many methodological approaches to measuring the quality of a therapist–patient interaction. However, whatever scales or methods are used, the overall message from studies is that the therapeutic alliance really does make a difference. A meta-analysis by Horvath and Simonds[5], bringing together 20 data sets, found that there was a significant difference in patient outcomes. Further and more recent meta-analyses have reached the same conclusion.[6] Studies looking at specific modalities of therapy have demonstrated the importance of the therapeutic alliance in CBT, interpersonal psychotherapy, pharmacotherapy, and even in placebo groups receiving no formal therapy.[7,8]

Box 16.2 The first consultation

The results of an experimental study in the UK have shown that patients even pay great attention to how psychiatrists introduce themselves in the very first consultation. Providing information about what psychiatrists do, how long the consultation is likely to take, and what the potential outcomes might be, seems to have a substantial impact on a patient's perception of the psychiatrist and on the therapeutic alliance.

Source data from: British Journal of Psychiatry, 202, Priebe, S.; Palumbo, C.; Ahmed, S.; Strappelli, N.; Gavrilovic, J.J.; Bremner, S. How psychiatrists should introduce themselves in the first consultation: an experimental study, p. 459–62, Copyright (2013) The Royal College of Psychiatrists.

Although most studies have looked at the impact of the therapeutic alliance in psychotherapy, there are a number of reviews and studies demonstrating the importance of the alliance between health professionals and patients in other areas. Non-attendance at appointments, disengagement, and non-concordance with medication are significant therapeutic concerns. Frank and Gunderson[9] and Mitchell and Selmes[10] have shown a positive relationship between the alliance and treatment adherence. Similarly, Johansson and Eklund[11] have shown that the 'degree of helpfulness' perceived by the patient is a positive predictor of attendance at future appointments.

Interestingly, those studies which use patient and clinician perceptions of the quality of the therapeutic alliance as a predictor of outcomes tend to find that the patient's perceptions are more important, which again stresses how essential it is to listen to and address the concerns of our patients.

So the answer to the question of whether the therapeutic alliance makes a difference to outcomes is that it really does seem to matter. This would back up the common-sense perception that health professionals share that forming positive, meaningful, and trusting relationships with patients is an essential part of the job we do (see Box 16.2).

Building a good therapeutic alliance

The therapeutic alliance is a two-way relationship and requires engagement and responsibility from the patient and/or carer as well as from health professionals. However, there are many things that we, as health professionals, can do to help improve engagement with our patients (see Table 16.1).

Four groups of techniques to improve the therapeutic alliance have been described[12]:

1 Supportive—affirming the patient's experience
2 Exploratory—open questions, seeking clarification
3 Experiential and affect-focused—exploring and facilitating patients' feelings and emotions
4 Engaged and active relationship—active involvement, with feedback.

Table 16.1 Tips for building a therapeutic alliance

Things to do	Things to avoid
◆ Smile appropriately, make eye contact, use body language to convey that you are hearing.	◆ Not talking about the difficult things; we often avoid talking about areas where it is difficult to build a shared understanding (e.g. hallucinations and delusions).
◆ Listen to your patient and respond to what they tell you.	
◆ Be alert to your patient's non-verbal communication.	◆ Using professional terms or jargon; wherever possible, mirror the language used by the patient.
◆ Empathize with your patient - respond in a human way (think 'how would I react if told that a friend or colleague had just been given this bad news?'); likewise, use humour where appropriate.	◆ Looking rushed or preoccupied with other things—in a busy clinic, it is all too easy to forget the person in front of you when there are conflicting demands of teaching students, looking for information in guidelines, or searching through patient records.
◆ Address patient's concerns and take such concerns seriously.	
◆ Explain the rationale for medication or psychotherapy.	◆ Using too many closed questions. Focusing on the psychopathology or 'check-listing' symptoms can blind us to the context and possibly bigger issues. The key is getting the right balance between closed and open questions. This often involves starting with open questions and showing the patient you are actively listening to them, and moving towards closed questions later in the interview. Of course, the balance will always depend on the nature of the encounter—for example, a patient who tends to be more discursive or someone presenting with mania may need more closed questions, at an earlier stage.
◆ Ask your patients how they think and feel about their illness and symptoms.	
◆ Talk about side-effects from medication.	
◆ Allow your patients time to reach decisions.	
◆ Remember it is fine to disagree - be open about areas where there are differences in how you choose to understand the problem, seek to understand the patient's point of view, and concentrate on finding goals and tasks where there is shared agreement.	
◆ Be aware of the counter-transference and transference in your interaction with a patient. Be aware also of how you feel about the patient in an interview—this is an important indicator of the quality of the therapeutic alliance, and our own emotions towards patients (or what patients say about us) can signal potential problem areas that need addressing or that could spiral out of control if we are not careful.	◆ Judging your patients. Instead, try to understand and empathize with their point of view. If you do not understand something, ask them to explain.

The beginnings and endings of sessions and longer therapeutic relationships are especially important times for developing and maintaining the therapeutic alliance. At the early stages of treatment, a collaborative approach aimed at developing a shared understanding of the problem, goals, and management plan is essential. As sessions end, it is important to recheck with your patients—are they happy with what has been discussed? Do they have further questions or concerns? Do they understand the plan?

Explaining and discussing the rationale for treatment and the reasons for the next appointment help to improve both patient engagement with the treatment plan and attendance at the next appointment.

How to improve?

As we progress through our careers, lists of what we should and should not do in our encounters with patients can seem too simplistic. The interview and relationship we develop with our patients is the bread and butter of psychiatry, and it is what we do every day of our working lives. Speaking and listening to patients is a complex, nuanced, and subtle art, and as we progress, it becomes increasingly difficult to boil down our hard-earned wisdom to generalisms.

However, it is dangerous to assume that having acquired a certain level of experience, we know it all or cannot improve further on our communication skills. So, how can experienced clinicians and health professionals keep improving? There are two key steps that we should all integrate into our everyday practice: *feedback* and *reflection*.

Feedback has consistently been shown to be one of the most powerful interventions for changing behaviour.[13] As we progress through medical training, we often make use of role play and simulation to get constructive feedback on our interactions in clinical or therapeutic situations. These are important tools, and as we become more senior, seeking feedback from real-life encounters with patients is increasingly essential (and, unless we make a habit of it early in our careers, it risks becoming something that we do reluctantly, if at all).

One source of feedback is from our colleagues—other health professionals. Many health organizations offer structured tools to collect feedback from colleagues (e.g. the Mini-Peer Assessment Tool[14] which, in the UK, is essential for annual appraisal). When collecting feedback from others, explain why you are doing so, stress that you want constructive feedback to help you improve, choose a range of colleagues from different professional groups (from the cleaner to the consultant—everyone is important), and avoid choosing just the people you know will give you positive feedback.

To bring this principle of seeking feedback into the patient interaction, you may want to invite colleagues, particularly those experienced in medical education, to observe you with patients and to offer structured advice after the consultations. Try to make sure that the feedback you receive is immediate (as far as possible), structured, and makes specific recommendations for what you could do differently. These are factors that research has shown can improve the impact that feedback has on our behaviour.[15]

A second, and perhaps the most important source of feedback, is that received from the patients and carers. Patient experience and satisfaction has been shown to predict clinical effectiveness and outcomes—the more we listen to our patients and act to improve their satisfaction, the better our services.[16-18] This hinges on the therapeutic relationship. Collecting direct feedback from our patients is a crucial way of getting information on the quality of the therapeutic alliances we establish and of helping us to improve those alliances.

In recent years, there has an increasing recognition of and emphasis on the importance of patient feedback. In the UK the General Medical Council (GMC) has implemented a programme of 'revalidation' for all doctors, regardless of seniority, and collecting patient feedback forms is an essential part of this. There are also online tools available (e.g. 'I Want Great Care') for patients and carers to rate and review doctors, providing open, transparent, and timely feedback to doctors and healthcare organizations.[19] The emphasis on patient feedback is particularly important given that there is evidence that patient perceptions of the therapeutic alliance are one of the most useful measures of the quality of the alliance and predict patient outcomes and engagement.

Feedback is well and good, but how should we respond to comments and suggestions we seek from patients and colleagues? Reflective practice is the key to this, and obtaining feedback enables us to reflect. Kolb's cycle of reflective practice [20] still provides the best model for how to reflect. This describes a cycle in which learners gain concrete experience, observe and reflect (this is where feedback is important), conceptualize, and then actively experiment and integrate learning into practice.

Conclusions

The therapeutic alliance—a key part of our relationships with patients—is the cornerstone of all clinical practice. We can distinguish the therapeutic alliance from transference and counter-transference as a conscious, agreed 'pact' between the health professional and patient or carer. There is now plenty of evidence showing that the therapeutic alliance matters and that it has a real impact on patient outcomes. This chapter has summarized a number of key tips to help improve the therapeutic alliances we build with our patients. In particular, beginnings and endings of consultations are crucial points where a bit of extra thought and attention can help shape a positive alliance. Finally, the key 'take home message' is that we can all improve our communication and relationships with patients by seeking, reflecting on, and acting on feedback from colleagues and, especially, from patients.

References

1 **Hughes P, Kerr I**. Transference and countertransference in communication between doctor and patient. *Adv Psychiat Treat* 2000; **26**:57–64.

2 **Horvath AO, Luborsky L**. The role of the therapeutic alliance in psychotherapy. *J Consult Clin Psychol* 1993; **61**:561–73.

3 **Bordin ES**. The generalizability of the psychoanalytic concept of the working alliance. *Psychotherapy* 1979; **16**(3):252–60.

4 **Luborsky L**. Helping alliances in psychotherapy: the groundwork for a study of their relationship to its outcome. In: *Successful Psychotherapy* (ed. Cleghorn JL). New York: Brunner/Mazel; 1976, p. 92–116.

5 **Horvath AO, Simmonds BD**. Relation between working alliance and outcome in psychotherapy: a meta-analysis. *J Consult Clin Psychol* 1991; **38**:139–49.

6 **Ardito RB, Rabellino D**. Therapeutic alliance and outcome of psychotherapy: historical excursus, measurements, and prospects for research. *Frontiers Psychol* 2011; **2**:Article 270.

7 **Castonguay LG, Goldfried MR, Wiser S, Raue PJ, Hayes AM**. Predicting the effect of cognitive therapy for depression: a study of unique and common factors. *J Consult Clin Psychol* 1996; **64**(3):497–504.

8 **Krupnick JL, Sotsky SM, Simmens S, et al**. The role of the therapeutic alliance in psycho-therapy and pharmacotherapy outcome: findings in the National Institute of Mental Health Treatment of Depression Collaborative Research Program. *J Consult Clin Psychol* 1996; **64**(3):532–9.

9 **Frank A, Gunderson J**. The role of the therapeutic alliance in the treatment of schizophrenia: relationship to course and outcome. *Arch Gen Psychiat* 1990; **47**:228–36.

10 **Mitchell AJ, Selmes T**. Why don't patients take their medicine? Reasons and solutions in psychiatry. *Adv Psychiat Treat* 2007; **13**:336–46.

11 **Johansson H, Eklund M**. Helping alliance and early dropout from psychiatric out-patient care: the influence of patient factors. *Soc Psychiat Psychiat Epidem* 2006; **41**:140–7.

12 **Yakely J**. Psychodynamic psychotherapy: developing the evidence base. *Adv Psychiat Treat* 2014; **20**:269–79.

13 **Norcini J**. The power of feedback. *Med Educ* 2010; **44**:16–7.

14 **Archer JC, Norcini J, Southgate L, Heard S, Davies H**. Mini-PAT (peer assessment tool): a valid component of a national assessment programme in the UK? *Adv Health Sci Educ* 2008; **13**:181–92.

15 **Cooper J, Robinson P**. The argument for making large classes seem small. *New Dir Teach Learn* 2000; **81**:5–16.

16 **Doyle C, Lennox L, Bell D**. A systematic review of evidence on the links between patient experience and clinical safety and effectiveness. *BMJ Open* 2013; **3**:e001570. DOI:10.1136/bmjopen–2012–001570.

17 **Jha KA, Orav J, Zheng J, Epstein AM**. Patients' perception of hospital care in the United States. *N Engl J Med* 2008; **359**:1921–31.

18 **Black N, Varaganum M, Hutchings A**. Relationship between patient reported experience (PREMs) and patient reported outcomes (PROMs) in elective surgery. *BMJ Qual Saf* 2014. DOI:10.1136/bmjqs–2013–002707.

19 **Bardach NS, Asteria-Peñaloza R, Boscardin WJ, Dudley RA**. The relationship between commercial website ratings and traditional hospital performance measures in the USA. *BMJ Qual Saf* 2013. DOI:10.1136 /bmjqs–2012–001360.

20 **Kolb DA**. Experiential learning: experience as the source of learning and development. 1984, Englewood Cliffs, NJ: Prentice Hall.

Chapter 17

Managing psychiatric emergencies

Hussien Elkholy, Ahmed A. Abd Elgawad,
Nagendra Bendi, and Julian Beezhold

Introduction

One of the most common difficulties that face psychiatrists in their early years of training is dealing with emergency situations in psychiatry. Psychiatry is usually perceived
as the medical specialty that focuses on 'talking' the patient through his or her problems. However, this is often not the situation. Thus, a psychiatrist must grasp both the
knowledge of a good physician and the skills of a competent psychiatrist.

Most of the psychiatric textbooks classify psychiatric emergencies into 'suicide' and
'others'. For the sake of simplicity and a more practical approach, psychiatric emergencies can be divided into three categories:

1 Medical emergencies in psychiatric settings (e.g. medication side-effects, myocardial infarction, ketoacidosis, seizures)

2 Psychiatric emergencies in medical settings (e.g. agitation, violence, delirium)

3 Psychiatric emergencies in psychiatric settings (e.g. suicide, violence, panic,
   conversion)

In this chapter, we will go through some of the aforementioned emergencies, covering the basic knowledge and skills that an early career psychiatrist should have.

Medical emergencies in psychiatric settings

It is always important to bear in mind that psychiatry is a branch of medicine. Before
you become a psychiatrist, you will have completed your basic training as a physician.
However, unfortunately, as time goes by, we tend to remember less and less of our basic
training.

Medical emergencies in psychiatric settings include the following:

♦ Medication side-effects:
  • acute extrapyramidal side-effects (EPSE) (e.g. acute dystonia, acute akathisia)
  • neuroleptic malignant syndrome (NMS)
  • serotonin syndrome
  • lithium toxicity
  • arrhythmias (e.g. QTc prolongation, torsade de pointe)

- General medical conditions:
  - central nervous system
  - renal
  - respiratory
  - hepatic
  - cardiac
  - metabolic (e.g. diabetic ketoacidosis, hyperglycaemic coma)
  - vascular (e.g. deep venous thrombosis)
- Drug and alcohol intoxication and withdrawal

As this book is not intended to cover basic medical training, we advise early career psychiatrists to ensure that they maintain competence in core skills such as how to read an ECG (Electrocardiogram), basics of CPR (cardio-pulmonary resuscitation), and management of seizures.

Medication side-effects

Neuroleptic malignant syndrome (NMS)

NMS is a rare but potentially fatal side-effect of antipsychotics. It is essentially a syndrome of sympathetic over-activity due to antagonizing dopaminergic activity. NMS can also be seen with other drugs such as antidepressants (selective serotonin reuptake inhibitors may contribute to NMS as they are also indirect dopamine antagonists) and lithium.

Risk factors There are several factors that might increase the risk of developing NMS, including:

- Using high-potency antipsychotics
- Recent or rapid dose increase
- Sudden withdrawal of anticholinergics
- Organic brain disease
- Parkinson's disease
- Dehydration
- Hyperthyroidism.

Diagnosis

- *Clinical presentation*: ill patient, fever, diaphoresis, rigidity (lead pipe), disturbed conscious level, fluctuating blood pressure, and tachycardia
- *Laboratory tests*: elevated creatine kinase (usually more than 1000 IU/L), leukocytosis, and altered liver function tests

Complications NMS complications are common and severe, even fatal. They include:

- *Metabolic*: dehydration and electrolyte imbalance
- *Renal*: acute renal failure (due to rhabdomyolysis)

- *Cardiac*: arrhythmias, including torsade de pointe, cardiac arrest, myocardial infarction, and cardiomyopathy
- *Respiratory*: respiratory failure from chest wall rigidity, aspiration pneumonia, pulmonary embolism
- *Vascular*: deep venous thrombosis, thrombocytopenia, and disseminated intravascular coagulation
- Seizures from hyperthermia and metabolic derangements
- Hepatic failure

Treatment The following treatment procedure should be observed:[3]

- Upon suspicion, stop antipsychotics immediately (also stop lithium and antidepressants if used).
- Monitor vital signs.
- Transfer to a medical unit immediately, to start treatment:
  - Rehydration—insensible fluid loss from fever and from diaphoresis should also be considered. If CK (creatine kinase) is very elevated, intravenous fluids with urine alkalinization may help prevent renal failure from rhabdomyolysis.
  - Dantrolene is a direct-acting skeletal muscle relaxant which is effective in treating malignant hyperthermia. Doses of 1–2.5 mg/kg IV are typically used in adults and can be repeated to a maximum dose of 10 mg/kg/day. It will help to reduce heat production and rigidity. Usually, its effects appear within minutes of administration.
  - Bromocriptine (a dopamine agonist) is prescribed to restore lost dopaminergic tone. Doses of 2.5 mg (through nasogastric tube) every 6–8 hours are titrated up to a maximum dose of 40 mg/day. Continuation of bromocriptine for 10 days after NMS is controlled is recommended, then tapered slowly.
  - Sedation with benzodiazepines and artificial ventilation, if required.
  - Apomorphine, L-dopa, and carbamazepine have also been used.

Serotonin syndrome

Serotonin syndrome is due to increased serotonin activity in the central nervous system (CNS).[1] It usually presents with the classic clinical triad:

- Mental status changes (agitation, confusion)
- Autonomic hyperactivity (tachycardia, fever, and excessive sweating)
- Neuromuscular abnormalities (rigidity and increased reflexes).

Diagnosis Serotonin toxicity can vary from a mild form, up to becoming life-threatening. The initial symptoms include akathisia, agitation, tremor, tachycardia, autonomic instability (usually hypertension), increased bowel sounds, diarrhoea, mydriasis, and altered mental status. The patient may be feverish. On examination, increased reflexes and clonus may be induced.

Causes Several drugs are implicated in the production of serotonin syndrome and examples include:

- Selective serotonin reuptake inhibitors (SSRIs)
- Serotonin and norepinephrine reuptake inhibitors (SNRIs)
- Bupropion
- Tricyclic antidepressants
- Monoamine oxidase inhibitors (MAOIs)
- Anti-migraine medications (e.g. triptans, carbamazepine, valproic acid)
- Pain medications (e.g. meperidine, tramadol)
- Lithium
- Illicit drugs (e.g. LSD, Ecstasy, cocaine, amphetamines)
- Herbal supplements (e.g. St John's wort)

Treatment The following treatment procedure should be observed:[3]

- The first thing to do is to stop, immediately, the medications involved and to hospitalize the patient. Most cases of serotonin syndrome typically resolve within 24–72 hours after stopping the offending drug(s). However, administration of oral cyproheptadine (5-HT and histamine H_1 antagonist) may be helpful. An initial dose of 4–12 mg, followed by up to a maximum dose of 32 mg/24 hours, in four divided doses, can be given.
- Additionally, supportive measures (e.g. control of fever, sedation, intubation, ventilatory support) and good monitoring should be done.
- Benzodiazepines can be used to treat agitation and/or seizures.

Differentiating serotonin syndrome from NMS Serotonin syndrome and NMS share some clinical features[2] which make it a bit confusing to reach the diagnosis. Both syndromes may present with fever (>40°C), elevated blood pressure, tachycardia, diaphoresis, and disturbed conscious level.

It is important to take a good history of medication usage since, although there might be some overlap with causative medications, this will generally help to pinpoint the corresponding, suspected syndrome (e.g. using antipsychotics or any dopamine antagonist will raise the suspicion of NMS). Also, the onset in NMS is variable and can take 1–3 days, while in serotonin syndrome, it usually occurs in less than 12 hours.

There is increased muscle tone in both syndromes: NMS usually presents with 'lead pipe' rigidity in all muscle groups, while for serotonin syndrome, there is often increased tone in lower extremities. In NMS, the reflexes are diminished, in contrast to serotonin syndrome which shows hyperreflexia and clonus. Other differentiating clinical features include dilated pupils in serotonin syndrome (normal in NMS), and increased bowel sounds in serotonin syndrome (normal or decreased in NMS). Finally, to diagnose NMS, there should be marked CK elevation (usually above 1000 IU/L).

Other differential diagnoses for serotonin syndrome and NMS As both serotonin syndrome and NMS produce fever, they must be differentiated from other causes of hyperthermia.[1] Differential diagnoses of hyperthermia syndromes in psychiatry include:

- Neuroleptic malignant syndrome
- Serotonin syndrome
- Malignant (or lethal) catatonia
- Anticholinergic toxicity syndrome
- Malignant hyperpyrexia
- Parkinsonism–hyperpyrexia syndrome
- Infections: encephalitis, meningitis, septicaemia
- Thyrotoxicosis
- Overdoses with sympathomimetics and other drugs
- Alcohol or drug withdrawal delirium

Extrapyramidal side-effects

Extrapyramidal side-effects are caused by dopamine blockade or depletion in the basal ganglia, which produces a picture similar to idiopathic pathologies of the extrapyramidal system. The extrapyramidal symptoms include acute dystonic reactions, tardive dyskinesia, Parkinsonism, akathisia, and neuroleptic malignant syndrome.

Extrapyramidal symptoms can develop acutely or occur late after starting the medication. Acute forms of extrapyramidal side-effects include acute dystonia and acute akathesia (Table 17.1).

Lithium toxicity

Lithium toxicity mostly occurs with blood levels above 1.5 mmol/L.

Diagnosis It should be suspected when any patient on lithium starts exhibiting any of the following:[3]

- *Gastrointestinal symptoms*: anorexia, nausea, vomiting, and diarrhoea
- *Nervous system*: muscle weakness, drowsiness, dysarthria, coarse tremors, ataxia, and muscle twitching

In levels above 2 mmol/L, other symptoms (including disturbed conscious level, disorientation, seizures, and coma) may occur. Eventually, death may result.

Risk factors Risk factors for lithium toxicity include:

- Dehydration
- Over-exercise
- Salt-free diet
- Drug interaction (e.g. ACE (angiotensin converting enzyme) inhibitors, diuretics (especially thiazides), NSAIDs (non-steroidal anti-inflammatory drugs), carbamazepine)

Basically, any drug or condition that increases serum lithium or decreases sodium level might predispose to lithium toxicity.

Table 17.1 Different forms of acute extrapyramidal side-effects

	Acute dystonia	**Acute akathisia**
Definition	Uncontrolled muscle spasm in any part of the body	A subjectively unpleasant state of inner restlessness
Mechanism	Dopaminergic *hyperactivity* in basal ganglia (occurs when central nervous system levels of antipsychotic drugs begin to fall between doses)	Dopaminergic *hypoactivity* caused by an extensive (>80%) decrease in dopamine (D2) receptor stimulation.
Clinical picture and diagnosis	◆ Abnormal movements due to contraction of muscles ◆ Usually very painful ◆ Include oculogyric crisis, torticollis, blepharospasm ◆ Most serious are the pharyngeal dystonias as they may result in difficulty in breathing	◆ Subjective feeling of restlessness ◆ And/or objective signs of restlessness ◆ Can occur with antipsychotics, antidepressants, and sympathomimetics
Management	◆ Management of life- threatening conditions (e.g. ensure patent airway in case of laryngospasm) ◆ Anticholinergic drugs given orally, IM, or IV depending on the severity of symptoms ◆ IV or IM diphenhydramine ◆ IV diazepam	◆ Reduce the dose ◆ Control using other drugs such as beta-blockers (propranolol 30–80 mg/day) and/or benzodiazepines ◆ Consider changing the medication if the above methods fail

Treatment Treatment is as follows[4]:

◆ Patients with suspected lithium toxicity should be hospitalized and observed for at least 24 hours.

◆ Lithium should be stopped or the dose reduced upon suspicion.

◆ Lithium levels should be monitored immediately and then every 6–12 hours, depending on the presentation.

◆ The diagnosis of lithium toxicity is made on clinical grounds. Serum level is not always a good guide as a therapeutic level does not exclude toxicity. This is because individuals vary in their susceptibility, and also because lithium absorption from the gastrointestinal tract and release from intracellular stores may be prolonged.

◆ In mild cases, ensure good hydration, electrolyte balance, and ECG monitoring.

◆ In severe cases, forced alkaline diuresis can be used. If serum lithium levels are greater than 3 mmol/L, haemodialysis should be considered. Haemodialysis should also be used in cases of coma or shock, or when conservative measures have failed.

Arrhythmias in psychiatry

Causes ECG changes have been recorded with many psychiatric medications. Some of the medications have been associated with serious arrhythmias. Moreover, psychiatric patients, like any individuals, are liable to heart disease. Thus, as mentioned earlier in the chapter, it is recommended that a psychiatrist should maintain basic knowledge about how to interpret an ECG.

In this chapter, the focus is on those ECG changes related to several psychotropic medications. As these medications block cardiac potassium channels, they lead to prolongation of the QT interval, which is linked to serious ventricular arrhythmias (namely, torsade de pointe) which may be fatal. There is some evidence that the risk of arrhythmia is related to QTc interval (QT corrected for heart rate) prolongation beyond a certain limit (440 ms for men; 470 ms for women), and the risk increases significantly with QTc values above 500 ms.

Medications that increase the risk of QTc prolongation As mentioned earlier, different psychiatric medications have been associated with ECG changes. Focusing on QTc prolongation[3], it is worth noting that the effect of medications on QTc differs.

♦ *No effect:* antipsychotics (aripiprazole); antidepressants (SSRIs—except citalopram, mirtazepine); antiepileptics and mood stabilizers (carbamazepine, gabapentin, lamotrigine, valproate)

♦ *Low effect:* antipsychotics (amisulpride, sulpride, clozapine, olanzapine, risperidone); antidepressants (citalopram, bupropion, venlafaxine, trazodone); mood stabilizers: (lithium)

♦ *Moderate effect:* antipsychotics (chlorpromazine, quetiapine, ziprasidone); antidepressants (tricyclic antidepressants)

♦ *High effect:* antipsychotics (pimozide, haloperidol, sertindole)

Non-psychotropic medications involved in QTc prolongation

♦ *Antibiotics:* erythromycin, clarithromycin, and ampicillin

♦ *Antimalarials:* chloroquine, mefloquine, and quinine

♦ *Antiarrhythmics:* quinidine and amiodarone

♦ *Others:* amantadine, cyclosporin, diphenhydramine, and tamoxifen

Management of QTc prolongation

♦ *QTc < 440 ms (men) or 470 ms (women):* no action required unless abnormal T-wave morphology

♦ *QTc > 440 ms (men) or 470 ms (women) but < 500 ms:* consider reducing dose or changing the drug, repeat ECG, and consult a cardiologist if needed

♦ *QTc > 500 ms:* stop the drug and refer to a cardiologist immediately

Drug and alcohol intoxication and withdrawal

Table 17.2 is a summary of what to look for if intoxication or withdrawal is suspected. Further information about substance abuse and management should be obtained from

Table 17.2 Differences between intoxication and withdrawal of different substances of abuse

Substance	Intoxication	Withdrawal
Alcohol	◆ Slurred speech ◆ Loss of co-ordination ◆ Unsteady gait (swaying and falling) ◆ Decreased alertness ◆ Disinhibition (e.g. talking loud, annoying others, inappropriate sexual or physical behaviour) ◆ Red watery eyes ◆ Flushed face ◆ Stupor or coma ◆ Respiratory depression in severe intoxication	◆ Tremors ◆ Diaphoresis ◆ Sleeplessness ◆ Gastrointestinal upset ◆ Anxiety ◆ Craving for alcohol ◆ Seizures (grand mal) may occur ◆ In around 5% of patients, *delirium tremens* may set in
Benzodiazepines	◆ Slurred speech ◆ Inco-ordination ◆ Unsteady gait ◆ Nystagmus ◆ Impairment in attention or memory ◆ Behavioural changes, including inappropriate sexual or aggressive behaviour, mood lability, impaired judgement ◆ Stupor or coma	◆ Autonomic hyperactivity ◆ Increased tremors ◆ Insomnia ◆ Nausea or vomiting ◆ Transient visual, tactile, or auditory hallucinations or illusions ◆ Psychomotor agitation ◆ Anxiety (most prominent) ◆ Grand mal seizures ◆ Kinaesthetic hallucinations reported occasionally
Amphetamines	◆ Tachycardia or bradycardia (arrythmias may be fatal) ◆ Pupillary dilation ◆ Elevated or lowered blood pressure ◆ Nausea or vomiting ◆ Psychomotor agitation or retardation ◆ Confusion, seizures, dyskinesias, dystonias, or coma ◆ Psychological effects such as elevated mood, changes in sociability, anxiety, impaired judgement ◆ Psychosis	◆ Dysphoric mood, sometimes with suicidal ideation ◆ Fatigue ◆ Vivid, unpleasant dreams ◆ Hypersomnia ◆ Increased appetite ◆ Psychomotor retardation ◆ Pupils may be smaller

(*continued*)

Table 17.2 (continued) Differences between intoxication and withdrawal of different substances of abuse

Substance	Intoxication	Withdrawal
Cocaine	◆ Increased energy ◆ Heightened self-esteem ◆ Elevated mood ◆ Agitation ◆ Impaired judgement ◆ Tachycardia ◆ Hypertension ◆ Mydriasis ◆ Sensation of bugs crawling beneath the skin (formication) has been reported ◆ Psychosis	◆ Dysphoria ◆ Anhedonia ◆ Anxiety ◆ Irritability ◆ Hypersomnia ◆ Intense cravings for cocaine with lack of many physical withdrawal symptoms
Opioids	◆ Elevated mood ◆ Psychomotor agitation or retardation ◆ Pupillary constriction (if pupillary dilation is seen, this suggests overdose so severe that it leads to anoxia) ◆ Drowsiness or coma ◆ Impairment in attention or memory	◆ Dysphoric mood ◆ Nausea or vomiting ◆ Muscle aches ◆ Lacrimation or rhinorrhoea ◆ Pupillary dilation, piloerection (goose flesh), and sweating ◆ Insomnia ◆ Diarrhoea ◆ Yawning ◆ Fever
Cannabis	◆ Elevated mood ◆ Sensation of slowed time ◆ Social withdrawal ◆ Conjunctival injection ◆ Increased appetite ('munchies') ◆ Impaired motor co-ordination ◆ Dry mouth ◆ Tachycardia ◆ Psychosis	◆ Irritability ◆ Insomnia ◆ Anorexia ◆ Mild nausea

other textbooks. However, as psychiatric emergencies are the focus of this chapter, special attention will be given to delirium tremens.

Delirium tremens is a severe form of alcohol withdrawal. It is a toxic confusional state manifested by clouded consciousness, autonomic hyperactivity (tachycardia, hypertension, sweating, and fever), vivid hallucinations, and marked tremors. Symptoms usually peak 72–96 hours after last alcohol consumption.

Risk factors for delirium tremens

- Severe alcohol dependence
- Past experience of delirium tremens
- Older age
- Co-occurring acute medical illness
- Long history of alcohol dependence
- Severe withdrawal symptoms at presentation
- Withdrawal seizures

Management of delirium tremens It is of utmost importance to detect delirium tremens as early as possible and to transfer the patient to a medical ward to start management:[3,5]

- Hospitalization is a must
- Monitor the vital signs closely
- Correct electrolyte imbalance and treat concomitant medical problems (e.g. infections)
- Ensure adequate hydration
- Benzodiazepines:
  - Usually used for 5–7 days
  - Chlordiazepoxide 25–100 mg orally, every 6 hours (IV use is not recommended), to control agitation, tremors, and increased vital signs *or*
  - Lorazepam 1–2 mg orally or IM or IV, every 4 hours for the first day, then decrease; better choice for the elderly and medically compromised (liver cirrhosis) *or*
  - Diazepam 5–10 mg IV, every 3–4 hours, then titrate dose and frequency according to patient's response.
- Thiamine: 200–300 mg IM daily, for 3–5 days, as a prophylaxis for Wernicke's encephalopathy
- Magnesium sulphate: 1 g IM, every 6 hours, for a total of four doses, for patients who suffered post-withdrawal seizures.

Psychiatric emergencies in medical settings

Common psychiatric emergencies in medical settings include:

- Organic—delirium/acute confusional states
- Agitation (aggression and violence)
- Catatonia
- Mood disorder
- Deliberate self-harm/suicide
- Substance misuse

In this chapter, we will focus only on the first three.

Delirium

Delirium, also known as acute confusional state, is one of the most common disorders encountered by psychiatric trainees in acute hospital wards.[6] It is extremely common in the medical and surgical ward environment (10–20%) [7] and is often mistaken for psychiatric illness due to the presentation. Patients with dementia are particularly vulnerable in this regard. While potentially reversible, delirium may lead to death if untreated—hence why it is a medical emergency.

Delirium (ICD-10, F05) is an illness with a group of symptoms. It is characterized by the rapid onset of symptoms (within hours or days), with altered levels of consciousness, global cognitive impairment, fluctuating course, perceptual abnormalities (especially visual hallucinations), and an underlying physical cause usually evident.

The fifth edition of the *Diagnostic and statistical manual of mental disorders* (DSM-5)[8] gives the diagnostic criteria for delirium as follows:

◆ Disturbance in attention (e.g. reduced ability to direct, focus, sustain, and shift attention) and awareness.

◆ Change in cognition (e.g. memory deficit, disorientation, language disturbance, perceptual disturbance) that is not better accounted for by a pre-existing, established, or evolving dementia.

◆ The disturbance develops over a short period (usually hours to days) and tends to fluctuate during the course of the day.

◆ There is evidence from the history, physical examination, or laboratory findings that the disturbance is caused by a direct physiological consequence of a general medical condition, an intoxicating substance, medication use, or more than one cause.

Differential diagnoses for delirium

While it is not exhaustive, the list includes:

◆ Dementia (Alzheimer's, vascular, Lewy body)
◆ Schizophrenia and other psychoses
◆ Depression
◆ Mania

Risk factors for delirium

The various risk factors for delirium[9] include:

◆ Older age
◆ Cognitive impairment (past or present) and/or dementia
◆ Current hip fracture
◆ Any severe physical illness
◆ Polypharmacy
◆ Infection/inflammation post surgery
◆ Metabolic disorder (liver/renal failure, hypoglycaemia)

- Endocrine causes (e.g. diabetic ketosis, hypothyroidism, hyperthyroidism, adrenal or pituitary insufficiency, Cushing syndrome, hyperparathyroidism)
- Drugs (withdrawal/toxicity, anticholinergics).

Management of delirium

National Institute for Health and Care Excellence (NICE) guidelines stipulate that:

- If delirium is suspected, carry out a clinical assessment based on the *Diagnostic and statistical manual of mental disorders* criteria or short confusion assessment method (short CAM) to confirm the diagnosis. In critical care or in the recovery room after surgery, CAM-ICU should be used.
- If there is difficulty distinguishing between delirium, dementia, or delirium superimposed on dementia, treat delirium first.

Finding the cause of delirium is the absolute, first priority in its management. The psychiatric management of delirium is outlined in Box 17.1.

Box 17.1 Psychiatric management of delirium

General

1 Identify the underlying causes of the delirium
2 Address the underlying aetiology of the delirium
3 Assess the safety of the patient
4 Ongoing assessment of the mental state
5 Psycho-education regarding risk factors to carers

Environmental

1 Reduce the level of stimulation on the ward (preferably in a side room)
2 Address any sensory impairments like vision or hearing
3 Ensure physical safety of the ward surroundings
4 Provide environmental cues (easily visible clocks, calendars, etc.) that facilitate orientation
5 Ensure good lighting
6 Ensure same staff provide care to increase familiarity
7 Cognitive supportive measures: re-orientation, reassurance, and information

Biological treatments

1 Antipsychotic treatment should be reserved for those patients who put their own or others' safety at risk, and for when de-escalation techniques fail.

> **Box 17.1 Psychiatric management of delirium (continued)**
>
> 2 Haloperidol (or newer antipsychotic medications like olanzapine) is commonly used.
>
> 3 Start at a low dose and titrate cautiously, alongside treatment of the underlying cause.
>
> 4 Monitor with ECG.
>
> 5 Benzodiazepine is to be used cautiously; special indications for its use include Parkinson's disease, Lewy body dementia, etc., where antipsychotics are contraindicated.

Agitation

Agitation is a non-specific mixture of comparatively unrelated behaviours characterized by often intense subjective emotional and/or physical feelings of discomfort that may pose a risk to the safety of the patient or others.

Agitation can be seen in a number of clinical situations, such as dementia, substance intoxication/withdrawal, psychotic disorders, affective disorders, anxiety disorders, personality disorders, pervasive developmental disorders like autism, learning disabilities, and/or as a medication side-effect. Agitation can be caused by many medical problems, including delirium. Hence, it is essential for the assessment to be comprehensive, with identification and ongoing management of any medical problems. The risk of violence toward him/herself or toward other people is an important determinant of further management.

Management of agitation

Prior to any pharmacological intervention, the initial management of agitation[3,10] involves non-drug approaches including de-escalation techniques or talking down, time out, observation, stimulus reduction, etc.

With regard to pharmacological treatment, most rapid tranquilization guidelines suggest:

1 Always first consider non-pharmacological interventions.

2 Always offer oral medication before considering parenteral administration.

3 Always use the lowest likely effective dose.

4 Benzodiazepines (lorazepam) are the most common first choice. Major side-effects include respiratory depression and respiratory arrest.

5 Antipsychotics can be used either in conjunction with benzodiazepines or as an alternative.

6 Oral antipsychotic options include: olanzapine 10 mg; quetiapine 100–200 mg; risperidone 1–2 mg; haloperidol 5 mg.

7 When IM treatment is considered, evidence-based options are: lorazepam 1–2 mg; promethazine 50 mg; olanzapine 10 mg; aripiprazole 9.75 mg; haloperidol 5 mg.

8 Seek expert advice if these measures fail.

Catatonia

Catatonia is a complex psychomotor syndrome with motor, affective, and behavioural features which can be manifested across a wide range of neuropsychiatric and non-psychiatric medical conditions. The symptoms include motor immobility—catalepsy/waxy flexibility, stupor, motor excitement, negativism/mutism, posturing, sterotypies, mannerisms, echolalia or echopraxia. Similar to delirium, catatonia is a marker of severe underlying medical or psychiatric illness.

In DSM-5, catatonia is not recognized as a separate disorder, but is associated with psychiatric conditions such as schizophrenia (catatonic type), bipolar disorder, post-traumatic stress disorder, and depression. It may also be seen in some general medical conditions such as encephalitis, autoimmune disorders, and metabolic disturbances.

Management of catatonia

1 Inpatient treatment[11] is usually a must as the patient will need continuous monitoring of vital signs and continuous care and support.

2 Parental nutrition might be needed.

3 The underlying cause should be treated promptly.

4 Best evidence in terms of symptomatic relief is for benzodiazepines (lorazepam).

5 Treatment with electroconvulsive therapy (ECT) may be indicated, if catatonic symptoms do not resolve, and can be life-saving (e.g. with severe mania).

6 The use of antipsychotics in patients with catatonic symptoms depends on the cause.

Psychiatric emergencies in psychiatric settings

Suicide is still a major and serious health issue,[12,13] and its importance comes from being a preventable cause of death. Thus, understanding suicide causes and risk factors are essential for proper identification of people at risk, and also for prevention of death.

Suicide is a complex phenomenon, and suicidal behaviour usually occurs along a continuum of suicidal ideation, suicidal plan, suicidal attempt, and, ultimately, death by suicide (Box 17.2).

Box 17.2 Suicide: definition of terms

◆ *Suicidal ideation*: thoughts of serving as the agent of one's own death.

◆ *Suicidal intent*: subjective desire for a self-destructive act to end in death.

◆ *Suicidal attempt*: self-injurious behaviour with a non-fatal outcome, accompanied by evidence that the person intended to die.

◆ *Suicide*: self-inflicted death with evidence that the person intended to die.

Suicide differs from deliberate self-harm, which is defined as self-inflicting of painful, destructive, or injurious acts *without* intent to die.

Epidemiology of suicide

◆ In the UK, overall deaths due to suicide were 6054 persons at 2011, with the suicidal rate equal to 11.8 per 100,000.

◆ In the USA, 30,000 (12.5 per 100,000) deaths are attributed to suicide each year.

◆ Suicide rates reach more than 25 per 100,000 persons in Scandinavia, Switzerland, and Germany; but are less than 10 per 100,000 persons in some Arabic countries.[12–14]

Risk factors for suicide

These include *biopsychosocial risk factors, environmental risk factors, and socio-cultural risk factors.*[12,13]

Biopsychosocial risk factors

1 Demographic features

◆ Sex: males commit suicide four times more often than females; however, females attempt suicide more often than males. Men's higher rate of completed suicide is related to the *methods* they use: firearms, hanging, or jumping from high places. Women more commonly take an overdose of psychoactive substances or a poison.

◆ Age: suicide increases with age, with a major significant spike in adolescents and young adults. The peak age range is from 45 years in males and from 55 years in females; older persons attempt suicide less often than younger persons, but are more often successful.

◆ Race: more frequent among the white population.

◆ Marital status: widowed, divorced, or single marital statuses have more risk.

◆ Occupation: suicide is higher among unemployed persons; physicians, dentists, artists, lawyers are considered at higher risk. Among physicians, *psychiatrists* are at greater risk.

2. Mental illness

◆ Almost 95% of all suicidal persons have a diagnosed mental disorder.

◆ Also, psychiatric patients' risk for suicide is 3–12 times that of non-patients.

◆ Patients who commit suicide tend to be relatively young.

◆ Among inpatients, suicidal risk increases in the first week of admission, and then it declines to reach, after 4–5 weeks, the same risk level as of the general population.

◆ Discharged patients are at increased risk of suicide for 3 months after discharge.

Depression:

◆ The most common diagnosis associated with suicide.

◆ More patients with depressive disorders commit suicide early in the illness than later.

♦ Preoccupation with death, sense of hopelessness, helplessness, and social isolation enhance suicidal tendencies among depressed patients.

Schizophrenia:

♦ Up to 10% of schizophrenic patients die by committing suicide.

♦ Suicidal behaviour in schizophrenic patients usually occurs out of poor judgement, from obeying ordering auditory hallucination, or to escape persecutory delusions. Also, development of depressed symptoms, with feelings of helplessness and hopelessness, could raise the risk of suicide.

Delirium and dementia:

♦ 5% of suicide cases occur with mental illness due to dementia and delirium.

♦ The conditions of memory loss, disorientation, hallucinations, and delusions, together with poor judgement, may lead to suicidal behaviour.

Alcohol and other substance dependence:

♦ Up to 15% of all alcohol-dependent persons commit suicide.

♦ Heroin-dependent patients have a suicidal rate 20 times that of the general population.

♦ Suicide can occur in any phase of use—intoxication, withdrawal, and with chronic usage.

♦ Depression, impulsiveness, aggressiveness, and criminal behaviours are factors that contribute to suicide; also, experiencing a number of major losses in life is another factor.

Other mental disorders:

♦ Anxiety disorders, obsessive compulsive disorders, and phobic disorders.

♦ Eating disorders.

Personality disorders: especially cluster B personality disorders

3 Some major physical illnesses: chronic diseases with disability or disfigurement have more risk for depression and suicide.

4 History of trauma or abuse.

5 A previous suicide attempt is considered the most important risk factor for suicide.

6 Family history of suicide.

Environmental risk factors

These refer to major stressful life events like the loss of a loved one, a job, or money, and relational or social loss.

Socio-cultural risk factors

♦ Lack of social support

♦ Isolation

♦ Stigma associated with help-seeking behaviour

- Barriers to accessing mental health and substance abuse treatment
- Certain cultural and religious beliefs
- Exposure to and influence of others who have died by suicide (e.g. through media).

Management of suicide

Management and treatment should encompass the following:[12,13]

1 General rules
   - All suicide threats should be taken seriously, even if they seem manipulative.
   - Deal with patients in an empathetic manner; also, physicians should remain calm and uncritical.
   - Ensure privacy while asking the patient about suicide.
   - Collateral information from family members or friends about the incident of suicide is essential.
   - Close observation using special nursing to protect the patient; do not allow sharp instruments, tissue, or medications in the patient's room.
   - Suicide has legal implications; documentation of every step of management is a must.

2 Assessment of seriousness
   - Previous past history of serious attempts
   - Presence of mental illness before the attempt
   - High-risk group (male gender, old age, single)
   - Lack of social support
   - Planning and precautions taken by the patient to prevent being rescued
   - The use of a serious method (e.g. shooting, hanging, jumping from a height).

3 Assessment of mental state
   - History: recent stressful life events; drug intake (medical/psychotropic)
   - Past history of medical illness, psychiatric disorder
   - Positive family history

4 Hospitalization—*essential for persons at high risk of suicide*
   - Patient has mental illness.
   - Suicidal attempt has occurred, with the lethal method still present; or lethal weapons are available to the patient.
   - Patient has persistent plan or intent for suicide.
   - Patient took many precautions to avoid rescue or discovery.
   - Distress is increased after the suicidal attempt, or patient regrets still being alive.
   - Patient is male, >45 years of age, especially with new onset of psychiatric illness.
   - Patient has limited social support, including lack of a stable living situation.

- ◆ Patient has impulsive behaviours, severe agitation, poor judgement, or refuses help.
- ◆ Patient has had a recent change in mental status which requires further investigation within the hospital setting.

5 Electroconvulsive therapy, r.TMS (repetitive transcranial magnetic stimulation), and deep brain stimulation may be used, especially in severe depression.

6 Drug therapy: medication (antidepressants, antipsychotics, anxiolytics, or mood stabilizers) is given according to the cause and the physical condition of the patient after the attempt.

7 Psychotherapy: CBT (cognitive behavioural therapy), IPT (interpersonal psychotherapy), or DBT (dialectical behaviour therapy) may be used.

References

1 **Ahuja N, Cole A**. Hyperthermia syndromes in psychiatry. *Advances in Psychiatric Treatment* 2009; **15**:181–91.

2 **Bienvenu OJ, Neufeld KJ, Needham DM**. Treatment of four psychiatric emergencies in the intensive care unit. *Critical Care Medicine* 2012; **40**:2662–70.

3 **Taylor D, Paton C, Kapur S**. *The Maudsley prescribing guidelines* (10th edn). UK: Informa Healthcare; 2009.

4 **Ferrier N, Ferrie LJ, Macritchie KA**. Old drug, new data: revisiting . . . lithium therapy. *Advances in Psychiatric Treatment* 2006; **12**:256–64.

5 **Sadock BJ, Sadock VA**. *Kaplan and Sadock's pocket handbook of clinical psychiatry* (5th edn). USA: Lippincott, Williams & Wilkins; 2010.

6 **Puri B, Treasaden I**. *Emergencies in psychiatry*. USA: Oxford University Press; 2008.

7 **Semple D, Smyth R**.(eds.) *Oxford handbook of psychiatry* (3rd edn). USA: Oxford University Press; 2013.

8 American Psychiatric Association. *Diagnostic and statistical manual of mental disorders* (5th edn). Arlington, VA: American Psychiatric Publishing; 2013.

9 National Clinical Guideline Centre/NICE. *Delirium: diagnosis, prevention and management. NICE clinical guidelines*. London: National Clinical Guideline Centre; 2010.

10 NICE. *Violence and aggression: short-term management in mental health, health, and community settings*. NICE; 2015. Available at: https://www.nice.org.uk/guidance/ng10

11 **Rajagopal S**. Catatonia. *Advances in Psychiatric Treatment* 2007; **13**:51–9.

12 **Sadock BJ, Kaplen HI, Sadock VA**. *Kaplen and Sadock's synopsis of psychiatry: behavioral sciences/clinical psychiatry* (10th edn). USA: Lippincott, Williams & Wilkins; 2007.

13 American Psychiatric Association. *APA practice guidelines for the assessment and treatment of patients with suicidal behaviors*. APA; 2004.

14 **Scowcrof E**. *Suicide statistical report 2014: including data for 2010–2*. UK: Samaritans; 2014. Available at: http://www.samaritans.org/sites/default/files/kcfinder/files/research/Samaritans%20Suicide%20Statistics%20Report%202014.pdf

Chapter 18

Building ties in the community for patients with mental illness

Daniele Carretta, Giuseppe Carrà,
Massimo Clerici, and Reinhard Heun

Community psychiatry: origins, definition, strengths, and limitations

The end of asylums and the birth of community psychiatry

Community psychiatry is a term that indicates an approach to the treatment of mental disorders aimed not only at caring for individuals suffering from mental illnesses through interventions that allow them to stay and live a decent life in their home environment, but also at promoting and protecting the mental health of the general population.

Community psychiatry was born in the 1960s, as a consequence of the massive protests that rose against asylums in Western countries. These asylums were large facilities, often hosting hundreds of mentally ill individuals for long-term residential treatment, and usually located outside towns, largely secluded from the outer world and patients' former communities and social lives. Patients admitted to asylums were totally prone to institutional rules, with poor or no attention to their individual needs.[1] During the 1950s, the asylum model of mental healthcare had come to a crisis because of several weaknesses such as the lack of adequate treatment, poor living conditions, poor financial resources and training, professional isolation of staff and sometimes scarce sanitary conditions.[2]

The struggle for more humane care of mental disorders was widely supported by the massive protests against all forms of authoritarianism that took place in the 1960s, and was further favoured by the development of the first antipsychotic drugs (phenotiazines) and outpatient treatment initiatives. This synergy facilitated the end of the asylum era, and its replacement with less restrictive and less humiliating forms of mental healthcare. The process initially took place in the most developed countries, namely in the United States of America and Europe, and subsequently in many other countries, although at a different pace, depending on local social and economic factors.[3]

The abolishment of large psychiatric institutions led to the development of treatment strategies that allowed users to maintain contacts with their home community, so-called 'community psychiatry'. Box 18.1 contains a definition of community psychiatry.[4]

Box 18.1 Definition of community psychiatry

Community psychiatry studies and implements 'principles and practices aimed at promoting mental health for a local population'. Its main aim is to promote patients' recovery, not only regarding clinical symptomatology (clinical recovery) but also in terms of personal effectiveness in living in the community (personal recovery). For this purpose, community psychiatry is committed not only to treating mental illness, but also to strengthening patients' personal resources and their social networks. Treatment programmes should be evidence-based and, whenever possible, agreed with patients.

Source data from: Thornicroft G, Szmukler G, Mueser KT, Drake RE, Community Mental Health, in Drake RE, Szmukler G, Mueser KT, Thornicroft G. Introduction to community mental health care. Copyright (2011) Oxford University Press.

From a practical perspective, community psychiatry treats mental illness without long-term admission to closed psychiatric facilities, but by allowing patients to stay and live a decent life in their home environment. For this purpose, community mental healthcare relies on the co-ordinated activity of various services and facilities such as community mental health centres, day hospitals, and staffed or non-staffed residential facilities. Indeed, even after deinstitutionalization, residential treatment maintains some of its importance. Community psychiatry relies on hospitals and other inpatient settings for three purposes: short admissions for acute mental healthcare, rehabilitation, and long-term accommodation for the most severely ill and disabled patients. The most salient features of the main instruments for community clinical practice will be discussed in this chapter.

Efficacy, strengths, and limitations of community psychiatry

Evidence on the efficacy and efficiency of community mental healthcare has been accumulating in the last 20 years. One of the most extensive studies was carried out in the United Kingdom, between 1985 and 1998, by the Team for the Assessment of Psychiatric Services (TAPS). It evaluated the consequences of discharge of 1166 long-stay patients (more than one year of hospitalization) from two psychiatric hospitals in London. The vast majority of people were referred to staffed houses, and a large proportion of these reported an improvement in their quality of life, within new, less restrictive settings and with larger social networks, although psychiatric symptoms and social skills often remained unchanged.

A prospective evaluation carried out by the TAPS among a subset of 670 patients discharged from hospital found that 84% of the sample were satisfied with deinstitutionalization and the new community life.[5] Moreover, patients acquired significant community skills, such as using public transport and accessing public facilities (cinemas, pubs, etc.), as well as domestic skills (namely, caring for their personal and common space and purchasing food). However, while the community skills remained stable for all the five years of follow-up, the domestic ones tended to decrease after the first year. The authors hypothesized that the aging of the sample may have contributed to this decline. A recent review about the effectiveness of community mental healthcare confirmed that deinstitutionalization often brought an improvement in quality of life and better social functioning, especially if rehabilitation in everyday skills was offered to patients both before and after discharge.[6]

Financially, the TAPS evaluation showed that there are no significant differences in costs between psychiatric hospital services and community care,[7] but the improvement in patients' conditions and quality of life makes community mental healthcare a more cost-effective option.[2] However, despite its positive impact on patients' life courses, de-institutionalization and community psychiatry have shown some limitations.

First of all, where deinstitutionalization has been implemented without planning adequate outpatient services (i.e. outpatient clinics), people discharged from mental hospitals, as well as the most severely ill new patients, receive neither adequate treatment nor social care, and so face clinical worsening, social drift, and homelessness. The same effect may be the result of the fact that community mental healthcare usually has to assist many individuals, affected by disorders that widely vary in severity and disability. Therefore, a considerable amount of time and resources has to be dedicated to a great number of people with less severe disorders, with the risk of neglecting the minority with the most severe disorders.[8]

Second, despite community psychiatry allowing patients to live in their community, the most disabled patients rely on staff support for many (if not all) of their needs. Therefore, there is a risk of creating what has been defined as a 'virtual asylum'—namely, a situation in which new, chronically disabled patients live in the community, but depend entirely on mental healthcare.[7] This may raise the phenomenon of explicit social control that conflicts with the aim of community psychiatry.[1] A higher risk is that what happened in asylums may be reproduced for those patients in long-term residential facilities because of their disability or forensic needs. The increase in number of these patients has been called reinstitutionalization or transinstitutionalization, to stress this risk and the similarities with institutionalization.[1]

Nonetheless, community mental healthcare is mainstream in many countries, especially for the most disabled and disadvantaged individuals. Therefore, psychiatrists should know related activities and techniques, and be involved in its implementation and relevant research.

Practicing community psychiatry

Community psychiatry works according to some principles,[9] which will be summarized and discussed with some suggestions for their effective implementation.

Synergy between medical science and recovery philosophy

The daily practice of community psychiatry must take into account the so-called 'recovery dimension', an expression that describes the struggle that mental health patients go through to maintain or achieve their priorities in their most important life domain.[10] The clinician should take into account what is important for patients and how to best preserve it, agreeing the most effective treatments with them. On the other hand, an authoritarian or paternalistic approach to treatment risks bringing patients back to a 'virtual asylum' and a poor clinical outcome.[7]

Practical suggestions

- Assess patients' opinions and expectations about their quality of life.
- Whenever possible, agree treatment with patients that does not compromise their quality of life.
- Assess patients' recovery through appropriate and validated instruments.

A population view

Clinicians should have appropriate knowledge of the characteristics of the populations they care for. Community psychiatry should aim at discovering the current needs of populations and developing specific intervention programmes.[11] Clinical practice should be enriched with an approach aimed at discovering patients' activities and daily experiences.

Practical suggestions

- Research information about the population that lives near and attends mental health facilities.
- Ask patients about their daily life, their activities, and the socio-economic context of their life. Observe their life environment and their daily routine, and speak with their significant others (with patients' consent).
- Take into account patients' socio-economical situation when prescribing treatments. For example, do they have enough money to buy medicines or to take the bus to the mental healthcare facilities?

Mental health promotion and prevention of mental illness: individual and population level

Mental health promotion implies the implementation of strategies to help people maintain or acquire their psychosocial well-being and their capability of coping with adversities. Prevention reduces the probability of harm to mental health. It can be primary, if directed against risk factors for mental health; secondary, if aimed at protecting people exposed to potential harm to their mental health; and tertiary (i.e. treatment to reduce the risk of relapse).

The needs of mental health promotion and prevention may be different according to age, gender, and other specific features of target populations.

Practical suggestions

- Assess patients' daily life. Unhealthy lifestyles or socio-economic disadvantage may arouse stressful situations that might trigger a clinical relapse, as well as cause other health or social problems (such as HIV infection due to intravenous drug use or liver cirrhosis due to alcoholism).

- Material support or psychotherapy may be useful to overcome difficult periods of life (which should be detected in the clinical interview).
- Promote initiatives for educating the general population about mental health, early recognition of mental health problems, and appropriate help-seeking strategies.[12]

Long-term (often lifelong) treatment perspective

Community psychiatry services usually care for patients throughout their whole life. This means that patients' lifestyle and health needs will vary across time, and that elderly mental health patients will face several problems related to aging, such as anxiety or depression, cognitive impairment and dementia, or other neurological and physical problems.[13] Moreover, due to increased life expectancy, a rise in the number of older people developing age-related mental disorders is expected.[14]

Practical suggestions

- Modify interventions according to patients' age (for instance, take into account their co-morbidities and concomitant pharmacological therapies for somatic co-morbidities when prescribing medications).
- When evaluating psychopathological symptoms in elderly patients, assess if they may be due to a co-morbid condition, a metabolic problem, or medications.[15]
- Screen older patients for cognitive impairment and dementia. Mini Mental State Examination (MMSE) is practical and has proved to be useful in detecting cognitive impairment in middle-aged and older patients affected by schizophrenia.[16] It is also important to bear in mind that depression and negative symptoms (for psychosis) may worsen a patient's cognitive performance.[15]

Team-based services

As living in the community means that patients have to face several different problems, community psychiatry relies on a multidisciplinary approach, with mental healthcare teams composed of various different professionals who support patients in the most critical aspects of their life. A typical mental healthcare team includes psychiatrists for pharmacological treatment and general medical care supervision, psychologists for psychotherapy, nurses for support with daily mental health issues, and social workers for job support and access to welfare measures.

The main setting of community psychiatry practice is the community mental health centre,[17] which is the outpatient facility that houses the community mental healthcare team. This is the setting for visits, psychotherapy, and other activities. Moreover, as stated before, team members can reach users in their home environment for assessment, counselling, help in daily activities, or crisis intervention.

Practical suggestions

- Each team member should provide and share his or her experiences and opinions about a patient's clinical situation. This does not mean that members must become interchangeable; rather, that each member should combine their specific competencies and contribution with those of other members.[18] Working as a team is also useful to prevent professional burnout, especially when working with the most severely ill patients.[19]

◆ The mental healthcare team also interacts with many other services, including non-mental healthcare services (e.g. general practitioners, emergency room staff) and non-health care services (e.g. the criminal justice system, patients' employers). Therefore, regular and clear communication is essential to avoid gaps in treating and supporting fragile individuals,[17] as well as to increase patients' adherence and satisfaction, though less for symptoms and social functioning.[20]

◆ It may be useful to establish simple protocols to facilitate communications and referral of patients (e.g. from schools to community psychiatry services for the early treatment of the onset of mental disorders).

Case study 1

John was an 18-year-old high-school student who began to behave strangely. He missed several school days, and reduced the time spent with his friends. He spent a lot of time at home, playing on his computer or watching television. His school marks, which had been quite good, began to fall. He quarrelled several times with his professors and school mates, and began to dress bizarrely.

Thanks to some informative meetings held by the local community mental health service with John's professors, he was referred to an early intervention team for assessment of the possible onset of a psychotic disorder. John's parents were sceptical about it, but they met the local community mental health team who gave them information about the possible severity of John's condition.

It is important to remember that an early referral for assessment and treatment of a possible psychotic onset has a favourable effect on prognosis, as the longer is the period of untreated illness, the more severe is the harm for patients, as mental illness prevents them from reaching properly the developmental milestones in their life (e.g. completing schools, acquiring adequate social skills).

Cost effectiveness

Cost effectiveness is important in relation to both community mental healthcare and also the clinical practice of mental healthcare.

Firstly, according to the previously described results of the TAPS study, there was little difference between the cost of an asylum-based model of mental healthcare and a community-based one. However, the better outcomes observed with the latter make the community-based model a more cost-effective one.[2]

Secondly, the aim of providing mental healthcare for a whole population, with limited funds, implies that resources should be rationally distributed. For instance, it could be necessary not to prescribe the most promising treatment for some patients (such as a new, expensive antipsychotic), with the aim of saving resources to ensure adequate treatment for many other patients.[21] This is especially important as community psychiatry often cares for patients with the most disabling mental disorders or with very low incomes. As such patients often rely on social welfare to fund their treatment, saving resources to care for them may be a priority. Indeed, community psychiatry has a strong commitment to social justice, as caring for people by taking into account their socio-economic situation means also helping them to face material adversities.[4]

Practical suggestions

♦ Always keep in mind the financial situation of patients when prescribing treatments and medications. Economic stability is in fact related to higher health status, health literacy, attention to preventive care, and capability of buying medications.[21] Therefore, additional attention may be necessary when dealing with the most deprived patients.

♦ Make sure to grant an adequate, acceptable, and accessible service to everyone, with specific initiatives to care for the most severely ill patients and for individuals belonging to neglected populations (e.g. ethnic minorities, homeless).[4]

Community care of the most severely ill patients

Although living in the community offers more opportunities to people with mental health problems for a satisfying quality of life, it exposes them to the risk of a poor quality of life as the result of the synergy of patient disability and hostile environmental factors (Fig. 18.1).

Many individuals suffering from mental disorders experience severe disability and the need for long and intensive treatment. This condition has been defined as 'severe mental illness' or 'severe mental disorder', an expression that, irrespective of diagnosis, identifies patients with a poor clinical course, who require a high commitment by several professional and non-professional caregivers, including psychiatric services, families, and welfare agencies. There are many definitions of severe mental illness, with scarce consistency between them, but they all usually make reference to the prolonged duration and significant disability which lead to relevant difficulties in living in the community.[22]

The disability associated with mental disorders may have many causes, such as positive, negative, and cognitive symptoms of schizophrenia; relationship problems

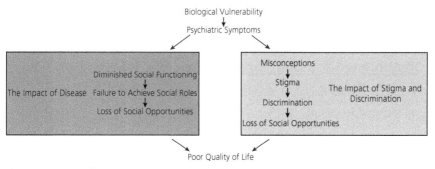

Fig. 18.1 Impact of psychiatric diseases, stigma, and discrimination

Adapted from Cogn Behav Pract, 5(2), Corrigan PW, The impact of stigma on severe mental illness, p. 201–22, Copyright (1998), with permission from Elsevier.

associated with personality disorders; poor self-efficacy; and bizarre behaviour. There-fore, severe mental disorders may not allow for appropriate integration into society,[23] increasing the risk of social drift, exclusion from social contexts, financial disadvan-tage, and (at times) contiguity with deviant environments. On the other hand, it is important not to overlook the personal assets and resources on which patients can rely when aiming for their personal goals, as well as the support they can receive from their significant others and their wider home community.[17]

The following provides a brief overview of some effective ways of treating severely ill patients.

Case management

Case management involves the allocation of a member of a community mental health-care team for long-term support of a specific (and usually severely ill and disabled) patient.[17] The most widely implemented model of case management is the 'Clinical Case Model'. According to this model, the case manager is responsible for connecting patients to community services, as well as in helping them to cope with their disability and in supporting their families.

Case management requires close and prolonged contact with patients and their life environment, which implies the establishment of a stable, trustful, and supportive rela-tionship.[24] The main aspects of case management are summarized in Box 18.2.

Box 18.2 Main tasks of case management

Co-ordination

+ Facilitate continuity of care among different interventions and services.
+ Monitor the implementation of interventions.

Health promotion and prevention

+ Help users in identifying their personal goals and resources.
+ Help users in identifying stressors or other risk factors for clinical relapse or social drift.

Treatment (not usual)

+ Psychoeducational interventions.
+ Social skills training.

Source data from: Schizophrenia Bull, 24(1), Mueser KT, Bond GR, Drake RE, Resnick SG. Models of community care for severe mental illness: a review of research for case manage-ment, p. 37–74, Copyright (1998) Oxford University Press; Hosp Community Psych., 40, Kanter J. Clinical case management: definition, principles, components, p. 361–68, Copy-right (1989) Oxford University Press.

Residential treatment: acute mental healthcare, rehabilitation, and accommodation

According to the principles of community care, treatment of acute conditions should take place at outpatient facilities (e.g. mental health centres, day hospitals) or at the patient's home. However, patients who require ongoing observation and care are admitted to specific hospital wards, sometimes with compulsory measures.

Rehabilitation can take place in long-term residential facilities, where patients with adequate psychopathological compensation and adherence to treatment can take part in individualized programmes. However, the most disabled patients may not be able to participate in rehabilitation programmes because of their severity of illness, old age, or co-morbidities. These patients are usually in residential care facilities, with or without medical assistance. In the latter case, staff are responsible only for the patients' basic needs (e.g. preparing meals, supporting the regular taking of medications).[8]

Apart from clinical requirements, modern residential treatment must take into account the need to allow patients to maintain their social contacts.

Crisis and outreach interventions

After deinstitutionalization, it became clear that, even if community mental health centres, semi-residential facilities, and some residential institutions could adequately take care of the majority of patients, there were a minority who needed a more intensive approach (due to the severity of their symptomatology, scarce consciousness of illness, poor adherence, and a high rate of co-morbid addiction or physical illness). Many of these patients were incapable of or unwilling to access community mental healthcare facilities, but the severity of their conditions caused them to be frequently admitted to accident and emergency wards for psychiatric or non-psychiatric health issues. Therefore, since the 1970s, community psychiatry has developed special interventions for those patients who cannot be appropriately cared for and followed up by regular mental healthcare practice.[7] The most important initiatives for these 'difficult' patients are Assertive Community Treatment (ACT) and Crisis Resolution Teams (CRT), described in Table 18.1.

Compulsory treatment

Not all psychiatric symptoms are egodystonic. It happens quite often, especially with the most severe mental disorders, that patients have no insight of their mental illness and refuse treatment. In cases of acute decompensation, this condition can expose them, and their significant others, to high risks. Thus, compulsory treatment, administered against a patient's will, is considered. In psychiatry, treatment can be residential (with compulsory admission to a hospital) or non-residential (i.e. community compulsory treatment). Research about its efficacy is scarcely informative, due to methodological and theoretical issues. However, it may be useful in those situations in which protecting a patient from his own symptomatology is crucial (e.g. persecutory delusions, suicidal or homicidal intent). At the one-year follow-up of a cohort of patients compulsorily admitted to hospital, only 15% were readmitted involuntarily.[25]

Table 18.1 Assertive Community Treatment and Crisis Resolution Teams

Assertive Community Treatment (ACT)	Crisis Resolution Teams (CRTs)
◆ Multidisciplinary team, often including a psychiatrist, a psychologist, a nurse and social workers, that usually reaches patients at home or in their life environment, providing care and support in that context	
◆ Low user to staff ratio (e.g. 1:10) and caseloads shared across clinicians	
◆ 24-hour coverage	
◆ Most interventions provided in the community	
◆ Usually involved in patients' long-term treatment	◆ Care for acute decompensation of mental disorders or intolerable psychosocial stressors
	◆ Some act as gate-keepers for admission to acute mental healthcare wards

Source data from: Štrkaljlvezić S, Mužinić L, Filipac V. Case management—a pillar of community psychiatry. Psychiat Danub, 2010; 22(1): 28–33; Hasselberg N, Grâve RW, Johnson S, Šaltytâ-Benth J, Ruud T. Psychiatric admissions from crisis resolution teams in Norway: a prospective multicentre study. BMC Psychiatry, 2013; 13(117):.17; Mueser KT, Bond GR, Drake RE, Resnick SG. Models of community care for severe mental illness: a review of research for case management, Schizophrenia Bull., 1998; 24(1): 37–74.

Please note: even if case management, ACT, and CRTs have proven to be effective, there is evidence that the full implementation of these interventions is not necessary if their main characteristics are already offered by standard, established community mental healthcare, as happens in countries such as United Kingdom and Italy.[7]

Compulsory treatment has been criticized as its coercive nature may hamper the therapeutic relationship. However, several examples indicate that this does not happen if treatment is carried out according to good clinical practice. Treatment conditions during the first week of admission and an empathic, supportive therapeutic relationship with the patient have been shown to play a key role in helping patients to maintain a positive relationship with their carers and to understand their need for care at the moment of admission. Usually, only a minority of patients do not understand why such a measure has been taken.[26,27]

Practical suggestions

◆ Always try to explain to patients their need for care; also tell them when they are highly decompensated.

◆ Do not tell lies to patients to encourage them to go to hospital (e.g. telling them that they are only going to be visited by an orthopaedic consultant for their back pain).

◆ Do not promise patients that you will never impose a compulsory treatment order, but ensure, through your daily clinical practice, that you reach agreement with them on each step of treatment and, if necessary, explain to them that should they not be able to make decisions themselves, you will have to do that for them.

Case study 2

Catherine was a 45-year-old woman with a borderline personality disorder who was placed, by her psychiatrist, on the waiting list for admission to a day hospital, due to severe depressive symptomatology. While waiting for a place, Catherine phoned her psychiatrist, telling him that she did not want to live anymore and that she had just taken all her medications in order to kill herself. The psychiatrist sent the police and the emergency services to her home. Then, the woman was taken to hospital and admitted to the psychiatric ward under a compulsory treatment order. This action made her very angry towards her psychiatrist. However, the psychiatrist managed to re-establish a positive and supportive relationship with her and, after some weeks, she apologized to the psychiatrist for her anger as she had since understood that, at that time, she had needed help.

Specialized mental health services

This term refers to mental healthcare interventions for specific populations, such as patients with eating disorders, those with co-morbid substance use disorders (dual diagnosis), pregnant women, and early intervention teams for psychosis. Their use is recommended for those countries with the highest level of resources, but should still take into account local needs and resources as well as treatment gaps.[20]

Employment and occupational support

Unemployment is part of the burden of disability associated with severe mental disorders. More than two thirds of users with severe mental illness (SMI) think that finding a job is one of the primary targets in their life, but only 15% have one.[28] Many people with SMI rely on social welfare measures for their income. Having a job can help them in ameliorating their quality of life, in terms of both material benefits and self-esteem.[8] Therefore, supporting employment is a core element of community mental health services, with vocational rehabilitation programmes including 'train then place' models that provide a preliminary assessment of a patient's working capability, followed by pre-occupational training, and then research of an appropriate job. On the other hand, 'place then train' models, such as individual placement and support (IPS) models, support people with SMI in first finding a job in the competitive community labour market, and then in delivering and maintaining that job. Such models provide support that is tailored to patients' specific needs, assessing skills and preferences during the phase of job finding and, once the job has been obtained, with on-site job coaching or specific skills training.

The IPS model seems more successful than 'train then place' models, although many of the jobs found in IPS programmes are part-time and low income, and about a third of patients who start a job, subsequently lose it.[29]

Finally, there are programmes for those people who are not able to find or keep a job in a competitive environment. These initiatives allow them to get acquainted with the requirements of a competitive job setting, through activities scheduled according to their treatment programme and disability and designed to avoid excessive distress. Work Integration Social Enterprises (WISEs), in particular, are social firms providing employment for individuals with disabilities and offering products or services. Every member receives a full market wage and all workers share the same rights and duties. WISEs usually offer services such as gardening, cleaning, or maintenance work, as well as work in manufacturing.[30]

Psychoeducation and peer support

To help patients to be accepted fairly in the society in which they live,[7] mental health community services need to consider relevant social capital (i.e. the system of norms, shared beliefs, and networks that make a society capable of pursuing shared objectives).[31] Minorities and those facing difficulties in accepting the widely acknowledged social norms may be marginalized and excluded from society. Social inclusion of community mental healthcare patients can be improved by psychoeducation, in which patients and their significant others are taught to understand the symptoms of their mental illness and to appropriately manage them, using narrative models and cognitive behavioural techniques such as problem solving and role playing.[32]

Psychoeducation has been successfully implemented for schizophrenia and bipolar disorder, improving patients' self-management of their illness, as well as reducing the burden of care for their families.[33] Since members of patients' social networks often do not have sufficient awareness of mental healthcare, staff of primary healthcare services and police officers may benefit from psychoeducation, as inadequate comprehension and acceptance of SMI may undermine patients' well-being and their potential recovery.

However, patients with mental illness can themselves constitute social capital. They share difficulties and experiences, which make them able to effectively support each other, with peer support services in community psychiatry providing a recovery-oriented environment and developing the capacity of caring for their members.[34] It is however very important, before organizing peer-support initiatives, to assess if participating patients are really capable of supporting their peers.

Training in community psychiatry

Training in modern psychiatry should dedicate significant resources to teaching the fundamental principles of community psychiatry, as in many parts of the world it is the most usual approach to chronic and disabling mental disorders.[35]

According to various authors, a good training programme should include some of the specific competencies summarized in Box 18.3.

Box 18.3 Core elements of a reliable training programme in community psychiatry

Development of personalized treatment plans, agreed, whenever possible, with patients

- Ethical appropriateness of clinical practice
- Consideration of patients' cultural and spiritual background in assessment and treatment
- Tailoring assessment work to patients' characteristics, taking into account both areas of need and readiness to commitment and change, to properly support patients in self-management and recovery

Box 18.3 Core elements of a reliable training programme in community psychiatry (continued)

◆ Giving information taking into account individual needs (language or cognitive problems), and collection of informed consent when needed

Dealing with complex questions within a multidisciplinary team

◆ Capability of acting as a team member and also of having a leadership role

◆ Development of multidisciplinary treatment plans, which should integrate all staff contributions into the care programme

◆ Integration of pharmacological treatment with other treatments, such as individual or group psychotherapy or psychoeducational interventions

◆ Implementation of case management activities

◆ Consideration of substance use disorders and of developmental and physical health issues in treatment programmes and strategies for establishing regular consultations with caring professionals and services

Integration and co-ordination of clinical practice within health systems

◆ Knowledge of health systems and development of joint strategies, together with other agencies, according to main principles of community mental health

◆ Requirements and strategies to develop health delivery services and to integrate them with mental healthcare services and policies

Teaching and development of research plans

◆ Provision of adequate teaching of the theoretical bases and clinical practice guidelines for community psychiatry

◆ Techniques of leading a supervision of learners' clinical practice

◆ Critical evaluation of healthcare literature

◆ Capability of developing community-based research plans and integrating them in multidisciplinary research initiatives

Source data from: Hogan MF. Transforming mental health care: realities, priorities, and prospects. Psychiatr Clin North Am. 2008; 31:1–9.

Fiorillo A, Calliess IT, Sass H. How to Succeed in Psychiatry: a Guide to Training and Practice. In: Carrà G, Sciarini P, Nolan F, Clerici M. Training in community psychiatry, Copyright (2012) John Wiley & Sons Ltd.

Community psychiatry in fact comes into contact with highly complex systems, so it is important that relevant staff have as much knowledge as possible.

Moreover, the complexity faced by community psychiatry requires a strong effort in developing methodologically appropriate research strategies[7] that focus initially on finding valid and accepted definitions for services, in order to allow appropriate comparisons and syntheses between different delivery models and populations.[36]

Conclusions

This chapter aimed at providing an overview of the main aspects of community psychiatry, with the objective of helping practicing clinicians in developing a basic knowledge of its main aspects. People with SMI should be able to live a satisfying life in the community, but this opportunity, although close to them, is frequently denied by the burden of their disability and stigma. Therefore, community psychiatry should not only take care of patients but should also stimulate and support society in developing a healthier environment for the most mentally ill. With this approach, community psychiatry could act as a mediator that allows patients and their families to live the adequate life that deinstitutionalization has promised them.[3]

Acknowledgement

Carlo Beccarelli for graphics of Figure 18.1.

References

1 **Chow WS, Priebe S**. Understanding psychiatric institutionalization: a conceptual review. *BMC Psychiat* 2013; **13**:169.

2 **Thornicroft G, Tansella M**. Balancing community-based and hospital-based mental health care. *World Psychiat* 2002; **1**(2):84–90.

3 **Muijen M**. Mental health services in Europe: an overview. *Psychiat Serv* 2002; **59**(5):479–82.

4 **Drake RE, Szmukler G, Mueser KT, Thornicroft G**. Introduction to community mental health care. In: *Community mental health* (eds. Thornicroft G, Szmukler G, Mueser KT, Drake RE). Oxford: Oxford University Press; 2011.

5 **Leff J, Trieman N**. Long stay users discharged from psychiatric hospitals: social and clinical outcomes after five years in the community. The TAPS Project 46. *Brit J Psychiat* 2000; **176**:217–23.

6 **Kunitoh N**. From hospital to the community: the influence of deinstitutionalization on discharged long-stray psychiatric users. *Psychiat Clin Neuros* 2013; **67**:384–96.

7 **Killaspy H**. From the asylum to community care: learning from experience. *Brit Med Bull* 2007; 79–80:245–58.

8 **Davis L, Fulginiti A, Kriegel L, Brekke JS**. Deinstitutionalization? Where have all the people gone? *Curr Psychiat Rep* 2012; **14**:259–69.

9 **Thornicroft G, Tansella M**. *Better mental health care*. Cambridge: Cambridge University Press; 2009.

10 **Sklar M, Groessl EJ, O'Connell M, Davidson L, Aarons GA**. Instruments for measuring mental health recovery: a systematic review. *Clin Psychol Rev* 2013; **33**:1082–95.

11 **Caplan G, Caplan R**. Principles of community psychiatry. *Comm Ment Hlt J* 2000; **36**(1):7–24.

12 **Min JA, Lee CU, Lee C**. Mental health promotion and illness prevention: a challenge for psychiatrists. *Psychiatry Investig* 2013; **10**:307–16.

13 **Vink D, Aartsen MJ, Schoevers RA**. Risk factors for anxiety and depression in the elderly: a review. *J Affect Dis* 2008; **106**:29–44.

14 **Blevins D, Morton B, McGovern R**. Evaluating a community-based participatory research project for elderly mental healthcare in America. *Clin Interv Aging* 2008; **3**(3):535–45.

15 **Felmet K, Zisook S, Kasckow JW**. Elderly users with schizophrenia and depression: diagnosis and treatment. *Clin Schizoph Related Psychoses* 2011; **4**(4):239–50.

16 **Moore DJ, Palmer BW, Jeste DV**. Use of the Mini Mental State Exam in middle-aged and older outusers with schizophrenia. *Am J Geriat Psychiat* 2004; **12**:412–9.

17 **Mueser KT, Bond GR, Drake RE, Resnick SG**. Models of community care for severe mental illness: a review of research for case management. *Schizophrenia Bul.* 1998; **24**(1):37–74.

18 Ministry of Health. Report of the Working Party on Social Workers in the Local Authority Health and Welfare Services. London: Her Majesty Stationery Office; 1959.

19 **Fothergill A, Edwards D, Burnard P**. Stress, burnout, coping and stress management in psychiatrists: findings from a systematic review. *Int J Soc Psychiat* 2004;**50**: 54–65. DOI: 10.1177/0020764004040953.

20 **Thornicroft G, Tansella M**. Components of a modern mental health service: a pragmatic balance of community and hospital care. *Brit J Psychiat* 2004; **185**:283–90.

21 **Everett A, Huffine C**. Ethics in contemporary community psychiatry. *Psychiat Clin N Am* 2009; **32**:329–41.

22 **Wiersma D**. Needs of people with severe mental illness. *Acta Psychiat Scand* 2006; **113**(429):115–9.

23 **Corrigan PW**. The impact of stigma on severe mental illness. *Cogn Behav Pract* 1998; **5**:201–22.

24 **Ivezić Štrkalj S, Mužinić L, Filipac V**. Case management—a pillar of community psychiatry. *Psychiat Danub* 2010; **22**(1):28–33.

25 **Sheehan KA**. Compulsory treatment in psychiatry. *Curr Opin Psychiatry* 2009; **22**:582–6.

26 **Luciano M, Sampogna G, Del Vecchio V, Pingani L, Palumbo C, De Rosa C, Catapano F, Fiorillo A**. Use of coercive measures in mental health practice and its impact on outcome: a critical review. *Expert Rev Neurother* 2014; **14**:131–41.

27 **Priebe S, Katsakov C, Amos T, et al**. Users' views and readmissions 1 year after involuntary hospitalisation. *Brit J Psychiat* 2009; **194**(1):49–54.

28 **Hogan M**. Transforming mental health care: realities, priorities and prospects. *Psychiat Clin N Am* 2008; **31**(1):1–9.

29 **Tenhula WN, Bellack AS, Drake RE**. Chapters 12.13: Schizophrenia: Psychosocial approaches. In: *Kaplan & Sadock's comprehensive textbook of psychiatry* (9th edn) (eds. Sadock BJ, Sadock VA, Ruiz P). Philadelphia: Lippincott Williams & Wilkins; 2009.

30 **Warner R, Mandiberg J**. An update on affirmative businesses or social firms for people with mental illness. *Psychiat Serv* 2006; **57**(10):1488–92.

31 **Putnam RD**. The strange disappearance of civic America. *Am Prospect* 1996; **7**:1–18.

32 **Lukens EP, McFarlane WR**. Psychoeducation as evidence-based practice: considerations for practice, research and policy. *Brief Treat Crisis Interv* 2004; **4**(3):205–25.

33 **Chien WT, Leung SF, Yeung FKK, Wong WK**. Current approaches to treatments for schizophrenia spectrum disorders, part II: psychosocial interventions and patient-focused perspectives in psychiatric care. *Neuropsychiatr Dis Treat* 2013; **9**:1463–81.

34 **Mahlke CI, Krämer UM, Becker T, Beck T**. Peer support in mental health services. *Curr Opin Psychiat* 2014; **27**:276–81.

35 **Carrà G, Sciarini P, Nolan F, Clerici M**. Training in community psychiatry. In: *How to succeed in psychiatry: a guide to training and practice* (eds. Fiorillo A, Calliess IT, Sass H). Hoboken: John Wiley & Sons, Ltd.; 2012.

36 **Roberts E**. A review of economic evaluations of community mental health care. *Med Care Res Rev* 2005; **62**(5):503–43.

Chapter 19

Practical strategies to fight stigma in mental health

Sara Evans-Lacko, Petra C. Gronholm,
Ahmed Hankir, Luca Pingani,
and Patrick Corrigan

Definitions of and concepts related to stigma and discrimination

Stigma is related to exclusion from civil society, increased risk of contact with the criminal justice system, victimization, poverty, homelessness, less access to physical healthcare, and reduced life expectancy. Historically, the word 'stigma' was used in ancient Greek (500 BC) to mean 'puncture' or 'brand'. In particular, it referred to the process by which a person found guilty of significant crimes (theft or murder) or belonging to a low social class (specifically, slaves) was marked or branded by an iron point at the top of a wooden stick.[1] This way, the person could be immediately identified by others in the community, who were also warned against having any kind of relationship with that person.

Although the term stigma has ancient origins, it was only in the twentieth century that the term was introduced in the psychological and sociological literature. Erving Goffman, a Canadian sociologist, introduced the concept of stigma and analysed the phenomenon in his two most famous papers—*Asylums: essays on the social situation of mental patients and other inmates*[2] and *Stigma: notes on the management of spoiled identity*.[3] According to Goffman, stigma is an attribute considered undesirable and unpleasant by society and which differentiates the person from other members of the community that he/she should be part of. Thus, a person with such an attribute is regarded as someone marked and discredited.

Although Goffman is still often cited, Link and Phelan have further developed the definition of stigma, to reflect advances in research, by referring to 'the co-occurrence of its components—labelling, stereotyping, separation, status loss, and discrimination'.[4] Stereotypes are widely held beliefs concerning the habits, behaviours, and characteristics that are associated with people with mental illness. Prejudice, instead, is the automatic emotional response to the stereotype (for example, 'people with schizophrenia are dangerous and so I am afraid of them!'). This affective response (attitude) in turn leads to behaviour adopted to preserve and protect from possible consequences that might arise from the stereotype (for example, 'they are dangerous and should be excluded from the community').[5]

The consequences of stigmatization against people with mental illness are dramatic and are often considered to be as important as the illness itself. Stigma can undermine many of the life goals of people with severe mental illness through reduced participation in higher education, employment, and relationships, and lower levels of well-being and empowerment. It is therefore essential that young physicians and early career psychiatrists are aware of the impact of stigma.[6–9]

Types of stigma

There is a rich literature discussing and developing concepts pertaining to stigma. Van Brakel describes five types of stigma: public stigma, structural stigma, self-stigma, felt or perceived stigma, and experienced stigma.[10] Label avoidance has been highlighted as an additional critically important type of stigma.[11] Table 19.1 defines each of these types of stigma and provides an example for each of them.

Table 19.1 Definitions and examples of different types of stigma

Type of stigma	Definition	Examples
Public stigma	The reaction that the general population has to people with mental illness[12]	'I would not want to live next door to someone who has been mentally ill' (one in eight people in England agree)[13]
		'I think that being prone to violence is a distinguishing feature of people with mental illness' (36% of people in England agree)[13]
Structural stigma	Regulations, laws or institutions which systematically discriminate against or disadvantage people with mental illness[14]	HB-5639 State of Michigan: increases discrimination by prohibiting mental health agencies from operating within 1000 feet of a school's property line[14]
		Sensationalist headlines of newspapers ('Get violent crazies off our streets')[15]
		Laws which prohibit individuals with mental illness from being elected to office or serving on a jury
Self-stigma	The decrease of self-esteem and self-efficacy, as a result of the internalization of stigma of mental illness by the person with a mental illness[16]	'At first I thought I was crazy and I was like okay, do I have a mental illness?... 'cause my mom, she has a mental illness of paranoid schizophrenic, and I was thinking I'm going to turn out like her; I didn't want that to happen'[17]
		'Believing I'll be sick forever and useless and never able to do what I want to do and will never amount to anything because I have a mental illness'[18]

(continued)

Table 19.1 (continued) Definitions and examples of different types of stigma

Type of stigma	Definition	Examples
Felt or perceived stigma	The stigma that people with a (potentially) stigmatized mental health condition fear or perceive to be present in the community or society [10]	Fear that others would associate taking antidepressant medications with being under narcotic effects[19] Not applying for a job for fear of being discriminated against
Experienced stigma	Experience of actual discrimination and/or participation restrictions on the part of the person affected[10]	Treated differently by the other members of the family[20] 'I have been shunned or avoided when it was revealed that I am a consumer'[21]
Label avoidance	Not seeking out or participating in mental healthcare in order to avoid the egregious impact of a stigmatizing label[22,23]	'I feel ashamed about my diagnosis and therefore avoid using mental health treatments' 'I feel embarrassed about having a diagnosis of depression and so hide my medication or peel the label off the bottle'

How can we stop stigma?

Corrigan describes three different strategies for overcoming stigma towards people with mental illness: protest, education, and contact.[24] Protest aims to eliminate negative stereotypes in public statements, media reports, or advertisements.[25] The second strategy, education, is characterized by providing evidence-based information about mental illness or by demonstrating how false beliefs (e.g. most murderers have schizophrenia) are represented in society. The literature suggests this approach may be most successful with people who already know someone with a mental illness or have some knowledge about mental illness.[25] The third strategy involves direct contact with people with a psychiatric disorder. Contact has been recognized as one of the most effective ways to fight stigma:[26,27] it reduces anxiety and also allows the checking, *in vivo*, of the invalidity of one's own prejudices.[7] Given the range of types of stigma (as shown in Table 19.1), it is important to target anti-stigma work at the type we seek to eradicate. We now discuss how these strategies have been used and evaluated in actual interventions.

What are the best anti-stigma interventions?

In Europe, research on stigma and social exclusion in relation to people with mental illness has been increasing over recent years. A systematic mapping of the literature showed that the number of published articles has increased significantly over the past five years; however, the majority of papers are characterized by descriptive research, with few studies of anti-stigma interventions or underlying social mechanisms.[28] Further understanding of social mechanisms is important to forming the basis for future interventions to reduce stigma and promote inclusion.

There are recent systematic reviews which identify effective interventions for reducing stigma. Pettigrew and Tropp[29] reviewed more than 515 studies, including 713 independent samples of which 66 focused on mental illness; meta-analysis focusing on mental illness showed that greater intergroup contact was associated with a reduction in prejudice and a small to moderate effect size of r = 0.18. A more recent review by Corrigan and colleagues examined anti-stigma approaches specific to mental illness which incorporated elements of education, protest, or contact.[27] Personal contact interventions yielded the greatest effect size for adults, while education was most effective among adolescents. Although studies which incorporated protest were associated with a lower effect size, there were fewer studies which evaluated these kinds of interventions. Additionally, when comparing across strategies, it is important to consider the aims of the intervention in relation to the outcome measures. Population attitude measures may be less relevant for anti-stigma work involving protest, as these interventions may be better at engaging policymakers, changing the representation of people with mental illness in the media, or suppressing discriminatory behaviours. Finally, a systematic review by Clement and colleagues focused specifically on mass media strategies and showed that mass media interventions may reduce prejudice; while fewer studies have investigated their effects on discrimination.[30]

Reducing public stigma through nationwide campaigns

Stigma and discrimination against people with mental illness reflect the cultural beliefs present in society and thus, efforts towards reducing public stigma could also foster a more favourable social context for people with mental illness. In 1996, the World Psychiatric Association initiated several national and regional efforts through the 'Open the Doors' programme (http://www.openthedoors.com/english/index.html) which aimed to reduce public stigma, specifically in relation to people with schizophrenia.[31] Shortly after, other national initiatives were launched including the pioneering 'Like Minds, Like Mine' in New Zealand in 1997 (http://www.likeminds.org.nz/; see Fig. 19.1),[32] 'Beyond Blue' in Australia in 2000 (http://www.beyondblue.org.au/), 'See Me' in Scotland in 2002 (http://www.seemescotland.org.uk/; see Fig. 19.2), and 'Time to Change' in England in 2009 (http://www.time-to-change.org.uk/)—all of which are ongoing. More recently, interest in large, national campaigns has increased, especially in Europe, and there are now at least 21 anti-stigma campaigns across European countries and regions.[33]

As efforts have grown and been evaluated, it is possible to begin to distil a set of 'best practice principles' for campaigns. For example, based on evidence from existing anti-stigma interventions, Corrigan has identified five principles for strategic stigma change: consumer contact, and contact that is targeted, local, credible, and continuous[34] (see Table 19.2). Continued rigorous evaluation of these programmes will help us further refine this framework and our understanding of the mechanisms by which stigma is reduced. Several large-scale evaluations have now been published which contribute towards this understanding.

Evaluation of 'Beyond Blue', Australia's national depression initiative, suggests that the programme has contributed towards improved mental health literacy for

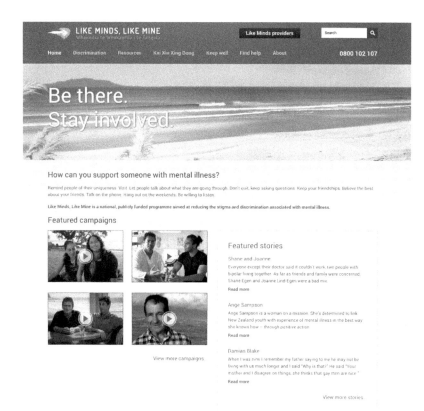

Fig. 19.1 Screenshot of the New Zealand 'Like Minds, Like Mine' campaign website.

Reproduced from Like Minds, Like Mine, http://www.likeminds.org.nz/, with permission.

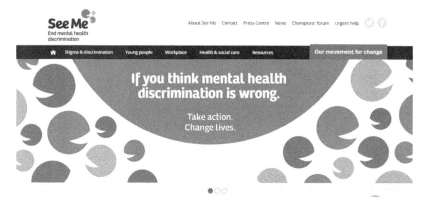

Fig. 19.2 Screenshot of the Scotland 'See Me' campaign website.

Reproduced from See Me, http://www.seemescotland.org.uk/, with permission.

Table 19.2 Principles for strategic stigma change

♦ **Contact:** Consumer/service user contact which involves direct personal interaction between people with and without mental illness, is fundamental to stigma change

♦ **Targeted:** Contact is more effective when it is targeted at key groups

♦ **Local:** When developing interventions, local factors such as geographic region and socio-demographic factors should be considered

♦ **Credible:** Contact is most effective if it demonstrates recovery and incorporates and represents the aims of the intervention

♦ **Continuous:** Ongoing efforts are needed and are more effective than one-off interventions

Source data from: Psychiatr Serv, 62(8), Corrigan PW. Best practices: strategic stigma change (SSC): five principles for social marketing campaigns to reduce stigma, p. 824–6, Copyright (2011) American Psychiatric Publishing.

depression and other mental illnesses.[35,36] In Scotland, there has been a significant reduction in the proportion of respondents agreeing that people with mental illness are dangerous, and a significant increase in willingness to interact with someone who has a mental illness[37,38] Evaluation of England's 'Time to Change' programme showed modest but significant improvements in intended behaviour and a positive trend for attitudinal improvement.[13] Moreover, awareness of the campaign was associated with better knowledge, attitudes, and intended behaviour.[39] There was also a significant increase in the proportion of service users who reported having experienced no discrimination during the previous year.[40] Economic evaluation has also demonstrated that national anti-stigma programmes represent potentially cost-effective, and low-cost strategies for reducing the impact of stigma on people with mental health problems.[41,42]

Altogether, evidence supports the effect of gradual change among the public alongside anti-stigma campaigns. There are, however, some challenges in the evaluation of these programmes. Randomized controlled trials are not usually feasible and identifying an appropriate, non-exposed control group is a significant challenge when evaluating such large-scale national interventions. Smaller-scale controlled experiments would allow for a control group but these would not tell us about the campaign's potential to work in real life as a national programme and the indirect effects which may result in relation to the intervention. Thus, it is important when evaluating programmes to consider, for example, long-term effects, dose–response relationships or multiple measures, and/or methods, in order to triangulate findings when randomized controlled trials are not possible. Finally, secular trends (e.g. economic recession) should be accounted for to the extent possible.[43]

Target groups

Public anti-stigma interventions may be aimed broadly at the general population (see Fig. 19.3) or may focus on a specific target group (see Fig. 19.4). Target groups could be identified as important by service user groups either because of their high levels of contact with service users (e.g. general practitioners, psychiatrists, teachers), or because they are people in positions of power (e.g. employers, landlords), or because they represent potential for changing the future (e.g. young people).[44] Additional

Myth: People with mental illness can't work.
Fact: You probably work with someone with mental illness.

You can help. Find out how at time-to-change.org.uk

Fig. 19.3 Example from the 'Time to Change' campaign in England, targeted at the general public.

Reproduced from Time to Change, http://www.time-to-change.org.uk/, with permission.

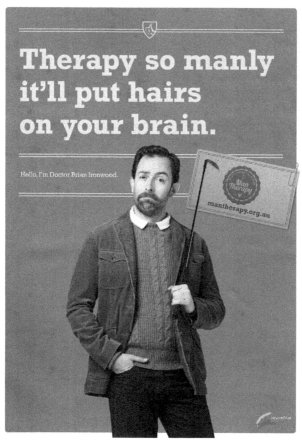

Fig. 19.4 Example of an advertisement from the 'Beyond Blue' campaign in Australia, specifically targeted at men.

Reproduced from Beyond Blue, http://www.beyondblue.org.au/, with permission.

considerations may include readiness for change, availability of methods for reaching the group, and whether there are other interventions which are already working with the group. Existing interventions may be an advantage if the plan is to tailor or adapt available evidence-based interventions to a new context; however, if there are already several ongoing efforts with a certain group, it may be worth considering what can be done with other, less active groups.

Interventions to reduce self-stigma and increase empowerment

As reducing public stigma is a slow and complex process, interventions which aim to reduce self-stigma among people with mental illness and/or to improve stigma coping are also needed. As long as public stigma persists, these strategies may be helpful for reducing the harm associated with negative public beliefs and actions against people with mental illness. Mittal and colleagues identified 14 studies evaluating interventions aimed at reducing self-stigma among people with mental illness.[45] Although most studies were pilot or exploratory studies, eight of the fourteen demonstrated a significant reduction in self-stigma, representing a promising avenue for future research.

While previous interventions tended towards educational approaches,[46,47] recent efforts have also incorporated features such as cognitive restructuring. Narrative enhancement cognitive behavioural therapy (NECT) is a group-based therapy which combines psychoeducation, cognitive restructuring to challenge negative self-beliefs, and narrative therapy which explores ways to enhance one's narratives or life story. Using a quasi-experimental design, evaluation of NECT provides preliminary support for reduction of self-stigma in three of four subscales following completion of the intervention, in comparison with a control group.[48]

'Ending Self-stigma' is a nine-session group programme that combines cognitive behavioural exercises, discussion, sharing of experiences, group support, skills training, and problem solving for people with serious mental illness.[49] An initial pilot evaluation suggested that following the intervention, participants had lower self-stigma and greater perceived social support and recovery orientation, though there was no control group.

A third intervention, 'Coming Out Proud', is a three-session, manual-based, peer-led group intervention developed around the idea that disclosure or 'coming out' can reduce self-stigma. The intervention aims to empower participants to make a personal decision about their own disclosure. A pilot randomized controlled trial[50] suggested that the intervention was effective in reducing stigma stress, disclosure-related stress, secrecy, and an improvement in perceived benefits of disclosure. There was no significant reduction in self-stigma or empowerment.

Young people: an important target group for anti-stigma interventions

The foundations for maintained adult fears, avoidance, and disrespect—elements central to continued stigma and discrimination—are argued to be present already at an early age.[51] As such, children and adolescents have been identified as one key target population for stigma change.[52,53]

Stigmatizing attitudes and beliefs in children

Negative conceptualizations of mental illness are present already from a very young age. It is suggested that as early as in kindergarten, children have established a preferential hierarchy where individuals labelled as 'mentally ill' are considered with more fear, distrust, disgust, and aversion relative to a 'normal' person or members of other 'deviant' groups (e.g. physically handicapped individuals). This negative reaction was even stronger for individuals labelled 'crazy'.[54] A similar finding was provided by a study that reported how, already when aged 8–9 years, children seemed to have developed negative beliefs, suggesting that individuals with mental health problems are undesirable and should thus be avoided, even though they lacked a clear understanding of exactly what mental illness is or what characterizes individuals affected by such difficulties.[55]

A further striking insight of how negatively the concept of mental illness is perceived among children is provided in a study by Rose and colleagues.[56] In this qualitative study, 14-year-old students in England were asked to shout out the kinds of words or phrases that might be used to describe someone experiencing mental health problems. This exercise generated 250 labels. Tellingly, of these, 70% were negative and 30% neutral, whereas no positive terms or phrases were suggested. The most frequently occurring terms (mentioned by three or more pupils) are listed in Table 19.3.

If unchallenged, negative attitudes towards and beliefs regarding mental illness often persist, as remarkably similar, from early childhood onwards.[53,57]

Table 19.3 The words and terms occurring most frequently among 14-year-old school students to describe a person experiencing mental illness

Disturbed	Weird	Stress
Nuts	Depressed	Violence
Confused	Different	Brain dead
Psycho	Freak	Demanding
Spastic	Odd	Demented
Crazy	Problem	Dinlo
Depression	Retard	Distressed
Disabled	Scary	Embarrassed
Mad	Div	Flid
Unpredictable	Dumb	Frustrated
Insane	Ill	Isolated
Loony	Loneliness	Sad
Mental	Loony bin	Strait jacket
Schizophrenia	Psychiatric	Wheel chairs
Thicko	Screw loose	

Sources of stigma in young people

The fact that very young children already report negative attitudes towards and beliefs regarding individuals with mental illness could be considered to reflect deep-rooted and pervasive societal beliefs and perspectives that young people have taken on.

Nearly half of the 250 labels for mental illness suggested by school children[56] reflected popular derogatory terms, illustrating how easily children and adolescents might pick up on prejudicial descriptions and attitudes in relation to mental illness prevalent in their social context. Another likely key influence on children's and adolescents' perceptions about mental health is stigmatizing attitudes that their parents might hold.[58,59] Also, the media can influence young people's views. A review of portrayals of mental illness in children's films, TV programmes, video games, and so on, concluded that these provided children with pervasive depictions of people with psychiatric disorders as unattractive, villainous, and dangerous, and were frequently coupled with the use of offensive slang and negative labels.[51] This was seen to facilitate rejection of peers with mental health problems, and also to encourage insensitivity and a lack of empathy from young children in relation to mental illness. Also, newspapers have been reported to influence negative opinions regarding mental illness amongst adolescents.[60]

Importance of anti-stigma efforts among young people

Anti-stigma campaigns which primarily target adults sideline derogatory perspectives nurtured among young people. Anti-stigma efforts directed towards children and adolescents could shape sensitive and empathic attitudes towards individuals affected by mental illness, which might be easier than modifying and challenging well-formed and

Box 19.1 School-based anti-stigma strategies

Schools provide a useful context for anti-stigma work among young people. Many such programmes have been developed; within these, strategies have included, for instance, puppetry[63] and story books[64] for younger children, and educational interventions building on drama, quizzes and games,[65] and inclusive dialogue[66] for older students.

School-based anti-stigma strategies vary and can be categorized into protest, education, and contact-driven programmes.[24] A systematic review on school-based anti-stigma efforts reported that nearly all programmes included an educational component. At times, the interventions were education-focused only, but some also combined this with contact-type elements. A few programmes were based purely on contact; whereas no strategies based on the principle of protest were identified.[67]

There is suggestive evidence that a curriculum employing strategies of social contact with individuals with mental health problems could foster empathy, which in term could facilitate social inclusion, inclusiveness, and reduced discrimination.[67] However, we need additional, methodologically rigorous research to better understand the effectiveness of school-based anti-stigma interventions and the most effective components to fight stigma among school-age persons.

firmly entrenched negative and discriminatory beliefs and perspectives in adulthood.[52] Furthermore, as children's conceptions of the world are still developing, this age group has been suggested to be particularly vulnerable to taking on or becoming affected by stigmatizing messages they are exposed to.[51,56] This perspective serves to further highlight the need for specific efforts to target stigma among young people.

Through targeting prejudice about and discrimination towards people with mental illness early on, it might be possible to foster future generations of adults for whom stigma of mental illness has never developed or is muted[61,62] (see Box 19.1 for school-based intervention examples).

'The Wounded Healer': an effective anti-stigma intervention targeted at the medical profession

Quis custodiet ipsos custodes? Who will watch the watchmen?

Despite the perception that doctors should be 'invincible', mental illness is more common among doctors than among the general population.[68–70] In the United Kingdom, between 10% and 20% of doctors become depressed at some point during their career.[71] Suicide rates are also high, with 400 doctors lost to this cause of death every year in the United States alone.[72] Mental health problems may present early on during medical school;[73,74] however, doctors and medical students have low levels of help-seeking, often only presenting to mental health services once a crisis arises. Fear of stigmatization has been identified as a critical factor contributing towards secrecy and symptom concealment.[75]

Stigma towards people with mental illness among healthcare professionals

Many service users report that medical practitioners could benefit from anti-stigma programmes. The 2008 'Stigma Shout' survey of almost 4000 people (and their carers) using mental health services throughout England asked participants, 'From which groups of people do you personally experience most stigma and discrimination?' Healthcare professionals were among the highest in the ranking, with the percentage of respondents for each specialty and the position on the 'league table' as follows: general practitioners (23%, sixth); psychiatrists (19%, ninth); and accident and emergency staff (17%, eleventh).[76]

The consequences of healthcare professionals having stigmatizing views towards people (including doctors) who have mental illness can be tragic. Daksha Emson, a brilliant trainee psychiatrist with bipolar affective disorder, killed herself and her daughter in October 2000. An independent inquiry into her death concluded that Dr Emson was the victim of stigma within the National Health Service. The inquiry team consequently called for a wider understanding of mental illness in order to help end the taboo and secrecy associated with it.[77]

The 'Wounded Healer' and autobiographical narrative

Carl Jung used the term the 'Wounded Healer' as an archetypal dynamic to describe a phenomenon that may take place in the relationship between the analyst and the analysed.[78] It remains a powerful archetype in the healing arts. Jung discovered this archetype in relation to himself; for him, 'it is his own hurt that gives a measure of his power to heal'.[79]

Autobiographical narratives of the 'Wounded Healer' are gaining popularity among doctors with mental health challenges, both as an effective form of adjunctive therapy and as a means to campaign against stigma.[80] It is with the immediacy and authenticity of the first-person narrative that the mental illness memoir creates a vivid account of human existence in the 'Kingdom of the Sick'.[81] Reading autobiographical narratives of psychopathology sufferers can 'augment' and 'embellish' service providers' and the general public's humanity by offering precious qualitative insights into minds afflicted with mental illness.[78] Narratives also provide an opportunity to illustrate the influence that stigma can have on people's attitudes and behaviours towards mental illness, and thus facilitate empathy towards people who experience mental illness. There may be something about the medical–scientific stance that can 'de-humanize' medical practitioners; narratives could enable doctors to re-engage with their humanity and, consequently, better understand patient's feelings and emotions.

Box 19.2 provides one such first-person narrative account, and describes how this has come to form the basis of an anti-stigma lecture delivered to future medics in training. In this case, a presentation from a peer with experience of mental health treatment may have a greater impact on attitudes of future health professionals, in line with the support for social contact interventions, as discussed previously in this chapter.

Box 19.2 The first-person narrative of Dr Ahmed Hankir

'In order to restore the human subject at the centre, the suffering afflicted fighting human subject, we must deepen the case history into a narrative or tale.' (Reproduced from Sacks O. The Man Who Mistook His Wife For A Hat: And Other Clinical Tales, p. 243, Copyright (1998) Simon and Schuster)

I spent my formative years in the Middle East. Lebanon at the time was just recovering from a brutal and bloody civil war. I will never forget my first foray into a Palestinian refugee camp. I remember meeting children whose parents were killed as a result of an explosion, and they were consequently rendered orphans. Despite their tragedy and as well as being homeless and hungry (they had no benefactor to provide for them and they would survive off scraps of food if and when they could find any), they had broad smiles adorning their innocent faces.

This exposure to the catastrophic consequences of conflict made me realize just how fortunate I was relative to so many others. Even to this day, whenever I am feeling low, I still remind myself of the hardship that these children had to endure, and this helps to put things into perspective for me.

I returned to England when I was 17. I took the year out in order to work and earn some money, since I was completely dependent on myself. With no skill-set and a qualification from Lebanon that was not recognized, I started off as a janitor cleaning floors. These were challenging times indeed. However, I was fully aware that I had been given a decent shot at life. I just had to focus, be patient, and work hard.

Box 19.2 The first-person narrative of Dr Ahmed Hankir (continued)

After my first year, I enrolled into a sixth form college. I was, however, still independent and so I had to work full-time hours to sustain myself. This posed a constant threat to obtaining the grades necessary to enter medical school. Despite the challenges I faced, I obtained straight As and I was granted admission into medical school.

In 2006, when I was a third-year medical student, reports started trickling in about a war that was being waged upon Lebanon. A full-blown mania then ensued (sometimes an appropriate response to reality is to go insane):

◆ Grandiloquent ideas

◆ Racing thoughts, 'Knight's move' thinking evident

◆ Pressurized speech

◆ Increased amounts of energy (subjective 11/10)

The aftermath of mania is invariably melancholia; I started to sink into the murky depths of a depressive illness, a depression too dreadful to describe. I was experiencing low mood which was pervasive and ubiquitous, irregular/disturbed sleeping patterns, feelings of worthlessness and utter guilt, an inability to concentrate, and a bleak outlook for the future.

By far the worst aspect of the experience was being labelled with mental illness and the stigmatizing effects this had on me. I was ostracized by my so-called friends.

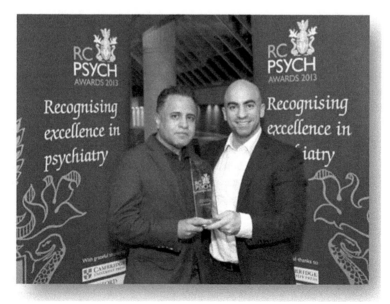

Fig. 19.5 Dr Rashid Zaman FRCPsych (left) and Dr Ahmed Hankir (right). Following treatment, Dr Hankir made a full recovery from his mental illness and went on to receive the 2013 Royal College of Psychiatrists' Foundation Doctor of the Year Award.

Reproduced with permission from the Royal College of Psychiatrists.

Box 19.2 The first-person narrative of Dr Ahmed Hankir (continued)

Social exclusion had a profoundly deleterious effect on me. I was sinking deeper and deeper into the darkness.

I developed suicidal ideation whilst in extremis. However, as a practicing Muslim, I was aware that suicide is strictly forbidden in Islam. Thus I resisted acting upon any impulse to end my own life.

Convalescence

I convalesced in 2010 and I have been in full remission ever since. I qualified from medical school in 2011 and was appointed National Institute for Health Research Academic Clinical Fellow in Psychiatry with Manchester University in 2013.

Ever since my recovery, I have been actively campaigning to stamp out the stigma associated with mental health challenges, particularly in the medical profession. I co-authored a publication entitled, '*The Wounded Healer' mental illness in the medical profession and the role of the health humanities in psychiatry*[80] and have since then designed, developed, and delivered an anti-stigma lecture (adapted from the publication) to five different universities across the United Kingdom.

The feedback that I received has been exceptionally positive, suggesting that we can engage students in anti-stigma efforts: 96% of respondents would recommend the talk to a colleague, 93% agreed that the talk made them realize that medics who suffer from a mental illness can go on to recover and achieve their goals, and 76% agreed that their views towards mental health issues were more positive after the talk.

Countering stigma and negative attitudes starts with the individual, by challenging our own prejudices and preconceptions. Being more accepting of doctors who experience mental health challenges will help to reduce stigma and result in better outcomes.

Conclusion

Stigma and discrimination are pervasive phenomena which exert a negative influence, through a multitude of ways, on the lives of many individuals affected by mental illness. Both specifically targeted interventions and nationwide campaigns have been found effective for reducing stigma and discrimination against people with mental illness. Anti-stigma work targeting specific groups, such as young people and healthcare staff, or strategies which empower individuals facing discrimination, are likely to play a key role in reducing the impact of stigma. Interventions building on the principle of contact frequently show promise, and we need to consider how to incorporate personal stories and narratives to build awareness at national and local levels. National strategies can help engage influential stakeholders, but it is also critical that we increase empowerment and local involvement through local grass-roots activities.

As we further our understanding of the mechanisms which facilitate and maintain stigma, we also need to further develop and refine the strategies we use to fight stigma and discrimination. This will require robust evaluation and thoughtful consideration of the methodological challenges in determining the long-term impact of anti-stigma work. Improving attitudes, reducing levels of discrimination, and increasing social inclusion for individuals affected by mental illness pose a significant challenge. However, with thoughtful, systematic, and comprehensive strategies, achieving change is possible, albeit this is likely to be a slow and gradual process.

Acknowledgements

PG currently receives funding support from the National Institute for Health Research (NIHR) Mental Health Biomedical Research Centre at South London and Maudsley NHS Foundation Trust and King's College London. The views expressed are those of the author(s) and not necessarily those of the NHS, the NIHR, or the Department of Health. SEL currently holds a Starting Grant from the European Research Council.

References

1 **Pianigiani O**. *Vocabolario etimologico della lingua italiana*. Rome: Albrighi e Segati; 1907.

2 **Goffman E**. *Asylums: essays on the social situation of mental patients and other inmates*. New York: Anchor Book Edition; 1961.

3 **Goffman E**. *Stigma: notes on the management of spoiled identity*. Englewood Cliffs, NJ: Prentice-Hall; 1963.

4 **Link BG, Phelan JC**. Conceptualizing stigma. *Annu Rev Sociol* 2001; **27**(1):363–85.

5 **Corrigan PW, Shapiro JR**. Measuring the impact of programs that challenge the public stigma of mental illness. *Clin Psychol Rev* 2010; **30**(8):907–22.

6 **Rüsch N, Corrigan PW, Heekeren K, et al**. Well-being among persons at risk of psychosis: the role of self-labeling, shame, and stigma stress. *Psychiatr Serv* 2014; **65**(4):483–9.

7 **Evans-Lacko S, Brohan E, Mojtabai R, Thornicroft G**. Association between public views of mental illness and self-stigma among individuals with mental illness in 14 European countries. *Psychol Med* 2012; **42**:1741–52.

8 **Lasalvia A, Zoppei S, Van BT, et al**. Global pattern of experienced and anticipated discrimination reported by people with major depressive disorder: a cross-sectional survey. *Lancet* 2012; **381**: 55–62.

9 **Lee S, Tsang A, Breslau J, et al**. Mental disorders and termination of education in high-income and low- to middle-income countries: epidemiological study. *Br J Psychiatry* 2009; **194**:411–7.

10 **Van Brakel WH**. Measuring health-related stigma—a literature review. *Psychol Heal Med* 2006; **11**(3):307–34.

11 **Corrigan PW, Watson AC**. The paradox of self-stigma and mental illness. *Clin Psychol Sci Pract* 2006; **9**(1):35–53.

12 **Corrigan PW, Watson AC**. Understanding the impact of stigma on people with mental illness. *World Psychiatry* 2002; **1**(1):16–20.

13 **Evans-Lacko S, Henderson C, Thornicroft G**. Public knowledge, attitudes and behaviour regarding people with mental illness in England 2009–12. *Br J Psychiatry Suppl* 2013; **55**:s51–7.

14 **Corrigan PW, Watson AC, Heyrman ML, et al**. Structural stigma in state legislation. *Psychiatr Serv* 2005; **56**(5):557–63.

15 'Get the violent crazies off our streets'. *New York Daily News* 1999; 11–19.

16 **Watson AC, Corrigan P, Larson JE, Sells M**. Self-stigma in people with mental illness. *Schizophr Bull* 2007; **33**(6):1312–8.

17 **Kranke DA, Floersch J, Kranke BO, Munson MR**. A qualitative investigation of self-stigma among adolescents taking psychiatric medication. *Psychiatr Serv* 2011; **62**:893–9.

18 **Peterson D, Barnes A, Duncan C**. *Fighting shadows. self-stigma and mental illness*. Auckland: Mental Health Foundation of New Zealand; 2008.

19 **Interian A, Martinez IE, Guarnaccia PJ, Vega WA, Escobar JI**. A qualitative analysis of the perception of stigma among Latinos receiving antidepressants. *Psychiatr Serv* 2007; **58**(12):1591–4.

20 **Thornicroft G, Brohan E, Rose D, Sartorius N, Leese M**. Global pattern of experienced and anticipated discrimination against people with schizophrenia: a cross-sectional survey. *Lancet* 2009; **373**:408–15.

21 **Wahl OF**. Mental health consumers' experience of stigma. *Schizophr Bull* 1999; **25**(3):467–78.

22 **Ben-Zeev D, Young MA, Corrigan PW**. DSM-V and the stigma of mental illness. *J Ment Health* 2010; **19**(4):318–27.

23 **Clement S, Schauman O, Graham T, et al**. What is the impact of mental health-related stigma on help-seeking? A systematic review of quantitative and qualitative studies. ***Psychol Med*** 2015; **45**:11–27.

24 **Corrigan PW, River LP, Lundin RK, et al**. Three strategies for changing attributions about severe mental illness. *Schizophr Bull* 2001; **27**:187–95.

25 **Rüsch N, Angermeyer MC, Corrigan PW**. Mental illness stigma: concepts, consequences, and initiatives to reduce stigma. *Eur Psychiatry* 2005; **20**(8):529–39.

26 **Evans-Lacko S, London J, Japhet S, et al**. Mass social contact interventions and their effect on mental health related stigma and intended discrimination. *BMC Pub Heal* 2012; **12**(1):489.

27 **Corrigan PW, Morris S, Michaels P, Rafacz J, Rüsch N**. Challenging the public stigma of mental illness: a meta-analysis of outcome studies. *Psychiatr Serv* 2012; **63**:963–73.

28 **Evans-Lacko S, Courtin E, Fiorillo A, et al**. The state of the art in European research on reducing social exclusion and stigma related to mental health: a systematic mapping of the literature. *Eur Psychiatry*. 2014; **29**:381–9. DOI:10.1016/j.eurpsy.2014.02.007.

29 **Pettigrew TF, Tropp LR**. A meta-analytic test of intergroup contact theory. *J Pers Soc Psychol* 2006; **90**:751–83.

30 **Clement S, Lassman F, Barley E, et al**. Mass media interventions to reduce mental health-related stigma: Cochrane protocol. *Cochrane Data Syst Rev* 2013; **23**;7:CD009453. doi: 10.1002/14651858.CD009453.pub2.

31 **Warner R**. Local projects of the World Psychiatric Association programme to reduce stigma and discrimination. *Psychiatr Serv* 2005; **56**(5):570–5.

32 **Vaughan G, Hansen C**. 'Like Minds, Like Mine': a New Zealand project to counter the stigma and discrimination associated with mental illness. *Australas Psychiat* 2004; **12**(2):113–7.

33 **Borschmann R, Greenberg N, Jones N, Henderson RC**. Campaigns to reduce mental illness stigma in Europe : a scoping review. *Die Psychiatr* 2014; (January):43–50.

34 **Corrigan PW**. Best practices: strategic stigma change (SSC). Five principles for social marketing campaigns to reduce stigma. *Psychiatr Serv* 2011; **62**(8):824–6.

35 Jorm AF, Christensen H, Griffiths KM. Changes in depression awareness and attitudes in Australia: the impact of beyondblue: the national depression initiative. *Aust NZ J Psychiat* 2006; **40**:42–6.

36 Yap MB, Reavley NJ, Jorm AF. Associations between awareness of beyondblue and mental health literacy in Australian youth: results from a national survey. *Aust NZ J Psychiat* 2012; **46**(6):541–52.

37 Dunion L, Gordon L. Tackling the attitude problem. The achievements to date of Scotland's 'See Me' anti-stigma campaign. *Ment Heal Today* 2005; Mar:22–5.

38 Mehta N, Kassam A, Leese M, Butler G, Thornicroft G. Public attitudes towards people with mental illness in England and Scotland, 1994–2003. *Br J Psychiat* 2009; **194**:278–84.

39 Evans-Lacko S, Malcolm E, West K, et al. Influence of Time to Change's social marketing interventions on stigma in England 2009–11. *Br J Psychiat Suppl* 2013; **55**:s77–s88.

40 Corker E, Hamilton S, Henderson C, et al. Experiences of discrimination among people using mental health services in England 2008–11. *Br J Psychiat Suppl* 2013; **55**:s58–s63.

41 Evans-Lacko S, Henderson C, Thornicroft G, McCrone P. Economic evaluation of the anti-stigma social marketing campaign in England 2009–11. *Br J Psychiat Suppl* 2013; **55**:s95–101.

42 McCrone PR, Knapp M, Henri M, McDaid D. The economic impact of initiatives to reduce stigma: demonstration of a modelling approach. *Epidemiol Psychiatr Soc* 2010; **19**(2):131–9.

43 Evans-Lacko S, Corker E, Williams P, Henderson C, Thornicroft G. Effect of the Time to Change anti-stigma campaign on trends in mental-illness-related public stigma among the English population in 2003–13: an analysis of survey data. *Lancet Psychiatry* 2014; **1**:121–128.

44 Corrigan PW. Target-specific stigma change: a strategy for impacting mental illness. *Stigma: Psychiat Rehab J* 2004; **28**: 113–121 28(2/9).

45 Mittal D, Sullivan G, Chekuri L, Allee E, Corrigan PW. Empirical studies of self-stigma reduction strategies: a critical review of the literature. *Psychiatr Serv* 2012; **63**(10):974–81.

46 McCay E, Beanlands H, Zipursky R, et al. A randomised controlled trial of a group intervention to reduce engulfment and self-stigmatisation in first episode schizophrenia. *Adv Ment Heal* 2007; **6**(3):212–20.

47 Link BG, Struening EL, Neese-todd S, Asmussen S, Phelan JC. On describing and seeking to change the experience of stigma. *Psychiatr Rehabil Ski* 2002; **6**(2):201–31.

48 Roe D, Hasson-Ohayon I, Mashiach-Eizenberg M, Derhy O, Lysaker PH, Yanos PT. Narrative enhancement and cognitive therapy (NECT) effectiveness: a quasi-experimental study. *J Clin Psychol* 2014; **70**(4):303–12.

49 Luckstead, A, Drapalski, A, Calmes, C, Forbes, C. DeForge, B, Boyd J. Ovid: ending self-stigma. Pilot evaluation of a new intervention to reduce internalized stigma among people with mental illnesses. *Psychiatr Rehabil J* 2011; **35**:51–4.

50 Rüsch N, Abbruzzese E, Hagedorn E, et al. Efficacy of Coming Out Proud to reduce stigma's impact among people with mental illness: pilot randomised controlled trial. *Br J Psychiatry* 2014; **204**:391–7.

51 Wahl OF. Depictions of mental illnesses in children's media. *J Ment Heal* 2003; **12**(3):249–58.

52 Wahl OF. Children's views of mental illness: a review of the literature. *Psychiatr Rehabil Ski* 2002; **6**(2):37–41.

53 Hinshaw SP. The stigmatization of mental illness in children and parents: developmental issues, family concerns, and research needs. *J Child Psychol Psychiat* 2005; **46**(7):714–34.

54 **Weiss MF**. Children's attitudes toward the mentally ill: a developmental analysis. *Psychol Rep* 1986; **58**(1):11–20. DOI:10.2466/pr0.1986.58.1.11.

55 **Adler AK, Wahl OF**. Children's beliefs about people labeled mentally ill. *Am J Orthopsychiat* 1998; **68**(2):321–6.

56 **Rose D, Thornicroft G, Pinfold V, Kassam A**. 250 labels used to stigmatise people with mental illness. *BMC Health Serv Res* 2007; **7**:97. DOI:10.1186/1472-6963-7-97.

57 **Weiss MF**. Children's attitudes toward the mentally ill: an eight-year longitudinal follow-up. *Psychol Rep* 1994; **74**(1):51–6.

58 **Jorm AF, Wright A**. Influences on young people's stigmatising attitudes towards peers with mental disorders: national survey of young Australians and their parents. *Br J Psychiat* 2008; **192**(2):144–9.

59 Time to Change Report. *Parents still lost for words where mental health is concerned.* September 2013. Available at: http://www.time-to-change.org.uk/news/parents-still-lost-words-where-mental-health-concerned

60 **Dietrich S, Heider D, Matschinger H, Angermeyer MC**. Influence of newspaper reporting on adolescents' attitudes toward people with mental illness. *Soc Psychiat Psychiatr Epidemiol* 2006; **41**(4):318–22.

61 **Corrigan PW, Watson AC**. How children stigmatize people with mental illness. *Int J Soc Psychiat* 2007; **53**(6):526–46. DOI:10.1177/0020764007078359.

62 **Gale F**. Tackling the stigma of mental health in vulnerable children and young people. In: *Mental health interventions and services for vulnerable children and young people* (ed. Vostanis P). London, Philadelphia: Jessica Kingsley Publishing; 2007, pp. 58–79.

63 **Pitre N, Stewart S, Adams S, Bedard T, Landry S**. The use of puppets with elementary school children in reducing stigmatizing attitudes towards mental illness. *J Ment Heal* 2007; **16**(3):415–29.

64 **Shah N**. Changing minds at the earliest opportunity. *Psychiatr Bull* 2004; **28**(6):213–5.

65 **Essler V, Arthur A, Stickley T**. Using a school-based intervention to challenge stigmatizing attitudes and promote mental health in teenagers. *J Ment Heal* 2006; **15**(2):243–50.

66 **Lindley E**. Inclusive dialogue: the way forward in anti-stigma mental health education? *J Public Ment Health* 2012; **11**(2):77–87.

67 **Schachter HM, Girardi A, Ly M, et al**. Effects of school-based interventions on mental health stigmatization: a systematic review. *Child Adolesc Psychiat Ment Heal* 2008; **2**(1):18.

68 **Carson AJ, Dias S, Johnston A, et al**. Mental health in medical students. A case control study using the 60 item General Health Questionnaire. *Scott Med J* 2000; **45**(4):115–6.

69 **Dyrbye LN, Thomas MR, Shanafelt TD**. Systematic review of depression, anxiety, and other indicators of psychological distress among US and Canadian medical students. *Acad Med* 2006; **81**(4):354–73.

70 **Fox FE, Rodham KJ, Harris MF, et al**. Experiencing 'the other side': a study of empathy and empowerment in general practitioners who have been patients. *Qual Health Res* 2009; **19**(11):1580–8.

71 **Firth-Cozens J**. A perspective on stress and depression. In: *Understanding doctors' performance* (eds. Cox J, King J, Hutchinson A). Oxford: Radcliffe Publishing; 2006, pp. 22–5.

72 *American Foundation for Suicide Prevention. Facts and Figures* http://www.afsp.org./understanding-suicide/facts-and-figures.

73 **Vaz RF, Mbajiorgu EF, Acuda SW**. A preliminary study of stress levels among first year medical students at the University of Zimbabwe. *Cent Afr J Med* 1998; **44**(9):214–9. Available at: http://europepmc.org/abstract/MED/10101425. Accessed 9 April 2014.

74 **Ibrahim N, Al-Kharboush D, El-Khatib L, Al-Habib A, Asali D**. Prevalence and predictors of anxiety and depression among female medical students in King Abdulaziz University, Jeddah, Saudi Arabia. *Iran J Pub Heal* 2013; **42**(7):726–36.

75 **Semple D, Smyth R**. *Oxford handbook of psychiatry* (2nd edn). Oxford: Oxford University Press; 2008, pp. 279–317.

76 Time to Change. *Stigma shout: service user and carer experiences of stigma and discrimination*. London: Time to Change; 2008.

77 Authority NELSH. *Report of an independent inquiry into the care and treatment of Daksha Emson and her daughter Freya*. London; 2003.

78 **Burns L, Burns E**. *Literature and therapy: a systemic view*. Karnac: London; 2009.

79 **Stevens A**. *On Jung*. Oxford: Oxford University Press; 1994.

80 **Hankir A, Zaman R**. Jung's archetype, 'The Wounded Healer', mental illness in the medical profession and the role of the health humanities in psychiatry. *BMJ Case Rep* 2013; Jul: 12.

Chapter 20

Working with families of patients with mental illness

Valeria Del Vecchio, Gaia Sampogna,
Bino Thomas, Tamas Kurimay,
and Lisa Dixon

Case study

Mark was a 19-year-old single, university student who lived with his parents. Mark's family requested treatment on his behalf because they felt that he had been out of control for about three months. His relatives described a change in his behaviour beginning approximately one year before and coinciding with the end of his first love affair. Since then, Mark had shown obvious mood swings, been verbally violent and agitated, and started to smoke marijuana regularly. His situation considerably worsened about four weeks ago, when he became suspicious of his relatives, convinced that they wanted to harm him; he believed that the television was spying on him. Things became completely unmanageable three days before the first contact with mental health professionals, when he destroyed furniture in his family's house and kicked in the television.

During this period, Mark's parents were very frightened and felt alone. They did not talk to anybody about the situation because they were worried about the negative comments they thought their friends would make. Ultimately, Mark's neighbours called the emergency services and he was forcibly taken to the hospital.

At the time of admission, Mark was agitated and physically threatening, with a labile affect. He was primarily elevated and angry. He was involuntarily admitted to a locked ward and then started pharmacological treatment with antipsychotic medications and benzodiazepines. After approximately two weeks, the agitation began to diminish, and Mark was transferred to an open ward. Mark's parents still did not want to inform their friends and other relatives about Mark's situation as they worried about being blamed for causing his mental problems.

At the end of the involuntary admission, the pharmacological therapy was supplemented with psychoeducational family intervention. During this intervention, together with his parents, Mark discussed the drug misuse and gradually developed some insight into the possible role of marijuana as a precipitating factor of his psychotic symptoms. His family was also supported with weekly family consultation sessions.

Introduction

There was a time when the families of individuals diagnosed with severe mental disorders were excluded from the care of their relatives. In the past, relatives were even considered 'responsible' for mental illness.[1] According to the psychoanalytic tradition, many mental disorders were caused by inadequate parenting skills. In 1948, Freida Fromm-Reichman proposed the 'schizophrenogenic mother' concept[2] and, in 1950, Gregory Bateson proposed the 'double bind theory'.[3] Both theories have been widely accepted for many years by the scientific community.

Such theories reinforced the idea that the involvement of families in patients' care could lead to a worsening of their clinical condition. The shift of mental healthcare from the hospital to the community has resulted in the recognition and acceptance of the major role played by families in the recovery process of their relatives who are living with mental illness.

After deinstitutionalization, many people diagnosed with a severe mental illness were simply discharged to families who were not prepared to cope with the situation. Some family members reluctantly accepted this responsibility, having established other priorities in their own lives, whereas other families had unrealistic expectations and were unable to handle psychotic behaviours or to maintain household stability. When patients returned to live with their families, family members reported high levels of stress and of practical and psychological burden.[4]

While patient care has always been the clinician's priority, a wealth of evidence showing that relatives' experiences can have an impact on patient health and well-being[5] underscores the importance of family support as being a clinical priority, too. In fact, in everyday psychiatric practice, mental health professionals inevitably deal with families; for example, when asking about family histories of previous medical and psychiatric disorders, and assessing patients' and family members' high-risk behaviours (suicide attempts, addiction, etc.). In clinical practice, there is the need to provide evidence-based biopsychosocial treatments including pharmacotherapy, psychotherapy (i.e. family therapy—as one of the modalities of psychotherapy), and family interventions. The family, as the first socializing agent, serves as both a site for better understanding the origin of mental disorders and as a resource to facilitate the patient's recovery.

The family is a systemic and networked unit, which mental health professionals need to utilize. To help patients with severe mental disorders and their family members it is necessary to have some concept about healthy family functioning and the marital and family life-cycle model. According to Keitner et al., healthy family functioning is defined as the ability to accomplish tasks that are important for the family's well-being, to adapt to changing circumstances, and to balance the individual and the family system. A family may have areas of healthy and unhealthy functioning.[6]

The marital and family life-cycle model, which includes a series of longitudinal stages that mark a family's life over time, is an effective concept for understanding which tasks, roles, and relationships in families change over time. Carter and McGoldrick[7] created a frequently used family life-cycle model that divides the life cycle into six distinct stages. There are two key ideas behind the notion of the family life cycle: families have to adapt their organization to match the tasks associated with different stages of the life cycle; and the time of transition and change is particularly stressful and during this period symptoms are most likely to arise. The concept of the family life cycle may help in understanding the family burden and in planning the therapeutic intervention.

Moreover, the need for caring by the significant others (relatives) is an important element, not only for the clinical practice but also as an ethical issue.[8] Caring is a transgenerational phenomenon, and from this perspective, the role of a psychiatrist is to facilitate the mutual care among family members, including the patient.[8]

Relatives can greatly benefit from professional support for a number of reasons. In fact, the sudden increase of caregiving responsibilities can result in relatives feeling overwhelmed, which can lead them to experience anxiety or depression.[9] Family interventions like psychoeducation, which promote understanding of the mental disorder, result not only in improved interpersonal relationships, but also in improved treatment participation. Moreover, establishing open lines of communication with family members allows mental health professionals to provide support to relatives, and treatments or referrals if necessary, resulting in improved patients' care.

Although in the last decades, the family structure has been significantly modified by demographic, economic, and professional changes,[10] relatives are still highly involved in the care of patients with mental disorders. Additionally, families can play a crucial role in preventing relapses and in facilitating pathways to care for patients.[11]

Characteristics of the family context

Research on the relationship between the family environment and the long-term outcome of people with severe mental disorders has led to the identification of family burden, expressed emotions (EE), and coping strategies as key issues to understand when working with relatives of such patients.[5]

As early as 1966, Grad and Sainsbury (1966)[12] defined family burden (see Box 20.1) as 'any negative impact to the family caused by caring for ill member'. Family burden was subsequently dichotomized into objective and subjective burden.[13] According to Hoenig and Hamilton (1966), objective burden is any event or activity associated with negative caregiving experiences, whereas subjective burden refers to psychological reactions to caregiving. In particular, objective burden includes the practical consequences of taking care of someone with an illness, such as difficulties with social relationships, family life, leisure activities, and finances. Subjective burden includes feelings of anxiety, guilt, sadness, anger, pain, loss, and depression. Several studies[14-16] have pointed out that high levels of family burden reduce patients' and relatives' quality of life, increase patients' relapses and hospitalizations, and increase relatives' incidence of physical and psychological disorders.

Box 20.1 Definition of family burden

Family burden: practical and psychological difficulties related to care for a relative suffering from a long-term disease.

Box 20.2 Definition of expressed emotions

Expressed emotions: aspects of communication of family members. Expressed emotions encompass five components: emotional over-involvement, critical comments, hostility, positive remarks, and warmth.

Box 20.3 Definition of coping strategies

Coping strategies: specific efforts, both behavioural and psychological, that people adopt to manage stressful events. Coping strategies are grouped into emotion-focused and problem-oriented.

Expressed emotions (EE) refers to the observed aspects of communication from family members towards a person with a mental disorder that have a great impact on patients' outcome.[17] The five elements of EE are given in Box 20.2.[17]

Coping is a multidimensional construct referring to the thoughts and behaviours that people engage to manage, tolerate, or reduce internal or external demands that are exceeding an individual's resources.[18] Coping strategies (see Box 20.3) are grouped into emotion-focused and problem-oriented. Several studies[14,19,20] carried out with relatives of patients with severe mental disorders show that problem-oriented coping strategies are adaptive, while emotion-focused coping are viewed as maladaptive and tend to be associated with increased family distress.

Assessment instruments to explore the family context

Many assessment instruments have been developed to explore the family context. A selection of these is shown in Table 20.1.

Table 20.1 Assessment tools for exploring the family context

Assessment instrument	Explored areas	Description
Experience Caregiving Inventory (ECI)	Caregiver's subjective experience	Self-compiled questionnaire of 66 items, grouped in 10 subscales: difficult behaviours, negative symptoms, stigma, problems with mental health centre, effects on family, need to provide support, dependency, loss, positive personal experience, good aspects of relationship
Family Coping Questionnaire (FCQ)	Coping strategies	Multiple-choice questionnaire of 34 items, grouped in 11 subscales: social involvement, maintenance of social interests, positive communication, seek for information, talking with friends, collusion, coercion, avoidance, resignation, alcohol/drugs use, spiritual help
Brief-COPE	Coping strategies	Self-compiled questionnaire of 24 items, grouped in 14 subscales: self-distraction, active coping, denial, substance use, use of emotional support, use of instrumental support, behavioural disengagement, venting, positive reframing, planning, humour, acceptance, religion, self-blame
The Camberwell Family Interview (CFI)	Expressed emotions	90-minute semi-structured interview, divided in five subscales: emotional over-involvement, critical comments, hostility, positive remarks, warmth

(continued)

Table 20.1 (continued) Assessment tools for exploring the family context

Assessment instrument	Explored areas	Description
Five-Minute Speech Sample	Expressed emotions	Semi-structured interview, lasting 5 minutes, based on CFI
Family Problems Questionnaire (FPQ)	Family burden	Multiple-choice questionnaire of 57 items grouped in five subscales: objective burden, subjective burden, criticism, positive attitudes, received help
Perceived Family Burden Scale (PFBS)	Family burden	Self-reported questionnaire of 24 items grouped in two subscales: objective and subjective burden
Involvement Evaluation Questionnaire (IEQ)	Family burden	32-item questionnaire divided into four subclasses: tension, supervision, worrying, urging
McMaster Family Assessment Device (FAD)	Family functioning	Multiple-choice questionnaire of 60 items grouped in seven subscales: global functioning, problem solving, communication skills, family roles, affective responsiveness, affective involvement, behaviour control
Questionnaire of Family Functioning (FF)	Family functioning	24-item questionnaire, used to evaluate family functioning before a family psychoeducational intervention
Needs and Burden Assessment Questionnaire (ABC)	Relatives' opinions and needs; subjective and objective burden	Self-compiled questionnaire of 34 items grouped in three subscales: relatives' opinions on quality of care, needs for information, family burden
Social Network Questionnaire (SNQ)	Relatives' social network	Multiple-choice questionnaire of 15 items grouped in four subscales: social contacts, practical support, psychological support, support of partner
Family Environment Scale (FES)	Social involvement of family members	Self-compiled questionnaire of 90 items

Supporting family members

Clinical studies on the prognosis of major mental disorders show the importance of the involvement of family members and friends in producing positive outcomes. In the last 10 to 15 years, the active involvement of family members in the treatment of patients with a severe mental disorder has improved patients' outcomes, following a reduction of the family burden and improvement of communication skills.[1] Moreover, in recent years, there has been a growing awareness to go beyond 'illness' outcomes of individuals with mental illness and to place a greater emphasis on supporting service users and relatives through the process of recovery.[21] Several family intervention approaches have been developed for optimal management of patients with severe mental disorders, and these have many characteristics that are consistent with the growing recovery movement in mental health in that they are community-based, emphasize achieving personally relevant goals, work on instilling hope, and focus on improving natural supports. Family interventions can be understood as being entirely in accord with a recovery orientation, although they were developed well before the recovery model.[21]

The different approaches may vary in format or participants, basic premises, treatment modalities, and expected outcomes, but all are based on the same model of the stress–vulnerability theory proposed by Zubin and Spring (1977).[22]

Family intervention models

Many approaches have been developed to meet the needs of relatives of patients with severe mental disorders and to improve the family context. These models include psychoeducational family intervention, systemic family therapy, family counselling, family education, family support, and advocacy groups, among others. Table 20.2 summarizes the main models of family intervention. Family psychoeducation has proven to be particularly effective in reducing patient relapse, reducing family burden, and strengthening coping strategies of family members, when administered as an integrated treatment alongside drug therapy.[23] This intervention provides psychological support, knowledge, and information on the disorder, and practical strategies to manage critical situations and family conflicts.

Table 20.2 Main models of family interventions

Model	Participants	Background	Aims
Psychoeducational family intervention	Family, with or without the patient; single or multi-family groups	High levels of expressed emotion and family burden; poor coping strategies	Reduction of relapses and hospitalizations; improvement of family burden
Systemic family therapy	All family members	Dysfunctions in the family system	Symptom reduction; systemic change
Family consultation	The whole family or single family member	Consulting on family problems	Resolution of problems
Family education	Multi-family groups led by trained relatives	Improvement of relatives' knowledge about the illness	Reduction of family distress and family burden
Family support	Multi-family groups led by professionals or trained family members	Experience sharing with people facing similar difficulties	Improvement of relatives' quality of life and reduction of the levels of self-stigma
Advocacy group	Family members	Mutual help among people with similar problems	Reduction of isolation and loneliness

Psychoeducational family intervention

- It is the most effective available family intervention. International guidelines[24,25] suggest providing a psychoeducational family intervention together with pharmacological treatment to people with severe mental disorders.

- This approach, originally developed to meet the needs of families of patients with schizophrenia, has been adapted recently to other major mental disorders, such as depression, bipolar disorder, eating disorders, and obsessive compulsive disorder.

- Different models of family psychoeducation intervention exist. The most successful approaches are the single-family intervention[26] and the multi-family intervention.[27] Other approaches include 'needs-based cognitive behavioural family psychoeducation' (the intervention developed by Anderson and Hogarty and adapted to the American context), the behavioural approach of R. Liberman (1970), and the family intervention for problem solving developed by I. Falloon.[23,26]

- The common aim of all these approaches is to reduce relapses and improve the quality of life for patients and their relatives. Their therapeutic goals include:

  1) providing information to patients and their relatives about symptoms, course, and treatment of the disorder;

  2) improving communication styles within the family;

  3) enhancing family problem-solving skills and coping strategies;

  4) encouraging family members to achieve personal goals.

- These various approaches differ in some aspects such as:

  1) the composition of the group participating in the meetings (uni- or multi-family);

  2) the involvement of the patient;

  3) the setting in which it is provided (during hospitalization, at the mental health centre, or at the patient's home);

  4) the duration of treatment (from a minimum of 6 months to a maximum of 2 years);

  5) the type of mental health professionals conducting the intervention;

  6) the focus on communication skills and problem-solving strategies.

- The most effective interventions should be scheduled as one session every 15 days, for at least 6 months, with the involvement of the patient.

- Research on the different family psychoeducational models has not resulted in determining which one is superior to the others. However, the Falloon model is the most frequently adopted approach when the intervention is provided in an individual format, while the McFarlane approach represents the most frequently used group model.[23]

- The recovery model is embodied in the family psychoeducational intervention goals of equipping family members and patients with information, skills,

---

Box 20.4 Aims of psychoeducational family interventions

1 Increasing personal skills to successfully deal with stressful situations
2 Rebalancing the biological aspects associated with the disease
3 Increasing family strengths on which an individual can rely
4 Increasing family abilities to deal with stressful situations
5 Reducing stressful situations for the patient
6 Improving the quality of life of patients and their families

---

problem-solving strategies, and ways to optimize 'natural supports' to more effectively address the real-life challenges of living with mental disorders.[28]

◆ Despite the efficacy, family psychoeducational interventions (see Box 20.4) are not routinely provided to patients with severe mental disorders. Reasons for the low level of dissemination include organizational problems for mental health professionals (lack of resources, lack of staff, heavy workload), lack of training, too structured an intervention, difficulties in involving families, and lack of consideration of patients' and relatives' preferences.

The Falloon model of psychoeducational family intervention

◆ The Falloon model includes 10–12 weekly sessions (although the total number of sessions may vary depending on a patient's clinical status). Sessions last 60–90 minutes and require the active participation of all family members, including the patient, who is assigned the role of 'expert'.

◆ The approach developed by Ian Falloon (1988)[26] consists of six phases:
  1) family engagement;
  2) individual assessment;
  3) family assessment;
  4) informative sessions;
  5) communication skills;
  6) problem-solving skills and achieving personal goals.

◆ Each session is ideally divided into three phases: a first phase, dedicated to introducing the topic of the session; a second phase on the main topic of the session (the so-called 'teaching phase'); and a final phase, during which the most important aspects discussed during the meeting are summarized. The final phase ends with the 'homework'.

◆ Between one session and another, family members are invited to organize a 'family meeting', without the participation of the mental health professional, to analyse the topics previously discussed during the session, the progress made, and the problems encountered.

Phases of the Falloon psychoeducational family intervention

1 **Family engagement** Mental health professionals should provide patients and relatives with all information on the intervention, explaining the content, purpose, and procedures. It is important to emphasize that the intervention provides psychological support, which aims to improve the quality of life of the patient and of his/her family members. Moreover, it should be clearly stated that this approach has a high efficacy and does not interfere with the other treatments the patient is receiving.

2 **Individual assessment** Each family member is assessed through an interview which investigates their health status, knowledge and opinions about mental disorders, family burden, coping strategies, quality of life, and social and family relationships. This phase ends with the identification of 'personal goals', which must be easily achievable in 3–6 months and related to the personal life of each family member.

3 **Family assessment** At the end of the individual assessments, the mental health professionals should explore how the family interacts, communicates, and discusses problems. During this phase (family assessment), the professional should only observe the interaction, without intervening.

4 **Informative sessions** Informative sessions are focused on:

1) clinical features of the disease, including onset and course, symptoms, prognosis, risk factors;

2) available pharmacological treatments, their side-effects, strategies to manage them, contraindications, duration of treatment, risk factors for relapse;

3) early warning signs, with the identification of user-specific signs, and compilation of an ad hoc schedule.

5 **Communication skills** The objective is to improve the communication skills of participants, especially during stressful situations.[18] In particular, communication skills are:

1) to express pleasant feelings;

2) to make positive requests;

3) to express unpleasant feelings;

4) active listening.

Mental health professionals should explain the importance of communication skills, using practical examples provided by family members themselves.

6 **Problem-solving strategies** Problem solving and goal achievement involves the use of a six-stage model:

1) pinpoint the problem or goal;

2) list all possible solutions;

3) highlight likely consequences;

4) agree on the 'best' strategy;

5) plan and implement;

6) review results.

Family members should be invited to choose problems or goals that can be easily achieved in a short time.

Systemic family therapy

- The central focus of systemic therapy is on the system rather than the individual. Patients are seen as part of a system, and their symptoms and dysfunctional behaviours are considered the consequence of an 'ill system'. The family system is characterized by dysfunctional organization and by miscommunication.

- According to this approach, difficulties are analysed as arising in the relationships, interactions, language, and behavioural patterns that develop between individuals within a family system, rather than in individuals themselves.[29]

- The therapist should act on the different components of the 'system' family, trying to improve communication and to restore family balance.

- Systemic therapy is one of the most widely applied psychotherapeutic approaches in the treatment of children and adolescents. According to a recent review, systemic therapy is efficacious for the treatment of internalizing disorders (including mood disorders, eating disorders, and psychological factors in somatic illness). There is some evidence for it also being efficacious in mixed disorders and anxiety disorders.[30]

- It is open to families, couples, and individuals.

- It is particularly indicated in psychosomatic disorders, phobic disorders, eating disorders, and depression and other mood disorders.

Family consultation

- An individual approach that aims to provide support, information, and practical advice on how to deal with the patient and manage crisis situations, that is available to single family members or the family as a whole. Patients are usually not involved in family consultation.

- The intervention is usually provided by a mental health professional, but can also be administered by trained family members.

- It is a short-term approach: a few sessions on specific topics.

- This model differs from a strictly educational model by offering specific advice and problem-solving assistance. Unlike the formal structure and group format of family education, consultation focuses on immediate needs and agendas. Consultation may be useful for families, particularly if it is offered at the time of initial diagnosis and thereafter on an as-needed basis.

- The end of the intervention is decided by professionals and family members together.

- It is suitable for family members of patients with eating disorders, depression, and anxiety.

Family education

◆ It contains the same didactic components as family psychoeducational interventions and is usually offered to different families in a group setting, without the patient.

◆ It is designed to help key relatives or caregivers to understand and cope with the illness.

◆ Family education is shorter than psychoeducational family interventions.

◆ This approach is primarily designed to provide information about diseases to family members.

◆ It is often offered by professionals, but also by well-trained family members using manual-based materials.[31]

Family support

◆ Non-clinical intervention, the primary goal of which is to offer information and support to family members of patients with severe mental disorders. It is usually provided in a group setting.[1,5]

◆ Groups are usually conducted by adequately trained family members. Mental health professionals are often invited to sessions, but their presence is not necessary. The intervention is usually conducted in 'neutral' settings such as houses, schools, or other places easily accessible.

◆ This approach is open to anyone who has a family member with a serious mental disorder.

◆ Usually, relatives' groups are homogenous based on patient's diagnosis. The duration is short, being one to twelve sessions, once a week.

◆ It is particularly suitable for family members of patients with depression, anxiety disorders, or eating disorders.

Advocacy groups and self-help groups

◆ Self-help and support groups for people and families dealing with mental illnesses are becoming increasingly common.

◆ Family members join a relatives' group where they can meet other people who are in a similar situation. These groups are usually indicated for relatives wanting to share their experiences.

◆ Although they are not led by a professional therapist, these groups are therapeutic in nature because members give ongoing support to each other.

◆ Members of groups share frustrations and successes, referrals to qualified specialists and community resources, and information about what works best when trying to recover. They also share friendship and hope for themselves, their loved ones, and others in the group.

◆ Associations of users and carers are playing a more active role in the field of mental health care.[32]

◆ Being part of these groups is helpful for families advocating for better mental health research and treatment.

'Family to family' model

◆ In the USA, the National Alliance for Mental Illness (NAMI) has developed the 'family to family' (FTF) approach—a new model of family intervention, led by family members.[33]

◆ FTF is an educational course for the family, caregivers, and friends of individuals living with mental illness.

◆ The course consists of 12 sessions, lasting 2.5 hours each, and free of cost. The course is led by trained family members of individuals living with mental illness and it provides critical information and strategies related to caregiving.

◆ Several studies provide evidence that FTF is effective in improving problem-oriented coping strategies, levels of knowledge, and empowerment of families of persons with mental disorders. Moreover, all the significant benefits of FTF were sustained at 9 months after the end of the programme, without any additional booster sessions or support.[34]

◆ FTF was designated as an evidence-based practice in 2013 by the American Substance Abuse and Mental Health Administration (SAMHSA).

How to increase the family's involvement in patient care

◆ Consider that every family is different. Although this is self-evident, it is the starting point for good communication with family members and caregivers.

◆ Recognize ways in which families are organized and the roles that different family members may play for the patients. Clinicians need to be sensitive to who in the family are the central figures in the patients' life.[35]

◆ Consider that family roles and expectations with regard to patients obviously differ among parents, children of various ages, siblings, and more distant relatives.

◆ Develop a collaboration with the family (have a positive first contact, interviewing to uncover both the patient's and family's history and needs).

◆ Consider that some families might reject the support or education group. It is important to remain patient, polite, and tolerant throughout, and to continue to offer contact if it is felt to be appropriate. For example, some families wish for privacy and distance; mental health professionals must remain sensitive both to the wishes of families and of the patient. Also be aware that these wishes may change: so continue to offer options.

◆ Offer information about mental disorders (e.g. answer questions about mental disorders, help families understand the long course of the disease), considering that a lack of knowledge, combined with stigma regarding mental disorders, often leaves family members feeling profoundly isolated in dealing with the many challenges related to their relative's disorder. It is important to keep in mind that family members may have varying levels of knowledge on mental disorders and to avoid making assumptions about what they may or may not know.[35]

◆ Help families in the service system to use and co-ordinate patients' care with psychiatric nurses, psychologists, social workers, and all other mental health professionals.[6]

◆ Listen to families and treat them as equal partners in treatment planning and delivery; help family members to participate in developing the treatment plan; inform family members about the different roles of mental health professionals; support family members during a patient's relapse/readmission; and provide an explicit crisis plan.[8]

◆ Assess the family's strengths and limitations in being able to support the patient, and evaluate the family context in terms of family burden, expressed emotions, and coping strategies. Subsequently, propose to the patient and family members a family intervention and organize training for mental health professionals in order to carry out such an intervention.

◆ Enhance family communication and problem-solving skills, and encourage the family to expand their social network.

◆ Provide (in the mental health centres and in outpatient and inpatient units) some specific programmes for supporting family members. Such programmes should be co-ordinated by adequately trained mental health professionals or family members in order to provide a forum for family members to learn about their relative's disorder.[35] Remember that family intervention skills need to be part of formal residency programmes in psychiatry, which is not yet the case in general medicine.

◆ Promote (in the local mental health centre) the organization of self-help groups, and periodically evaluate how they work.

◆ Adapt family interventions to different families' needs and socio-cultural backgrounds.

◆ Promote the patients' participation in innovative programmes such as REORDER (Recovery-oriented Decisions for Relatives Support), that use a shared decision-making process to improve relatives' involvement in patients' care. REORDER is tailored according to patients' preferences for family involvement, focusing on the mental health recovery goals of the patient. In the USA, participation in REORDER led to marked increases in family participation and improved outcomes.[36]

Advantages of involving family members

For mental health professionals

◆ Improving relationships with colleagues and users, in particular as regards the exchange of information

◆ Increasing knowledge on the patient's family background

◆ Improving professional skills, such as regarding setting time limits for meetings with family members and issues of confidentiality

For patients

- ◆ Reducing the number of relapses and hospital admissions
- ◆ Improving quality of life
- ◆ Improving compliance to pharmacological treatments

For family members

- ◆ Reducing family burden
- ◆ Strengthening social network
- ◆ Improving coping strategies, knowledge about the disorder, communication skills
- ◆ Improving quality of life

References

1 **Lefley HP**. *Family psychoeducation for serious mental illness*. London: Oxford University Press; 2009.

2 **Fromm-Reichmann F**. Notes on development of treatment of schizophrenia by psychoanalytic psychotherapy. *Psychiatry* 1948; **11**:263–27.

3 **Bateson G**. Toward a theory of schizophrenia. In: *Double bind: the foundation of the communicational approach to the family* (eds. Sluzki CE, Ransom DC). New York: Grune and Stratton; 1976, pp. 3–32.

4 **Brown GW**. Measuring the impact of mental illness on the family. *Proc Roy Soc Med* 1966; **59**:18–20.

5 **Galinker I**. *Talking to families about mental illness. What clinicians need to know*. New York: Norton & Company; 2011.

6 **Keitner GI, Kurimay T, Wilson AK**. Advances in family research and intervention. In: *Advances in psychiatry (2nd volume)* (ed. Christodoulou G). World Psychiatric Association; 2005, pp. 127–37.

7 **Carter B, McGoldrick M**. Overview: the changing family life cycle—a framework for family therapy. In: *The changing family life cycle* (2nd edn) (eds. Carter B, McGoldrick M). Boston: Allyn and Bacon; 1989, pp. 3–29.

8 **Kurimay T, Kelemen G**. Ethical practice and issues of power. In: Distance education for family therapy. Counselling and supervision (eds. Lask J, Dallos R, Kurimay T, Etenyi Z). Budapest: European Training Foundation; 1999, pp. 228–58.

9 **Perlick DA, Rosenheck RA, Miklowitz DJ, et al**. Caregiver burden and health in bipolar disorder: a cluster analytic approach. *J Nerv Ment Dis* 2008; **196**:484–91.

10 **Luciano M, Sampogna G, Del Vecchio V, et al**. The family in Italy: cultural changes and implications for treatment. *Int Rev Psychiatr* 2012; **24**:149–56.

11 **Thomas B**. Treating troubled families: therapeutic scenario in India. *Int Rev Psychiatr* 2012; **24**:91–8.

12 **Grad J, Sainbury P**. Problem of caring for the mentally ill at home. *Proc Roy Soc Med* 1966; **59**:20–3.

13 **Hoenig J, Hamilton MW**. The schizophrenic patient in the community and his effect on the household. *Int J Soc Psychiatr* 1966; **12**:165–76.

14 **Magliano L, Fiorillo A, Malangone C, De Rosa C, Maj M**. Patient functioning and family burden in a controlled, real-world trial of family psychoeducation for schizophrenia. *Psychiatr Serv* 2006; **57**:1784–91.

15 **Luciano M, Del Vecchio V, Giacco D, De Rosa C, Malangone C, Fiorillo A**. A 'family affair'? The impact of family psychoeducational interventions on depression. *Expert Rev Neurother* 2012; **12**:83–91.

16 **Fiorillo A, Sampogna G, Del Gaudio L, Luciano M, Del Vecchio V**. Efficacy of supportive family interventions in bipolar disorder: a review of the literature. *It J Psychopath* 2013; **19**:134–42.

17 **Leff JP, Vaughn CE**. *Expressed emotions in families*. New York: Guildford Press; 1985.

18 **Lazarus RS, Folkman S**. *Stress appraisal and coping*. New York: Springer: 1984.

19 **Moon E, Chang JS, Choi S, et al**. Characteristics of stress-coping behaviors in patients with bipolar disorders. *Psychiatr Res* 2014: **218**:69–74. DOI: S0165–1781(14)00274–1.

20 **Kate N, Grover S, Kulhara P, Nehra R**. Relationship of caregiver burden with coping strategies, social support, psychological morbidity, and quality of life in the caregivers of schizophrenia. *Asian J Psychiatr* 2013; **6**:380–8.

21 **Glynn SM, Cohen AN, Dixon LB, Niv N**. The potential impact of the Recovery Movement on family interventions for schizophrenia: opportunities and obstacles. *Schizoph Bull* 2006; **32**:451–63.

22 **Zubin J, Spring B**. Vulnerability: a new view on schizophrenia. *J Abnorm Psych* 1977; **86**:103–26.

23 **Fiorillo A, Galderisi S**. *Family based approaches for schizophrenia patients. Encyclopedia of schizophrenia*. London: Springer Healthcare; 2011, pp. 112–8.

24 NICE guidance: http://guidance.nice.org.uk/CG155/Guidance

25 American Psychiatric Association (APA) Practice Guidelines: http://psychiatryonline. org/guidelines.aspx

26 **Falloon IRH**. *Comprehensive management of mental disorders*. Buckingham, UK: Buckingham Mental Health Service; 1988.

27 **McFarlane WR, Link B, Dushay R, Marchal J, Crilly J**. Psychoeducational multiple family groups: four-year relapse outcome in schizophrenia. *Fam Proc* 1995; **34**:127–44.

28 **Lucksted A, McFarlane W, Downing D, Dixon L, Adams C**. Recent developments in family psychoeducation as an evidence-based practice. *J Mar Fam Ther* 2012; **38**:101–21.

29 **Selvini Palazzoli M, Cirillo S, Selvini M, Sorrentino AM**. *Family games: general models of psychotic processes in the family*. Norton: New York; 1989.

30 **Retzlaff R, Von Sydow K, Beher S, Haun MW, Schweitzer J**. The efficacy of systemic therapy for internalizing and other disorders of childhood and adolescence: a systematic review of 38 randomized trials. *Fam Proc* 2013; **52**:619–52.

31 **Solomon P**. Moving from psychoeducation to family education for adults with serious mental illness. *Psychiatr Serv* 1996; **47**:1364–70.

32 **Fiorillo A, Luciano M, Del Vecchio V, et al**. Priorities for mental health research in Europe: a survey among national stakeholders associations within the ROAMER project. *World Psychiatr* 2013; **12**:165–70.

33 **Schiffman J, Kline E, Reeves G, et al**. Differences between parents of young versus adult children seeking to participate in family-to-family psychoeducation. *Psychiatr Serv* 2014; **65**:247–50.

34 **Lucksted A, Medoff D, Burland J, et al**. Sustained outcomes of a peer-taught family education program on mental illness. *Acta Psychiatr Scand* 2013; **127**:279–86.

35 **Dixon L, Murray-Swank A, Stewart B**. Working with families. In: *Textbook of hospital psychiatry* (eds. Sharfstein S, Dickerson F, Oldham J). Washington, DC: American Psychiatric Publishing, Inc.; 2009, pp 245–52.

36 **Dixon LB, Glynn SM, Cohen AN, et al**. Outcomes of a brief program, REORDER, to promote consumer recovery and family involvement in care. *Psychiatr Serv* 2014; **65**:116–20.

Chapter 21

Informed consent in research settings

Julian Beezhold, Michael J. Wise,
Defne Eraslan, and Marianne Kastrup

Definition

In this chapter, we will address informed consent in research using a definition from the 2014 European Union (EU) Clinical Trials Regulation, this being the law governing clinical trials conducted in the 28 member states:

> 'Informed consent' means a subject's free and voluntary expression of his or her willingness to participate in a particular clinical trial, after having been informed of all aspects of the clinical trial that are relevant to the subject's decision to participate or, in case of minors and of incapacitated subjects, an authorization or agreement from their legally designated representative to include them in the clinical trial.[1]

Introduction

Informed consent in research settings symbolizes voluntary participation and it is a crucial issue because it gives necessary and important information to the participants. Informed consent includes the knowledge about the research and its possible risks. The aim of getting informed consent is to be sure that the participant knows all of processes and is able to decide whether she or he wants to be a part of the research.[2] The role of informed consent is indispensable when it comes to ethical and legal requirements of research. There is some debate over how much technical information should be communicated to the subjects, and recently, some authors have supported the participant's right of having limitless information about the research.[3]

Informed consent has three components; information, decisional capacity, and voluntarism. The information includes the structure and aim of the study, its possible positive and negative effects, and opportunities for the participant. This is a very problematic area, with a wide range of views regarding the level of detail required. Over recent decades, there has been a seismic shift away from providing minimal information towards providing a large amount of very detailed information. Decisional capacity includes the factors—mental and physical—that enable participants to be able to decide. Decision making gives the opportunity to the participants to decide whether they want to be part of the research. Voluntarism basically states that the participant is autonomous.[4]

Another dimension that particularly affects psychiatry is that of conducting research with participants who may have impaired capacity to consent to that research. This is a particularly important issue as those people who, as a result of their condition, become unable to consent, also have a right to benefit from advances in scientific knowledge that may contribute to better treatments and outcomes for them. Simply excluding these vulnerable groups (such as those suffering from dementia) from any research is not a realistic option as it could hamper efforts to improve treatments. All modern codes for research conduct have safeguards for this eventuality. The exact procedure for obtaining authorization to proceed, as distinct from consent from the subject, varies from jurisdiction to jurisdiction, and will continue to do so under the 2014 EU Clinical Trials Regulation.

Historical context

There had been relatively little attention paid to the issue of informed consent in research settings for many years. There was a general assumption that doctors did well and that they knew best, including regarding the ethics and process of research. The Second World War was the event that changed this, decisively and dramatically. During the War, there were multiple reports of doctors conducting experiments, both without consent and also of dubious scientific value, on human subjects who were prisoners in concentration camps. Following the end of the War, and as a result of these activities, 23 doctors were tried at Nuremberg for war crimes, in what was known as the 'Doctors Trial'. The judges in the case realized that there was a need for an ethical framework governing medical research. They proceeded, in their verdict in 1947, to set out ten principles for ethical research that became known as the Nuremberg Code (Box 21.1).[5]

Box 21.1 The ten principles of the Nuremberg Code

1 'The voluntary consent of the human subject is absolutely essential. This means that the person involved should have legal capacity to give consent; should be so situated as to be able to exercise free power of choice, without the intervention of any element of force, fraud, deceit, duress, over-reaching, or other ulterior form of constraint or coercion; and should have sufficient knowledge and comprehension of the elements of the subject matter involved, as to enable him to make an understanding and enlightened decision. This latter element requires that, before the acceptance of an affirmative decision by the experimental subject, there should be made known to him the nature, duration, and purpose of the experiment; the method and means by which it is to be conducted; all inconveniences and hazards reasonably to be expected; and the effects upon his health or person, which may possibly come from his participation in the experiment. The duty and responsibility for ascertaining the quality of the consent rests upon each individual who initiates, directs or engages in the experiment. It is a personal duty and responsibility which may not be delegated to another with impunity.

Box 21.1 The ten principles of the Nuremberg Code (continued)

2 The experiment should be such as to yield fruitful results for the good of society, unprocurable by other methods or means of study, and not random and unnecessary in nature.

3 The experiment should be so designed and based on the results of animal experimentation and a knowledge of the natural history of the disease or other problem under study, that the anticipated results will justify the performance of the experiment.

4 The experiment should be so conducted as to avoid all unnecessary physical and mental suffering and injury.

5 No experiment should be conducted where there is an a priori reason to believe that death or disabling injury will occur; except, perhaps, in those experiments where the experimental physicians also serve as subjects.

6 The degree of risk to be taken should never exceed that determined by the humanitarian importance of the problem to be solved by the experiment.

7 Proper preparations should be made and adequate facilities provided to protect the experimental subject against even remote possibilities of injury, disability, or death.

8 The experiment should be conducted only by scientifically qualified persons. The highest degree of skill and care should be required through all stages of the experiment of those who conduct or engage in the experiment.

9 During the course of the experiment, the human subject should be at liberty to bring the experiment to an end, if he has reached the physical or mental state, where continuation of the experiment seemed to him to be impossible.

10 During the course of the experiment, the scientist in charge must be prepared to terminate the experiment at any stage, if he has probable cause to believe, in the exercise of the good faith, superior skill and careful judgement required of him, that a continuation of the experiment is likely to result in injury, disability, or death to the experimental subject.'

Reproduced from Trials of War Criminals before the Nuremberg Military Tribunals under Control Council Law. 2, p. 181–2, Copyright (1949) U.S. Government Printing Office.

In 1964, at its general assembly in Finland, the World Medical Association adopted a much more detailed code for research ethics that became known as the 'Declaration of Helsinki'. This has had updates and revisions over the years, with the current version having been adopted in Fortaleza, Brazil, in 2013. The paragraphs dealing with informed consent are reported in Box 21.2.[6]

Both the Nuremberg Code and the Declaration of Helsinki place heavy emphasis on the importance and the necessity of informed consent when conducting research. These two documents have informed many other codes that deal with informed consent in research, and one can see the principles echoed and reflected, for example, in the 2014 EU Regulation No. 536/2014 on Clinical Trials.[1]

Box 21.2 'Declaration of Helsinki' of the World Medical Association

25 Participation by individuals capable of giving informed consent as subjects in medical research must be voluntary. Although it may be appropriate to consult family members or community leaders, no individual capable of giving informed consent may be enrolled in a research study unless he or she freely agrees.

26 In medical research involving human subjects capable of giving informed consent, each potential subject must be adequately informed of the aims, methods, sources of funding, any possible conflicts of interest, institutional affiliations of the researcher, the anticipated benefits and potential risks of the study and the discomfort it may entail, post-study provisions and any other relevant aspects of the study. The potential subject must be informed of the right to refuse to participate in the study or to withdraw consent to participate at any time without reprisal. Special attention should be given to the specific information needs of individual potential subjects as well as to the methods used to deliver the information.

   After ensuring that the potential subject has understood the information, the physician or another appropriately qualified individual must then seek the potential subject's freely-given informed consent, preferably in writing. If the consent cannot be expressed in writing, the non-written consent must be formally documented and witnessed.

   All medical research subjects should be given the option of being informed about the general outcome and results of the study.

27 When seeking informed consent for participation in a research study, the physician must be particularly cautious if the potential subject is in a dependent relationship with the physician or may consent under duress. In such situations the informed consent must be sought by an appropriately qualified individual who is completely independent of this relationship.

28 For a potential research subject who is incapable of giving informed consent, the physician must seek informed consent from the legally authorised representative. These individuals must not be included in a research study that has no likelihood of benefit for them unless it is intended to promote the health of the group represented by the potential subject, the research cannot instead be performed with persons capable of providing informed consent, and the research entails only minimal risk and minimal burden.

29 When a potential research subject who is deemed incapable of giving informed consent is able to give assent to decisions about participation in research, the physician must seek that assent in addition to the consent of the legally authorised representative. The potential subject's dissent should be respected.

> **Box 21.2 'Declaration of Helsinki' of the World Medical Association (continued)**
>
> 30 Research involving subjects who are physically or mentally incapable of giving consent, for example, unconscious patients, may be done only if the physical or mental condition that prevents giving informed consent is a necessary characteristic of the research group. In such circumstances the physician must seek informed consent from the legally authorised representative. If no such representative is available and if the research cannot be delayed, the study may proceed without informed consent provided that the specific reasons for involving subjects with a condition that renders them unable to give informed consent have been stated in the research protocol and the study has been approved by a research ethics committee. Consent to remain in the research must be obtained as soon as possible from the subject or a legally authorised representative.
>
> 31 The physician must fully inform the patient which aspects of their care are related to the research. The refusal of a patient to participate in a study or the patient's decision to withdraw from the study must never adversely affect the patient–physician relationship.
>
> 32 For medical research using identifiable human material or data, such as research on material or data contained in biobanks or similar repositories, physicians must seek informed consent for its collection, storage and/or reuse. There may be exceptional situations where consent would be impossible or impracticable to obtain for such research. In such situations the research may be done only after consideration and approval of a research ethics committee.'
>
> Reproduced from World Medical Association. Declaration of Helsinki—Ethical Principles for Medical Research Involving Human Subjects, Updated (2013).

Regulation 536/2014 is the current European law governing clinical research on medicinal products by which all 28 member states are bound. It has effectively taken the principles for informed consent and ethical procedures into a research context, and codified these into statute law. The 2014 Regulation replaces an earlier 2001 version. There are still ongoing controversies regarding this law and how it applies to informed consent. One is the view that the law allows for too much interpretation on the part of member states with respect to the informed consent process, with many commentators feeling that it should be more prescriptive. A second controversy is that 536/2014 allows for research participants to sign consent that allows for unspecified future research use of their subject data that has been obtained from the original consented trial. There have been some strong critical voices, such as Katrin Fjeldsted (President of the Standing Committee of European Doctors), opposing this on the grounds that research participants should consent to each use of the data.[7]

The importance and necessity of informed consent

Informed consent is crucial while looking at research from legal, ethical, and administrative perspectives. The legal perspective, while country-specific, claims that participants have the right to know what will be done to them. They need to have sufficient information to be able to make an informed choice before participating in the research. This gives the participants autonomy before enrolling into the research. The legal concept of informed consent is practical and takes place as a standard procedure in researches. The ethical perspective is an essentially theoretical one; however, in practice, it ensures respect for participants has been maintained and that they have been treated in a morally defensible manner.

From the administrative perspective, informed consent has four important components:

1) there must be a valid decision maker (whether the participant or a surrogate);

2) the researcher should disclose necessary information to the participant;

3) the participant should be able to understand and retain necessary information;

4) the participant should decide without any pressure being placed on them.[8]

Some medical journals require the additional considerations that the results of the trial are communicated to the participants, and that the trial is registered. The latter reduces the risk of publication bias and selective reporting. Stemming from the Declaration of Helsinki, it is increasingly a requirement that every research study involving human subjects must be registered in a publicly accessible database, before recruitment of the first subject. In some countries, ethical approval by research oversight committees is a prerequisite.[9]

Due to the impact of psychological and psychiatric illnesses, decision making can be a challenging process in this patient group. Public prejudice and pressure on these patients does not make things easier. As a result of this, ethical principles, especially around informed consent, become more important when planning and carrying out research with this group.[10]

Problems with informed consent in psychological and psychiatric research

Informed consent can be considered as a safeguard for participants before taking part in research. It favours voluntary participation and decreases the possibility of a negative reaction from the public to scientific research. The risk factors should be explained to the participants, as detailed and precisely as possible Words such as 'harm' or 'risk' have different meanings for different settings and different individuals. Emotionally charged words may inadvertently change their opinions. Although it is not possible to know all the risks and harm factors in research, the researchers should give as much information as they can.[11]

In psychiatric research, informed consent becomes even more important because the mental status of the participants may be altered. Ethical councils should review and validate the research rationale and methodology, and the informed consent procedure.[12] As Appelbaum[13] claims, even though these requirements are present, voluntary participation might be threatened by issues such as poverty and personal dependency of the patients.

The most crucial aspect of informed consent relates to decision making. Decision-making capacity is so important and inevitable that it cannot be ignored in psychological and psychiatric research. The essential point regarding informed consent and decision making of psychologically handicapped patients is to be sure that they have an understanding of the consent, despite their illness.

Dunn and Jeste[14] found that patients with schizophrenia were good at answering dichotomous questions, but had problems with ordering choices according to priorities. Nonetheless, there was little difference between them and healthy participants in terms of understanding and retaining information necessary to the consent process.

The capacity for decision making and understanding required for informed consent is more sensitive and essential for people who have mental illnesses. Cognitive evaluations are important assessments that might determine the validity of informed consent. Inability of the patient to make decisions might cause problems in relation to informed consent and, in this situation, proxy consenters might be used for psychological and psychiatric treatment and research in certain jurisdictions.[15]

There are a number of different issues relating to informed consent for research that remain subjects of debate and controversy. These include the meaning of 'informed', the issue of research on population data banks, and research on particularly vulnerable groups such as those lacking the capacity to consent (e.g. children, patients with dementia, severely disturbed patients, patients with learning disability).

The exact meaning of 'informed' can be problematic in two ways. The first is that there is huge potential for, or even an inevitability of, misunderstanding. An example of this is the 'therapeutic misconception' highlighted by Appelbaum, whereby research subjects in treatment trials tend to assume, despite explanation and information, that even in randomized placebo-controlled trials, they will be given an experimental treatment that is active and is based on their personal and individual needs.[16] The corollary of this is an inadequate understanding among participants of the reality that they may receive placebo only. Participants appear to assume that they will personally benefit from their research treatment; although there is some truth in that, as the effects of observation bias show that the measurements required in research will themselves result in improved care.

Secondly, there is ample evidence that it is very hard to demonstrate adequate levels of understanding and recall sufficient to meet legal tests for informed consent, especially when relaying highly complex technical and scientific issues to a lay audience. Indeed, the overwhelming focus in the informed consent process is on the provision of information, with little, if any, attention paid to the participant's level of understanding of this information. This is the embodiment of an issue regarding 'informed consent' more generally—namely, that there is a tension between, on the one hand, the amount of time and effort required to ensure that each participant has an adequate understanding of all the information required to give informed consent, and, on the other hand, that achieving this, including documenting the necessary evidence, is a practical impossibility in many clinical and research situations because of time and cost constraints. The resultant dilemma is that the process of obtaining proper, verifiable, informed consent is likely to be so long, complex, and expensive that it would defeat the object of the consent.

The debate regarding data banks revolves around the issue of whether separate and specific individual informed consent should be required for every research project that accesses (often anonymized) subject data that forms part of this registry or data collection. There is also a related issue regarding whether consent in these situations should be 'opt in' (whereby the participant has to actively indicate agreement for participation) or 'opt out' (whereby individuals have to actively indicate their refusal to participate). Views on these issues range widely, depending on the relative value placed on the sometimes competing ethical principles of autonomy (what is best for oneself) and the common good (what is best for the wider society). These perspectives can differ according to whether care is a social good or privately provided.

How to improve practice about informed consent in psychiatric research

The definition of informed consent includes voluntariness, decision making, autonomy, and being informed (especially about the possible risks). In addition to these characteristics, the researcher should take care when balancing the prevention of possible risks with reaching his or her aims. However, there is no study which does not include any risk. Better informed consent will be achieved if participants have the opportunity to make decisions freely and voluntarily. Although decision making should be easy and practical, the researcher should try to be sure to give enough information for better decision making. The decision-making process also offers legal protection to both the researcher and the participants. Another important point relates to the capacity and comprehension of the participant with regard to the decision procedure. One of the ways a researcher can be sure of their comprehension is by repeating the question and interpreting their answer to a series of questions.[8] However, it has also been stated that to respect autonomy, capacity requires 'understanding, [but] not wisdom'.[17]

The list of qualifications for informed consent should include the following important points:

1) participating in the research on a voluntary basis;

2) having information about the design, the possible results of participating, and risks of the study.

As repeatedly explained and emphasized, decision making, and the capacity and ability of participants to make decisions, plays an efficient, essential, and legal role within the study. Informed consent in psychiatry necessitates accurate information that the patient can understand.[10] It remains to be seen whether provision of the results of the study to participants will become a research norm,[18] although some journals now require this in order to consider a paper for publication.

Conclusions

Informed consent requires voluntarism, information disclosure, and decisional capacity. Well-developed informed consent requires understanding, knowledge about the study, the ability to make decisions, logical reasoning, and understanding of the significance of the decision. The right to withdraw, without jeopardizing existing care, should also be emphasized.[15]

Readers should also keep in mind that the standards and process used when obtaining informed consent for research are culturally determined and are also particular to the time in which they are developed. Culture is a dynamic entity undergoing constant change. These changes, along with technological advances, mean that there will no doubt be further changes to the way in which informed consent is dealt with in research settings. As researchers, we should endeavour to be vigilant for the need for such change, and proactive in agreeing and implementing any changes.

References

1 European Commission (Public Health). *Clinical trials—EU Regulation No. 536/2014*. Available at: http://ec.europa.eu/health/human-use/clinical-trials/regulation/index_en.htm

2 **Shahnazarian D, Hagemann J, Aburto M, Rose S**. *What is informed consent? Informed consent in human subjects research*. Office for the Protection of Research Subjects. University of Southern California, Los Angeles: 2013. Available at: http://oprs.usc.edu/files/2013/04/Informed-Consent-Booklet-4.4.13.pdf

3 **Kottow M**. The battering of informed consent. *J Med Ethics* 2004; **30**:565–9.

4 **Roberts LW**. Informed consent and the capacity for voluntarism. *Am J Psychiatr* 2002; **159**:705–12.

5 Trials of war criminals before the Nuremberg military tribunals under Control Council Law No. 10. Washington, DC: Library of Congress; 1949. Available at: http://www.loc.gov/rr/frd/Military_Law/NTs_war-criminals.html

6. World Medical Association. *Declaration of Helsinki—ethical principles for medical research involving human subjects, update 2013, Fortaleza (Brazil)*. Available at: http://www.wma.net/en/30publications/10policies/b3/index.html

7 **Fjeldsted K**. EU substantially weakens informed consent in clinical trials regulation. *The Parliament Magazine*; 23 April 2014. Available at: https://www.theparliamentmagazine.eu/printpdf/851

8 **Hall DE, Prochazka AV, Fink AS**. Informed consent for clinical treatment. *Can Med Associat J* 2012; **184**:533–40.

9 National Health Service—Health Research Authority. *Trial registration to be condition of the favourable REC opinion from 30 September 2013*. Available at: http://www.hra.nhs.uk/news/2013/09/10/trial-registration-to-be-condition-of-the-favourable-rec-opinion-from-30-september/#sthash.5jzzZ5a1.dpuf

10 **Hanon C, Eraslan D, Mathis D, Donovan AL, Kastrup MC**. The role of ethics in psychiatric training and practice. In: *How to succeed in psychiatry* (eds. Fiorillo A, Calliess IT, Sass H). Chichester, UK: John Wiley; 2012, pp. 259–72.

11 **Lindsey RT**. Informed consent and deception in psychotherapy research: an ethical analysis. *Counsel Psychol* 1984; **12**:79–86.

12 **Helmchen H**. Ethics of clinical research with mentally ill persons. *Eur Arch Psychiat Clin Neurosci* 2012; **262**:441–52.

13 **Appelbaum PS**. Can a theory of voluntariness be a priori and value-free? *Am J Bioethics* 2011; **11**(8):17–8.

14 **Dunn LB, Jeste DV**. Problem areas in the understanding of informed consent for research: study of middle-aged and older patients with psychotic disorders. *Psychopharmacology* 2003; **171**:81–5.

15 **Gupta UC, Kharawala S**. Informed consent in psychiatry clinical research: a conceptual review of issues, challenges, and recommendations. *Perspect Clin Res* 2012; **3**:8–15.

16 **Appelbaum PS, Roth LH, Lidz C**. The therapeutic misconception: informed consent in psychiatric research. *Int J Law Psychiat* 1982; **5**:319–9.

17 British Medical Association. *Medical ethics today. The BMA's handbook of ethics and law* (3rd edn). Wiley Blackwell: Chichester; 2012.

18 **Partridge A, Winer P**. Sharing study results with trial participants: time for action. *J Clin Oncol* 2009; **27**:838–9.

Chapter 22

Ethics and clinical practice in psychiatry

Julio Torales, César Ruiz-Díaz, and Dinesh Bhugra

Introduction

Ethical practice is at the heart of clinical practice, irrespective of the medical specialty. It is absolutely vital that both the society within which clinical practice occurs and clinicians agree on ethical matters. A major aspect of professional values lies in ethical practice.

As in other fields of medicine, ethical analysis in psychiatry can centre on many different activities, the aim of which is always to generate behaviour in accordance with societal customs, cultural norms, individual values and beliefs, and respect for human dignity.[1] Among these activities, clinical practice is one of the most visible.

However, psychiatry has not reached a universal consensus concerning an optimal theoretical framework for ethical decision making in clinical practice, although many theories have been considered.[2] In order to avoid confusion for the clinician, and instead of pursuing a single theoretical framework for ethics in psychiatry, all psychiatrists should garner the strengths of all the available compatible approaches in a synergistic way, in order to make sense of ethics and to practice ethically.

There are two main ethical traditions in Western thought relevant to psychiatry. One is the deontological tradition, usually associated with Kantian philosophy, and variously expressed in the ethics of obligations and of convictions. The other tradition is teleological, because the main emphasis is placed on the consequences of actions and the attendant responsibility of actors and agents. Clinicians are more often invited to reflect upon their responsibility towards other people than to show allegiance to a certain belief, although it may be said that each and every instance of ethical decision making partakes of one or both of the aforementioned traditions.[1]

No psychiatrist should be obliged to do something against his or her conscience, and every person is expected to respect the dignity of human persons and not to harm them. Respect for autonomy and a duty of beneficence are two out of four ethical principles that underpin ethical reasoning in medicine; the other two are non-maleficence and respect for justice.[3] However, to be beneficent and 'to do good' is no obligation but, rather, the conquest of an autonomous moral agent endowed with the ability to empathize with others and think in terms of their larger good. This is sometimes called 'moral imagination' and is part of the implicit knowledge we would like every physician and psychiatrist to possess.[3,4]

Psychiatry differentiates itself from other medical specialties in the unique role of the therapeutic relationship in therapeutic outcome; the vulnerability of psychiatric patients; and the features of the psychiatric therapeutic project. However, increasingly, psychiatrists are being asked to carry out risk assessments (of the risk to the patients themselves or to others) and to manage risk accordingly, which raises certain specific ethical issues. Additional ethical issues are related to the stigma, discrimination, and prejudice experienced by patients with psychiatric illnesses and their informal and formal carers[5] Furthermore, some academics highlight that the special virtues required of the psychiatrist include compassion, humility, fidelity, trustworthiness, respect for confidentiality, veracity, prudence, warmth, sensitivity, humility, and perseverance.[6]

There are many documents from professional organizations on the topic of ethical practice. These include the *Good medical practice guide* (the UK's General Medical Council's guide to ethics, published in 2006) and the *Good psychiatric practice guide* (from the Royal College of Psychiatrists, published in 2004). The Royal College has produced other documents on ethical issues in psychiatry which can be consulted (see especially, the ones published in 2002 and 2006).

The main objective of this chapter is to outline the ethical framework for psychiatry and to present a few of the most common ethical issues in psychiatric practice, highlighting some ways to initiate ethical reasoning when dealing with them.

What is ethics?

Socrates once asked the question 'How should I live?'. The key aspect of the answer to this question is embedded in a 'good life'. By 'good', one does not mean 'not bad', but rather, some prevailing sense of value to a life. The foundations for an ethical life are provided by religion, for some, and by the concept of being a responsible member of a society, for others.[7]

The word 'ethical' itself has several connotations. Many confound the description of an act or a person as 'ethical' as meaning 'right' or 'lawful'. As such, to describe something as 'unethical' does not mean it to be illegal or even necessarily incorrect. To best understand ethics, one must understand the values from which these values emerge. Put simply, Socrates' question is best answered in the notion that living a good life is to live in accordance with a set of values. Such values may be handed down by divine command, may emerge as part of broader social values, or may be simply constructed by individuals in the course of their lives.[8,9]

Ethics should be the discourse of 'ought' and 'should' in clinical practice. Ethical reasoning is the process of thought and reflection that we engage in when we ask ourselves: 'What *ought* I to do in this situation? What *should* the good psychiatrist do now?'.[10] Ethics in psychiatry is a branch of medical ethics that is part of the larger domain of ethics, which has been a chapter of philosophy for thousands of years. From the very beginning, law (Hammurabi code) and ethics were at the heart of the medical profession, and essential ethical issues such as confidentiality and prioritizing the interests of the patients were already enshrined in the Hippocratic Oath, 2500 years ago.[11]

Table 22.1 Reasons why ethical dilemmas are part of everyday practice in psychiatry

Psychiatry is an empirically evolving discipline	One act of self-harm may indicate a high level of suicidality in one patient and not in another, but the current evidence base may make it difficult to tell which is which.
	Key message: ethical reasoning needs good-quality facts, but good doctors may interpret facts differently, so they will also deal with the ethical dilemmas differently.[10]
Many professionals are involved in psychiatry practice	An elderly, male inpatient with mild Alzheimer's disease wants to be treated at his home. His carers may take one view, his doctors another, his social worker and key nurse yet another.
	Key message: ethical reasoning comprises reflection on, and respect for, the different set of values, especially when there appears to be no way to resolve the difference.[10]
The duty to respect patient's autonomy and dignity	Mental disorders do not always compromise autonomy, so it may be hard to know if a patient's choices reflect their true will or if they are actually a product of an abnormal mental state. Furthermore, psychiatrists are the only doctors who can force patients to have treatment against their will.
	Key message: ethical reasoning involves the need to balance the psychiatrist's 'power' and the true wishes of every patient.[10]

Source data from: D. Bhugra, S. Bell, A. Burns, O. Howes, The complete psychiatrist, in Adshead G., Ethical reasoning in psychiatry, p. 17–24, Copyright (2010) Royal College of Psychiatrists.

Today, medical ethics are still part of ordinary clinical practice. In general medicine, ethical dilemmas often arise in difficult or life-threatening situations, or when there is a clash of values between the patient and the physician. However, ethical dilemmas in psychiatry are, for a number of reasons, part of everyday clinical practice (see Table 22.1).[10]

It is known that the more power medicine has, the more ethical rules it should have. This is part of the principle of professionalism. The problem is that technological advances in medicine are so rapid, with constantly evolving changes in diagnosis, management, and treatment, that ethical reasoning sometimes lags behind. Psychiatry is the only medical specialty that can deprive a person of liberty (letting aside the justice system). This is why it is essential for all psychiatrists to learn how to solve the multiple ethical dilemmas that each patient might (and will) bring to the table.[12]

Bioethical challenges in psychiatric clinical practice

Psychiatrists deal with human beings in conditions of high vulnerability, establishing relationships with people which are intimate but detached. That is, a psychotherapist or clinical psychiatrist should be in ownership of all relevant information about a person in order to be helpful, but at the same time, he or she should preserve the necessary detachment in order not to assume the role of a personal contact (mentor, lover, or friend) and to keep a scientific point of view.[1] Any intervention, if considered in the context of bioethics, should fulfil at least the three conditions outlined in Box 22.1.

> ## Box 22.1 Conditions to be fulfilled by any psychiatric intervention
>
> ◆ The intervention should be *appropriate* to the problem at hand.
> ◆ The intervention should be *good* in the sense that it does good to those who receive it but also to those who perform it.
> ◆ The intervention should be *just* in the sense that its outcomes can be generalized to the whole of society.
>
> Source data from: World Psychiatry, 5(3), Lolas F. Ethics in psychiatry: a framework, p. 185–187. Copyright (2006) John Wiley & Sons Ltd.

If the aforementioned conditions are completely fulfilled and kept in mind, along with respect for human rights and dignity, then everybody will understand that a good doctor recognizes the duty to inform patients and the right of patients to be informed in order to reach the goals of the scientific endeavour and of the healthcare professions.[1]

In addition to clinical practice, teaching is a context in which ethical conduct is imperative. Students should be acquainted with how to maintain confidentiality and privacy, avoid stigmatization, and abstain from personal involvement in the lives of those whom they treat. Learning by doing and learning by example—two key strategies in psychiatric teaching—demand mindful effort on the part of faculty members.[1,13] A brief note on teaching ethics in psychiatry is presented later in this chapter.

Like all doctors, psychiatrists, too, have obligations and duties towards patients and their families and carers, as well as towards fellow members of the profession and colleagues. Declared or undeclared conflicts of interest, which the individual may or may not be consciously aware of, may lead to material or status gains. Prestige and the need for career advancement may sometimes clash with honesty and friendly relations with peers, and may create conflicts which are difficult to acknowledge. These and other challenges are especially important for psychiatric practice. Thus, it is necessary to devise ways in which teaching of traditional ethics is complemented by the dialogical enterprise called 'bioethics', for it is in the context of deliberation and discussion where tolerance and understanding of diversity can improve the art of healing and curing.[1] This also includes reflexive thinking and reflective practice.

An ethical framework for psychiatry

An ideal ethical framework for psychiatry should provide clear guidelines as well as flexibility in the face of unique clinical circumstances. Furthermore, ethical deliberation has to cover the search for features that constitute moral action, as well as traits of character that are morally laudable.[14]

A potential way forward in doing this has its provenance in a key premise of David Hume that states that ethical behaviour derives primarily from sentiment, not reason. The natural motivation of human beings is to act benevolently, although this inclination is constrained by societal circumstances (e.g. scarce resources, increased competitive nature of certain societies). This prompts a need to establish rules of justice. Moral guidelines therefore originate from matters of the heart, and are eventually adopted as societal norms. Reason enables us to understand an ethical dilemma, but sentiment determines what is fair and unfair. In this way, David Hume's theory allows for a balance between rule- and character-based theories by granting significance to 'moral' emotions which are then applied to derive or modify moral rules.[2,15]

Care ethics is a contemporary framework that derives from Hume. Interpersonal relating is a cardinal aspect of ethical decision making. The associated psychological dimension (the notion of 'heart' as expressed in the capacity to extend care to others) is placed at the centre of ethical thinking. Moral and psychological development are intimately bound together, as emotional sensitivity 'positively reinforces our responses to the good of cooperation, trust, mutual aid, friendship and love, as well as regulating responses to the risk of evil'.[2,16] Furthermore, trust emerges as paramount in this schema, particularly in its relation to vulnerability. This suits the psychiatrist well as this 'vulnerability' is ever present. An appropriate moral attitude, in response, is to contribute to a 'climate of trust' in our relationships with others. Promoting trust is complemented by other virtues such as acting thoughtfully, being considerate, willing to listen, and not forcing one's views on others. This is comparable to doing to others as we would have them do to us, if roles were reversed. Other qualities that enhance the promoting of a climate of trust include patience, tact, honesty, and discretion.[16]

Does the care ethics theory, centred on trust, better serve the psychiatrist who grapples with moral dilemmas than other classical theoretical approaches?[2] Some would argue that the proposed approach does in fact help, but not on its own. Instead, it needs to be complemented by a more structured framework that allows the psychiatrist to resort to a set of guiding principles, like the ones set up by *principlism* (a theory that fulfils this requirement because it is inherently flexible and pragmatic).

According to principlism, there exist, between universal values and practical norms of conduct, prima facie principles. Furthermore, some authors have introduced the idea that the principles behind moral reasoning in research and clinical practice with human subjects can be subsumed under general headings such as *autonomy, beneficence, non-maleficence*, and *justice*. An extensive body of literature has given currency to the utility of formal principles in dealing with case analysis. It should be noted, however, that the term 'formal' in this context means that each of the principles may have different expressions or contents in different cultures. Autonomy, for example, although grammatically univocal, is different in an Islamic society and a secular community, and, while highly appreciated in some regions of the world, may have a different worth in others. This does not imply relativism, but suggests that some degree of cultural sensitivity is vital for an adequate understanding of the contents of each formal principle and the details of its extension and impact in a particular community.[1,17]

Another characteristic that should be noted refers to the relative significance of the principles when applied to particular cases or situations. Although useful, codes of ethics do not indicate which principle should be given priority or predilection in a given situation. More often than not, true ethical dilemmas start from a clash between principles (for instance, when to prefer autonomy over beneficence, or vice versa). Deciding on priorities is one of the responsibilities of an ethics committee, along with adequate assessment of the risks and benefits of research or healthcare interventions.[1]

Ethical dilemmas in clinical practice

On the one hand, psychiatrists face similar ethical challenges as their medical colleagues, and their responses may have direct consequences for patients, their families, and society. However, on the other hand, issues related to mental healthcare (e.g. competence, lack of capacity, compliance, threat and history of self-harm or of harm to others, involuntary treatment) suggest that ethics for psychiatry differ from those enshrined in the principles of bioethics and applicable to all fields of medicine.[2,5] Box 22.2 summarizes the most common ethical dilemmas in psychiatry.[10]

Capacity to consent and refusal to treatment

Here, the ethical dilemma centres around the question of whether the person really has a mental disorder that is affecting their thinking, or whether they are just thinking in ways that other people do not like. At present, psychiatric patients are the only patients who do not have a right to refuse treatment for their disorder. They can refuse medical treatment for physical disorders, if they are deemed to have capacity to refuse; but although they have capacity, they cannot refuse treatment for mental disorders.[10]

The current evidence shows that diagnosis means very little in terms of capacity; it cannot be assumed that everyone with schizophrenia is incapable of making decisions for themselves. Rather, psychiatrists should assess each case on its own merits.[18]

Forced treatment and detention

What should psychiatrists do when faced with a patient who is clearly mentally ill but refusing treatment? This ethical dilemma is one of the most common in the mental health system. Most countries have developed legislation within a framework that allows psychiatrists to detain people against their will for treatment of their mental illness. In some countries, the legislation allows for enforceable involuntary treatment.

The ethical dilemma could be sorted out if a competent psychiatrist is thoughtful about his or her duty to help the patient, and his or her duty to do no harm and to act justly. Although the patient is too ill to consent, he or she must be treated with respect.

Box 22.2 Most common ethical dilemmas in psychiatry

- ◆ Capacity to consent and refusal to treatment
- ◆ Forced treatment and detention
- ◆ Consent to disclosure
- ◆ Professional boundary violations

Source data from: D. Bhugra, S. Bell, A. Burns, O. Howes, The complete psychiatrist, in Adshead G., Ethical reasoning in psychiatry, p. 17–24, Copyright (2010) Royal College of Psychiatrists.

Patients who are forced into treatment against their will may feel distressed; it is a key part of the psychiatrist's therapeutic duty of beneficence to attend to those feelings, as well as treating the patient's disorder.[10]

Special attention should be paid to the fact that psychiatrists could detain patients solely for the benefit of other people (usually for the prevention of some anticipated harm). However, it is impossible to know if the harm would have happened if one had not detained the patient. Here, the ethical dilemma raises a question: How many of us would like to be detained in hospital on the basis of possible harm that we might do in the future?[10]

Consent to disclosure

The dilemma begins with consent. If the patients consent to their material or data being disclosed to another person, then there is no dilemma. However, all doctors have the obligation to talk about the issue with the patient and to inform them of what they propose to tell the other person. A more likely everyday situation is when the psychiatrist wants to breach confidentiality but does not want to tell the patient, either because they suspect that the patient would decline consent to disclosure and/or they think that telling the patient would be hazardous in some way. Most often these situations arise when the psychiatrist thinks that the patient represents a risk to themselves or others, and that by disclosing information about the patient, harm can be prevented. These are difficult situations for every psychiatrist because they involve a breach of confidentiality without consent. An ethical justification to this violation of autonomy is the benefit obtained by the prevention of serious harm to others.[19] The issues of confidentiality vary tremendously across cultures. In many cultures, patients will be accompanied by family friends and acquaintances who will all know what is being decided and discussed. Under these circumstances, issues related to confidentiality have to be in line with socio-cultural contexts.

The UK's General Medical Council has taken the view that is justifiable for doctors to breach patient confidentiality in order to prevent harm to others, especially when those others are actually identifiable and there is good evidence that the breach really will reduce the risk.[20] An ethical approach here would be to advise the patient, during the first therapeutic meeting, that the psychiatrist could breach confidentiality in situations of possible harm to others, but that he or she will discuss those breaches with the patient if at all possible.

Professional boundary violations

Boundary violations occur when aspects of one's personal identity sneak into the professional space and/or there is abuse of the power differential between the patient and the doctor.[7,9,10] In psychiatric practice, professional boundary violations are common, because patients are especially vulnerable in relation to their psychiatrists. These violations not only include sexual boundary violations, but also financial misconduct, dilemmas to do with receiving gifts, and inappropriate self-disclosure (such as sharing personal details about oneself with the patient).

It is necessary to repeat and reinforce that it is ethically unjustifiable to have sexual relationships with patients at any time, even if the patient seems disposed to such. Sexual relationships with ex-patients could be considered inappropriate, if not ethically questionable.

Patients value genuine warmth, humanity, and empathy[10] in their psychiatrists, and these personal characteristics could enhance therapeutic outcomes. Nevertheless, psychiatrists should be aware that if these aspects of personal identity are not carefully monitored, then they may act as possible triggers for boundary violations. Empathy involves reflecting on a patient's emotional experience from their point of view, while sympathy involves a sharing of the psychiatrist's personal information. Sympathy, per se, is not always inappropriate; however, it carries more risk than empathy and it could lead to minor boundary violations.[21]

All psychiatrists are at potential risk of becoming involved in boundary violations if they are not careful. The best advice is to pay attention to any anxiety that one has about relationships with certain patients, and to look for counsel and guidance in a mentor or trusted colleague.

A note on teaching ethics in psychiatry

The teaching of ethics could be part of the general teaching of medical ethics, or could be specific to students, trainees, and other health professionals working in psychiatry. Teaching ethics is about, first of all, asking questions and debating clinical cases. This approach is generated from the premise that there is often no ideal solution for an ethical dilemma, only the least bad, that is finally chosen after long discussion and analysis.[11,12]

Table 22.2 briefly presents the minimum four parts that a curriculum for the teaching of ethics in psychiatry should contain.[11]

Students must also learn that no research can be conducted without the approval of the ethics committee, even when it is a simple case note or epidemiological study. On the same note, no teaching with patients can be done without their expressed agreement, and no written clinical material should be used without being sure that the identity of the patient is preserved in the teaching group. Finally, teachers should encourage students to read textbooks and articles on ethics in psychiatry on a regular basis, as another way of progressing in the field.[11]

Table 22.2 Parts of a curriculum for the teaching of ethics

First part: historical context	The first part should offer a historical perspective of psychiatry and include:
	1) history of the creation of the asylums in the 16th and 17th centuries in Europe and the Americas;
	2) the act of Philippe Pinel and Jean-Baptiste Pussin when they removed the chains of the patients in Bicêtre Hospital in Paris;
	3) the political abuse in psychiatry in the ex-Soviet Union and in South Africa in the 1960s and 1970s.[11]
Second part: declarations and codes	The second part should include explanation of the Madrid Declaration of the World Psychiatric Association and other guidelines and codes developed by national and international non-governmental organizations.[23,24]

(continued)

Table 22.2 (continued) Parts of a curriculum for the teaching of ethics

Third part: clinical dilemmas	The third part should deal with the main ethical questions that psychiatry has to deal with, namely:
	1) informed consent;
	2) hospitalization against the will of the patient;
	3) access to medication in needy psychotic patients;
	4) stigmatization of mental patients, including by some colleagues;
	5) relationship to the pharmaceutical industry;
	6) patients' human rights, including a special attention to the human rights of patients in prison.[11]
Fourth part: case studies	The fourth part should comprise case studies. These could be written, videotaped, presentations of actual patients, or verbal reports by the teacher or the students. This part is the most important one, and should comprise at least half of the teaching time.[11]

Conclusions

There are many other ethical dilemmas in the clinical practice of psychiatry that both senior and junior psychiatrists will need to be aware of, apart from those presented in this chapter. Taking into account that psychiatrists have to come up with solutions to ethical dilemmas in their everyday practice, they have an overarching duty to make the best-quality decisions they can, so they can be the best psychiatrists they can be.[10]

Ethical reasoning is a capacity that psychiatrists and their medical colleagues engage with and will hopefully continue to develop throughout their working lives. Sometimes, ethical dilemmas will pose real challenges for any psychiatrist. In order to overcome the challenges, he or she must always reflect on the issues presented in Box 22.3.[10]

All psychiatrists should take into account that ethical reflection and reasoning needs equal consideration of the ethical principles and codes involved, as well as the

Box 22.3 Issues for reflection

- What are the facts of the case? Does everyone agree with the facts?
- What are the areas of uncertainty?
- What is the 'should' question?
- What other ethical perspectives need to be taken into account?

Source data from: D. Bhugra, S. Bell, A. Burns, O. Howes, The complete psychiatrist, in Adshead G., Ethical reasoning in psychiatry, p. 17–24, Copyright (2010) Royal College of Psychiatrists consequences of any decision. Furthermore, psychiatrists need to be aware that the ethical reasoning process may lead them to the conclusion that their own position, no matter how heartfelt, may not be the most convincing.

Education in medical ethics has the main objective to create virtuous doctors and to provide a way for doctors to deal with ethical dilemmas in practice.[22] Virtuous psychiatrists are born after reflecting on their own personal stories, professional decisions, and particular identities. However that, as Gwen Adshead and others have said, is another story.[10]

References

1 **Lolas F**. Ethics in psychiatry: a framework. *World Psychiatry* 2006; **5**(3):185–7.

2 **Bloch S, Green S**. An ethical framework for psychiatry. *The British Journal of Psychiatry* 2006; **188**:7–12.

3 **Beauchamp T, Childress J**. *Principles of biomedical ethics* (5th edn). Oxford: Oxford University Press; 2001.

4 **Lolas F**. Bioethical narratives: toward the construction of social space for moral imagination. *Int J Bioethics* 1996; **7**:53–5.

5 **Radden J**. Notes towards a professional ethics for psychiatry. *Australian and New Zealand Journal of Psychiatry* 2002; **36**:52–9.

6 **Radden J**. Psychiatric ethics. *Bioethics*, 2002; **16**(5):397–411.

7 **Robertson M**. *An overview of psychiatry ethics*. New South Wales: Health Education and Training Institute; 2009, pp. 1–84.

8 **Robertson M, Walter G**. Overview of psychiatric ethics II: virtue ethics and the ethics of care. *Australasian Psychiatry* 2007; **15**(3):207–11.

9 **Robertson M, Walter G**. Overview of psychiatric ethics I: professional ethics and psychiatry. *Australasian Psychiatry* 2007; **15**(3):201–6.

10 **Adshead G**. Ethical reasoning in psychiatry. In: *The complete psychiatrist* (eds. Bhugra D, Bell S, Burns A, Howes O). London: Royal College of Psychiatrists; 2010, pp. 17–24.

11 **Moussaoui D**. Ethical issues in teaching Psychiatry. In: *Teaching psychiatry: putting theory into practice* (eds. Gask L, Coskun B, Baron B). Chichester: Wiley-Blackwell; 2011, pp. 19–25.

12 **Carmi A, Moussaoui D, Arboleda-Florez J**. *Teaching ethics in psychiatry: case vignettes*. UNESCO Chair in Bioethics, Haifa/World Psychiatric Association's Psychiatry Committee on Ethics; 2005.

13 **Lolas F**. *Bioethics*. Santiago de Chile: Editorial Universitaria; 1999, p. 45.

14 **Veatch R**. (1998) The place of care in ethical theory. *Journal of Medicine and Philosophy* 1998; **23**:210–24.

15 **Hume D**. *An enquiry concerning the principles of morals*. Indianapolis: Hackett; 1983.

16 **Baier A**. Demoralization, trust and the virtues. In: *Setting the moral compass* (ed. Calhoun C). New York: Oxford University Press; 2004, pp. 176–88.

17 National Commission for the Protection of Human Subjects of Biomedical and Behavioral Research. *The Belmont Report: ethical principles for the protection of human subjects in research*. Washington: US Government Printing Office; 1978.

18 **Palmer B, Dunn lN, Appelbaum P, et al**. Correlates of treatment-related decision making capacity among middle aged and older patients with schizophrenia. *Articles of General Psychiatry* 2004; **61**:230–6.

19 **Adshead G, Sarkar S**. Ethical issues in forensic Psychiatry. *Psychiatry* 2004; **3**:5–16.

20 General Medical Council. *Good medical practice*. London: GMC; 2006.

21 **Sarkar SP**. Sexual boundary violations in psychiatry and psychotherapy: a review. *Advances in Psychiatric Treatment*, 2004; **10**:312–20.

22 **Eckles RE, Meslin EM, Gaffney M, et al**. (2005). Medical ethics education: where are we? Where should we be going? A review. *Academic Medicine*, **80**, 1143–52.

23 World Psychiatric Association. *Madrid declaration on ethical standards for psychiatric practice*; 2008. Available at: http://www.wpanet.org/detail.php?section_id=5&category_id=9&content_id=48 (accessed 14 April 2014).

24 **Moussaoui D, Murthy S**. (2005). *Declarations and codes of ethics related to psychiatry and mental health*. World Health Organization (EMRO)/World Psychiatric Association; 2005.

Chapter 23

Mental healthcare in the transition from child and adolescent to adult psychiatry: what a psychiatrist cannot ignore

Mariana Pinto da Costa, Ana Moscoso,
and Giovanni de Girolamo

Introduction

The transition from adolescence into adulthood is an important developmental stage for all young people. Yet, it may be especially challenging for those with mental disorders, their families, and the care systems.[1] Adolescence is a risky period for the emergence of serious mental disorders, substance misuse and other risk-taking behaviours, along with poor engagement with health services. Nevertheless, mental health provision is often inconsistent during this period, showing that there is room for improvement in the care provided, towards giving appropriate attention to individuals during their twenty-year-long journey from puberty to adulthood.[2] Relevant findings on life experiences and the current needs for mental health services, during this transition period, are presented in this chapter.

Epidemiology

Epidemiological estimates are vastly variable, ranging from high[3] to much lower rates.[4] However, they all point out the importance of giving proper care from an early age. Current global epidemiological data reports the overall prevalence of mental disorders and their onset (Box 23.1). A systematic analysis of the global disease burden for young people aged 10–24 years revealed that the main cause of years lost due to disability (YLD) were neuropsychiatric disorders.[5] The birth cohorts give clear evidence that a considerable proportion of mental disorders are already manifest in adolescence. Moreover, half of all mental health disorders with a life course occurred first between the ages of 7 and 24 years.[6]

While determining the magnitude of these disorders, challenges in assessment appear, since the currently used diagnostic categories often lack the integration of cultural perspectives, raising additional difficulties in identifying co-morbidities. Moreover, a diagnostic shift has been occurring over time. This happens as the scale of the impact

Box 23.1 Epidemiological data

◆ Up to 20% of children and adolescents suffer from a disabling mental disorder.

◆ Suicide is the third leading cause of death among adolescents.

◆ Up to 50% of all adult mental disorders have their onset in adolescence.

and burden of these disorders is documented according to different perspectives based on discrepant views. For instance, two children with the same diagnosis can have different degrees of impairment depending on family support and culture.[7]

Course of disorders with onset in infancy and adolescence

A prospective study[8] was carried out aiming to recognize how often common mental disorders persist from adolescence into young adulthood, and the demographic, behavioural, and disorder-related characteristics that predict the continuation of such disorders. This study identified that about one third of men and more than half of women had a prominent episode of depressive and anxiety symptoms at least once during mid to late adolescence, with the highest risk period being from adolescence until young adulthood. For those with one single episode of less than six months' duration, persistence into young adulthood was substantially lower than in those with longer-lasting or recurrent episodes (see Box 23.2). The level of continuity dropped sharply during the late twenties, raising the possibility of further resolution for many whose disorder had persisted into their early twenties.

Child mental health needs are intersectorial and children with mental health problems are often first seen in education, social services, or juvenile justice systems.[9] In fact, 10% of the costs to society emerge from the health sector, and the rest are from education, social welfare, family care, and the welfare system.[10]

A follow-up study (n = 142) into adulthood of children with antisocial behaviours showed that the costs of public services were ten times higher than for children without these problems. These high long-term costs related not only to direct medical care but also to crime, foster and residential care, and state benefits.[11,12] During transition from childhood to adulthood, different concerns appear to be related to mental disorders (Box 23.3). First, the importance of 'a place' and of a community in the healthy development of an individual is hindered in conditions of displacement.[13,14] Second,

Box 23.2 Predictors of mental illness continuity into adulthood

◆ Longer duration of mental health disorders in adolescence (>6 months)

◆ Being a girl

◆ Background of parental separation or divorce

Box 23.3 Contextual concerns

- Displacement
- Soldiering and prostitution
- HIV/AIDS
- Substance abuse
- Violence and abuse
- Youth suicide

in low-income countries, where it is known that children may be forced to become child soldiers or to have sex, there are reports of children suffering from post-traumatic stress disorder.[15] The psychological consequences of child labour in such countries are also complex, with children having to assume, prematurely, adult roles within their families. Third, there is the fact that 3.3 million children under 15 years of age are living with HIV.[16] These children and adolescents may also suffer from neuropsychological dysfunctions which go largely untreated. Frequently, they live as orphans and are quite vulnerable because of the loss of parental figures, malnutrition, and disengagement from society.[7] Fourth, substance abuse in children and adolescents is very common worldwide,[7] with its consequent serious impact on morbidity and co-morbidities. Illicit drugs and psychoactive substances not defined as drugs of abuse are used by youths, regardless of economic circumstances or religious prohibition. Fifth, exposure to violence is frequent with increased levels of substance use.[17] Evidence shows that physical and sexual abuse are a risk factor for mental disorders.[2] Lastly, worldwide, suicide is the second leading cause of death in the 15–19 years age group,[18] with 200,000 adolescents and young adults committing suicide each year.[19]

Standpoints from child and adult psychiatry

Despite their commonalities, child psychiatry differs at several levels from adult psychiatry. Historically, child psychiatry emerged when the world began to acknowledge, during the 1930s and 1940s, that children were more than just little adults.[20] During the past half-century, childhood itself has been specifically subdivided and now includes infancy, toddlerhood, pre-school, school-age, and adolescence.[21]

At a policy level, in many countries, child and adolescent mental health services (CAMHS) and adult mental health services (AMHS) were planned separated.[22] Hence, it is common for CAMHS to be historically linked with educational and social departments, while AMHS were historically linked to health or justice departments (the latter referring mostly to drug dependency units in some European countries). These different linkages can generate structural differences, designed to address different clinical needs, which should not be ignored during the child/adolescent to adult transition.

At a CAMHS level, there are inevitably close links with school, family, and social services, which work interdependently with CAMHS. These partners are often the main source of referrals and also important bodies to approach when additional clinical information or treatment measures are required. This is especially the case in relation to school and family, where the young person spends a great part of the day. School and place of learning is so important that it is common to find psychopedagogists operating within a CAMHS, and the role of the family and of family dynamics are key factors for the development of any young person. Besides, minors are under the responsibility of parents or other caregivers and, on the whole, family involvement in care is mandatory at CAMHS.

Patients seen in CAHMS have usually a different profile from those seen in AMHS. Depending on age, they can present with disorders similar to adults, and have reached the threshold for a specific disease. It is also common to follow patients who might be suffering the impact of abuse or neglect, despite having or not a specific diagnosis.[22]

Transitional services

Transitional phases are known to be a risk factor for mental health problems, bringing periods of vulnerability. This highlights the importance of providing care in this stage in a smooth, consistent, and effective way.

Transition should give a young person a sense of maturity and hope for the future,[23] while providing continuity of care into adulthood. Yet, unfortunately, this transitional process often does not meet the needs of young people, being abrupt and inadequate, and having as a cut-off point, age rather than development or readiness. The consequences of this failing transition[23] might be a reliance on crisis services, getting 'lost' to services, and an interruption to recovery.

Improved services for this transitional period should reflect the latest evidence (Box 23.4 and Table 23.1)[24,25] and take into account the life changes of young people, supporting them in these changes, rather than adding complexity and discontinuity.

Services should use age 'windows' to decide the optimal time for the transition to adult psychiatry, rather than having a strict age cut-off point. A crisis should be

---

Box 23.4 Requirements for a successful transition process

+ Timing of transition must be appropriate
+ Should involve a period of preparation and education
+ Young person and their families and carers should be involved
+ Should be co-ordinated and continuous
+ Should meet the needs of a wide-range of young persons
+ Needs to incorporate the common concerns of all young persons
+ Should be supported by effective communication channels and information flow
+ Should have appropriate managerial and administrative support

Table 23.1 Criteria for continuity in the transition pathway

Information continuity	Evidence that a referral letter, summary, or case notes were transferred
Relational continuity	Period of parallel care, of joint working between CAMHS and AMHS
Team continuity	At least one meeting, prior to transfer of care, involving the service user and/or carer and a key professional from both CAMHS and AMHS
Long-term continuity	Engaged with AMHS 3 months post transition or appropriately discharged by AMHS following transition

Source data from: Collis F, Finger E, Owens K. Review of Transitions to Young Adult Clinics. Final Report— Attachment 6: Literature Review, Copyright (2008) Ipsos-Eureka Social Research Institute; Br J Psychiatry, 197, Singh SP, Paul M, Ford T, Kramer T, Weaver T, McLaren S, et al. Process, outcome and experience of transition from child to adult mental healthcare: multiperspective study, p. 305–12, Copyright (2010).

a relative contraindication for transition, which should be planned and proceed in times of stability.[25] Particularly between 17–21 years, young people can require support as they are in transition from secondary education to employment or training, and from living at home with parents and family to independent living. Providing consistent and specialized mental health support across this age group is crucial. In addition, being accessible, flexible, and focused on individual needs is a key factor for success.

There is growing concern about the well-being of adolescents with serious emotional disturbances as they transit into adulthood, particularly those who have received public child services.[26] In general, young people and their parents report that services that could support their transition into adulthood are either not available or not appealing.[27] Adolescents with serious emotional disturbances are found in all public child systems, and many adolescents with psychiatric disorders receive no mental health services at all.[28] Smooth transitional processes are particularly important in children and young people with complex needs and co-morbid disorders, including alcohol and drug problems, or those who are vulnerable or do not have strong family supports.

There are different types of services[26] supporting young people transiting into adulthood, and living independently or in congregate housing. Examples are shown in Box 23.5. Such support might include onsite staff support or supervision; an administrator-identified 'wraparound' approach (for all adolescents and not just those specifically in transition); vocational assessment, counselling, or coaching; support groups or supported employment; training of independent living skills and assistance in finding living accommodation; efforts focused on assisting performance at high school or college; advocacy or leadership training or peer-mentoring programmes; specialized knowledge about transition issues to professionals, systems, young people, or their families; and assertive community treatments for adolescents.

Box 23.5 Types of transition services

- ◆ Supervised or supported housing
- ◆ Specialized *wraparound* approaches
- ◆ Standard *wraparound* approaches
- ◆ Vocational support
- ◆ Independent living preparation
- ◆ Supported education
- ◆ Peer leadership/mentoring
- ◆ Transition specialist
- ◆ Assertive community treatment

Obstacles to transition

Coming from a child psychiatrist. It can be difficult to end a strong relationship with a patient and their family after several years. Child psychiatrists are sometimes tempted to extend the follow-up of some patients, especially the ones with a greater investment in terms of time and resources (such as during psychotherapy) or those with developmental disorders and other pathologies that might be difficult to treat in AHMS services.

Coming from an adult psychiatrist. Not having access to previous medical records from CAHMS can be an obstacle. It can as well be perceived not having much experience with diagnostic categories often seen at CAHMS and seldom at AMHS, such as autism spectrum disorders and ADHD (attention deficit hyperactivity disorder).

Coming from the adolescent. Very often, complaints come from the patient: the fear of the unknown, the fear of losing a privileged relationship, and a certain resistance to the creation of a new therapeutic alliance. Ultimately, the adolescent can feel he or she is being abandoned at this critical phase, and often there can be an aggravation of the disorder.

Coming from parents. Very often, parents share the complaints of adolescents, who they perceive as being unable to be autonomous or to cope in adult facilities. They might also consider that their opinion will be less taken into account in an adult facility, while in reality, it will be as relevant as before.

Evidence from the TRACK study (Transitions of care from Child and Adolescent Mental Health Services to Adult Mental Health Services), carried out in individuals in transition, revealed that transfer failed more often because of young people's or parents' refusal to accept referral to adult services and CAHMS clinicians' failure to refer, rather than AMHS refusal to accept referrals.[29] However, these results should be interpreted cautiously, since they are geographically specific and field studies are needed to 'track' specific difficulties.

Pathways to referral

Starting with the child and adolescent psychiatrist, the adoption of a personal style favouring autonomy (to see the patient alone, to respect confidentiality) might be the first step to preparing for transition. This will also prepare parents, who are important, but progressively secondary, elements. The topic of transition should feature prominently in consultations with the adolescent and his or her family well in advance (months or years) of the event. This will aid preparation.

The experience at AMHS is inevitably different, which can be positive. Adult psychiatrists are typically better placed to answer the questions of young adults (such as those relating to autonomy, life, jobs). It is important to provide useful information about the new service and to be familiar with how the AMHS work, to avoid confusion and mistakes.

Interestingly, the TRACK study highlighted the differences between transfer and transition from child to adult psychiatric services. Accordingly, transfer of care from one healthcare provider to another is often understood as a suboptimal version of the process of transition, implying that the latter is a truly therapeutical engagement that involves the patient and both teams. Nevertheless, the results show that many individuals were transferred successfully to AMHS without good transition. Whether or not transfer needs to be matched with transition, and to which extent, remains a point for debate.[29]

The study showed that the service boundary for transition ranged from 16 to 21 years, with a mean age of 18.1 years. Diagnostically, half of them were suffering from emotional or neurotic disorders, a quarter from neurodevelopmental disorders, and 22% from serious mental disorders. Other disorders included substance abuse, conduct disorders, eating disorders, and emerging personality disorders.[25] Despite most of the users from CAMHS needing transfer to AMHS, a significant proportion (one third in this study) were not properly referred. Those with neurodevelopmental, emotional, neurotic, or emerging personality disorders were most likely to fall through the CAMHS–AMHS gap. Those with a severe and enduring mental illness, a hospital admission, and on a medication were more likely to make a transition to AMHS. Having social risks also predicted transition of care.

A pilot study led by the European Federation of Psychiatric Trainees (EFPT) and the Early Career Psychiatrists' Committee of the European Psychiatric Association (ECPC-EPA) addressed this issue from the providers' perspective.[30] In this study, 166 European adult and child psychiatrists were questioned about transition in their own country. Results showed that good communication between teams, services being close to each other, joint case-based discussions, and shared (electronic) files were highlighted as a possible powerful tool for improving transition. In contrast, lack of time and different paradigms of practice were pointed out as major restraints to good communication.

In conclusion, the integration of youth mental health programmes, including those within the health sector (such as reproductive and sexual health) and outside this sector (such as education), is highly recommended to guarantee a safe transition from CAMHS to AMHS for those who need care continuity.[2]

References

1 Vander Stoep A, Beresford SA, Weiss NS, McKnight B, Cauce AM, Cohen P. Community-based study of the transition to adulthood for adolescents with psychiatric disorder. *Am J Epidemiol* 2000; **152**:352–62.

2 Patel V, Flisher AJ, Hetrick S, McGorry P. Mental health of young people: a global public-health challenge. *Lancet* 2007; **369**:1302–13.

3 Copeland W, Shanahan L, Costello EJ, Angold A. Cumulative prevalence of psychiatric disorders by young adulthood: a prospective cohort analysis from the Great Smoky Mountains Study. *J Am Acad Child Adolesc Psychiatry* 2011; **50**:252–61.

4 Frigerio A, Rucci P, Goodman R, et al. Prevalence and correlates of mental disorders among adolescents in Italy: the PrISMA study. *Eur Child Adolesc Psychiatry* 2009; **18**:217–26.

5 Gore FM, Bloem PJ, Patton GC, et al. Global burden of disease in young people aged 10–24 years: a systematic analysis. *Lancet* 2011; **377**:2093–102.

6 Kessler RC, Berglund P, Demler O, Jin R, Merikangas KR, Walters EE. Lifetime prevalence and age-of-onset distributions of DSM-IV disorders in the National Comorbidity Survey Replication. *Arch Gen Psychiatry* 2005; **62**:593–602.

7 Belfer ML. Child and adolescent mental disorders: the magnitude of the problem across the globe. *J Child Psychol Psychiatry* 2008; **49**:226–36.

8 Patton GC, Coffey C, Romaniuk H, et al. The prognosis of common mental disorders in adolescents: a 14-year prospective cohort study. *Lancet* 2014; **383**:1404–11.

9 Burns BJ, Costello EJ, Angold A, et al. Children's mental health service use across service sectors. *Health Aff (Millwood)* 1995; **14**:147–59.

10 Knapp M. Schizophrenia costs and treatment cost-effectiveness. *Acta Psychiatr Scand Suppl* 2000; **407**:15–18.

11 Scott S, Knapp M, Henderson J, Maughan B. Financial cost of social exclusion: follow up study of antisocial children into adulthood. *BMJ* 2001; **323**:191–5.

12 Knapp M, McCrone P, Fombonne E, Beecham J, Wostear G. The Maudsley long-term follow up of child and adolescent depression: 3. Impact of comorbid conduct disorder on service use and costs in adulthood. *Br J Psychiatry* 2002; **180**:19–23.

13 Fullilove MT. Psychiatric implications of displacement: contributions from the psychology of place. *Am J Psychiatry* 1996; **153**:1516–23.

14 Sampson RJ, Raudenbush SW, Earls F. Neighborhoods and violent crime: a multilevel study of collective efficacy. *Science* 1997; **277**:918–24.

15 Singh S. Post-traumatic stress in former Ugandan child soldiers. *Lancet* 2004; **363**:1648.

16 Joint United Nations Programme on HIV/AIDS (UNAIDS). *Global report: UNAIDS report on the global AIDS epidemic*, 2013. Available at: http://www.unaids.org/en/resources/campaigns/globalreport2013

17 Vermeiren R, Schwab-Stone M, Deboutte D, Leckman P, Ruchkin V. Violence exposure and substance use in adolescents: findings from three countries. *Pediatrics* 2003; **111**:535–40.

18 Patton GC, Coffey C, Sawyer SM, et al. Global patterns of mortality in young people: a systematic analysis of population health data. *Lancet* 2009; **374**:881–92.

19 Greydanus DE, Calles J. Suicide in children and adolescents. *Prim Care* 2007; **34**:259–73.

20 Musto D. Prevailing and shifting paradigms: a historical perspective. In: *Lewis's child and adolescent psychiatry* (eds. Martin A, Volkmar F). Philadelphia: Wolters Kluwer; 2007, pp. 11–7.

21 **Sondheimer A, Rey JM**. Ethics and international child and adolescent psychiatry. In: *IACA-PAP e-textbook of child and adolescent mental health* (ed. Rey JM). Geneva: International Association for Child and Adolescent Psychiatry and Allied Professions; 2012, pp. 1–28.

22 **Lamb C, Murphy M**. The divide between child and adult mental health services: points for debate. *Br J Psychiatry Suppl* 2013; **54**:s41–4.

23 **Conway SP**. Transition for paediatric to adult-orientated care for adolescents with cystic fibrosis. *Disabil Rehabil* 1998; **20**:209–16.

24 **Collis F, Finger E, Owens K**. *Review of transitions to young adult clinics. Final report—attachment 6, literature review*. Ipsos-Eureka Social Research Institute; 2008.

25 **Singh SP, Paul M, Ford T, et al**. Process, outcome and experience of transition from child to adult mental healthcare: multiperspective study. *Br J Psychiatry* 2010; **197**:305–12.

26 **Davis M, Sondheimer DL**. State child mental health efforts to support youth in transition to adulthood. *J Behav Health Serv Res* 2005; **32**:27–42.

27 **Adams J, Nolte M, Schalansky J**. Who will hear our voices? In: *Transition to adulthood: a resource for assisting young people with emotional or behavioral difficulties* (eds. Clark IB, Davis M). Baltimore: Paul H. Brookes Co.; 2000, pp. 181–93.

28 **Costello EJ, Janieszewski S**. Who gets treated? Factors associated with referral in children with psychiatric disorders. *Acta Psych Scand* 1990; **81**:523–9.

29 **Paul M, Ford T, Kramer T, Islam Z, Harley K, Singh SP**. Transfers and transitions between child and adult mental health services. *Br J Psychiatry Suppl* 2013; **54**:s36–40.

30 **Moscoso A, Jovanovic N, Martina RK**. Transition from adolescent to adult mental health services in Europe from the provider's perspective. *Lancet Psychiatry* 2015; vol. 2 (9):779–780.

Chapter 24

How to responsibly prescribe psychotropics

Martina Rojnic Kuzman, Defne Eraslan, and Jerzy Samochowiec

Case study

Amanda is a psychiatric trainee in Europe. On duty last night, she admitted a new patient. The patient, E.F., aged 35, worked as an architect and was accompanied by his wife, who found him wandering around neighbourhood gardens, looking for cameras planted by people he thought were after him. He was anxious, frightened, paranoid, and hearing the voices of his persecutors. His wife confirmed that his problems started five years ago, with a similar but much shorter and less pronounced psychotic episode. After the introduction of olanzapine 10 mg daily, later in combination with fluvoxamine 100 mg/day, his psychotic symptoms subsided and he regained the premorbid level of functioning. However, as he gained significant weight, E.F. stopped taking the medication after six months. Two years ago, he was hospitalized because of a new psychotic episode and was treated with unusually high daily doses (10 mg) of risperidone, which he took for a year and then stopped using, as he was feeling well. Three months ago, he started to develop odd behaviours, suspiciousness, and hallucinations. Amanda admitted the patient to the ward and gave him risperidone (2 mg).

When her supervisor asked for the treatment plan, Amanda responded that the patient was psychotic but wanted to get treatment. She acknowledged the efficacy and side-effects of treatment, and problems of non-adherence to treatment. Thus, she suggested trying a medication that had proven efficient, with no significant side-effects. Amanda started with a low dose and planned to increase it to the same level as before, complementing the diagnostic procedure with therapeutic drug monitoring (due to the possible ultra fast hepatic metabolism of the patient). She also suggested switching to a depot form of risperidone, to improve adherence to treatment, or to paliperidone, to avoid extensive hepatic drug metabolism (if proven so by drug monitoring). To improve adherence, she recommended complementing pharmacological treatment with psychosocial interventions.

Case study discussion points

- Are the side-effects of the effective treatment significant for the treatment outcome?
- Why do some patients need unusually high doses of drugs?
- Why did the patient need a high dose of risperidone, but not of olanzapine?
- What is the role of fluvoxamine for olanzapine metabolism?
- When should depot medications start?
- When should therapeutic drug monitoring be used?
- What is the role of adherence to treatment for the treatment outcome?

Introduction

The introduction of pharmacotherapy has revolutionized the field of psychiatry when it comes to the major psychiatric disorders such as schizophrenia, bipolar disorders, or major depression. This applies to many drugs (such as chlorpromazine, haloperidol, and, later on, clozapine) used for the treatment of schizophrenia, lithium for the treatment of bipolar disorders, and tricyclics for the treatment of depression. The availability of these drugs, besides the tremendous steps forward in the treatment of major psychiatric disorders, has profoundly influenced the concepts of mental illness as well as the perception of psychiatry in society. In the case of chlorpromazine, which became available in psychiatric practice in 1952, its effectiveness was reflected in the dramatic transformation of psychiatric wards. The discovery that chlorpromazine blocks dopamine receptors shaped the concepts of development of schizophrenia toward biological causes. Because of this success, chlorpromazine led to the development of neuropsychopharmacology and many other drugs.[1] New agents that were added to these drug groups, especially the new generations of antipsychotics and antidepressants, brought more progress in the pharmacotherapy of these disorders due to their more favourable pharmacokinetic and side-effect profiles.[2,3] In fact, such newer medications quickly become widespread, even beyond their use in psychiatry.[4]

With the newer medications available, the expectations from patients, families, co-workers, as well as doctors, about treatment for major disorders, changed as well. While in the past, psychiatry was expected to 'remove' the dangerous patients from society, nowadays, psychiatry is expected to integrate patients into society and restore them to their previous level of functioning.[5–7] However, to achieve this ambitious goal, a skilled

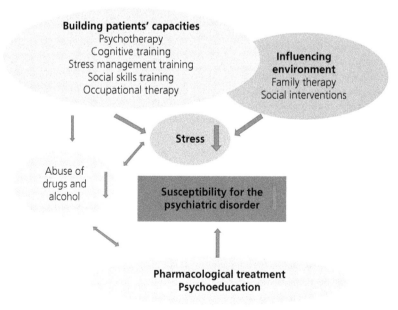

Fig. 24.1 General principles for the treatment of major psychiatric disorders.

psychopharmacologist must always acknowledge that even in the treatment of major psychiatric disorders, psychopharmacology, as the basic treatment, should always be accompanied by other treatment methods (Fig. 24.1).

Factors influencing the choice of medication

Psychopharmacological treatment forms the basic treatment for major psychiatric disorders. In this chapter, we shall discuss how to responsibly prescribe medications for these disorders, following the principle that 'the best pharmacotherapy is highly individualized'. To plan such tailor-made treatments, many illness-related, person-related, and drug-related factors should be taken into account (Fig. 24.2).

Personal factors and environment

A patient's diagnosis is obviously the leading factor in determining the choice of medication. When a diagnosis is made, usually the choice of the main medication will be made following the approved indications of the drug. There are a number of guidelines based on research and clinical practice that aim to help clinicians in determining the correct medication based on the diagnosis.[8-14] However, the majority of guidelines make recommendations on medication class, instead of specific members of that class. For example, using SSRIs (selective serotonin reuptake inhibitors) is recommended as the first-line treatment for depression.[9] In clinical practice, however, it is clear to most prescribers that SSRIs are very different from one another, even if belonging to the same pharmacological class.[3,15]

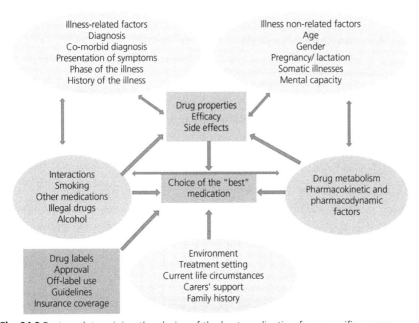

Fig. 24.2 Factors determining the choice of the best medication for a specific person.

Since there are still no psychiatric medications that would treat the cause of psychiatric illness, the determination of a psychiatric diagnosis is not enough to make a choice of medication. Thus, the next factor in determining the choice of a specific drug is the symptomatology the patient presents. While some authors recommend focusing on the leading symptoms, others recommend focusing mainly on the atypical symptoms, which are usually the most persistent (e.g. anxiety or sleep problems in depression).[16] A helpful approach is to focus, at first, on those symptoms that the patient defines as the most burdening, 'fine tuning' the treatment along the way, according to the patient's subsequent needs. Life-threatening symptoms such as suicidality, aggression, or intoxications present themselves as psychiatric emergencies and require the utmost attention while choosing medication, during any phase of the illness.

Further factors include eventual co-morbid disorders, which are rather prevalent among psychiatric patients.[17] In these cases, the use of medication which is compatible with all co-morbid disorders is strongly recommended. The chosen medication should not lead to the improvement of one condition, while worsening another. Attention should be paid to other somatic illnesses and other medications a person is taking, due to the possible influence of psychiatric drugs on somatic conditions and the possible interaction between drugs.

Other personal factors, like age and gender, need to be taken into consideration. The psychiatrist must always keep the Hippocratic principle of *primum non nocere* in mind. For example, some of the drugs that significantly increase prolactin levels can disrupt the menstrual cycle and induce galactorrhoea, which is a very annoying side-effect for women in their reproductive years. Children and older patients require usually lower doses of medications in order to avoid side-effects, due to their different pharmacokinetic properties.

The environment of the patient generally plays a less important role in the choice of medication, but on some occasions it may be very important. For example, a combination of psychiatric symptomatology (i.e. poor insight or reduced mental capacity), personality characteristics (e.g. unreliability), psychiatric history (e.g. previous accounts of relapses due to interruption of medication use), combined with an unsupportive environment (e.g. parents with poor insight or no caregivers at all) may lead to a high probability of non-adherence, and this may determine the choice of a specific formulation of the drug (e.g. depot formulations).

Drug properties

Clinical properties and interactions

As mentioned earlier, a drug is given specifically with the intention to treat a condition and/or to reduce symptoms. Thus, choosing the appropriate medication means matching the supposed mechanism of pathophysiology and the mechanism of action of a certain drug. For instance, an antipsychotic is supposed to reduce the positive symptoms of schizophrenia which are associated with hyperactivity of the dopaminergic mesolimbic pathway. Thus, antipsychotics work as D2 antagonists. However, negative schizophrenia symptoms are usually associated with hypoactivity of the dopaminergic mesocortical pathway. Thus, when treating the negative symptoms of schizophrenia, the psychiatrist should consider using other antipsychotics or lower doses than those usually preferred for treating primarily positive symptoms.

Apart from different pharmacodynamic profiles, there are very significant differences in pharmacokinetic properties among psychiatric drugs. This fact becomes even more important when the pharmacokinetic processes are slower due to impaired hepatic or renal functioning. In these cases, the usual dose should be decreased significantly.

However, even with normal hepatic function, caution is needed where multiple drugs with similar metabolic pathways are used. In fact, the majority of psychiatric drugs are metabolized through the liver and some have very potent effects on the liver metabolic system (Table 24.1). For example, concomitant use of CYP3A4

Table 24.1 Hepatic CYP450 metabolism of psychiatric drugs

	CYP1A2	CYP2C19	CYP2D6	CYP3A4
Inductor	Smoking; carbamazepine	St John's wort		Carbamazepine; St John's wort
Major metabolic pathway— inhibition of enzymes will significantly increase drug levels in blood	Clozapine Olanzapine Quetiapine Paroxetine Sertraline Chlorpromazine Agomelatine Caffeine Duloxetine Fluvoxamine	Clozapine Olanzapine Quetiapine Citalopram Diazepam Fluoxetine Moclobemide Clomirpramine Amitripltiline Sertraline	Risperidone Haloperidole Ziprasidone Iloperidone Aripiprazol Zuclopentixol Fluphenazine Sertindole Clorpromazine Mirtazapine Nortripliline Clomirpramine Amitripltiline Maprotiline Venlafaksine Citalopram Fluoxetine Fluvoxamine Mianserine Paroxetine Pregabaline	Clozapine Quetiapine Ziprasidone Aripiprazol Sertindole Haloperidol Buprenorphine Busprirone Citalopram Midazolam Trazodone Zolpidem Zolpicone
Inhibitor	Fluvoxamine	Fluvoxamine	Fluvoxamine Paroxetine Fluoksetine Duloxetine Bupropion Moclobemide	Fluvoxamine

inductors or CYP3A4 inhibitors with the main drug (which is metabolized through CYP3A4) may respectively increase or decrease the metabolism of the main drug, thus, in turn, lowering or increasing blood concentrations of the drugs (Table 24.1). In some cases, this may lead to potentially lethal effects (e.g. in patients using the anticoagulant drug warfarin, which is extensively metabolized through the CYP450 enzymes).

Thus, the metabolism of all drugs that the patient is taking should be always checked and compared with the metabolism of the psychiatric drug you want to prescribe. Indeed, therapeutic drug monitoring (TDM), including the quantification of serum or plasma concentrations of medications for dose optimization and respective pharmacogenetics, has proved a valuable tool for patient-matched psychopharmacotherapy (Table 24.2).

Table 24.2 When to use therapeutic drug monitoring in psychiatry

Possible clinical indication	Which psychiatric drugs to monitor
◆ Suspected complete or partial non-adherence (non-compliance) to medication ◆ Lack of clinical improvement under recommended doses ◆ Clinical improvement but presence of adverse effects under recommended doses ◆ Combination treatment with a drug known for its interaction potential or suspected drug interaction ◆ Recurrence under adequate doses ◆ Patients with pharmacokinetically relevant states or co-morbidities, children, elderly patients, pregnant women, hepatic or renal insufficiency, cardiovascular disease ◆ Dose optimization after initial prescription or after dose change	*Level 1—strongly recommended*: amitriptiline, clomipramine, imipramine, nortriptiline, amisulprid, clozpine, haloperidol, fluphenazine, olanzapine, perazine, pherpenazine, thioridazine, lithium *Level 2—recommended*: aripiprazole, chlorpromazine, flupentixol, paliperidone, quetiapine, risperidone, sulpiride, setindole, ziprasidone, desipramine, desvanlafaxin, duloxetin, escitalopram, flouxetine, fluvoxamine, maprotiline, mirtazapine, milnacipram, sertraline, venlafaxine, trazodone, carbamazepine, lamotrigine, valproic acid, carbamazepine, clonazepam, gabapentin, donepezil, buprenorphine, methadone, levomethadone, naltrexone, methylphenidate, dexmethylphenidate *Level 3—useful*: bupropion, mianserine, moclobemide, paroxetine reboxetine, iloperidone, pimozid, levomepromazine, zotepine, zuclopentixole, pregabalin, topiramate, buspirone, galantamine, rivastigmine, memantine, acaprostate, disulfiram, biperiden, modafininil *Level 4—potentially useful*: agomelatin, asenapine, alprazolam, bromazepam, clorazepam, midazolam, diazepam, lorazepam, nitrazepam, oxazepam, temazepam, triazolam, zolpidem, zolpicom

Drug labels

Right after the discovery of the first psychiatric drugs, only their clinical effects were known. Their mechanisms of action have been unravelled only over the last decades. Traditionally, psychotropics were classified based on their clinical effects as antipsychotics, antidepressants, antimanic drugs, anxiolytics, etc. However, in clinical practice, especially newer generations of drugs are now being used for a significantly extended range of indications than those originally intended. For example, almost all newer antipsychotics have also been tested in clinical trials and approved for the treatment of mania in bipolar disorders, while two of them (quetiapine, aripiprazole) are also labelled for the treatment of the depressive phase of bipolar disorder or of treatment-resistant depression. Most SSRIs have been tested in clinical trials and then approved for the treatment of anxiety disorders and obsessive compulsive disorder.[16]

At the same time, the last two decades have brought progress in the discovery of cellular mechanisms which challenge the older receptor-based concepts of the neurobiology of major psychiatric disorders. Although one can argue that despite the new knowledge, we are not much closer to the discovery of the causative agents of psychiatric disorders, it is also true that new research has exposed evidence for disturbed brain circuits that are expressed as a cluster of symptoms. With this concept, the lines that distinguish one diagnosis from another become blurred and a psychiatric illness is seen as a specific collection of endophenotypes which share common bases with other psychiatric disorders.[18] When the complex interaction of the biological base of the illness and the environment enters the picture, its outcome can rarely be labelled with one lifelong diagnosis.

With the blurring of borders between diagnoses and the emergence of the symptom-dimension treatment approach to psychiatric disorders,[19] one can get the impression that psychiatric medications have a very wide range of overlapping treatment indications and that psychiatrists treat all diagnoses in the same way (e.g. a person suffering from schizophrenia with post-psychotic depression, or a person with schizoaffective disorders, or a person with bipolar depression may all get the same treatment—a newer-generation antipsychotic, like olanzapine, and an SSRI, like paroxetine—and it may work in all three cases). Depending on its dosage, quetiapine can be used to treat severe insomnia, bipolar depression, cyclothymia, and schizophrenia. However, exactly the opposite is also true. With more and more available medications that can be effectively used in different disorders, a personalized treatment plan is possible.

To facilitate the choice of the optimal drug for a patient, a number of guidelines issued by international or national professional associations exist.[10–14] In most countries, such guidelines are not legally binding, but they do serve as professional guidance for clinicians and may affect reimbursement. In the majority of cases, these guidelines are flexible enough to allow a personalized approach for the 'unusual' cases, where augmentation strategies or modified treatment strategies are needed.

Off-label use

Off-label use is the use of pharmaceutical drugs for an unapproved indication, age group, dosage, or form of administration. Off-label use is legal unless it violates specific ethical guidelines or safety regulations, but it does carry differences in legal liability. For a drug to acquire 'labelled' use, it should be approved by a national or international agency for use in

> ## Box 24.1 Summary of product characteristics
>
> ◆ Therapeutic indications
> ◆ Posology
> ◆ Contraindications
> ◆ Special warnings and precautions for use
> ◆ Interaction with other medicinal products
> ◆ Undesirable effects

a certain dose for a specific indication. For example, in the European Union, the European Medication Agency (EMA) approves drugs for prescription use and continues to regulate the pharmaceutical industry's promotional practices; the Food and Drug Administration (FDA) does the same in the United States of America. In the majority of countries, this approval process is a very strict and costly administrative procedure, requiring a well-defined protocol which shows that a drug has been tested in all preclinical and clinical stages for a certain indication in a certain dose range. The 'summary of product characteristics' for a certain drug specifies its main characteristics, as listed in Box 24.1.

Drug marketing authorization in a given country implies that the drug has been authorized for its intended use. A deviation from guidelines in the summary of product characteristics (including the use of the drug in an unapproved age group, for an unapproved indication, and in an unapproved dosage) constitutes an off-label use. Every decision to use a drug in an off-label way should always be preceded by a risk to expected benefit assessment (Table 24.3).

In general, off-label prescriptions are legal and allowed in all countries. In some countries, off-label use is regulated by an official body, while in others, it is generally accepted as long as it better serves the patient's needs and is supported by some evidence or experience to demonstrate its safety and efficacy, as in the UK.[20] There is an extensive body of evidence to show that off-label use of many pharmaceutical products is a common practice in many countries worldwide. American statistics show that 60% of prescription neuroleptics in the USA are recommended for disorders not listed in product characteristics. Off-label prescribing and the use of drugs for indications that have not received regulatory approval, is common, occurring with up to 21% of prescribed drugs.[21] Although the absence of regulatory approval for a treatment indication does not mean a drug is harmful in that circumstance, off-label use is suspected to be an important determinant of preventable adverse drug events. However, there has not been any systematic investigation of the risks and benefits of off-label use beyond single drugs.[22]

In addition, little is known about the factors that contribute to off-label prescribing that may determine systematic differences in treatment outcome. The paucity of knowledge is in part related to the methodological challenges of measuring off-label use and its effects.[23] In most settings, treatment indication is not a required element of prescription. The indication for treatment needs to be inferred by reviewing either health problems documented in the patient's chart or diagnostic codes entered in

Table 24.3 How to use a drug in an off-label way

Factor	Rationale	Action
Professional experience	Clinical work is a constant learning process, thus clinical experience is an important element in every clinical decision-making process. This is often the first step in the decision-making process, but should be accompanied by others.	Gain experience in the field; present your case to your senior colleagues and ask for their expert opinion.
Current body of medical knowledge (standards/ guidelines)	Clinical guidelines are often more flexible in drug indications and may provide clinical 'approval/ support' for your choice of medication than drug labels (e.g. you may find that drugs have already been approved for the specific indication in other countries and supported by international guidelines, although the indication was not approved in your country).	Consult the existing guidelines on the topic (national and international).
Scientific papers and reports	Clinical guidelines are usually formed based on the scientific literature and clinical reports. Thus, guidelines for the use of novel drugs or treatment approaches beyond their original indications may not exist. Thus, scientific literature may provide you with the only evidence for the off-label use.	Consult the available scientific literature on the topic.
Legal responsibility	If a drug is used consistently with the summary of product characterization, the manufacturer will bear all the legal responsibility. In off-label use, the responsibility is born by the prescribing doctor.	Document that this way of drug use was justified and consistent with state of the art medical knowledge.
Patient's wishes	The therapeutic alliance should rely on partnership in the treatment process, which means that both patients and doctors participate in the decision- making process and assume responsibility.	Obtain patient's written consent.

physician surveys. For off-label use, the reason for treatment is, therefore, difficult to discern. Inclusion of treatment indications as a required field of an electronic prescription has been proposed as one method of addressing this problem and enhancing pharmacological surveillance. A study by Eguale et al. in 2012 was the first to take advantage of the inclusion of treatment indication in an electronic health record (EHR) to evaluate off-label use and assess drug, patient, and physician factors that influence off-label prescribing. A total of 650,237 electronic prescriptions were written between January 2005 and December 2009, and a total of 253,347 unique patient and drug indication combinations were identified once repeated prescriptions were removed, representing 50,823 patients, 113 physicians, and 684 drugs. Overall, 11% of drugs were prescribed for an off-label indication and 79% of off-label use lacked strong scientific evidence.

The highest proportion of off-label prescribing occurred with central nervous system drugs (26.3%), anti-infective agents (17.1%), and ear/nose/throat medications (15.2%). Among central nervous system drugs, the highest proportions of off-label use were for anticonvulsants (66.6%), antipsychotics (43.8%), and antidepressants (33.4%). Indications that were most likely to be treated with off-label drugs included nocturnal leg pain and benign positional vertigo, for which 100% of the drugs prescribed were off-label.[23]

Physicians with evidence-based orientation were less likely to prescribe off-label, and this effect was increased for drugs prescribed off-label without strong scientific evidence. This observation implies that physicians who give emphasis to evidence-based medicine base their treatment decisions not only on data from drug regulatory bodies but also on the overall evidence available from different sources (including peer-reviewed publications, clinical guidelines, and recommendations from professional societies). Currently, there is an effort to educate physicians on the level of evidence and appropriate off-label uses, with the aim of linking off-label use with rigorous outcome evaluation and with the physician being an active participant in evidence development.[24,25] Connecting drugs with their treatment indications and providing evidence to support off-label use at the time of prescribing would be one way of addressing scientifically unsupported off-label use.[26]

Treatment in the acute phase

All major psychiatric illnesses share similar temporal dynamics, as they are all long-term illnesses, characterized by alternating periods of acute symptoms and their remission. In the majority of cases of major psychiatric disorders, a cycle of relapses and remissions is repeated many times, until reaching a chronic phase.[9,27,28] Thus, treating psychiatric disorders is like a long-distance run, and different phases of the illness frequently need different treatment approaches.

Usually, treatment starts in the acute phase of the illness. The treatment goal in this phase is the reduction of symptoms. The drugs of choice for a particular patient will be selected following the process depicted in Fig. 24.2. The dose should be increased gradually, over days, for the majority of medications, although some may need more caution than others due to their wide therapeutic range.

Patients should be monitored frequently (on a daily to weekly basis) to assess the therapeutic response and the emergence of acute side-effects. Apart from the clinical examination, there a number of helpful scales aimed at objectively assessing the treatment response and based on the measurement of the severity of symptoms at several time points. These scales include the positive and negative symptoms severity scale (PANSS) for schizophrenia[29] and the Hamilton scale for depression (HAMD).[30] The frequency of evaluation of the treatment response varies among disorders and medication groups. For example, in most studies of schizophrenia and affective disorders, or in other disorders treated with antidepressants, the first measurement may occur in the third week, with the second one in the sixth week. However, for some medications that require very slow dose increases (e.g. lamotrigine), it is usually necessary to wait longer, even for many weeks or months.[10-14] Depending on the reduction of the initial score on the scales, a treatment response can be defined as full, partial, or no response.[31] A summary of the acute-phase treatment approach is given in Fig. 24.3.

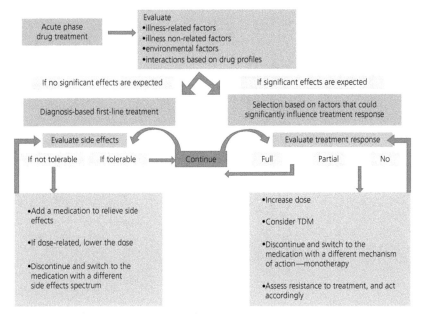

Fig. 24.3 Acute-phase treatment approach.

In the case of non-response to the first treatment in the acute phase, at least one more trial of another medication in monotherapy, at a dose within the therapeutic range, is recommended.[10–14] Although there are differences in existing criteria, if a response to treatment is still not obtained, the disorder can be regarded as resistant to treatment. However, in determining drug effectiveness, a common mistake seems to be that of sub-dosing.[32] A study by Tsutsumi et al., in 2011, revealed that in almost 50% of cases where doctors switched to another antipsychotic because of effectiveness, the dose of the 'non-effective' antipsychotic was below the recommended therapeutic range. In the case of further treatment inefficiency, therapeutic strategies may include:

1) the use of the most effective medications for 'treatment resistance' (such as clozapine in schizophrenia);

2) the addition of a complementary medication;

3) the addition of other treatment methods (such as electroconvulsive therapy (ECT); exemptions include some clinical presentations, such as catatonia, where ECT can be considered as first-line treatment;[33]

4) eventual addition of experimental treatment (Fig. 24.4).

Contrary to what is recommended by most guidelines and clinical studies, polypharmacy is widespread in psychiatric practice.[34,35] As a result, there is a lack of naturalistic studies where more than one medication is applied. Although the rationale behind polypharmacy is clearly not in line with guidelines (Table 24.4), in some cases, the patient will positively benefit from the addition of another medication[36] even before treatment resistance is established. Whenever adding a new compound, however, a

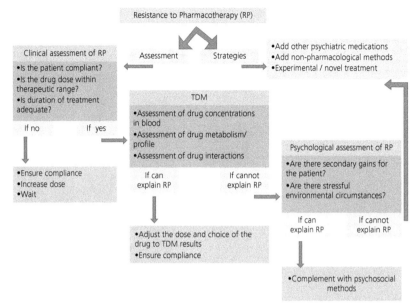

Fig. 24.4 Management of resistance to pharmacotherapy.

Table 24.4 The rationale for polypharmacy

Rationale	Example
The addition of medications to counteract the side-effects of the primary medication that needs to be used for a longer period in doses that cause side-effects	Addition of anticholinergic medication to counteract the effects of antipsychotics that cause extrapyramidal effects
'Treatment ineffectiveness' of the main medication used in monotherapy in acute states	The concomitant use of haloperidol with another medication for the treatment of aggression
Fast relief of acute symptoms during the prolonged period needed to obtain treatment response from medication	Concomitant use of sedatives with antidepressants (e.g. SSRIs) for sleeping difficulties in depression in the first three weeks of SSRI treatment
Complex symptomatology requiring more than one drug type	Post-psychotic depression in patients treated with antipsychotics may require the addition of antidepressant; depression with psychotic features
Cross titration leads to remission or satisfactory treatment response or significant decrease of side-effects, and thus the treatment team decides to go on with both of the medications	During cross titration from quetiapine to risperidone, a good treatment response was observed, along with decreased hypotension, while with a further increase of risperidone, akathisia occurred, and thus the team decided to go with low doses of both antipsychotics

psychiatrist should be aware of the potential interactions. Thus, they should regularly re-evaluate the treatment regimens of their chronic patients to see if there are any medications that can be stopped.

Treatment in the stabilization phase

Clinical status

After the acute symptoms remit, the psychiatric illness often enters a phase of stabilization that usually requires 'maintenance' treatment. The goal of maintenance therapy is to keep the symptoms in remission and to help restore patients to their premorbid level of functioning. Pharmacotherapy, along with other approaches, is an essential part of the treatment plan in this illness management phase, as shown in Fig. 24.1.

During pharmacological maintenance treatment, psychiatrists should evaluate the patients periodically. Unfortunately, for the majority of patients with major psychiatric disorders, the illness course is characterized by alternating periods of acute illness and periods of remission.[28] Each period of acute illness lasts longer and requires higher doses/additional medication to achieve symptom remission, and is associated with further deterioration in the patient's mental state, ability to work, and social interactions. In fact, the duration of acute illness may be associated with loss of brain white matter.[37] Thus, treating acute illness and keeping the symptoms from relapsing with maintenance therapy may actually prevent further deterioration in some psychiatric disorders (especially schizophrenia).

A common reason for relapse is non-adherence.[38] Indeed, studies show that up to 50% of patients taking psychiatric medications do not use the medications as prescribed by their doctor.[39] Non-adherence is a common problem with psychiatric patients, and especially those with lack of cognitive insight.[40] This problem is largely solved among patients with schizophrenia and mood disorders by the introduction of depot formulations of drugs. The use of depot formulations is quite widespread, although variable, among countries. Moreover, with the newer generations of antipsychotics being introduced as long-acting injecting drugs, the indication for their use has become more widespread. Indeed, it has been recently reported that use of such drugs with younger people, and often in the early phase of their illness, is associated with a tendency to prevent relapses and relapse-associated further progression of the illness.[41]

However, evidence also shows that long-term administration of typical antipsychotics is also associated with the loss of white matter in the brain, although with a different pattern than that seen in schizophrenia.[42] Thus, the most beneficial pharmacological approach is treatment with the lowest possible dose of medications which successfully keep the symptoms in remission and have the least possible side-effects. In practice, in order to achieve this goal, the psychiatrist must plan regular visits and monitor for symptoms and side-effects. Whenever psychiatrists observe the worsening of symptoms, the action they take will depend upon the cause of relapse. The stabilization-phase treatment approach is depicted in Fig. 24.5. The duration of maintenance therapy is still a matter of debate, and differs among different recommendations and among different major disorders.

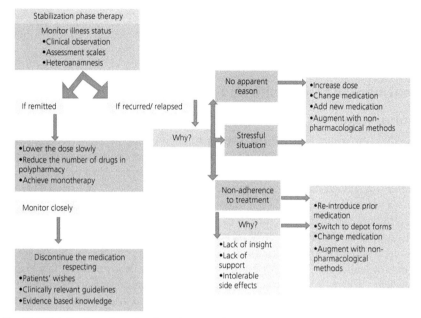

Fig. 24.5 Stabilization-phase treatment approach.

Side-effects

The World Health Organization defined an adverse reaction to a drug as 'noxious, unintended, and occurring at doses normally used in man for prophylaxis, diagnosis or therapy'.[43] Psychotropic drugs present a great variety of different types of adverse reactions, which in recent years have constituted a proving ground for the development of a new branch of clinical pharmacology concerned with the identification of adverse reactions, measurements of their incidence, and understanding of their mechanism. The monitoring of an acute side-effect to treatment usually involves clinical observation. In addition, there are a number of helpful scales aimed at objectively assessing the side-effects of antipsychotic treatment (e.g. the Simpson-Angus Scale (SAS)[44]).

The side-effects that occur in this later phase of treatment may, in some cases, be the same as in the acute phase (most commonly, weight gain), or there may be a different set of side-effects (tardive dyskinesia, metabolic disturbances, etc.). Thus, monitoring for side-effects is requested in any treatment phase. Usually, clinical check-ups, scales for the assessment of side-effects, and some laboratory measures are sufficient (Table 24.5).[45,46] Whenever a side-effect occurs, a psychiatrist should very carefully assess its origin, temporary dynamics, severity, and treatment options. When considering a pharmacological side-effect, the following strategies might be adopted:

1) decrease the dose;

2) withdraw the medication;

3) add a new medication (see Fig. 24.6).

Table 24.5 Assessment of side-effects during regular clinical check-ups

Somatic examination	Laboratory measurements
◆ Physical examination (e.g. skin, hair loss)	◆ Glucose in blood, cholesterol, HDL cholesterol, LDL cholesterol, triglycerides (with antipsychotics)
◆ Neurological examination (e.g. tremor, rigor, parkinsonism)	
◆ Heart and pulse rate, blood pressure	◆ Blood count (e.g. with clozapine, carbamazapine)
◆ Weight and body mass index	◆ Thyroid function (T4 and TSH) (with lithium)
◆ Waist circumference	◆ Kidney function (urea, creatine clirens) (with lithium)
	◆ ECG (with some antipsychotics e.g. aripiprazole, sertindole)

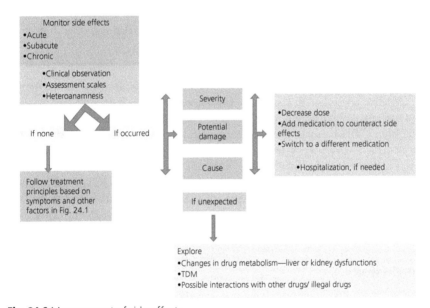

Fig. 24.6 Management of side-effects.

In most countries, the side-effects of drugs have to be reported to national or international regulatory drug agencies.

Non-pharmacological factors influencing treatment response

A skilled psychopharmacologist should be able to grasp all the factors that could modify the effects of the prescribed drug (Box 24.2).

At first defined as a simulated or otherwise medically ineffectual treatment for a disease or other medical condition, intended to deceive the recipient, it was later shown

Box 24.2 How to enhance the therapeutic effects of the prescribed medication

- Establish a good therapeutic alliance to decrease the chances of a 'nocebo' effect.
- Choose the medication appropriate for the patient's leading complaint.
- Stick to the *primum non nocere* principle (i.e. the patient's experience of side-effects should not outweigh the treatment effects).
- Regularly monitor the treatment response.
- Regularly monitor adherence (identification of full and partial non-adherence to medication).
- Re-evaluate the treatment plan (favouring an integrative approach which combines pharmacotherapy with psychosocial approaches such as psychotherapy, sociotherapy, or occupational therapy).
- Evaluate the influence of 'other' factors (such as family relations, work stress, partner relations, secondary gain).

that placebos can have real, measurable effects on physiological changes in the brain, and objective physiological changes.[47] The 'placebo effect' is part of the response to any active medical intervention and accounts for at least 30% of the effectiveness of a medication.[48] This is usually a welcome non-pharmacological effect. However, alternatively, a patient who disbelieves in a treatment may experience a worsening of symptoms, which is called the 'nocebo effect'. If a patient is paranoid and suspects that the treating psychiatrist is giving him or her poison, the nocebo effect will probably occur, irrespective of the objective drug effects. A good therapeutic alliance, where the patient and doctor are 'tuned in' to each other and where the patient trusts his or her doctor, prevents the nocebo effect.[49]

Conclusions

The non-availability of pharmacotherapy shaped the core of psychiatry throughout history, with regard to the major psychiatric disorders. It influenced concepts of mental illness and of psychiatric treatment, and the image of psychiatry in general. At present, the availability of psychotropics has led at least to the following consequences:

1) the perception that all major psychiatric disorders have a clear neurobiological basis;

2) recovery as an achievable treatment goal;

3) an ambiguous and wide-ranging perception of psychiatry by the medical community and the general population (from, at one extreme, the 'psychiatrist–psychopharmacologist' who is a prescriber and does not speak to patients through to, at the other extreme, the 'psychotherapist' who does not prescribe medications and only 'talks').

While the currently available psychotropics can be regarded as effective drugs, it is often cited that at last one third of patients with major psychiatric disorders do not achieve even moderate functional remission. This situation has led to a certain level of disappointment in psychopharmacological treatment and pointed out some of the controversies related to the current status of pharmacotherapy within psychiatry, such as:

1) the apparent lack of specific aetiology/pathogenetic process in choosing the drug;
2) the disproportion of monotherapy in treatment recommendations as opposed to the widespread use of polypharmacy in clinical practice;
3) the use of off-label medications;
4) the relative lack of success of new therapeutic approaches such as person-centred approaches based on genetics and pharmacogenomics;
5) the increased unnatural dichotomy between pharmacological and psychological treatment which replaced the biopsychosocial approach to mental illness.

Instead of sharing the disappointment and doubt in the efficacy of psychiatric drugs, we propose that responsible prescription of psychotropics can improve the functional outcome for patients. Appropriate strategies should encompass:

1) the choice of drugs, by acknowledging illness-related factors (i.e. personal illness), drug-related factors, and environmental factors;
2) the creation of a good treatment alliance;
3) the frequent evaluation of the effects of medication, including treatment response and side-effects;
4) the implementation of a comprehensive treatment plan, integrating psycho-pharmacology and a variety of psychosocial treatment methods.

Although such strategies may require more effort from psychiatrists and patients in the beginning, one should always remember that psychiatric treatment is a long-distance race and the winner is seen only at the end.

References

1 **Ban TA**. Fifty years chlorpromazine: a historical perspective. *Neuropsychiatr Dis Treat* 2007; **3**(4):495–500.
2 **Rang HP, Dale MM, Ritter JM**. Drugs used in affective disorders. In: *Pharmacology* (4th edn). Edinburgh, UK: Harcourt Publishers Ltd; 2001, pp. 550–65.
3 **Leucht S, Cipriani A, Spineli L, et al**. Comparative efficacy and tolerability of 15 antipsychotic drugs in schizophrenia: a multiple-treatments meta-analysis. *Lancet* 2013; **382**(9896):951–62.
4 **Greenberg PE, Kessler RC, Birnbaum HG, et al**. The economic burden of depression in the United States: how did it change between 1990 and 2000? *J Clin Psychiatry* 2003; **64**(12):1465–75.
5 Royal College of Psychiatrists. *Fair deal for mental health*. London: Royal College of Psychiatrists; 2008.
6 American Psychiatric Association. *Position statement on the use of the concept of recovery*. Washington DC: American Psychiatric Association; 2005.

7 College of Occupational Therapists. *Recovering ordinary lives: the strategy for occupational therapy in mental health services 2007–17*. London: College of Occupational Therapists; 2006.

8 Bauer M, Whybrow PC, Angst J, et al. World Federation of Societies of Biological Psychiatry (WFSBP) guidelines for biological treatment of unipolar depressive disorders. Part 2: maintenance treatment of major depressive disorder and treatment of chronic depressive disorders and subthreshold depressions. *World J Biol Psychiatry* 2002; **3**(2):69–86.

9 Bauer M, Pfennig A, Severus E, et al. World Federation of Societies of Biological Psychiatry (WFSBP) guidelines for biological treatment of unipolar depressive disorders. Part 1: update 2013 on the acute and continuation treatment of unipolar depressive disorders. *World J Biol Psychiatry* 2013; **14**(5):334–85.

10 Grunze H, Vieta E, Goodwin GM, et al. The World Federation of Societies of Biological Psychiatry (WFSBP) guidelines for the biological treatment of bipolar disorders: update 2012 on the long-term treatment of bipolar disorder. *World J Biol Psychiatry* 2013; **14**:154–219.

11 Hasan A, Falkai P, Wobrock T, et al. World Federation of Societies of Biological Psychiatry (WFSBP) guidelines for biological treatment of schizophrenia. Part 2: update 2012 on the long-term treatment of schizophrenia and management of antipsychotic-induced side effects. *World J Biol Psychiatry* 2013a; **14**(1):2–44.

12 Hasan A, Falkai P, Wobrock T, et al. World Federation of Societies of Biological Psychiatry (WFSBP) guidelines for biological treatment of schizophrenia. Part 1: update 2012 on the acute treatment of schizophrenia and the management of treatment resistance. *World J Biol Psychiatry* 2013b; **13**(5):318–78.

13 National Institute of Clinical Excellence. *Bipolar disorder NICE guideline: the management of bipolar disorder in adults, children and adolescents, in primary and secondary care*. NICE; 2006.

14 National Institute of Clinical Excellence. *NICE clinical guideline: psychosis and schizophrenia in adults. Treatment and management*. NICE; 2014.

15 Cipriani A, Furukawa TA, Salanti G, et al. Comparative efficacy and acceptability of 12 new-generation antidepressants: a multiple-treatments meta-analysis. *Lancet* 2009; **373**(9665):746–58.

16 Stahl S. *Stahl's essential psychopharmacology: neuroscientific basis and practical applications* (4th edn). Cambridge University Press New York; 2013.

17 Prados-Torres A, Calderón-Larrañaga A, Hancco-Saavedra J, Poblador-Plou B, van den Akker M. Multimorbidity patterns: a systematic review. *J Clin Epidemiol* 2014; **67**(3):254–66.

18 Le Strat Y, Ramoz N, Gorwood P. The role of genes involved in neuroplasticity and neurogenesis in the observation of a gene-environment interaction (GxE) in schizophrenia. *Curr Mol Med* 2009; **9**(4):506–18.

19 Barch DM, Bustillo J, Gaebel W, et al. Logic and justification for dimensional assessment of symptoms and related clinical phenomena in psychosis: relevance to DSM-5. *Schizophr Res* 2013; **150**(1):15–20.

20 General Medical Council. *Good practice in prescribing and managing medicines and devices, 2013*. Available at: http://www.gmc-uk.org/guidance.

21 Radley DC, Finkelstein SN, Stafford RS. Off-label prescribing among office-based physicians. *Arch Intern Med* 2006; **166**(9):1021–6.

22 Yank V, Tuohy CV, Logan AC, et al. Systematic review: benefits and harms of in-hospital use of recombinant factor VIIa for off-label indications. *Ann Intern Med* 2011; **154**(8):529–40.

23 **Dal Pan GJ**. Monitoring the safety of off-label medicine use. *WHO Drug Inf* 2009; **23**(1):21–22.

23 **Eguale, T, Buckeridge DL, Winslade NE, Benedetti A Hanley JA, Tamblyn R**. Drug, patient, and physician characteristics associated with off-label prescribing in primary care. *Arch Intern Med* 2012; **172**(10):781–8.

24 **Largent EA, Miller FG, Pearson SD**. Going off-label without venturing off-course: evidence and ethical off-label prescribing. *Arch Intern Med* 2009; **169**(19):1745–7.

25 **Gazarian M, Kelly M, McPhee JR, Graudins LV, Ward RL, Campbell TJ**. Off-label use of medicines: consensus recommendations for evaluating appropriateness. *Med J Aust* 2006; **185**(10):544–8.

26 **Maher AR, Maglione M, Bagley S, et al**. Efficacy and comparative effectiveness of atypical antipsychotic medications for off-label uses in adults: a systematic review and meta-analysis. *JAMA* 2011; **306**(12):1359–69.

27 **Judd LL, Akiskal HS, Schettler PJ, et al**. Psychosocial disability in the course of bipolar I and II disorders: a prospective, comparative, longitudinal study. *Arch Gen Psychiatry* 2005; **62**(12):1322–30.

28 **Wiersma D, Nienhuis FJ, Slooff CJ, Giel R**. Natural course of schizophrenic disorders: a 15-year follow-up of a Dutch incidence cohort. *Schizophr Bull* 1998; **24**(1):75–85.

29 **Kay SR, Fiszbein A, Opler LA**. The positive and negative syndrome scale (PANSS) for schizophrenia. *Schizophr Bull* 1987; **13**:261–76.

30 **Hamilton M**. A rating scale for depression. *J Neurosurg Psychiatry* 1960; **23**:56–62.

31 **Kane JM, Leucht S, Carpenter D, Docherty JP,** Expert Consensus Panel for Optimizing Pharmacologic Treatment of Psychotic Disorders. The expert consensus guideline series. Optimizing pharmacologic treatment of psychotic disorders. Introduction: methods, commentary, and summary. *J Clin Psychiatry* 2003; **64**(Suppl 12):5–19.

32 **Tsutsumi C, Uchida H, Suzuki T, et al**. The evolution of antipsychotic switch and polypharmacy in natural practice—a longitudinal perspective. *Schizophr Res* 2011; **130**(1–3):40–6.

33 **Leiknes KA, Jarosh-von Schweder L, Høie B**. Contemporary use and practice of electroconvulsive therapy worldwide. *Brain Behav* 2012; **2**:283–344.

34 **Zink M, Englisch S, Meyer-Lindenberg A**. Polypharmacy in schizophrenia. *Curr Opin Psychiatry* 2010; **23**(2):103–11.

35 **Gallego JA, Bonetti J, Zhang J, Kane JM, Correll CU**. Prevalence and correlates of antipsychotic polypharmacy: a systematic review and meta-regression of global and regional trends from the 1970s to 2009. *Schizophr Res* 2012; **138**(1):18–28.

36 **Goodwin G, Fleischhacker W, Arango C, et al**. Advantages and disadvantages of combination treatment with antipsychotics. ECNP Consensus Meeting, March 2008, Nice. *Eur Neuropsychopharmacol* 2009; **19**(7):520–32.

37 **Andreasen NC, Liu D, Ziebell S, Vora A, Ho BC**. Relapse duration, treatment intensity, and brain tissue loss in schizophrenia: a prospective longitudinal MRI study. *Am J Psychiatry* 2013; 1; **170**(6):609–15. Erratum in: *Am J Psychiatry* 2013; 1; 170(6):689.

38 **Emsley R, Chiliza B, Asmal L, Harvey BH**. The nature of relapse in schizophrenia. *BMC Psychiatr* 2013; **13**:50.

39 **Velligan DI, Weiden PJ, Sajatovic M, et al**. The expert consensus guideline series: adherence problems in patients with serious and persistent mental illness. *J Clin Psychiatry* 2009; **70**(Suppl 4):1–46.

40 **Drake RJ**. Insight into illness: impact on diagnosis and outcome of non-affective psychosis. *Curr Psychiatry Rep* 2008; (3)**10**:210–216.

41 **Leucht C, Heres S, Kane JM, Kissling W, Davis JM, Leucht S**. Oral versus depot antipsychotic drugs for schizophrenia—a critical systematic review and meta-analysis of randomised long-term trials. *Schizophr Res* 2011; **127**(1–3):83–92.

42 **Fusar-Poli P, Smieskova R, Kempton MJ, Ho BC, Andreasen NC, Borgwardt S**. Progressive brain changes in schizophrenia related to antipsychotic treatment? A meta-analysis of longitudinal MRI studies. *Neurosci Biobehav Rev* 2013; **37**(8):1680–91.

43 WHO. Technical Report No 498: International Drug Monitoring, The Role of National Centres. Geneva: The Institute; 1972.

44 **Simpson GM, Angus JW**. A rating scale for extrapyramidal side effects. *Acta Psychiatr Scand Suppl* 1970; **212**():11–9.

45 **Sadock BJ, Sadock V A**. *Kaplan and Sadock's synopsis of psychiatry: behavioral sciences/clinical psychiatry* (9th edn). Philadelphia: Lippincott Williams and Wilkins; 2003.

46 **De Hert M, Cohen D, Bobes J, et al**. Physical illness in patients with severe mental disorders. II. Barriers to care, monitoring and treatment guidelines, plus recommendations at the system and individual level. *World Psychiat* 2011; **10**(2):138–51.

47 **Jakovljevic M**. The placebo-nocebo response: controversies and challenges from clinical and research perspective. *Eur Neuropsychopharmacol* 2014; **24**(3):333–41.

48 **Rutherford BR, Roose SP**. A model of placebo response in antidepressant clinical trials. *Am J Psychiatry* 2013; **170**(7):723–33.

49 **Verhulst J, Kramer D, Swann AC, Hale-Richlen B, Beahrs J**. The medical alliance: from placebo response to alliance effect. *J Nerv Ment Dis* 2013; **201**(7):546–52.

Chapter 25

Dealing with aggressive and violent behaviours in psychiatric settings

Mario Luciano, Julian Beezhold, Nagendra Bendi, and Dinesh Bhugra

Case study

On an intensive care unit, Sam had been admitted under a compulsory treatment order. This was her sixth admission in five years, and she was really fed up and irritated by repeated admissions that took her away from her family. She tried to be compliant but another patient, who she knew well, had been shouting at her. Eventually, Sam lashed out and hit the patient. When trying to control her, two members of staff were also injured. The doctor tried to negotiate with her, frequently inviting her to talk about the reasons for her behaviour, but Sam continued to shout at him, several times trying to hit him. The doctor proposed to Sam that she should take a benzodiazepine, but she refused. Therefore, intramuscular administration was provided. Sam was continuously monitored by nurses until the sedative effects of the benzodiazepine ended. At this stage, the doctor tried to explain to Sam what had happened and to identify reasons for her behaviour.

Introduction

Although aggressive behaviours are easy to recognize, defining them may be more difficult. The difficulties lie in distinguishing between 'acceptable' aggressive behaviours which can occur when individuals are angry or frustrated, and violence, that can be defined, according to WHO, as 'the intentional use of physical force or power, threatened or actual, against oneself, another person, or against a group or community, that either results in or has a high likelihood of resulting in injury, death, psychological harm or deprivation'.[1] To understand this phenomenon, a clear distinction needs to be made between *natural* or *positive aggression*, which is aimed largely at self-defence, combating prejudices, or social injustice, and *pathological aggression*, which results when an individual's inner nature has become twisted or frustrated.

Epidemiological data

Violence risk prediction is a priority issue for mental health professionals working in psychiatric settings. Despite recent advances, actual risk assessment studies have, as yet, yielded neither accurate nor practical violence risk predictions. However, several studies have shown that aggressive episodes occur relatively frequently in inpatient psychiatric units and are associated with specific socio-demographic and clinical characteristics. Young age, unmarried status, unemployment, and low socio-economic status can be considered as more reliable socio-demographic predictors of aggressiveness; while gender has not consistently been found to represent a significant risk factor (although aggressive behaviours by males are more frequently reported).[2]

Until the early 1980s, it was believed that there was no essential difference in the incidence of aggressive behaviours between people affected by major mental health problems and the general population. Recent evidence does not confirm this, with data highlighting that people with mental disorders have a relative risk for violent acts that is two to five times higher than that of the general population. Approximately 10% of psychiatric patients, at admission, present with an episode of aggressiveness, and approximately 22.5% of them, have at least one episode of aggressiveness in their lifetime. In addition, about 40% of mental health professionals have been victim of an aggressive episode at least once in their professional life, and more than 50% of psychiatric trainees have to deal with aggressive behaviours.[3]

Violence committed by psychiatric patients represents an important and challenging problem in clinical practice, since violent behaviours may negatively influence treatment, staff dynamics, and relationships among patients. Some studies have highlighted an increase in the number of episodes of aggression in psychiatric settings over the last few decades, which may be explained by the increasing awareness and perception of violence among staff, changes in staff attitude and in psychiatry practice, a greater incidence of violence in society as a whole, and higher prevalence of drug- and alcohol-related disorders (that are more often associated with aggressive behaviours).[3]

Predictors of violent behaviours

There are various factors at play in the determination of violent and aggressive behaviours. These can be classified as patient-related factors (which will include illness diagnosis and personality aspects), environmental factors, and staff dynamics (Box 25.1). Patient- and setting-related factors have been classically considered the best predictors for aggressive behaviour. While, in the past, a strong association between violence and schizophrenia or personality disorders was overemphasized, the most recent literature suggests that a specific diagnosis in itself does not constitute a risk factor for violence. Rather, some specific symptomatological dimensions (such as thought disturbances, delusions, and hallucinations) have been consistently associated with violence among psychiatric patients. Among clinical-related variables, a previous history of violence or of detention, a higher number of previous compulsory hospitalizations, drug or alcohol abuse, and the presence of abuse in childhood seem to have a significant predictive value for violent behaviours.[4]

Some staff features and ward characteristics have also been found to be related to patients' violent acts. Aggressive behaviours have been reported to be more frequent in wards located in urban areas and in those that are overcrowded or have fewer beds. This can be explained by the fact that urban mental healthcare centres have often to face more severe social and clinical problems, such as drug abuse, homelessness, and poor social networks.[4]

Box 25.1 Most frequent risk factors for violent behaviours among psychiatric patients

Socio-demographic characteristics

- Male gender
- Younger age
- Being homeless
- Low socio-economic status
- Low educational level
- Personal history of abuse, impulsiveness, and crimes
- Living in aggressive families
- Hyperactivity
- Poor social skills

Clinical characteristics

- Mental retardation
- Delirium
- Cerebral damage
- Paranoid delusions
- Hallucinations
- Substance or alcohol abuse
- Personality traits associated with violence

Biological factors

- Low expression of gene for monoamino-ossidasi
- Low expression of gene for serotonin transporter
- Intrauterine exposure to cigarette smoke, alcohol, or substances

Ward- and staff-related characteristics

- Urban hospitals/services
- Locked-door ward
- Lower number of junior doctors
- Higher number of nurses in the team

Table 25.1 Psychiatric disorders most commonly associated with violent behaviours

Psychotic disorders	Violent behaviours are often the direct consequence of hallucinations or delusions, especially when illness insight is low or absent. However, spontaneous or random assault is often uncommon among patients with psychoses. Aggressive behaviours are more frequent among young males with a past history of violence and impulsivity and with poor adherence to pharmacological treatment.
Bipolar disorders	Aggressive behaviours are common within manic episodes, and mainly related to the irritable mood, especially when the patients' wishes are denied and in cases of co-morbid addictions.
Borderline personality disorder	In these patient populations, violent acts are often linked with difficulties to manage emotional instability, with the instability of social relationships, with dysphoria and chronic feeling of emptiness. Violent acts are more frequently directed toward the patients themselves.
Anxiety disorders	Aggression and agitation are associated with the feelings of the presence of an external danger and with lower self-esteem. Aggressive behaviours can occur more frequently in panic disorder, obsessive compulsive disorder, and post-traumatic stress disorder.

Violent behaviours and mental disorders

It must be noted that aggressive behaviour does not represent a disease entity, disorder, or syndrome in itself, but according to the current International Classification Systems (DSM-V and ICD-10), it is considered a 'symptom' commonly associated with many clinical conditions including alcohol and drug abuse, impulse control and conduct disorders, personality disorders, and psychotic and affective disorders (Table 25.1). While aggressive and violent behaviours cannot be considered a clinical entity, they may represent the inappropriate expression of a disease when they are not controlled by those who manifest them and when they interfere with patients' relationships.[5]

Violent behaviours and physical disorders

Several physical conditions can be associated with aggressive behaviours. The psychiatrist needs to be adequately trained in the detection and management of physical conditions most frequently reported to be associated with aggressive behaviours (Box 25.2). Co-morbid physical conditions can contribute to irritability and aggressive behaviour, especially if both the patient and the staff are unable to recognize underlying physical problems.[6]

Box 25.2 Physical conditions most frequently associated with aggressive behaviours

- Sepsis
- Brain ischaemia
- Metabolic imbalances
- Dementia
- Epilepsy
- Encephalitis
- Intellectual disabilities
- Brain cancers
- Parkinson's disease

Table 25.2 Early risk signs for violent behaviours

Physical changes	Behavioural changes
•Clenched teeth and jaws •Shaking •Muscle tension •Clenched fists •Rapid breathing •Staring eyes •Restlessness •Extreme paleness of face •Sweating/perspiring	•Loud speech or shouting •Pointing with the finger •Verbal abuse •Over-sensitivity to what is said •Standing too close •Aggressive posture •Problems with concentration •Stamping feet

Early warning signs of aggressive behaviours

Usually, aggressiveness is easy to detect from one's actions, words, and/or expressions. It is important that anyone who has to deal with these situations knows how to respond to the aggressive behaviour, avoiding both an aggressive response and reinforcement of patients' violent behaviours. It is essential to watch for, and detect, signals that are usually associated with an escalation of aggressiveness. Extreme signals of aggression might indicate that an individual is becoming increasingly agitated, suggesting a real risk of developing aggressive behaviours[7] (Table 25.2).

Recognition of aggressive behaviours

The recognition and management of aggressive behaviours requires adequate skills (Table 25.3), since they represent psychiatric emergencies, and should be resolved as quickly as possible. For these reasons, mental health professionals need to have a clear picture about what to do and how to co-ordinate the team.

Table 25.3 General rules for the recognition and management of aggressive behaviours

First ask yourself . . .	◆ What determined the violent behaviours?
	◆ Has the patient presented with aggressive episodes in the past?
	◆ How does the patient manage the stress and what resources does he/she have to cope with it—on and off the ward?
	◆ Does the patient have any dangerous objects with him/her?
	◆ Is the patient aware of what is happening and what they are doing?
	◆ What is the diagnosis?
Priorities to be addressed	◆ Collect as much information as possible (all available sources of information must be taken into account, such as the patient, relatives, clinical records).
	◆ Carry out a rapid medical screening to identify any possible physical causes for aggressive behaviours.
	◆ Collect all information about triggers and the circumstances that determined the violent act.
	◆ Carefully assess the psychopathological status to reach a diagnosis and to assess all the possible risks to the patient's safety and to evaluate available social support and possible useful resources to overcome the crisis.
Take care of ward organization	◆ Ensure that all members of staff who work in mental health settings receive adequate training. (This should include interpersonal skills, aggression management, and personal safety issues, with special emphasis on prevention and assessment of risks.)
	◆ Wards should be equipped with special rooms for interviewing patients that ensure privacy, while avoiding isolation of the staff.
	◆ Security guards trained in principles of human behaviour and aggression must be provided in all emergency rooms. (Their presence often reduces threatening or aggressive behaviours by patients, relatives, friends, or those seeking drugs.)

Phases of aggressive behaviours

Experts in the field typically see an episode of violence as a sequence of five steps: trigger; escalation; crisis; recovery; and post-explosion depression—the so-called 'aggression cycle'. Although this represents a clear, well-known model of violent behaviour, it has to be pointed out that the intensity, frequency, and duration of each phase in the aggression cycle may significantly vary among individuals. For example, one person's anger may escalate rapidly after a provocative event and, in a few minutes, reach the 'crisis phase'; while another person's anger may escalate slowly but steadily for several hours, before reaching the crisis; and one person may experience more episodes of anger and progress through the aggression cycle more often than another. However, all individuals, despite differences in how quickly their anger escalates and how frequently they experience anger, will undergo all five phases of the aggression cycle (Fig. 25.1).[8]

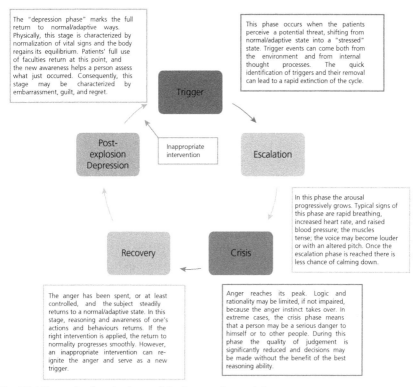

The "depression phase" marks the full return to normal/adaptive ways. Physically, this stage is characterized by normalization of vital signs and the body regains its equilibrium. Patients' full use of faculties return at this point, and the new awareness helps a person assess what just occurred. Consequently, this stage may be characterized by embarrassment, guilt, and regret.

This phase occurs when the patients perceive a potential threat, shifting from normal/adaptive state into a "stressed" state. Trigger events can come both from the environment and from internal thought processes. The quick identification of triggers and their removal can lead to a rapid extinction of the cycle.

Trigger

Post-explosion Depression

Inappropriate intervention

Escalation

Recovery

Crisis

In this phase the arousal progressively grows. Typical signs of this phase are rapid breathing, increased heart rate, and raised blood pressure; the muscles tense; the voice may become louder or with an altered pitch. Once the escalation phase is reached there is less chance of calming down.

The anger has been spent, or at least controlled, and the subject steadily returns to a normal/adaptive state. In this stage, reasoning and awareness of one's actions and behaviours returns. If the right intervention is applied, the return to normality progresses smoothly. However, an inappropriate intervention can re-ignite the anger and serve as a new trigger.

Anger reaches its peak. Logic and rationality may be limited, if not impaired, because the anger instinct takes over. In extreme cases, the crisis phase means that a person may be a serious danger to himself or to other people. During this phase the quality of judgement is significantly reduced and decisions may be made without the benefit of the best reasoning ability.

Fig. 25.1 Features of each phase of the 'aggression cycle'.

Assessment of violent behaviours

Personal history

♦ Investigate the presence of previous violent behaviours, contacts with the police, and the consequences of these behaviours in terms of health measures and legal services; consider all of the previous aggressive behaviours that did not require the intervention of public safety.

♦ Consider exposure to violence both as a victim and as a witness: the victims of abuse are, in turn, more frequently at risk of perpetrating abuse to others.

♦ Collect a detailed psychiatric history, including diagnoses received in the past, previous voluntary or involuntary hospitalizations, response to treatments, level of awareness of symptoms, reasons for failure of outpatient treatment, presence of sexual psychopathologies.

Circumstances

♦ Analyse the environmental components that contributed to the aggressive behaviour. Assess the quality of social relations; the patient's ability to establish social relationships; their level of dissatisfaction with lifestyle, work, and social relations. Try to determine if the patients have contact with groups at higher risk for violent behaviours.

 ◆ Try to determine if the aggressive behaviours were accidental or premeditated.

 ◆ Investigate the relationship between the patient and victim: if the victim was a relative, investigate their previous relationship.

Mental state

 ◆ Evaluate the possible presence of delusions, and if they are accompanied by fear and anxiety; do not underestimate the threats of the patient as well as his or her violent fantasies.

 ◆ Investigate the level of awareness of symptoms and the willingness to accept the proposed treatments.

 ◆ Inquire after the characteristics of the patient's personality, as well as his or her personal resources that can reduce the risk of further violent behaviours.

Environmental factors and aggressive behaviours

 ◆ Environmental factors are believed to be important determinants of disturbed/violent behaviours in psychiatric inpatient settings. A therapeutic environment is one that allows individuals to enjoy safety and security, privacy, dignity, choice and independence, without compromising the clinical objectives of the service. Comfort, noise control, light, colour, and space will all have an impact on the well-being of both staff and service users.

 ◆ The design of facilities should ensure uncrowded conditions for staff and patients. Rooms for privacy and protection, avoiding isolation, are needed; doors must be fitted with windows; security guards should be assigned to areas where there may be psychologically stressed patients (e.g. emergency rooms, psychiatric services); in crisis treatment areas and 'quiet rooms', furniture should be kept to a minimum and be fixed to the floor; and all potentially dangerous objects must be removed.

 ◆ Interview rooms for new patients or known aggressive patients should utilize a system which provides privacy but which may also permit other staff to see the patient's activity. In psychiatric units, 'time out' or seclusion rooms are usually needed. In emergency departments, agitated patients should be confined, safely, in dedicated rooms to protect themselves, other patients, and staff.

 ◆ Bright and effective lighting systems should be provided for all indoor building areas, grounds around the facility, and parking areas. A system for alerting security personnel when violence is threatened should be implemented in at-risk wards.

 ◆ Staff should not be alone with patients during examinations and an alarm system should be present in psychiatric units, mental health clinics, emergency rooms, or where drugs are stored. 'Panic buttons' are needed in medicine rooms, nurses' stations, stairwells, and activity rooms, as such preventive measures may reduce serious injury when a patient's aggressive or threatening behaviour (with or without a weapon) is escalating.

◆ Overcrowding in the emergency ward is considered a risk factor influencing the number of aggressive episodes. Bed occupancy should be decided at a local level and should not be exceeded, since overcrowding leads to tension, frustration, and overstretched staff.

◆ Mental health staff should be trained to manage aggressive behaviours. Staff should have the adequate skills needed to handle situations prone to violence (de-escalation and break-away techniques), to recognize potential sources of violence (verbal and non-verbal clues that the patient is stressed and may respond with violence or may not listen to directions or requests), and to deal with angry patients/residents/clients.

◆ Encourage staff members to take primary prevention steps to stop aggressive behaviours from escalating.

◆ Annual staff development sessions (refreshers) on techniques for managing violent behaviours should be provided.

Management of aggressive behaviours

The management of aggressive behaviours needs skilled mental health professionals who are able to establish a positive relationship with the patient, speaking in a calm and reassuring voice and trying to offer a way out of the situation (Table 25.4). The mental health professional should expressly refer to the person, calling him or her by name; use short sentences and simple terms; and be as less judgemental or aggressive as possible. It should be noted that when approaching a patient who is behaving aggressively, that patient will often become verbally aggressive. In this situation, it is important not to take the negative statements personally. In some cases, the use of time-out or other de-escalating techniques can be useful, while in others, the only possible intervention is the use of coercive measures such as pharmacological or physical restraint and seclusion.[9]

Treatment of aggressive behaviours

There is no one specific and effective treatment for aggressive behaviours. The intervention should consider the primary psychiatric disorder and should aim at removing causes that led to the aggressive behaviours. The intervention does not expire at the end of the crisis: engaging the patient in the post-explosion phase can be useful in further establishing a therapeutic alliance. Pharmacological and physical interventions, as well as seclusion, should be considered only in those cases where de-escalation and other strategies have failed[10] (Boxes 25.3–25.6 and Table 25.5).

In determining the interventions to apply, clinical needs, the safety of service users and others, and, where possible, advance directives should be taken into account. The selected intervention must be a reasonable and proportionate response to the risk

Table 25.4 How to manage an aggressive episode

Things to do	◆ Keep your own emotions under control. Stay calm and be genuine in your attempts to hear patients' issues.
	◆ Watch your body language; be aware whether your posture and gestures contradict what you are saying.
	◆ Align yourself with the person by focusing on a common goal.
	◆ Conflict avoidance skills include giving concessions to the patient, trying to engage them, giving choices on how to end the confrontation, and finding a joint solution.
	◆ Accompany the patient to a quiet, less stimulating room. Isolate the individual by getting him/her away from on-lookers who may encourage or incite the potential aggressor.
	◆ Embrace silence at times as an effective intervention that allows the individual to clarify their thoughts and restate the message.
	◆ Let the patient express grievances, but respond selectively. Clear up misconceptions and acknowledge valid complaints.
	◆ Set limits calmly but firmly.
	◆ Know your limitations and call for backup (panic button, silent alarm, or 'code white' message).
	◆ Try to explain to the patient that he/she is responsible for the behaviour, that it will be noted in their clinical records, and that it could have legal consequences. Make the patient realize that other people are frightened by their behaviour.
Things to avoid	◆ Do not let the patient get between you and the door. Never turn your back on him/her.
	◆ Make sure you have an escape route if the situation escalates.
	◆ Do not crowd the patient's space or try to make physical contact. Keep a distance of 1–2 metres from the potential aggressor. Calm, slow, deliberate movements signal to the angry person that the mental health professional is not going to harm him/her.
	◆ Do not try to talk when he/she is shouting. When you have the chance to say something. speak in a normal tone of voice. Check your paraverbal signs (tone, volume, rate, and rhythm of your speech) to ensure clarity by not contradicting the content of your words.
	◆ Do not argue or become defensive, confrontational, or judgemental. Use reflective questioning. Put the individual's statement in your own words and check with him/her to see if you have understood what he/she meant. Use open-ended sentences that provide openings for the disturbed person to verbalize feelings.
	◆ Do not react to any abusive statements. Communicate in simple sentences while showing your concern and offering realistic solutions (if appropriate).
	◆ Do not try to disarm the patient. If he/she has weapons (guns, knives, or other objects that could be used to injure), get away and call the police.
	◆ Do not show fear, anger, or anxiety: the patient may become even more violent and agitated.

Box 25.3 Benzodiazepines

◆ Frequently used as first-line treatments, to obtain rapid tranquillization of the patient. Their use in high doses or in combination with other hypno-sedatives (including alcohol and some illicit drugs) can increase the risk of respiratory depression.

◆ Benzodiazepines should be preferred when comprehensive information on the patient's clinical condition is not available.

◆ Among benzodiazepines, lorazepam has complete and rapid intramuscular absorption, and a shorter elimination half-life than many other benzodiazepines, which limits the risk of excessive sedation due to the cumulative effects of the drug; moreover, lorazepam has few interactions with other drugs and its metabolism does not require involvement of the cytocrome P450 system. For this reason, it represents the first choice for rapid tranquillization.

◆ The use of other benzodiazepines is complicated by their irregular intramuscular absorption rates and by the fact that they generate active metabolites that have a long half-life.

◆ Specific adverse effects contraindicating the use of benzodiazepines include loss of consciousness, respiratory depression or arrest, and cardiovascular collapse (in patients receiving both clozapine and benzodiazepines).

Box 25.4 Typical antipsychotics

◆ Haloperidol is one of the most frequently used antipsychotics and many authors suggest that this agent should be considered the first choice in the treatment of agitated patients. It can be administered orally, IM, or IV. When administered IM or IV, haloperidol has an onset of action within 30–60 minutes and a duration of effect of up to 24 hours.

◆ Important adverse effects associated with typical antipsychotics are: loss of consciousness, cardiovascular and respiratory complications and collapse, seizures, subjective experience of restlessness (akathisia), acute muscular rigidity (dystonia), involuntary movements (dyskinesia), excessive sedation, and neuroleptic malignant syndrome.

◆ Extrapyramidal side-effects are of major concern since they can significantly impact on patients' physical symptoms, and also because of their potential in augmenting patients' distress and medication refusal.

Box 25.5 Atypical antipsychotics

- This class of medication represents an effective and safer alternative to typical antipsychotics in the management of aggressive behaviours. After the resolution of an acute episode, they can be easily administered orally, promoting ongoing treatment.
- Olanzapine, ziprasidone, and risperidone are the most frequently used atypical antipsychotics.
- Olanzapine and ziprasidone have a faster onset of action when administered IM or IV.
- Risperidone has proven efficacy in adolescents with conduct disorders.
- As also happens with typical antipsychotics, prolongation of the QTc can occur with the use of these agents; therefore, their use in patients with a known history of cardiovascular disease should be avoided.
- The use of olanzapine IM in combination with benzodiazepine IM must be avoided because of the cumulative risk of respiratory depression and excessive sedation.

Box 25.6 Physical interventions

- Physical intervention should be avoided if at all possible; it should not be used for prolonged periods and should be brought to an end at the earliest opportunity.
- To avoid prolonged physical intervention, an alternative strategy, such as rapid tranquillization or seclusion (where available), should be considered.
- The use of coercive measures should be always performed by a team of professionals (comprising at least five members) and never by a single worker. During physical intervention, under no circumstances should direct pressure be applied to the neck, thorax, abdomen, back, or pelvic area.
- The overall physical and psychological well-being of the patient should be continuously monitored throughout the process.
- During physical intervention, one team member should be responsible for protecting and supporting the head and neck, where required; the team leader should take responsibility for leading the team through the physical intervention process and for ensuring that the airways and breathing are not affected and that vital signs are constantly monitored.
- The use of physical intervention should always be noted in the patient's clinical records.
- Seclusion should be for the shortest time possible and should be reviewed at least every two hours. The patient should be made aware of how frequently these reviews will take place.
- Patients in seclusion should be allowed to keep personal items, including those of religious or cultural significance, as long as they do not compromise their safety or the safety of others.

Table 25.5 Useful tips in the management of aggressive behaviours

Staff members should be given the greatest possible assistance in obtaining information to evaluate the history of, or potential for, violent behaviour in patients. They should be required to treat and/or interview aggressive or agitated clients in open areas where other staff may observe interactions but still provide privacy and confidentiality.	No employee should be allowed to work or stay alone in a facility or in an isolated unit. This is the case when the location is so solitude that they are unable to obtain assistance if needed, or in the evening or at night if the clinic is closed.
Referral systems and pathways to psychiatric facilities need to be properly developed to facilitate prompt and safe hospitalization of clients who demonstrate violent or suicidal behaviour. These methods may include: direct phone link to the local police, exchange of training and communication with local psychiatric services, and written guidelines outlining commitment procedures.	Staff should wear clothing which cannot be used to hit someone (such as low-heeled shoes, earrings, jewellery, or scarves).
Seclusion may be required to contain confused or aggressive clients. Although privacy may be needed both for the agitated patient and other patients, security and the ability to monitor the patient and staff is also required in any "quiet room".	All members of staff who work in mental health settings need to receive appropriate training in interpersonal skills, management of aggression, and personal safety. The training should be provided by experts; all members of staff should be provided with regular "refresher training" on these topics.

posed by the patient and to the effective resources available. Antipsychotics or ben-zodiazepines are often the drugs of choice for the treatment of aggressive behaviours. An oral therapy should be offered to the patient in order to maintain a therapeutic re-lationship. Intramuscular (IM) or intravenous (IV) formulations can be administered but only when there is a clear rejection of the treatment. If parenteral treatment proves necessary, the IM route should be preferred over IV for safety reasons. The patient should be transferred to oral routes of administration at the earliest opportunity.[11,12]

Conclusions

Although several papers and books have been published about management of ag-gressive behaviours, this topic still remains one of the most controversial issues in the mental health field. Clear predictive factors have not been identified and the major-ity of programmes to reduce the occurrence of aggressive behaviours have failed in their aims.

The management of patients' aggressive behaviours is even more cogent than in the past, since that their incidence and prevalence is continuously escalating due to the increasing of substance abuse disorders, changes in the organization of modern society, and as a consequence of the worldwide reduction in the number of hospital beds.

Key factors to properly managing the aggressive episodes are:

1) mental health professional related factors, such as skills in recognizing early warning signs for aggressive behaviours, knowledge of the main de-escalating techniques, and ability to work within a team;

2) environmental factors, such as the availability of separate rooms to manage aggressive episodes, of alarm systems, and of safety personnel in the wards;

3) policy factors, such as recognition of workplace violence risk and pledges to protect staff at work, details of managers' and employees' responsibilities and of the local prevention and reduction plans, and allocation of resources and appropriate authority to responsible parties[2] (Table 25.5).

On a research level, much has still to be done. The vast majority of research on this issue has come from Western countries, mainly Europe and the USA, and therefore a clear picture of what happens in low-income countries is still not available. Another important research gap relates to the ethical dilemma between the use of 'therapeutic' coercion for the treatment of aggressive behaviours and the loss of patients' dignity. Based on current knowledge, some suggestions have been provided for the implementation of involuntary treatments in clinical practice. Recommendations for good clinical practice in relation to involuntary hospital admission have been provided by the European Evaluation of Coercion in Psychiatry and Harmonization of Best Clinical Practice (EUNOMIA)NETWORK, an international study carried out in eleven European countries.[13,14] Larger international studies are needed to clarify how coercion is used in psychiatry in different contexts, how this practice can be improved, and, most importantly, if coercion is still necessary in psychiatry.

References

1 Krug GE, Dahlberg LL, Mercy JA, Zwi AB, Lozano R. *World report on violence and health.* Geneva: World Health Organization; 2002.

2 Luciano M, Sampogna G, Del Vecchio V, et al. Use of coercive measures in mental health practice and its impact on outcome: a critical review. *Expert Rev Neurother* 2014; **14**(2):131–41.

3 van Leeuwen ME, Harte JM. Violence against care workers in psychiatry: is prosecution justified? *Int J Law Psychiatry* 2011; **34**(5):317–23.

4 Husum TL, Bjørngaard JH, Finset A, Ruud T. A cross-sectional prospective study of seclusion, restraint and involuntary medication in acute psychiatric wards: patient, staff and ward characteristics. *BMC Health Serv Res* 2010; **6**:89.

5 Pacciardi B, Mauri M, Cargioli C, et al. Issues in the management of acute agitation: how much current guidelines consider safety? *Front Psychiatry* 2013; **7**(4):26.

6 Allen MH, Currier GW, Carpenter D, Ross RW, Docherty JP, Expert Consensus Panel for Behavioural Emergencies. The expert consensus guideline series. Treatment of behavioural emergencies. *J Psychiatr Pract* 2005; **11**(1):5–108.

7 Sethi D, Marais S, Seedat M, Nurse J, Butchart A. *Handbook for the documentation of interpersonal violence prevention programmes. Department of Injuries and Violence Prevention.* Geneva: World Health Organization; 2004.

8 **Powley D**. Reducing violence and aggression in the emergency department. *Emerg Nurse* 2013; **21**(4):26–9.

9 National Institute for Clinical Excellence. *Clinical practice guideline: 'Violence: the short-term management of disturbed/violent behaviour in psychiatric in-patient setting and emergency department'.* NICE; 2005.

10 World Health Organization. Mental health legislation and human rights (mental health policy and service guidance package). Geneva: World Health Organization; 2003.

11 **Marder SR**. A review of agitation in mental illness: treatment guidelines and current therapies. *J Clin Psychiatry* 2006; **67**(10):13–21.

12 **Topiwala A, Fazel S**. The pharmacological management of violence in schizophrenia: a structured review. *Exp Rev Neurother* 2011; **11**(1):53–63.

13 **Fiorillo A, Giacco D, De Rosa C, et al**. Patient characteristics and symptoms associated with perceived coercion during hospital treatment. *Acta Psychiatr Scand* 2012; **125**(6):460–7.

14 **Fiorillo A, De Rosa C, Del Vecchio V, et al**. How to improve clinical practice on involuntary hospital admissions of psychiatric patients: suggestions from the EUNOMIA study. Eur Psychiatry. 2011;**26**:201–7.

Chapter 26

Practical skills in old age psychiatry

Florian Riese, Cécile Hanon, Alexis Lepetit, and Linda Lam

Old age psychiatry in an ageing world

As a consequence of an ageing world population, the importance of old age psychiatry is steadily growing. More people are reaching the age of 65 (the age at which treatment in old age psychiatry begins in many countries) and life expectancy beyond 65 years is increasing. In internal medicine, geriatric patients already account for a large proportion of all patients. Psychiatry will likely follow this trend. Tomorrow's elderly will have lived in a culture where mental health problems are less stigmatized, and they may thus seek psychiatric treatment more frequently than did previous generations. Furthermore, there are often strong incentives that favour the expansion of old age psychiatric services: mental health problems such as cognitive decline or lack of energy contribute to an individual's loss of capacity for independent living and may make residential care necessary.

Interestingly, the 'silver tsunami' of increasing demand for old age services is not matched by an equal interest of physicians in the field.[1] Embracing old age psychiatry as a field of expertise therefore offers excellent career prospects. Even for psychiatrists who do not want to subspecialize in old age psychiatry, a sound knowledge in the field is essential, since exposure to the patient group is already high today and will only rise in the future.

Case study 1

A 77-year-old founder and chief executive officer of an engineering company is evaluated for participation as a healthy control subject in a research study on cognitive performance in the elderly. He claims not to be available for the next scheduled study visit, since he is going to be part of a climbing expedition to the Mount Everest Base Camp. A subsequent neuropsychological evaluation reveals deficits in several cognitive domains including complex attention and executive function. He is advised not to perform his climbing expedition but proceeds nonetheless.

The many facets of ageing and old age psychiatry

Case study 1 illustrates that the face of old age is moving away from how it was seen in the past. Consequently, the face of old age psychiatry is also changing. Today's old age patient spectrum reaches from high-functioning individuals who come for mental health check-ups to the multimorbid and terminally ill who need to be psychiatrically treated in medical high-tech environments such as intensive care units. Furthermore, practically every mental health issue that can be found in younger adults now has also to be specifically dealt with in the elderly. Due to the heterogeneity of its patient population, old age psychiatry has always emphasized an integrated and individually tailored model of health care.[2] Often, its treatment aim is the promotion of well-being and the stabilization of quality of life, which may require the use of preventive, curative, rehabilitative, and palliative measures. Old age psychiatrists therefore have to draw from a wider skill set than in the past, which includes the skills outlined within this chapter.

Building a relationship and communicating effectively

Case study 2

An 84-year-old woman is hospitalized for chronic disturbances of sleep and dependence on sleep medication. Upon admission, she is accompanied by her son and his wife, who organized the hospital stay and also provide most of the medical and psychiatric history. It is her first psychiatric admission. At the end of the intake interview, the patient's son and the psychiatrist shake hands and share their confidence in the success of the upcoming treatment. A nurse takes the patient to her room.

As in any other branch of medicine—especially when care for chronic conditions is required—the patient–doctor relationship is the key to successful treatment. In case study 2, a common mistake when dealing with elderly people is depicted: the main relationship is built with a family member, and not with the patient. Such behaviour is often driven by the apparent greater ease and efficacy of communication with a younger adult. However, it may also reflect implicit stereotypes about ageing, also referred to as

Table 26.1 DOs and DO NOTs when building a therapeutic alliance with an elderly patient

DO	DO NOT
Listen; be patient and leave the patient some time to respond; be genuinely interested in the person who sits in front of you.	Be condescending.
Know or research the historical context in which the patient has lived (war, migration, etc.)	Speak too quickly or softly.
Find a 'beacon of hope' (usually in the family) to promote recovery.	Be overly cautious when exploring suicidality.
Take time to explain both psychotherapeutic and pharmacological treatments.	Hesitate to ask questions about sexual dysfunction.
If pharmacological medication is prescribed, be very precise and careful with the name you use in order not to confuse the patient between generic and brand names.	Rush things—your patient has twice as many years of history to tell you than the average patient.

'ageism'.[3,4] Due to this, elderly people are often treated like children, who are unable to take decisions for themselves. Avoiding ageism requires listening to patients, following their treatment objectives, and, thereby, helping them to maintain autonomy and dignity (see Table 26.1). While a family's wishes for treatment may be justified and need to be taken into account, it is the patient who should lead whenever he or she has the capacity to do so. In addition, focusing on the caregiver burden and initiating measures to reduce it are often the way forward with the family.[5]

Formalized assessment of elderly patients

Case study 3

A 72-year-old woman is hospitalized in an old age psychiatric ward for treatment of persistent dysthymia. Two days after admission, the woman is found entertaining other patients and staff with stories from her time as a professional dancer on cruise ships. The patient visibly enjoys being the centre of attention. Further history taking reveals that the depressive symptoms started when osteoarthritis severely reduced the mobility of the patient. As a consequence, she had not been able to participate in her regular dance club.

The clues for what might be 'wrong' with an elderly patient are not always so clear as in case study 3 (i.e. physical impairment and lack of enjoyable social activities). Getting to know a patient takes time—usually more time than one has—but it is absolutely essential for devising a treatment plan. Therefore, it is recommended that formalized assessments of the most important psychiatric, general medical, and social health needs of the elderly are made[6] (see Table 26.2); the individual instruments used in different domains vary greatly among centres, with availability often dependent on language restrictions.

Using standardized assessment tools frees up time by not having to 'reinvent the wheel' for each assessment. Comprehensive geriatric assessments will also prevent you from overlooking important aspects of disease—like the impact of osteoarthritis in case study 3 or missing out on a hypoactive delirium. Finally, formalized assessment instruments can often be used to monitor the effect of therapeutic interventions, which is necessary for good psychiatric practice. Elderly patients who have undergone a comprehensive geriatric assessment also tend to achieve better treatment outcomes.[7]

From deficits to health priorities: devising a treatment plan

The greatest limitation of most currently available assessment tools is their focus on deficits, rather than on individual health needs. The assessment of a patient's needs and priorities should remain the main focus of an accurate evaluation and the time saved by using standardized instruments for assessment of deficits should be dedicated to such issues. For example, the patient in case study 3 might prioritize improving physical mobility over learning how to deal with depressive thinking. Consequently, physical

Table 26.2 Suggested domains, key questions, and standardized instruments for a comprehensive assessment in old age psychiatry

Domains	Key questions	Standardized instruments
Functional capacity	How well does the patient perform in daily life tasks? Does she/he need specific training, technical aids, or assistance?	- Katz Index of Independence in Activities of Daily Living - Lawton Instrumental Activities of Daily Living Scale
Fall risk/mobility	How high is the risk of falls in the patient? Is there need for motor training or walking aids?	- Timed Up and Go Test - Tinetti Test
Cognition/delirium	What is the cognitive status of the patient? How does that impact her/his functioning in daily life? Can workarounds be established (e.g. shopping lists)?	- Mini Mental State Examination - Montreal Cognitive Assessment - Confusion Assessment Method
Mood	Does the patient have symptoms of depression, grief, anxiety, or mania?	- Geriatric Depression Scale - Cornell Scale for Depression in Dementia
Medication/polypharmacy	Does the patient take unnecessary or inappropriate medications? Is she/he at risk for drug interactions?	- Check medications against Beers' list - Digital drug interaction databases
General medical health	Are all the physical conditions (e.g. kidney dysfunction, chronic heart disease) sufficiently managed? When has the female patient last seen a gynaecologist?	- Physical examination
Pain	Is the patient in pain?	- Visual Analogue Scale
Nutrition	Is the patient malnourished? How are meals organized? What kinds of food does she/he like?	- Mini Nutritional Assessment - Nutritional Health Checklist
Dentition	Does the patient have dental problems that cause nutritional problems or pain?	- Dental Screening Survey
Urinary incontinence	How are bladder and bowel function of the patient? Does she/he receive adequate treatment for incontinence (if necessary)?	- York Incontinence Perceptions Scale
Sensory function	Is the patient's hearing or vision impaired? Does she/he require technical aids? Is food still tasteful for her/him?	- Snellen Chart (for visual acuity) - Whisper Test - Hearing Handicap Inventory for the Elderly

(continued)

Table 26.2 (continued) Suggested domains, key questions, and standardized instruments for a comprehensive geriatric assessment in old age psychiatry

Domains	Key questions	Standardized instruments
Sexual function	Is the patient's sexual health impaired?	
Living situation	What are the living arrangements of the patient? Is there a lift in the building? How does the patient do the shopping?	
Social support	Who is part of the patient's social network? Who is aware of the patient's condition? Who can be involved in supporting the patient? Is there evidence for abuse or neglect?	
Financial matters	What is the financial situation of the patient? Is she/he entitled to social security? Will the patient be able to afford care in the future?	
Goals of care	What does the patient want from you as a psychiatrist (and from the treatment team)? What are her/his biggest problems and healthcare priorities? Does the current treatment plan follow the patient's priorities?	
Spirituality	Are the patient's spiritual needs addressed?	
Advance care preferences	Does the patient have an advance care directive? Is its contents known to family members and healthcare providers?	

therapy may be the immediate way forward. Even small improvements in physical mobility may vastly improve the patient's sense of self-efficacy and self-confidence, which will help in treatment for depression.

When devising a shared treatment plan, based on a patient's needs and priorities, one should make sure to set realistic, measurable goals and adequately communicate them to the patients and their carers. On the other hand, one should make sure that the 'big picture' is not lost among the tiny steps that are required on the way. Often, treatment planning requires you to 'think outside the box' of purely pharmaceutical treatment guidelines. However, do not mistake 'individualizing' a treatment plan for disregarding scientific evidence. Instead, a personalized approach means making the available evidence useful for patient decisions. This requires knowledge of the scientific literature and the ability to communicate it to the patient. For several conditions, there are now evidence-based decision aids that support the process of shared decision making.[8] The rewards are high—to eventually see a creative, tailor-made treatment plan working and helping a patient to get better is one of the most gratifying experiences a psychiatrist can have.

Choosing the right treatment setting and ensuring continuity of care

As mentioned in the beginning of this chapter, the patient population in old age psychiatry is highly heterogeneous. This translates not only into the need for individualized treatment plans but also individualized delivery of care ('patient-centred' or 'person-centred' care). For every patient, the psychiatrist should continuously reflect if the current therapy setting is adequate. Outpatient treatment often does not guarantee sufficient intensity of care, and it is difficult to install multiprofessional treatment teams and multicomponent interventions in this setting. On the other hand, inpatient treatment can facilitate the loss of self-care since many daily-life needs (e.g. regular meals) are simply taken over by institutional routines.

Ideally, patients should be treated within a flexible network of collaborating or integrated psychiatric services. Important components of such a network are outpatient clinics, inpatient facilities, day-care clinics, consultation/liaison services, and outreach teams. Access to psychotherapy should be possible throughout the network. Joint geriatric and psychiatric wards are rare but can be extremely helpful, for example when dealing with delirium.[9] On such joint wards, medical tasks can be distributed between geriatricians and psychiatrists (e.g. physical conditions and rehabilitation needs can be addressed by the geriatric specialist; see Fig. 26.1). Joint wards also facilitate access to certain diagnostic tools (e.g. echocardiography or abdominal ultrasound). In contrast, old age psychiatry should not be predominantly performed in so-called 'ageless wards', since the complex needs of elderly patients can best be addressed in specialized old age services.[10]

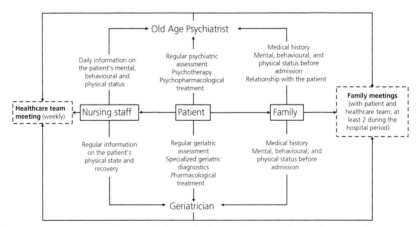

Fig. 26.1 Organization of care and flow of information on a joint geriatric/psychiatric ward. (In order to reduce the complexity of the figure, important care provider groups such as psychologists and physical therapists have not been depicted.)

Case study 4

A 64-year-old man is brought to an emergency department by the police who have found him sleeping in the streets, disoriented to time and place. Physical examination reveals multiple infected skin wounds, most prominently at the stump of the right leg, where a below-knee amputation has been performed in the past. The fit of the patient's prosthesis is inadequate, which he has remedied by applying some (now dirty) cotton pads. An X-ray examination indicates osteomyelitis on the ankle of the left foot. The patient insists on leaving the hospital immediately in order to 'report back to work as security guard in the airport'. Based on the presentation and previous medical records, a preliminary diagnosis of Wernicke's encephalopathy is made. The patient is involuntarily admitted to an old age psychiatry ward. Over the course of several weeks, the physical condition of the patient markedly improves, while the severe cognitive deficits remain unchanged. The patient is discharged to a residential care facility. Four days later, he does not return there from a walk in the afternoon.

Follow-up and continuity of care in old age psychiatry are sometimes taken for granted—especially when patients are transferred to residential care. As case study 4 illustrates, this is not always the case. Instead, reflection on the right treatment setting must continue beyond the period of immediate responsibility as the treating psychiatrist. Continuity of care can be facilitated by providing concise and relevant information on the treatment course and suggestions for the future care to the next care provider. Ideally, the psychiatrist remains available for consultation beyond discharge and active outreach is established to former patients. Integrated old age psychiatric services that provide inpatient, outpatient, consultation/liaison services, and community outreach are well suited to improve continuity of care. In case study 4, pre-scheduled follow-up phone calls or a liaison session in the residential care facility may have helped to avoid the patient's drop-out from care.

Liaising with other medical specialties and non-medical professionals

Ensuring continuity of care and addressing the varied health needs of elderly people often requires co-operation of the psychiatrist with other medical or non-medical professions. Even though such co-operation may sometimes appear time-consuming, it allows the mobilization of additional resources for the benefit of your patient. For example, referring to case study 4, the treating old age psychiatrist closely collaborated with an orthopaedic surgeon and an orthopaedic technician to improve the fit of the patient's prosthesis. On many occasions, it is the mental health conditions that determine the range of available treatment options (e.g. by limiting the patient's capacity to consent or to adhere to a treatment). Therefore, psychiatrists often have a key role in planning multidisciplinary care and might be uniquely qualified for the co-ordination of such care (see Box 26.1). As they are used to working in teams (often in a role as team supervisor), psychiatrists should have excellent communication skills and should feel at home both in the realms of psychological health and medical treatment. Therefore, instead of feeling threatened or burdened by today's reality of multidisciplinary care, it is better to embrace and even actively promote it. Taking over responsibility in a multidisciplinary care team will help psychiatrists to gain respect from other health professionals.

Box 26.1 Core competencies of interdisciplinary team members

1 Understanding their respective roles and responsibilities within the team

2 Establishing common goals for the team

3 Agreeing on rules for conducting team meetings

4 Communicating well with other members of the team

5 Identifying and resolving conflict

6 Shared decision making and executing defined tasks when consensus is reached

7 Providing support for one another, including the development of leadership roles

8 Being flexible in response to changing circumstances

9 Participating in periodic team performance reviews to ensure that the team is functioning well and that its goals are being met

Source data from: Partnership for Health in Aging Workgroup on Interdisciplinary Team Training, Position Statement on Interdisciplinary Team Training in Geriatrics: an Essential Component of Quality Healthcare for Older Adults, pp. 1–12. Copyright (2011) American Geriatric Society.

Multimorbidity and pharmacotherapy

Case study 5

A 79-year-old woman with chronic obstructive pulmonary disease, type 2 diabetes, osteoporosis, osteoarthritis, and hypertension is being treated according to the current clinical practice guidelines; thus, she needs to take 12 different medications, fractioned in 19 doses, at 5 different times during the day. Furthermore, she needs to adhere to 14 non-pharmacological recommendations—ranging from inspections of her feet to annual influenza vaccination.[11]

Case study 5 is an example of the complexity of treatment that arises from multimorbidity. Currently, most clinical guidelines focus on single diseases and fall short of providing guidance on how to prioritize treatments in the case of multiple co-morbidities. In this context, it often helps to refer to the patient's goals of care to reduce complexity. In cases of multimorbidity, getting a geriatric medicine consultation is also recommended if treatment in a joint old age psychiatry/geriatric ward or in a multidisciplinary team is not possible.

As a consequence of multimorbidity, polypharmacy may ensue. However, in pharmacotherapy for the elderly, often 'less is more'. Therefore, initiating pharmacotherapy in the elderly starts by critically reviewing the current medication. Algorithm-based medication reviews are effective in reducing inappropriate prescribing and medication-related problems.[12,13] Potentially inappropriate medications for elderly patients can be found in the Beers' list that every old age psychiatrist should be familiar with.[14] Medications may exert adverse effects for a variety of reasons, such as their anticholinergic potential, induction of orthostatic hypotension, or simply their lack of therapeutic benefit (e.g. primary preventive treatments in the very old).

After all unnecessary medications have been discontinued and the doses of all essential medications have been reviewed, the potential for drug–drug interactions must be evaluated for the remaining ones. Finally, when initiating a new pharmacological therapy in an elderly patient, 'start low and go slow'. Due to the changes in pharmacodynamics and pharmacokinetics, many medications behave differently than in younger patients. However, when necessary, do not forget to 'go far' in your treatment: a medication that is insufficiently dosed for fear of side-effects is useless (or even harmful).

Treating depression in the elderly

Case study 6

A 73-year-old woman is admitted to a psychiatric ward because she cannot cope with the recent diagnosis of advanced cancer in her husband. Her husband dies shortly after her admission. The woman blames herself for not being with her husband, 'when he needed me most'. She feels unable to resume her previous life and continuously asks the treating early career psychiatrist 'Please, doctor, help me: I want to die.'

Depressive states are common among the elderly. However, due to their atypical, often misleading symptomatology, the exact prevalence is difficult to determine, for many possible reasons (see Box 26.2). Still, from 2% to 5% of community-dwelling persons aged above 65 years suffer from depression, and the figure seems to be even substantially higher in long-term care facilities.[15] Furthermore, only a minority of depressed patients receive antidepressant treatment. Old age is an important risk factor for completed suicide.[16] So, in every depressed elderly patient, suicidality should be properly addressed and its treatment made the highest priority.

Another, often overlooked, form of self-harm in the elderly is self-neglect. It may manifest as insufficient food and fluid intake, neglecting personal hygiene, and insufficient use of medical or nursing care. The driving factors behind self-neglect are diverse (e.g. depression, cognitive impairment, social isolation, medical disease), but the condition is independently associated with increased mortality.[17,18] Like suicide, self-neglect is not to be simply considered an autonomous choice of a patient or 'his or her way of life', since it causes suffering and reduces quality of life. It should be considered a

Box 26.2 Characteristics of depression in old age

Compared to that of a young adult, depression in old age:

- is often associated with medical co-morbidity and polypharmacy
- often presents with physical symptoms (especially chronic pain)
- has a more chronic course
- is often more difficult to treat
- is often perceived as more 'normal'
- is easier to overlook.

possible symptom of severe depression—a potentially treatable condition. Self-neglect should therefore be recognized and discussed with the patient. When necessary, adult protective services (or similar institutions) must then be involved.

Notably, not every depressive syndrome in the elderly is caused by major depression: depressive symptoms may occur in the context of a cerebrovascular disease ('vascular depression') or as prodromal states of a dementia or as a consequence of medical diseases (e.g. hypothyroidism, sleep apnoea).

A very helpful conceptual model when planning treatment with a patient is the 'cycle of depression'.[15] Many patients (and also many medical professionals) perceive depression as a black block of rock that has come down on them. Splitting depression up into its components and showing the interdependence of such components may help in making it more manageable. When such a model is applied to the situation of the individual patient, it can also show the possible starting points for therapy, so that the cycle of depression can be turned around.

As in younger patients, the mainstays of treatment for depression in old age are pharmacotherapy and psychotherapy (see the following section). Among the pharmacological agents, selective serotonin reuptake inhibitors (SSRIs) (primarily citalopram, escitalopram, sertraline); serotonin-norepinephrine reuptake inhibitors (SNRIs) (venlafaxine, duloxetine); mirtazapine; and, among the tricyclic antidepressants, nortriptyline (due its relatively low anticholinergic side-effects) are suitable for elderly patients. For treatment of the most severe or therapy-resistant cases, electroconvulsive therapy (ECT) can be life-saving. ECT has been safely applied in patients up to 100 years of age.[19] ECT and other biological therapies, such as transcranial magnetic stimulation, should therefore not be discarded as treatment options just because a patient is elderly.

Psychotherapy for the elderly

Case study 7

An 87-year-old male is involuntarily hospitalized for violent behaviour against his wife (63 years old). She claims that the patient spends all the couples' money on prostitutes, which she cannot tolerate. This would often lead to fights, and the patient had pushed his wife away on several occasions. The patient confirms the accounts of his aggressive outbursts but also reveals that for several years he has been deeply in love with a 'tantra therapist'. The patient takes pride in his lifelong reputation as a 'womanizer' and recounts several 'adventures' from his times as an internationally acclaimed designer. According to the patient, his family physician had told him he was 'in such good shape that he would easily make it to 100 years'. The patient is now planning to start a new family with the tantra therapist.

Several psychotherapeutic modalities have proven efficacy in elderly patients, among them interpersonal therapy and cognitive behavioural therapy.[15] Old age is a period of life characterized by many changes, including those concerning physical abilities and social roles. The success of this 'journey of old age' depends on many different factors, most importantly, the psychological and social resources of a person (e.g. successful past problem-solving experiences, social network). In any case, old age requires constant adaptation by the individual and is a highly creative process. In contrast, if

Box 26.3 Frequent topics in old age psychotherapy

'Can I still behave in the same way I did 25 years ago? When I do, I run into more and more conflicts.'

'The dreams I have been chasing all my life have become obsolete and out of place. In fact, I never reached them. I wasted my life. Am I a failure? What can I hope for?'

'I am anyway going to die soon. Why should I change or even keep going?'

'I've already lost everything—my family, spouse, and friends! Even my children don't want anything to do with me. I am lonely.'

'I can't do anything because of physical impairments and pain. Nobody understands my situation.'

'When I still had a job, I was good for something. But now? When I offer my help at my former company, I only see eyes being rolled.'

'I did many things in my life of which I am deeply ashamed. Do I deserve the care that I get? Can I be forgiven?'

'My husband has dementia. I can't carry the burden of caring for him anymore. I am a bad wife.'

self-concepts are not modified (as illustrated by the persistent narcissistic attitude of the patient depicted in case study 7), suffering may result. In old age psychiatry, the therapist therefore often fulfils the role of an 'auxiliary ego' that induces self-reflection and stimulates a person to review his or her situation. Topics that frequently arise in psychotherapy for elderly patients are listed in Box 26.3. Especially in the beginning of psychotherapy, the patient may not be able to clearly specify his or her problems, or may even be unable to verbalize them at all.

Of course, the intensity and complexity of psychotherapy has to be adapted to the cognitive capacity of the patient—and may even be impossible in some cases. Beyond this limitation, psychotherapy is useful in many different situations in old age psychiatry, especially when treating depression.[20]

Treating the behavioural and psychological symptoms of dementia

Case study 8

An 84-year-old patient with advanced dementia is unable to maintain personal hygiene. Due to bladder incontinence, he requires regular change of absorbents and cleaning of the genital area. The patient frequently kicks and bites the nursing staff during the procedure. A 17-year-old nursing trainee now refuses to participate in the care of the patient. The head nurse of the residential care facility asks the liaison psychiatrist to discuss the issue during the next case conference.

Aggressive and/or disorganized behaviour is part of the behavioural and psychological symptoms of dementia (BPSDs).[21] Other common BPSDs include wandering, night-time agitation, and repetitive speech. Neuropsychiatric symptoms, such as apathy or depressed mood, are also frequently seen. Not only staff, but also family members and non-professional caregivers may be exposed to challenging and potentially violent behaviour which may be the main reason to seek psychiatric assistance. Exposure to

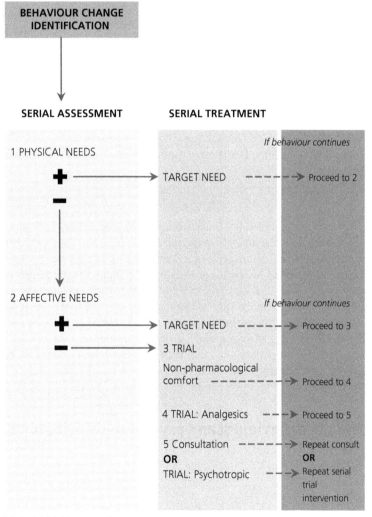

Fig. 26.2 Serial Trial Intervention.

violence may result in refusal to care (as in case study 8) and—if it persists—in elder abuse and neglect.[18,22] In response to violent behaviour, maintaining staff and family safety has the highest priority and represents a prerequisite for subsequent treatment. As with younger adults, where violent behaviour often occurs episodically under specific circumstances (e.g. under the influence of alcohol or drugs), trigger factors can often also be identified in the elderly. Even though the underlying condition for BPSDs may not be causally treated, it may thus still be possible to decrease their frequency or severity.

Several treatment algorithms for BPSDs have been proposed and empirically tested, among them the Serial Trial Intervention (see Fig. 26.2).[23,24] In case study 8, reorganization of the care routine may be effective in decreasing the aggressive behaviour. The process should include the involvement of more 'familiar' staff members, distracting the patient during the procedure, and speeding it up. The old age psychiatrist can guide the planning of such interventions and provide supervision during interdisciplinary case conferences.

If non-pharmacological measures are not successful, pharmacotherapeutic options should be considered. Antipsychotic medications are usually regarded as only second-line options and it is important to be acquainted with their adverse effects and be aware of their limited clinical effectiveness. Antipsychotic medications have been reported to be associated with increased mortality and adverse effects such as cerebrovascular events.[25] Alternatively, antidepressants may be used for some forms of BPSDs in Alzheimer's disease.[26,27]

Minimizing the use of restraints

Case study 9

A 76-year-old man develops atrial fibrillation in the context of hyperthyroidism. After hemi-thyroidectomy, post-operative bleeding necessitates two surgical revisions. Following the third surgery, the patient sees a 'moth flying through the room' and a 'multidimensional light sculpture' and becomes acutely confused. The patient is sedated with a benzodiazepine. Mechanical restraints are applied to allow medical treatment on the intermediate care unit. Five days later, the patient develops pneumonia and requires mechanical ventilation. The patient is finally discharged home after prolonged hospitalization and inpatient rehabilitation.

Chemical (i.e. pharmacologically induced sedation) or mechanical (e.g. fabric body holders) restraints are initiated in some cases of delirium to avoid immediate harm to self or others. However, they can lead to severe secondary complications like increased risk for pneumonia or prolongation of delirium—which themselves may lead to serious complications (as in case study 9; also see Box 26.4). Empirical evidence indicates that the 'culture of care' is a significant driver of restraint use and that educational interventions can significantly lower its frequency.[28] Therefore, all psychiatrists should actively work towards minimization of restraint use in their working environments.

If the use of restraints indeed cannot be forgone, it should be strictly limited to deal with a well-defined clinical syndrome, applied only for limited time periods, frequently monitored, and accurately documented. The application of restraints must be properly trained and regularly re-trained, in order to avoid harm to patients and staff.

> ## Box 26.4 Some possible negative outcomes of mechanical restraint
>
> ◆ Death or physical injury (e.g. choking/asphyxia, aspiration, thrombosis, dehydration, circulatory and skin problems, incontinence, injury from other patients)
>
> ◆ Prolonged behavioural symptoms, aggravated mental status (e.g. prolonged delirium, agitation, post-traumatic stress disorder, reactivation of traumatic experiences)
>
> ◆ Impaired future care (e.g. impaired therapeutic alliance with patient, ambivalence in treatment team)

In any case, the use of restraints must be thoroughly explained and eventually followed up by a discussion with all involved parties (family, staff, and (whenever possible) the patient). Written SOPs (standard operating procedures) for restraint are essential for minimizing errors and increasing transparency.

Dealing with the end of life

Case study 10

A 74-year-old man is brought to the psychiatric hospital for treatment of restlessness during the night. The family reports that the patient has had cognitive deficits 'for at least the last three to four years', but a diagnostic work-up of these deficits has not been performed. The intake examination and assessments give the picture of an advanced dementia syndrome. In the new environment of the psychiatric ward, the patient is disoriented to all dimensions. His behavioural symptoms worsen rapidly, he refuses medication, and his food and fluid intake is insufficient. Even one on one nursing for sustained periods cannot prevent repeated falls. The patient eventually dies—most likely from cachexia and dehydration—after 14 weeks of hospitalization. The patient's widow blames the treating old age psychiatrist for 'killing her husband'.

The condition of some patients will worsen even with the best possible medical care—and some will even die. In old age psychiatry, such cases are often related to dementia (as in case study 10), severe depression, or severe medical co-morbidity. A lot of distress to families and the treatment team can be prevented if end-of-life discussions are initiated in a timely way (e.g. sometime after a diagnosis of dementia has been made) and are not postponed to the terminal phase of a disease. End-of-life discussions should therefore be promoted by old age psychiatrists: they help families in advance care planning and may lead to written advance directives. The old age psychiatrist can facilitate such a process by providing examples from his or her practice, leading families to additional resources, and supplying facts about a disease (see Box 26.5). For example, burdensome and ultimately futile medical interventions (e.g. tube feeding in advanced dementia) occur less frequently if a family is informed about the limited prognosis.[29]

Box 26.5 General principles for dealing with end-of-life situations

- Talk about death, dying, and end-of-life care with your patient.
- Learn about the end-of-life care preferences of the patient. If appropriate, help the patient to establish a written advance care directive.
- Consider specific forms of psychotherapy for end-of-life care (e.g. dignity therapy).
- Decrease the suffering of the patient. Manage symptoms effectively. Avoid burdensome interventions.
- Support the family: explain what is happening, be accessible for questions.
- Treat the dying person with dignity and respect. Do not abandon the patient.
- Give room for spiritual, religious, or existential needs.
- Be culture-sensitive: end-of-life situations may be dealt with very differently in patients from other cultural backgrounds.
- Seek supervision and team support.

Following the concepts of palliative care, avoiding additional harm and reduction of suffering (e.g. by treating anxiety and pain) are the key principles of end-of-life treatment. Notably, palliative care does not necessarily end with the death of a patient, but may also involve supporting the family and the treatment team with their grief and feelings of guilt and inadequacy.

Conclusions

With all its complexity, old age psychiatry is a fascinating field to work in. In an ageing world, it also offers excellent career prospects. By adopting the specific skill set that is needed for dealing with mental health needs of elderly patients, psychiatrists can improve the care of this patient group.

References

1 Bartels SJ, Naslund JA. The underside of the silver tsunami—older adults and mental health care. *N Engl J Med* 2013; **368**(6):493–6.
2 Tinetti ME, Fried T. The end of the disease era. *Am J Med* 2004; **116**(3):179–85.
3 Jönson H. We will be different! Ageism and the temporal construction of old age. *Gerontologist* 2013; **53**(2):198–204.
4 Eymard AS, Douglas DH. Ageism among health care providers and interventions to improve their attitudes toward older adults: an integrative review. *J Gerontol Nurs* 2012; **38**(5):26–35.
5 Adelman RD, Tmanova LL, Delgado D, Dion S, Lachs MS. Caregiver burden: a clinical review. *JAMA* 2014; **311**(10):1052–60.

6 Elsawy B, Higgins KE. The geriatric assessment. *Am Fam Physician* 2011; **83**(1):48–56.

7 Ellis G, Whitehead MA, O'Neill D, Langhorne P, Robinson D. Comprehensive geriatric assessment for older adults admitted to hospital. *Cochrane Database Syst Rev* 2011; (7):CD006211.

8 Stacey D, Légaré F, Col NF, et al. Decision aids for people facing health treatment or screening decisions. *Cochrane Database Syst Rev* 2014; **1**:CD001431.

9 George J, Adamson J, Woodford H. Joint geriatric and psychiatric wards: a review of the literature. *Age Ageing* 2011; **40**(5):543–8.

10 Warner J, Jenkinson J. Psychiatry for the elderly in the UK. *Lancet* 2013; **381**(9882):1985.

11 Boyd CM, Darer J, Boult C, Fried LP, Boult L, Wu AW. Clinical practice guidelines and quality of care for older patients with multiple comorbid diseases: implications for pay for performance. *JAMA* 2005; **294**(6):716–24.

12 Garfinkel D, Mangin D. Feasibility study of a systematic approach for discontinuation of multiple medications in older adults: addressing polypharmacy. *Arch Intern Med* 2010; **170**(18):1648–54.

13 Patterson SM, Hughes C, Kerse N, Cardwell CR, Bradley MC. Interventions to improve the appropriate use of polypharmacy for older people. *Cochrane Database Syst Rev* 2012; **5**:CD008165.

14 The American Geriatrics Society's 2012 Beers' Criteria Update Expert Panel. American Geriatrics Society updated Beers' criteria for potentially inappropriate medication use in older adults. *J Am Geriatr Soc* 2012; **60**(4):616–31.

15 Unützer J, Park M. Older adults with severe, treatment-resistant depression. *JAMA* 2012; **308**(9):909–18.

16 Chan J, Draper B, Banerjee S. Deliberate self-harm in older adults: a review of the literature from 1995 to 2004. *Int J Geriatr Psychiatry* 2007; **22**(8):720–32.

17 Dong X, Simon M, Mendes de Leon C, et al. Elder self-neglect and abuse and mortality risk in a community-dwelling population. *JAMA* 2009; **302**(5):517–26.

18 Mosqueda L, Dong X. Elder abuse and self-neglect: 'I don't care anything about going to the doctor, to be honest . . .'. *JAMA* 2011; **306**(5): 532–40.

19 O'Reardon JP, Cristancho MA, Ryley B, Patel KR, Haber HL. Electroconvulsive therapy for treatment of major depression in a 100-year-old patient with severe aortic stenosis: a 5-year follow-up report. *J ECT* 2011; **27**(3):227–30.

20 Gould RL, Coulson MC, Howard RJ. Cognitive behavioral therapy for depression in older people: a meta-analysis and meta-regression of randomized controlled trials. *J Am Geriatr Soc* 2012; **60**(10):1817–30.

21 Lyketsos CG, Lopez O, Jones B, Fitzpatrick AL, Breitner J, DeKosky S. Prevalence of neuropsychiatric symptoms in dementia and mild cognitive impairment: results from the Cardiovascular Health Study. *JAMA* 2002; **288**(12):1475–83.

22 Lachs MS, Pillemer K. Abuse and neglect of elderly persons. *N Engl J Med* 1995; **332**(7):437–43.

23 Kovach CR, Logan BR, Noonan PE, et al. Effects of the Serial Trial Intervention on discomfort and behavior of nursing home residents with dementia. *Am J Alzheim Dis & Other Dem* 2006; **21**(3):147–55.

24 Gitlin LN, Kales HC, Lyketsos CG. Nonpharmacologic management of behavioral symptoms in dementia. JAMA. 2012 Nov 21;**308**(19):2020–9.

25 **Steinberg M, Lyketsos CG**. Atypical antipsychotic use in patients with dementia: managing safety concerns. *Am J Psychiatry* 2012; **169**(9):900–6.

26 **Banerjee S, Hellier J, Dewey M, et al**. Sertraline or mirtazapine for depression in dementia (HTA-SADD): a randomised, multicentre, double-blind, placebo-controlled trial. *Lancet* 2011; **378**(9789):403–11.

27 **Porsteinsson AP, Drye LT, Pollock BG, et al**. Effect of citalopram on agitation in Alzheimer disease: the CitAD randomized clinical trial. *JAMA* 2014; **311**(7):682–91.

28 **Köpke S, Mühlhauser I, Gerlach A, et al**. Effect of a guideline-based multicomponent intervention on use of physical restraints in nursing homes: a randomized controlled trial. *JAMA* 2012; **307**(20):2177–84.

29 **Mitchell SL, Teno JM, Kiely DK, et al**. The clinical course of advanced dementia. *N Engl J Med* 2009; **361**(16):1529–38.

Chapter 27

Management of intellectual disability

Sabyasachi Bhaumik, Reza Kiani, Shweta Gangavati, and Sayeed Khan

Case study

John is a 50-year-old gentleman with mild intellectual disability (ID) who has been referred to the specialist ID services as he has become increasingly housebound during the past year. John has always lived with his family, and following his mother's demise ten years ago, he has been looked after by his father. Before becoming housebound, he was known to have a good quality of life, with outdoor activities and regular access of community facilities. Despite having reasonable speech, John has never been very communicative with others and seldom initiates conversation.

John loves animals and has a specific interest in collecting toy trains. He is comfortable with his father but feels uncomfortable to speak in the presence of outsiders. He has a good relationship with his brothers. There is a tendency to being routine-bound and a history of persistent refusal to access healthcare facilities including visits to the dentist.

The current episode of becoming housebound was precipitated by a fall outside his home due to a slippery road surface, but unfortunately it has progressed to a stage where he is refusing to leave the house. His oral and personal hygiene have declined, and he has suffered from dental abscesses in the past. His biological functions are without major concerns, and there are no reports of significant mood swings or strange behaviours. His brothers are concerned about their father's welfare as he himself has mobility problems and has also to support John in his daily living activities. Previously, John has been treated with a selective serotonin reuptake inhibitor for his fears of leaving the house, but with little or no effect.

The family are concerned about John's high anxiety and his confinement. There are also concerns about his dental hygiene.

Questions (answers at end of the chapter)

1 What are the diagnostic possibilities for this case?
2 What are the likely physical health issues?
3 How will you support John with regards to addressing the issue of dental problems?
4 How will you support and plan his future care?
5 What other medications can be considered to manage his anxiety?

What is intellectual disability?

The term intellectual disability (ID) describes a lifelong heterogeneous condition and, as defined by the American Psychiatric Association,[1] it is based on three fundamental principles:

1 impairment of intellectual functioning (IQ <70);

2 significant impairment of adaptive skills; and

3 onset before 18 years of age.

The expression currently in use (ID) is synonymous with learning disability, mental retardation, or intellectual developmental disorders (IDD).

ID is an impairment of global mental abilities that impacts on adaptive functioning in three areas or domains. These domains determine how well an individual copes with everyday tasks and are the following:

1 the *conceptual domain* which includes skills in language, reading, writing, mathematics, reasoning, knowledge, and memory;

2 the *social domain* which refers to empathy, social judgement, interpersonal communication skills, the ability to make and retain friendships, and similar capacities;

3 the *practical domain* which refers to self-management in areas such as personal care, job responsibilities, money management, recreation, and organizing school and work tasks.

While ID is not age-specific, an individual's symptoms must begin during the developmental period, and diagnosis is based on the severity of deficits in adaptive functioning skills that include those listed in Table 27.1.

In the fourth edition of the *Diagnostic and statistical manual of mental disorders* (DSM)[1], the term 'mental retardation' was used, but in its most recent edition (DSM-5)[2], it has been changed to 'intellectual disability' (which refers more to an intellectual developmental disorder). The tenth edition of the *International classification of diseases* (ICD-10)[3] defines mental retardation as a condition of arrested or incomplete development of the mind that is especially characterized by impairment of skills manifested during the developmental period, which contributes to the overall level of intelligence (i.e. cognitive, language, motor, and social abilities). The ICD-10 also classifies ID into categories based on IQ, with a score less than two standard deviations below the population mean of 100 as the cut off (i.e. IQ <70)(see Table 27.2).

It is important to remember that the term ID represents a very heterogeneous group of individuals with a varying range of abilities from being completely dependent on

Table 27.1 Adaptive functioning skill areas

Communication	Health and safety
Self-direction	Functional academia
Leisure	Home living
Work	Social skills
Self-care	Community use

Table 27.2 Degrees of intellectual disability (ID)

Degree of ID	IQ	Mental age equivalent
Mild	50–69	9–12 years
Moderate	35–49	6–9 years
Severe	20–34	3–6 years
Profound	<20	<3 years

carers to being reasonably independent and needing only occasional support. In addition, readers are reminded that the term 'learning disability' is synonymous with ID but not with learning difficulties which include a range of reading, writing, and numeracy problems (e.g. dyslexia, specific scholastic disorders, specific language disorders).

It is often problematic to get an IQ assessment and, therefore, clinicians rely on the assessment of adaptive functioning in order to ascertain the degree of ID. Traditional measurements of IQ in children with developmental problems are not routinely carried out in many countries. Hence, there is a need to base subclassification on adaptive functioning rather than IQ measurement. In the absence of any IQ measurement, it is important that clinicians have a reasonable understanding of how to assess the degree of ID during the clinical assessment

How to clinically assess intellectual disability

The diagnosis of ID depends on a systematic assessment of both intellectual and adaptive functioning, but very often, an IQ assessment may not have been undertaken for the individual.

It is important to establish a diagnosis of ID and its degree when a clinician sees the person for the first time, as part of a detailed clinical assessment. Collateral history is important, and hence, when there is a suspicion of ID, one has to make sure that there are informants available (family, professional carers, or both) who can provide a detailed developmental history and an account of the person's current level of functioning. If the individual is presenting in a crisis, it is useful to assess premorbid functioning (best possible functioning) and also a typical day for that person (from waking up to going to bed), asking questions about each stage as to whether they need any prompting or assistance in carrying out activities. The pointers listed in Table 27.3 can assist with clinically determining the degree of ID.

Aetiology of intellectual disability

Where possible, every effort should be made to identify the cause of the ID as it may help in the assessment and management of the individual due to the specific association of physical and mental health problems with genetic disorders. For example, people with Down's syndrome have an association with hypothyroidism and dementia. Establishing the diagnosis also helps in understanding the long-term prognosis. However, it is not always possible to identify the underlying causes. There are various causes for an ID, which are broadly summarized in Table 27.4.

Table 27.3 Clinical assessment of degree of intellectual disability (ID) through adaptive functioning

	Mild IQ (69–50)	Moderate IQ (49–35)	Severe/profound IQ (34–0)
MENTAL AGE EQUIVALENCE	9 years–<12 years	6 years–<9 years	3 years–<6 years
PROPORTION	85% of the group	10% of the group	3–4% of the group
LANGUAGE ACQUISITION	Some delay in acquisition Most achieve the ability to use speech for everyday purposes	Slow in developing comprehension and use of language Eventual achievement is limited but variable	Acquire little or no communicative speech in early childhood years but may develop some speech during school-age period
EXPRESSIVE LANGUAGE	Most achieve the ability to use speech for everyday purposes, hold conversations, and engage in clinical interview Executive speech problems may persist and interfere with development of independence	From just enough language to communicate basic needs to simple conversations with limited vocabulary May learn to use manual signs to compensate	Limited to a few words only or absent speech May indicate choice through nodding or pointing
COMPREHENSION	Reasonable	Limited to simple instructions	Very limited understanding, if any
NON-VERBAL COMMUNICATION	Good	Limited	Rudimentary
SELF-CARE AND CONTINENCE	Most achieve full independence in washing, eating, dressing, as well as bladder and bowel control	Can attend to personal care with moderate assistance from carers Mainly continent	Achieve elementary skills only Full support of carers needed Mainly incontinent
INDEPENDENT LIVING	Full independence in practical and domestic skills possible May be able to cook simple meals; participate in household chores; operate common household appliances (television, telephone, microwave, washing machine, etc.)	Will need supervised living arrangements Limited mastery of domestic tasks; will require support and assistance Unlikely to shop or use public transport without support	Full 24-hour supervision required

(continued)

Table 27.3 (continued) Clinical assessment of degree of intellectual disability (ID) through adaptive functioning

	Mild IQ (69–50)	Moderate IQ (49–35)	Severe/profound IQ (34–0)
	May travel independently; do everyday shopping; and use money		
	Regression in skills is common under unusual social or economic stress		
ACADEMIC SKILLS	More likely to have left school without any qualifications; achievements up to approximately secondary school level; May learn to read, write, and do simple maths, but can have problems	More likely to have attended a special school; achievements unlikely beyond the second year of primary school May develop some reading, writing, and maths skills	Familiarity with the alphabet and simple counting. Simple sight reading of some words. May learn to copy write. Simple visuospatial skills
ADULT WORK	Capable of work demanding practical rather than academic skills	Simple practical work with supervision	Most not capable of this
MOTOR SKILLS	Normal mobility. Generally without problems with motor dexterity	Delayed but usually fully mobile	Frequent musculoskeletal abnormalities. Often severe restriction
SOCIAL AND EMOTIONAL DEVELOPMENT	Some immaturity is present which can make demands of marriage, child-rearing, or fitting in with cultural traditions and expectations difficult	Interaction may be as usual but difficulties in understanding social conventions may interfere with peer relationships	May be very limited. Autism common
ASSOCIATED DEFICITS	Organic aetiology identifiable in only a minority. Minimal sensorimotor impairment. Other deficits as in general population	Organic aetiology identifiable in a greater proportion. More frequent sensorimotor impairments with increase in CNS disorders like epilepsy	Organic aetiology frequently identifiable. Increased CNS disorders such as epilepsy and sensorimotor deficits including visual and hearing impairments
AUTISM AND OTHER PERVASIVE DEVELOPMENTAL DISORDERS	Present in varying proportions	Present in a substantial minority and can impact clinical picture and type of management needed	Increased prevalence affecting presentation and management

Table 27.4 Examples of aetiology of intellectual disability (ID)

Prenatal	Perinatal	Postnatal
Malnutrition:	*Traumatic birth delivery:*	Kernicterus
◆ Intrauterine growth retardation	◆ Brain haemorrhage	Meningo-encephalitis
Iatrogenic:	◆ Anoxia	Prolonged seizures
◆ Radiation	◆ Hypoxia	Hypoglycaemia
◆ Drugs		Lead poisoning
◆ Alcohol		Malnutrition
Intrauterine infections:		Hypothyroidism
◆ TORCH (toxoplasmosis, other, rubella, CMV, and herpes)		Neoplasm
Genetic syndromes:		Head trauma
◆ Angelman syndrome		Cerebrovascular incident
◆ Down's syndrome		Educational, social, and economic deprivation
◆ Fragile X syndrome		
◆ Lesch-Nyhan syndrome		
◆ Phenylketonuria		
◆ Prader-Willi syndrome		
◆ Tuberous sclerosis		
◆ Williams syndrome		

Epidemiology of intellectual disability

From an epidemiological perspective, ID prevalence rates vary according to the definitions and classification systems being used. Emerson and Hatton[4] estimate a prevalence of 2% of the adult population, with 0.47% of the adult population being users of specialist intellectual disability services (administrative prevalence). In a meta-analysis by Saxena et al.,[5] the overall prevalence (including all studies) is 10.37 per 1000 population. Harris et al.[6] report a prevalence of 1–3% globally. King et al.[7] reported that of all people with ID, 85% had mild, 10% moderate, 4% severe, and 2% profound ID. There is usually a male excess in the ID population, and the reasons include genetic disorders that tend to mainly affect men (e.g. fragile X syndrome).

Mortality in people with intellectual disability

People with ID have a shorter lifespan than the general population due to congenital malformations, neurological co-morbidities, and iatrogenic causes (often associated with polypharmacy). However, there are also other associated risk factors related to their environment and to barriers faced in accessing health services. All these might contribute to a reduced lifespan compared to the general population. Some deaths in acute care settings for individuals with ID may be potentially preventable if provision of good-quality care is ensured and professionals dealing with such individuals are trained appropriately to address the needs of people with ID.

A commonly employed measure in mortality studies is the standardized mortality ratio (SMR), which is the ratio of observed deaths in the population of interest to the expected deaths using the general population death rate. In 2009, a study [8] in a population of adults with ID found an all-cause SMR of 2.77 (95% confidence interval 2.53–3.03). The group that was particularly disadvantaged included those with congenital malformations and co-morbid disease of the nervous system (including epilepsy) and sensory organs, with their overall SMR noted to be 16.3. In another study that reviewed epilepsy[9], the SMR for men and women with ID and active epilepsy was noted to be 3.2 and 5.6, respectively. Sudden death in epilepsy (SUDEP) in patients with ID is a major cause for premature deaths in this population and SMR for SUDEP in males and females was 37.6 and 52.0 respectively.

Health problems in people with intellectual disability

People with ID experience more health problems than the general population as a whole. These health problems can be classified as physical and mental health problems.

Physical health problems

Major health problems include epilepsy, sensory impairment (visual and hearing), and mobility problems of varying degree. The health problems increase with increasing degree of ID. Secondary health issues may also arise due to underlying primary conditions or poor lifestyle choices (see Table 27.5). Common conditions like constipation,[10] if not identified and treated early, can lead to further health problems such as pain, nausea, faecal incontinence, anal fissures, haemorrhoids, and even rectal prolapse. There

Table 27.5 Physical health problems in people with intellectual disability (ID)

Physical health	Prevalence (%)[14]
Epilepsy	18
Visual impairment	2–67*
Hearing disorders	8–100*
Gastro-oesophageal reflux disease	48
Constipation	70
Fractures	32
Edentulous	23
Obesity	13–58

*Prevalence increases with age and is higher in people with Down's syndrome. The large variations are usually due to differences in methodology and settings of studies.

Reproduced from BMJ, 337, Schrojenstein Lantman-de Valk HMJ, Walsh PN, Managing health problems in people with intellectual disabilities, p. 1408–1412, Copyright (2008) with permission from BMJ Publishing Group Ltd

Table 27.6 Mental health problems in people with intellectual disability (ID)

Mental health problems	Prevalence (%)
Overall prevalence	40
Schizophrenia	3
Depression	4
Bipolar affective disorder	1.5
Dementia	20

is also a reported high prevalence of poor oral health including dental caries (58%). Hence, vigilance regarding health checks [11] is very important given the background problems of communication difficulties. Also, untreated physical health issues, with associated pain or discomfort, may present as challenging behaviour as these patients may not be able to verbalize these concerns.

Mental health problems

Similarly, psychiatric problems are three to four times more common in those with ID in comparison with the general population (see Table 27.6). Cooper et al.[12] found a lifetime prevalence of all mental health problems to be around 49.2%. Prevalence of dementia in people with Down's syndrome is at least three times higher than the general population, and schizophrenia is reported to be approximately two to three times that in the general population.

The prevalence of autism, which is characterized by qualitative impairment in social and communication domains, a deficit in imagination and empathy, along with repetitive speech or behaviour, is around 8–20% on average (based on different studies)[13], in comparison to around 1% in the general population.

Challenges in assessing health problems

Assessment of health co-morbidities in people with ID can be fraught with difficulties. Some people with intellectual disability due to communication difficulties may be unable to understand the significance of their symptoms and may not be able to report them early. Others may have a higher pain threshold due to their background sensory perception problems (something which can be seen also in individuals with autism). Medical specialists working in hospitals, if not appropriately trained, may struggle to carry out a proper assessment and reach a valid diagnosis for those with ID. The key barriers to accessing appropriate treatment modalities in general hospitals include lack of awareness of how this client group might present, negative attitudes of professionals toward this patient population, and communication difficulties.

Atypical presentation of symptoms

As already highlighted, any distress, either physical or psychological, could have an atypical presentation due to the underlying communication difficulties (Box 27.1).

Box 27.1 Common manifestations of underlying physical or psychological distress

- Refusal to eat or drink
- Withdrawal from daily activities
- Deterioration in baseline skills
- Challenging behaviour—head banging, bruxism, self-injury, aggression

Raising awareness of these issues through appropriate training for healthcare professionals and carers is therefore paramount to avoid *diagnostic overshadowing* (i.e. attributing the symptoms to the ID rather than actively investigating an underlying health issue) as well as a delayed diagnosis, leading to poor outcomes.

It is important to mention that, at times, reaching a diagnosis for a very unwell patient with ID might be extremely difficult due to the interface between physical and mental health problems, which often co-occur (see Box 27.2).

The challenges of obtaining a good history and performing a physical examination in people with ID can be overcome by having a good understanding of the communication principles in these individuals. It is important to be empathic and treat the person

Box 27.2 Case examples of the interface between physical and mental health problems in people with ID

Example 1: Consider the presentation of a patient with Down's syndrome with loss of skills, confusion, and self-isolation which can be related to a depressive disorder, dementia of Alzheimer's type, worsening visual/hearing impairment, and hypothyroidism, or a combination of two or more of these co-morbidities.

Example 2: Another example would be the atypical presentations of epilepsy. As various types of intractable epilepsy can be present in an individual at a given time, symptoms might be quite difficult to distinguish from those related to autistic stereotypes, movement disorders due to a primary neurological illness, arrhythmias, congenital cardiac diseases, or side-effects of medications.

Example 3: Delayed diagnosis of a visual or hearing impairment can lead to attributing symptoms, which can include challenging behaviour, to a mental illness or dementia. Working collaboratively with audiology services/optician and ophthalmology services is therefore extremely important in order to pick up these co-morbidities early on.

Example 4: Dental pain and gum pathology can present with drooling, face slapping, or refusal to eat or drink. Working jointly with a dentist is paramount to ensure that those with severe ID and autism receive an individually tailored treatment plan that is patient- friendly.

with respect and dignity, focusing on their abilities and using accessible information materials to improve their understanding. Sometimes, a clinician can only arrive at a provisional diagnosis for mental disorders and, only with the passage of time, do things become clearer and the working diagnosis finalized. It is important to identify the individual's normative pattern of behaviour and any shift from it due to illness, in order to establish an optimum target for treatment response. Observing the patient is key to identifying changes in behaviour and making a differential diagnosis.

General principles of management strategies

The provision of high-quality healthcare for people with ID should be an international priority. The World Health Organization carried out a survey [15] which suggests inpatient care, primary care, specialized services, and physical rehabilitation were available in most of the countries. The provisions were noted to be greater in high-income countries (80–90%) and lesser in low- income countries (60–70%). Primary healthcare provision was available in most of the countries, though the figures for low-income countries were noted to be 75% for children and adolescents and 70.3% for adults. Specialized services were noticeably less available for adults in South-East Asia (50%), Western Pacific (61.1%), and Africa (60.7%). Making reasonable adjustments for people with ID to access mainstream health services should be considered a priority if things are to improve.

For the majority of people with ID, regular health checks at the primary healthcare level can identify their health needs and can be followed by the provision of necessary treatment or signposting for access to treatment in secondary care.

When a patient is first referred to the specialist service, it is important that the clinician gathers appropriate information from all relevant sources including family, education, and day-care providers. Once the assessment and diagnostic process is completed, the results are shared with the patient and their family in a user-friendly format. The psychiatrist may need help from the speech and language therapist to facilitate this effectively.

The management plan should include a package of care provided by a team of multidisciplinary professionals (see Table 27.7) and consisting of culturally sensitive biopsychosocial components which address areas of both health and social care needs. Ideally, it should also include a clear plan for skills' development in the individual. Drug treatment for mental health problems is provided as per the evidence base that exists for the general population. However, caution should be exercised in relation to monitoring drug side-effects (through observation, interview, and carer feedback) as there may be a propensity for development of unacceptable side-effects which are not always reported due to communication difficulties. For this reason, starting drug treatment at a low dose and gradually titrating upwards is advised.

Depending upon the complexity of health needs, a *stepped-care approach* (see Fig. 27.1) might be beneficial, with basic health needs being met by primary healthcare workers or their equivalent (Table 27.8). With increasing complexity, it may be necessary to provide 'joined-up' care together with the nearest available mental health or

Table 27.7 Multidisciplinary team members working within the intellectual disability department and a summary of their main roles

Professionals	Summary of roles/responsibilities
Acute hospital liaison nurses	Based at the general hospitals, ensuring accessibility and reasonable adjustments
Community ID nurses	Monitoring mental health, administration of depot injection, Care Programme Approach co-ordination
Dietician	Advice on daily intake, healthy eating, and weight management including advice on food supplements
District nurses	Support with the management of diabetes, incontinence, and other medical problems in the community
Occupational therapists	Assessment of activities of daily living and independent living skills, assessment of falls, environmental assessment and adaptation, sensory assessment/ integration
Outreach learning disability nurses	Emergency support for the management of challenging behaviour in the community, behavioural assessment, and management strategies
Physiotherapists	Assessment and management of mobility problems
Primary care liaison nurses (formerly health facilitators)	Health facilitation, liaison with the primary care team (e.g. the general practitioners, the practice nurses, the district nurses), advice on completion of a health action plan
Psychiatrists	Assessment and management of mental health problems, autism, challenging behaviours, dementia, and epilepsy
Psychologists	IQ assessment, provision of psychological therapies (e.g. cognitive behaviour therapy)
Speech and language therapists	Assessment of swallowing and choking; developing an eating and drinking plan; assessment of communication and advice on developing a communication passport
Tissue viability nurses	Prevention and management of pressure sores

acute care service staff. In addition, input from social care is often beneficial for this group's extensive social needs. Inpatient care is needed for only very few individuals and may be provided in the secondary care setting, with appropriate support from the carers. It is therefore imperative to develop a co-ordinated and personalized care plan which includes input from all health professionals and social care. Stepping down from inpatient care to community care is another difficult transition time, which should be appropriately supported by the healthcare providers.

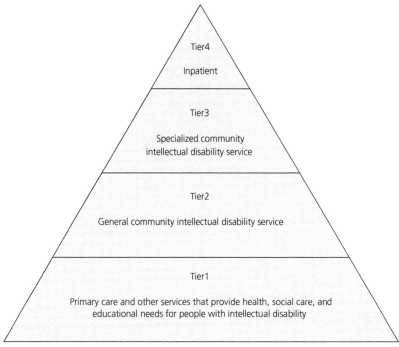

Fig. 27.1 Tiered/stepped model of care for learning disability services.

Source data from: Faculty of the Psychiatry of Learning Disability, Future role of psychiatrists working with people with learning disability, Royal College of Psychiatrists Faculty Report FR/LD/1, Copyright (2011), Royal College of Psychiatrists

Table 27.8 Outline of tiered/stepped-care approach

	Professionals involved	**Focus of involvement**	**Nature of involvement**
TIER 1	Primary healthcare and other mainstream services Social care	General healthcare e.g. annual health checks, epilepsy, anxiety disorder Educational and social needs e.g. appropriate residential placement, day-care arrangements, skills development	Virtually no input from the community ID team and psychiatrists apart from providing ad hoc advice or training if needed
TIER 2	General community ID services Psychiatrist	Less complex mental health needs e.g. one episode of depressive disorder—diagnosed, treated, and discharged back to primary care	Short-term involvement of specialist services
TIER 3	Specialized community ID services	More complex needs e.g. chronic mental illness with a relapsing and remitting course, dementia, challenging behaviour, pervasive developmental disorders, refractory epilepsy	Long-term involvement until patients are stabilized

Table 27.8 (continued) Outline of tiered/stepped-care approach

	Professionals involved	Focus of involvement	Nature of involvement
TIER 4	Specialist inpatient service including local assessment and treatment units up to secure forensic services	Very complex needs Risks cannot be contained or managed in the community and needing hospitalization for safe treatment e.g. depression with risk of suicide, severe aggression, florid psychosis	Long-term involvement until patients are discharged back into community

It should be emphasized that patients are likely to move from one tier to another as they deteriorate or improve with interventions made.

Service provision for people with intellectual disability

The recognition of ID happens usually within primary care services, where professionals are the first point of contact for most families. Subsequently, referrals from primary care to the child developmental clinic or community paediatric teams are not uncommon. Occasionally, an acute physical health crisis, such as childhood epilepsy, may lead to the recognition of the condition and trigger a referral to the specialist ID services.

In the Western world, unless the condition is evident at birth, help is usually sought during the early childhood period due to developmental delay, childhood epilepsy, poor social interaction, and delay in achieving scholastic skills. In addition, behavioural problems, insomnia, and incontinence can also trigger consultation with health services. In adulthood, the presence of epilepsy, mental health problems, and other chronic health problems are usually the reasons for seeking specialist service input.

Specialist ID services aim to provide care within the community setting for treatment of psychiatric disorders, epilepsy, and other long-term conditions. Many providers have provision for a short-term admission to an assessment unit to deal with acute mental health problems that pose a high risk. Such units may exist on their own, or these facilities may be provided within acute psychiatric settings. Institutional care is not considered to be the norm in Western countries; however, such care is still being provided in some countries where there is a paucity of health resources. Several reports of abuse and exploitation in institutional care have been published, and every effort is being made at present to replace institutional care, where possible, with the model of community care.

Health inequalities for people with ID have been reported from all over the world. Due to the complexity of the healthcare needs and the lack of communication, the quality of care received by this population leaves much to be desired. Avoidable mortality and morbidity due to poor care have raised concerns globally, and the emphasis has been on recognizing the basic principles of respect, dignity, and inclusion for the individuals in all healthcare settings. When treating such individuals, a personalized care pathway based approach, including the use of patient outcome and experience measures, has been found to be most useful.

In many countries, the prison population includes a substantial proportion of people with ID because of the failure to identify the condition during legal proceedings and lack of a diversion programme. Offending behaviours are not uncommon, especially in people with mild ID and those with autism spectrum disorder (ASD), and very often these are caused by a desire to please others, a high degree of suggestibility, any underlying mental health problems, and a lack of understanding of social norms and consequences of behaviour. In addition, a minority of people with ID may need secure-care provision because of the high risks they present with, and they may also benefit from locked or unlocked rehabilitation facilities.

Offenders with intellectual disability

It is reported that there is a higher prevalence of people with ID in the prison setting (Hassiotis et al.[16]) with figures ranging from 0.5% to 1.5% and up to 13%. Vaughan et al.[17] grouped forensic behaviours into physical assault, sexual assault against adults and children, property destruction, theft/burglary, and other behaviours (such as possession of a blade, abduction, cruelty to animals, and harassment).

Under law, a crime is generally defined by two components: *actus reus* (the act of crime) and *mens rea* (the intent to commit that crime). It is difficult to establish the latter in people with ID, especially in those with moderate to profound ID, and this is key to the legal perception of the difference between challenging behaviour and criminal behaviour. This can influence police decisions to caution or to arrest and convict, unless the criminal act is very serious.

People with ID, due to their limited communication and other co-morbidities, are likely to struggle in their journey through the criminal justice system without considerable additional support to understand the due process from the stages of arrest and interrogation to charging and sentencing. These individuals are also likely to experience greater difficulty coping in prison custody are vulnerable to bullying.[18] They are less likely to benefit from (or can even be excluded from) conventional prison treatment programmes that are generally designed for people with an IQ >80.[19]

Therefore, early identification and specialist evaluation cannot be overemphasized in order to determine these individuals' fitness to plead and to consider the options of non-custodial sentences and diversion routes such as hospital orders (with or without restriction orders), guardianship orders, and supervision and treatment orders. Forensic services for people with ID have staff with specialist skills and offer modified psychological therapies and offence-specific treatments for people with reduced cognitive abilities. This approach is also more rehabilitative and makes a difference to outcomes.

Ethical and social considerations

A person with ID is likely to face rejection and may often be socially isolated and segregated. The additional issues of mental health problems, epilepsy, and high dependency may also contribute to increasing the risk of discrimination, stigma, and exclusion. There is a high risk of potential abuse, and to safeguard the individual's interests, the ID services in the United Kingdom have adopted a model of advocacy which is available in most local authority areas. There are also teams located within health and social care settings dealing with safeguarding issues.

Conclusions and the way forward

Not all medical trainees need to become experts in the area of ID. However, it is expected that the majority will be able to identify the condition and will be fully aware of the risks of associated co-morbidities and their impact. (Table 27.9 lists organizations and websites that could be helpful with this.) They should also be fairly conversant about sign-posting when an ID is identified, and take the necessary steps toward reasonable adjustments when they are involved in providing care to these individuals.

Table 27.9 Useful organizations and websites

Organizations/websites	URL address link
American Association on Intellectual and Developmental Disabilities	http://aaidd.org/
Anticipatory Care Calendar	http://www.mccn.nhs.uk/userfiles/documents/Q4NAEDI%20dementia%20report%20mccn%20part1.pdf
Association for Persons with Developmental Disabilities and Mental Health	http://thenadd.org/
British Institute of Learning Disabilities	http://www.bild.org.uk/
Down's Syndrome Association	http://www.downs-syndrome.org.uk/
European Association of Intellectual Disability Medicine	http://www.mamh.net/
Improving Health and Lives Learning Disabilities Observatory	http://www.improvinghealthandlives.org.uk/
International Association for the Scientific Study of Intellectual and Developmental Disabilities	https://iassid.org/
Mencap	http://www.mencap.org.uk/
National Autistic Society	www.autism.org.uk
Palliative Care for People with Learning Disability	http://www.pcpld.org/
People with Profound and Multiple Learning Disabilities	https://www.mencap.org.uk/about-learning-disability/information-professionals/pmld
Royal College of Psychiatrists' Faculty of Psychiatry of Intellectual Disability	http://www.rcpsych.ac.uk/workinpsychiatry/faculties/intellectualdisability.aspx
See Ability	http://www.seeability.org/
Sense	http://www.sense.org.uk/
SUDEP Aware	http://www.sudepaware.org/
Australasian Society for Intellectual Disability (ASID)	http://www.asid.asn.au/

The specific evidence base for treatment of mental illness and challenging behaviour for people with ID is very small, and further research is needed in this area. One way ahead might be to consider inclusion of people with ID in future research proposals that are specifically aimed at assessing effectiveness and outcomes of interventions. Alternatively, research proposals that deal with the applicability of an intervention method that is already in use, with a strong evidence base in the general population, can be extrapolated to the population with ID (see Box 27.3).

Box 27.3 Ten key points in managing intellectual disability

1 ID is a condition that affects around 2% of the population and is characterized by a reduced IQ (<70), poor adaptive functioning, and difficulties in communication, arising before the age of 18.

2 ID may be caused by specific genetic conditions, infections, difficulties during pregnancy and labour, or poor socio-economic situation. However, for some individuals, no known cause can be established.

3 It is possible to determine the degree of ID through clinical assessment, without the use of an IQ test.

4 ID is a heterogeneous condition and includes those who may function independently with minimal support and those who may be totally dependent on others for care provision.

5 ID is commonly associated with mental health problems (three to four times that of the general population). About 20% of people with ID present with challenging behaviours, which may have multiple causative factors.

6 While taking a history, it is important to obtain collateral information from carers and to establish the person's pre-morbid baseline functioning level, so that treatment goals can be identified.

7 Interface between mental and physical health is very common in this population, often leading to diagnostic overshadowing. Mental health conditions, especially in those with impaired communication, can sometimes only be diagnosed through observation of behaviours.

8 Beware of the coexistence of physical conditions. Avoid polypharmacy where possible; 'start low, go slow' with medications. Review medications regularly and actively monitor for possible side-effects.

9 Individuals with ID have extensive health and social care needs, and hence joint working with multidisciplinary teams involving community nurses, speech and language therapists, occupational therapists, physiotherapists, and psychologists is the norm for their management.

10 The role of psychiatrists predominantly involves assessment, diagnosis, and management of mental disorders, dementia, pervasive developmental disorders, challenging behaviour, and epilepsy.

Answers to case study questions (at beginning of chapter)

1 The differential diagnosis includes agoraphobia, generalized anxiety disorder, high anxiety state related to a background of possible autism spectrum disorder.

2 Physical health issues: pain following the fall, poor dental health, possible visual impairment and other sensory issues, and mobility problems related to uneven surfaces.

3 Care staff or community nurses should support him during desensitization for the dental appointment. If dental problems are severe and need immediate attention, consider organizing a best- interest decision meeting and undertaking dental work under general anaesthesia.

4 Assessment by the multidisciplinary team (please refer to Table 27.3).

5 Other alternatives could be the use of propranolol for the management of anxiety.

References

1 American Psychiatric Association. *Diagnostic and statistical manual of mental disorders* (4th edn) (DSM-IV). Washington, DC: APA; 2000.

2 American Psychiatric Association. *Diagnostic and statistical manual of mental disorders* (5th edn) (DSM-5). Washington, DC: APA; 2013.

3 World Health Organization *The ICD-10 classification of mental and behavioural disorders.* Geneva: WHO; 1992.

4 **Emerson E, Hatton** C. People with learning disabilities in England: Centre for Disability Research Report, May 2008. Lancaster: CeDR; 2008.

5 **Pallab K, Maulik, MN, Mascarenhas CD, Mathers TD, Shekhar S**. Prevalence of intellectual disability: A meta-analysis of population-based studies. *Res Develop Dis* 2011; **32**:419–36.

6 **Harris JC.** *Intellectual disability: understanding its development, causes, classification, evaluation and treatment.* New York: Oxford University Press; 2006, pp. 42–98.

7 **King BH, Toth KE, Hodapp RM, Dykens EM.** Intellectual disability. In: *Comprehensive textbook of psychiatry* (9th edn) (eds. Sadock BJ, Sadock VA, Ruiz P). Philadelphia: Lippincott Williams & Wilkins; 2009, pp. 3444–74.

8 **Tyrer F, McGrother** C. Cause-specific mortality and death certificate reporting in adults with moderate to profound intellectual disability. *J Intellect Disabil Res* 2009; **53**:898–904.

9 **Kiani R, Tyrer F, Jesu A, et al**. Mortality from sudden unexpected death in epilepsy (SUDEP) in a cohort of adults with intellectual disability. *J Intellect Disabil Res* 2014;**58**:508–20.

10 **Coleman J, Spurling G**. Constipation in people with learning disability. *BMJ* 2010; **340**:c222.

11 **Hoghton M, Martin G, Chauhan U**. Annual health checks for people with intellectual disabilities. *BMJ*;2012 **345**:e7589.

12 **Cooper SA, Smiley E, Morrison J, Williamson A, Allan L**. Mental ill-health in adults with intellectual disabilities: prevalence and associated factors. *Br J Psychiatry* 2007; **190**:27–35.

13 **Bhaumik S, Tyrer F, Barrett M, Tin N, McGrother CW, Kiani R**. The relationship between carers' report of autistic traits and clinical diagnoses of autism spectrum disorders in adults with intellectual disability. *Res Dev Disabil*; 2010 **31**(3):705–12.

14 **Schrojenstein Lantman-de Valk HMJ, Walsh PN**. Managing health problems in people with intellectual disabilities. *BMJ* 2008; **337**:1408–12.

15 World Health Organization. *Atlas of global resources for persons with intellectual disabilities*. Geneva: WHO; 2007

16 **Hassiotis A, Gazizova D, Akinlonu L, Bebbington P, Meltzer H, Strydom A**. Psychiatric morbidity in prisoners with intellectual disabilities: analysis of prison survey data for England and Wales. *Br J Psychiatry*; 2011 **199**(2):156–7.

17 **Vaughan PJ**. Secure care and treatment needs of individuals with intellectual disability and severe challenging behaviour. *Br J Intellect Dis* 2003; **31**:113–17.

18 **Petersilia J**. Justice for all? Offenders with mental retardation and the California corrections system. *Prison J* 1997; **77**: 355–380.

19 **Talbot J**. *No one knows: offenders with learning difficulties and learning disabilities*. London: Prison Reform Trust; 2008.

Chapter 28

Managing child psychiatry

Felipe Picon, Patrick Kelly, and
Rutger Jan van der Gaag

Introduction

The emergence of child psychiatry as a specialty has its origins in the joint work between pedagogy, psychology, and philosophy in the late nineteenth century, undertaken by the German philosopher and psychiatrist Theodor Ziehen, working as a consultant at the school founded by Johannes Trüper.[1] In 1930, in the United States, Leo Kanner was the first to be considered a proper 'child psychiatrist'. He founded the first academic department of child psychiatry at the John Hopkins Hospital in Maryland and coined the term 'child psychiatry' for his book, published in 1935.[2] In 1937, at the Emma Pendleton Bradley Home (known today as the Bradley Hospital), in East Providence (Rhode Island), Dr Charles Bradley discovered the 'paradoxical' benefits of benzedrine to treat behavioural problems in children. This still represents one of the most important psychiatric therapeutic discoveries in (child) psychiatry and, especially, in the treatment of attention deficit hyperactivity disorder (ADHD).[3,4] Later on, the field evolved to become a recognized specialty within medicine in the USA in 1959, six years after the founding of the American Academy of Child Psychiatry, today known as the American Academy of Child and Adolescent Psychiatry (AACAP). Throughout the world, child and adolescent psychiatry is either a subspecialty within psychiatry or a medical specialty in its own right.

The evolution of child psychiatry continued with the beginning of paediatric psychopharmacology studies using, for example, antidepressants for separation anxiety disorder and antipsychotics for Tourette's disorder in the late 1970s[5] and many other medication options as adjuvants to psychological treatment in the following decades. Since then, developments in assessment (e.g. acknowledging autism as an innate developmental disorder), accuracy of diagnosis (e.g. refining classifications in a heuristic fashion based on solid empirical evidence), and effectiveness of treatment have continued to evolve.

Within child and adolescent psychiatry, an interesting range of subspecialties can be discerned, ranging from infant psychiatry to the specific interventions for children with learning disabilities, from psychopathology related to perceptual deficits (deafness, blindness, and combinations of them) to forensic child and adolescent psychiatry.

Even though child psychiatry cannot be considered a novel specialty, it is still an open field for discoveries and improvements in the fascinating area of developmental psychopathology—a unique field of research at the core of the nature–nurture debate. Professionals involved in neuroscience—dealing with genetics, the exploration of neurophysiological and psychological functioning of the brain, and with evidence-based psychotherapeutic approaches—are still greatly needed in the field of child psychiatry. Both developing[6] and developed countries[7] struggle with the shortage of child psychiatrists, and this is a challenge for future psychiatrists worldwide.

This chapter aims to elucidate some possible questions for early career psychiatrists who are considering pursuing a career in child psychiatry by presenting the differences in training when compared to adult psychiatry, exploring some challenges in the beginning of the profession, and showing the opportunities of the field. We hope this chapter will also inspire future psychiatrists to choose this specialty while, at the same time, demystifying some aspects of the profession for those residents that have already chosen child psychiatry as a career.

Comparing adult and child psychiatry

Considering that some evidence suggests that half of life-time cases of psychiatric disorders start before the age of 14,[8] the availability of child psychiatrists and of effective mental health services for children and adolescents, around the world, becomes of crucial importance for early recognition and treatment of such disorders. The possibility of being able to work with children who are starting to present symptoms, even before having fully consolidated disorders, besides being an important prevention opportunity, represents a source of great pleasure and enthusiasm for the profession. Of course, the expectations concerning prevention and cure of developmental disorders should be tempered by the fact that many child psychiatric conditions have a highly persistent character. However, early diagnosis can make a huge difference in terms of burden for the child and their environment (mainly, family and school), and early acknowledgement has a tremendous impact on the actual and future quality of life of the child. This perhaps represents one of the main characteristics of child and adolescent psychiatric practice, in comparison to that of adult psychiatry.

Another important difference in child psychiatric practice is the absolute need to have a broad range of interactive skills, to be adapted to the different stages of development of children and adolescents, without excluding the need to be well prepared to deal with adults too (e.g. parents, grandparents, and teachers). This is probably one of the features that may attract or repel young doctors when evaluating this career. It requires a psychological aptitude and willingness to deal with family systems, which is more relevant for daily practice in child psychiatry than in general adult psychiatry. Obviously, in many situations during the treatment of adults, it is necessary to involve other family members and other relevant adults, besides needing, in some cases, a combined approach that includes family therapy. However, in child psychiatry, the contact and dealings with parents are indeed the starting point of any treatment, because it is almost never the child who seeks out the child psychiatrist but, rather, the parents (either on their own initiative or following the recommendations of school staff, paediatricians, etc.). The main characteristics of adult versus child and adolescent clinical practice are detailed in Table 28.1.

Table 28.1 Characteristics of adult versus child psychiatric daily practice

Characteristic	Adult psychiatry	Child psychiatry
Stage of development	Although human development is continuous throughout the life span, the child has a more rapid pace of development. Although individual conditions may vary in different stages of adult development, no specific adaptation to life stages is required to propose a diagnosis.	A child goes through non-stop developmental changes, and a feature that might be a symptom in one age may be appropriate in another. Therefore, the stage of development has to be taken into consideration for the proposal of a diagnosis.
Psychopathology	Psychological functioning and symptoms are usually more stable over time.	Symptoms may be more volatile and change during further development.
		The onset of different developmental disorders occurs at different developmental stages (early onset: autism; toddler onset: anxiety disorders/behavioural disorders; childhood onset: ADHD, OCD; adolescent onset: eating disorders, depression, substance abuse, schizophrenia).
Communication	Usually, communication is predominantly verbal.	Children are usually less able to express their suffering in words and they do it more through behaviour.
Collateral information	Additional information is important, but not always crucial to diagnosis.	Since children often express their problems through behaviour and the environment is of great influence on the expression and reinforcement of (inadequate) behaviour, the collateral information from parents, other relatives, teachers, and other caregivers is essential in order to make a comprehensive diagnosis.
Search for treatment	Treatment is usually sought by the adult subject, and sometimes by a spouse or relative.	Children rarely seek help for themselves; it is usually a parent or another caregiver that seeks medical attention to deal with a disturbance in the observable behaviour of the child.

(*continued*)

Table 28.1 (continued) Characteristics of adult versus child psychiatric daily practice

Characteristic	Adult psychiatry	Child psychiatry
Family involvement	Adults do not always need the involvement of the family in the treatment.	The child's very existence and emotional development depend on the family or caregiver; therefore their role is very important at all stages of evaluation and treatment. The collaboration of the family (in its broadness and complexity) is crucial, and they need to be on board to give treatment a chance for success. (All family members should be involved: for example, in cases of divorce, both parents should be contacted.)
Environmental influences	Adults might become ill due to changes in the environment (family, work, etc.).	Children are very vulnerable to adverse environmental influences and greatly benefit from environmental protectiveness; some factors may predispose or precipitate disorders (e.g. abuse during childhood is a major risk for the future development of other disorders).
Psychopharmacotherapy	Usually, the adult gives (or not) their own consent to the use of medication, and the effects of psychotropics have been tested in a high number of controlled studies with adult samples.	Many medications for children and adolescents have not been adequately assessed in controlled studies and are often prescribed off-label, with the decision to use medication (or not) made with the parents' informed consent.
Diagnosis	Usually, the disorders present as full-blown clinical syndromes and characterization is more often straightforward.	Children often present with an atypical symptomatology or a variable clinical picture. The formal diagnosis takes a long period to complete and frequently, the child psychiatrist manages symptoms first. Thus, diagnosis in child psychiatry is a process more than a state.

Training in child psychiatry

In line with the dissimilarities in clinical practice, training in child psychiatry is also different from that for adult psychiatry, in order to prepare medical students for dealing with its specific features. Historically, there were proposals to split child psychiatry from general psychiatry, in the same way that paediatrics was separated from internal medicine, but generally, training in child psychiatry follows the training in adult psychiatry. In Table 28.2, the main training modalities for the child and adolescent psychiatrist are described.

Despite the advantages of the different models presented here, in most countries, a traditional training path is still the most prevalent one. Therefore, for most medical students considering a career in child psychiatry, the path still takes them through training in general psychiatry. Considering that in most countries, such training lasts for two and a half to three years, becoming a general psychiatrist is already, in itself, an effortful accomplishment. For those willing to continue on the road to become a child psychiatrist, there are some important challenges that need to be taken into consideration while transitioning from one training scheme to another (Table 28.3).

Table 28.2 Training in child psychiatry

Modality	Training characteristics
Traditional training	Traditional training in child psychiatry occurs after 2–4 years of training in general psychiatry and lasts 1–2 years, depending on the country in which it takes place.
Integrated training	Integrated training is the combination of general psychiatry and child and adolescent psychiatry. The schemes that follow this approach meet the requirements for training residency education for both general and child psychiatry and usually last 5–6 years.
Triple board	Triple board training consists of a sequence of paediatrics, general psychiatry, and child and adolescent psychiatry, with a total duration of 5 years. It was initiated in the USA in 1985, and was approved throughout the country in 1992, but still has few training centres. The aim of this type of formation was to train professionals with expertise in the three areas faster than in the traditional way.
Academic integrated training	This training integrates general and child psychiatry with training in the basic developmental sciences in order to increase the number and quality of child and adolescent psychiatrists in research careers.

Source data from: Martin A, Volkmar FR, Lewis M. Lewis's Child and Adolescent Psychiatry. Copyright (2007) Wolters Kluwer Health

Table 28.3 Challenges in transitioning from general psychiatry to child psychiatry

Challenge	Description
Initiation	When the resident reaches child psychiatry residency, he or she has already had at least three periods of initiation: medical school, internship, and general psychiatry specialistic training. Entering child psychiatry can generate the fear of losing the knowledge acquired in general psychiatry, besides having to cope with the relative frustration of starting from scratch again, as a beginner.
New skills	Trainees need to use non-verbal language, deal with patients at very different stages of development, and manage behaviours with patients who are much less able to deal with concepts and cognitive abilities than adults. They also need to be able to understand the complexity of generation boundaries, loyalties, and complex countertransferences; undo actions of 'incompetent' parents; and still serve as the authority for families, schools, judges, and social services. All these new skills are required early in training, adding difficulty during the transition.
Integrated approach	It is necessary to integrate the different groups that interact with the child, such as parents and family, caregivers, teachers, paediatricians and other medical specialists, psychologists, pedagogues, and other allied professionals. Usually, the child psychiatrist acts like a maestro, bringing together and organizing all the efforts to help the child, and requiring diplomatic and strategic competencies in order to act effectively in the best interest of the child.
Multi-theory approach	Child psychiatric practice requires the integration of different theoretical fields such as child development, phenomenological psychiatry, genetics, family therapy, cognitive behavioural therapy, psychodynamic understanding, neurosciences, epidemiology, and paediatric psychopharmacology. This approach emphasizes the integration of such different aspects within training.

Source data from: Martin A, Volkmar FR, Lewis M. Lewis's Child and Adolescent Psychiatry. Copyright (2007) Wolters Kluwer Health

Opportunities in child psychiatry

The job opportunities for the child psychiatrist are as rich as the complexity of the models that he or she has to integrate during daily practice. Many opportunities arise from the training of the child psychiatrist. In fact, after finishing training, the child psychiatrist can work in private practice, in general hospitals (either in a general outpatient clinic or in a specialized clinic), or as a paediatric consultant. Furthermore, the professional may become responsible for the supervision of psychiatric cases undertaken in community services, helping family physicians with discussion of cases and guidance on pharmacotherapy. We have listed and described the job settings available for child psychiatrists in Table 28.4, and their possible career focuses in Table 28.5.

Table 28.4 Child psychiatry job settings

Job setting	Description
Private practice	The child psychiatrist with his or her own private practice serves patients who seek help, either charging his honoraria directly or receiving it from health insurance companies. Often, child psychiatrists will team up with psychologists, specialized psychotherapists, and other relevant disciplines.
General outpatient clinics	In a general outpatient clinic, the child psychiatrist can assist patients with all sorts of disorders and mental health problems. The clinic will usually be held within a general health facility such as a hospital or a referral clinic.
Specialized outpatient clinics	Specialized outpatient clinics are usually dedicated to the assessment, diagnosis, and treatment of a specific disorder. Many specialized outpatient clinics are also dedicated to research in the specific disorder and often are held within university hospitals, mixing clinical assistance and clinical research.
Psychiatric inpatient units	Child psychiatrists are the key professionals to assist hospitalized patients in child psychiatric units. Such inpatient units can be located either in a general hospital or in psychiatric hospitals.
Paediatric inpatient unit consultation	The child psychiatrist conducts consultations at a paediatric unit when the child has a co-morbid psychiatric disorder or when there is suspicion that someone in the family has a psychiatric disorder that can threaten the physical health of the child (e.g. Münchausen's syndrome by proxy).
Community-based mental health centres	The child psychiatrist can either work within a community-based mental health team as a team leader or as a clinician, or can also act as a consultant for family physicians who are struggling with difficult psychiatric cases in the community. Nowadays, the consultation can also be done through telemedicine technology.
School consultation	When out of the home, children spend most of their time in school. Schools are frequently the environment in which many of the psychiatric symptoms will be spotted for the first time. It is also the place where bullying usually happens and where ADHD causes academic burden. Therefore, it is during a school consultation that the child psychiatrist is able to make preventive and environmental adjustments at the same time as helping his or her referred patient and also other students.
Forensic consultation	Child psychiatrists are often called to assist the judge in a judicial case involving a child. Forensic consultation may also be necessary in cases of legal dispute over a child in separated families, when child abuse has been perpetrated by one of the family members, and when the child or the adolescent is the offender.

(*continued*)

Table 28.4 (continued) Child psychiatry job settings

Job setting	Description
Universities	Child psychiatrists work in universities as professors in both general psychiatry and child and adolescent psychiatry departments. Occasionally, they can also act in other departments such as paediatrics, or even in the areas of education or psychology, depending on their specific training.
Research centres	Neuroscience research centres can hire child psychiatrists who possess a background in academic research and can therefore participate in the different areas of child psychiatry research (see also Table 28.7 for more details).
Government facilities	Child psychiatrists work within the government, either planning mental health policies or acting as advocates for the improvement of child psychiatric care and of mental health prevention policies and actions.

Table 28.5 Career focuses for the child psychiatrist

Career focus	Description
Broad-sense clinical practice	The child psychiatrist can use all the spectrum of therapeutic approaches, choosing them according to the needs of each patient and not being restricted to only one approach, such as psychopharmacology (e.g. using psychostimulants for ADHD, while only a psychotherapeutic approach is provided, for a child struggling academically due to emotional/psychological difficulties but not with a diagnosis of ADHD).
Psychopharmacology-centred clinical practice	In areas where there are many other skilled professionals using psychotherapeutic approaches, it is easier for the child psychiatrist to specialize in the psychopharmacological approach. This might also be a fulfilling choice within the profession.
Psychotherapeutic-centred clinical practice	Some child psychiatrists might also choose to focus predominantly on one specific type of psychotherapy, depending on aptitude, interest, and background. The main types of psychotherapy are evidence-based and include cognitive behavioural therapy, interpersonal psychotherapy, and systemic therapy (family therapy) or more traditional ones, like psychodynamic psychotherapy.
Child and adult psychiatry	Many child psychiatrists choose to continue seeing adult patients, instead of only focusing on children.
Academic	The academic focus happens when a child psychiatrist becomes a university professor of child and adolescent psychiatry, psychiatry, or a related field. An academic life can be time-consuming, but it is not incompatible with seeing patients. Many child psychiatrists are able to manage both focuses simultaneously, although it might be laborious and overwhelming, at times.

(continued)

Table 28.5 (continued) Career focuses for the child psychiatrist

Career focus	Description
Research	In some countries, child psychiatrists can choose to focus their efforts only in research, but in others, they need to combine research with clinical activities, due to the difficulties in funding research. This division can sometimes be difficult and may even become a source of problems, but many colleagues are successful in managing both areas simultaneously.
Political advocacy	The political work in defence of children's mental health is a challenging task. Child psychiatry needs advocates within governmental structures, and child psychiatrists, along with the families of patients, often perform that task. Structured institutions that help political advocacy are either professional associations (like AACAP and IACAPAP) or associations of families of patients with a specific disorder (like the National Autism Association). Child psychiatrists who become politicians can have this as their sole career focus, but most blend advocacy with their other activities.

Challenges in child psychiatry

Despite the several aforementioned attractive characteristics of the field of child psychiatry, it also holds many challenges. Future child psychiatrists have to be aware of stigma, so that they can be better prepared to deal with it. Accepting the idea that one's child has a mental health problem and taking them to see a psychiatrist is very often an extremely difficult situation for parents. Whenever parents have preconceived ideas about psychiatry, or child psychiatry, the situation becomes even harder. Besides parental stigma, there are other challenges that need attention, listed in Table 28.6.

Table 28.6 Challenges of child psychiatry

Challenge	Description
Parental stigma	Parental stigma happens when the child's parents show disapproval of or discontent with their child, due to the existence of a psychiatric disorder. This often presents in a subtle or veiled manner, but is always highly detrimental for the child's development. Parental stigma interferes directly with the evaluation and treatment of the child, as parents end up not seeking the help of a child psychiatrist.
Stigma in school	Stigma in the school environment is also highly detrimental to the healthy development of children. It can be veiled or explicit, and can be perpetrated by peers and, unfortunately, also by unprepared teachers. The overload that many teachers face in their daily routine impairs their ability to cope with children who show psychiatric symptoms that disturb the normal course of their classes. School approaches with children and teachers, carried out by the child psychiatrist, are extremely helpful because they may dissipate the tension and offer information on how to deal with the appearance of psychiatric symptoms in class.

(*continued*)

Table 28.6 (continued) Challenges of child psychiatry

Challenge	Description
Stigma within medicine	Unfortunately, stigma during the course of medical school also occurs. Often, professors of other specialties argue that psychiatry and, even more so child psychiatry, lacks objectivity and therefore does not deserve much attention. There are still medical school curricula that do not properly expose students to the practice of child psychiatry; therefore, students do not develop interest for the area.
Lack of professionals	Another challenge of child psychiatry is the lack of professionals, both in developing and developed countries. It is thought that the stigma attached to psychiatric disorders, the stigma towards the profession by medical colleagues in other specialties, the lack of opportunities for exposure to child psychiatry during medical school, and training in general psychiatry may represent some of the reasons that lead to this phenomenon.

Adapted from Psychiatr Clin North Am., 32(1), McCarthy M, Abenojar J, Anders TF. Child and adolescent psychiatry for the future: challenges and opportunities, p. 213–26. Copyright (2009) with permission from Elsevier

Research in child psychiatry

Another area that needs attention for future child psychiatrists is that of research. Child psychiatry has much to gain from the discoveries made by current global efforts to search for understanding of the developing brain. The growing number of publications in neuroimaging, the increasing capacity of analysis of DNA, and growing global neuroscientific collaboration make this field a fertile ground for young researchers. Those future child psychiatrists who have interest in a scientific career will certainly find satisfaction and professional challenge in child psychiatry research, since there is still much to be discovered about the brain and its dysfunctions. Hopefully, in the future, our therapeutical armamentarium will be more specific, individualized, faster, and with fewer side-effects.[9] The areas that need further development in child psychiatry research are summarized in Table 28.7.

Table 28.7 Areas of research in child psychiatry

Area	Description
Epidemiology	Epidemiological research of child psychiatric disorders is important worldwide in order to accurately map what is most troubling our youth, so that the preventive and therapeutic efforts can be best guided and become more effective.
Genetics	Gene–environment interaction mechanisms are of great importance and need constant attention and focus because they mediate the onset of child psychiatric disorders and the environmental factors (trauma, smoking, food additives, etc.).

(continued)

Table 28.7 (continued) Areas of research in child psychiatry

Area	Description
Neuroscience	Many different areas within neuroscience can be of extreme value for the field of child psychiatry. Considering the worldwide efforts to understand the brain, neuroscience is an umbrella category that holds advances that go from the discoveries in neuronal mechanisms made by novel technologies (e.g. optogenetics[10]) to the exploration of the animal connectome as a model for the future study of the human one.[11]
Neuroimaging	Neuroimaging approaches will also aid the quest for understanding of the normal and the disordered brain, applying minimally or non-invasive techniques to study the structure and function of children's brains.
Neuropsychology	Neuropsychology within child psychiatry also needs further development because it is an important tool to aid assessment of psychological processes and behaviours related to the disorders, and development of adequate treatments.
Psychopharmacology	Studies in psychopharmacology are always necessary as most current usage is still based on studies done with adults. Hopefully, in the future, we will be able to guide our prescription based on individual genomic knowledge, tailoring psychopharmacological treatments to each individual.
Psychotherapy	Evidence-based research with the different types of psychotherapy is mandatory to make the choice of modality more specific and effective.

Conclusions

Child psychiatry is an area of great opportunities and challenges. The opportunity to work with children and see their development being recovered with the various available therapeutic approaches is a source of great reward and fosters pleasure and enthusiasm in daily work. Working with families with children and adolescents with psychiatric disorders can be very difficult, but to be able to make them appreciate their improvement may represent an immeasurable reward. Scientific innovation and other potential future developments make us eager for the results of new studies and new discoveries. Just as the development of a child highlights new things every day, child psychiatry can also be seen in the same way, with great attractions and novelties, but also with difficult moments that require a considerable ability to cope, understand, and act. The daily practice of child psychiatry should be chosen by the early career psychiatrist based on their passion for child development, interest in novelty, and desire for constant improvement, because our children always deserve the best of us.

References

1 **Gerhard U-J, Schönberg A, Blanz B**. Johannes Trüper—mediator between child and adolescent psychiatry and pedagogy. *Z Kinder Jugendpsychiatr Psychother* 2008; **36**(1):55–63.

2 **Neumärker KJ**. Leo Kanner: his years in Berlin, 1906–24. The roots of autistic disorder. *Hist Psychiatry* 2003; **14**(54:2):205–18.

3 **Baumeister AA, Henderson K, Pow JL, Advokat C**. The early history of the neuroscience of attention-deficit/hyperactivity disorder. *J Hist Neurosci* 2012; **21**(3):263–79.

4 **Lange KW, Reichl S, Lange KM, Tucha L, Tucha O**. The history of attention deficit hyperactivity disorder. *Atten Def Hyp Disord* 2010; **2**(4):241–55.

5 **Werry JS**. An overview of pediatric psychopharmacology. *J Am Acad Child Psychiatry* 1982; **21**(1):3–9.

6 **Moraes C, Abujadi C, Ciasca SM**. Brazilian child and adolescent psychiatrists task force. *Revista Brasileira de Psiquiatria* 2008; **30**(3):294–5.

7 **Kim WJ**, American Academy of Child and Adolescent Psychiatry's Task Force on Workforce Needs. Child and adolescent psychiatry workforce: a critical shortage and national challenge. *Acad Psychiatry* 2003; **27**(4):277–82.

8 **Kessler RC, Berglund P, Demler O**. Lifetime prevalence and age-of-onset distributions of DSM-IV disorders in the National Comorbidity Survey Replication. *Arch Gen Psychiatry* 2005; **62**(6):593–602.

9 **Anders TF**. Child and adolescent psychiatry: the next 10 years. *Psychiatric Times*. Available at: http://www.psychiatrictimes.com/articles/child-and-adolescent-psychiatry-next-10-years [accessed 22 June 2014].

10 **Touriño C, Eban-Rothschild A, de Lecea L**. Optogenetics in psychiatric diseases. *Curr Opin Neurobiol* 2013; **23**(3):430–5.

11 **Oh SW, Harris JA, Ng L, et al**. A mesoscale connectome of the mouse brain. *Nature* 2014; **508**(7495):207–14.

Chapter 29

Liaison psychiatry—is it possible?

Silvia Ferrari, Annegret Dreher, Giorgio Mattei, and Albert Diefenbacher

Introduction

Liaison psychiatry, also known as consultation–liaison psychiatry (CLP), psycho-somatic medicine, or psychiatry of the medically ill, is a branch of psychiatry oper-ating at the interface of the somatic disciplines and psychiatry. It is dedicated to the care (and related training and research activities) of patients with medical–psychiatric co-morbidities. Despite this operative definition, CLP works in the conceptual and practical framework of the biopsychosocial paradigm, according to which the ten-dency to split somatic and psychosocial disorders and dysfunctions should be avoided, favouring a holistic approach to illness and well-being.[1]

CLP operates in a demanding area of contemporary medicine. This is due to epi-demiological factors (i.e. the high prevalence of somatization and so-called func-tional conditions, with their related massive impact on healthcare costs) and other reasons. The latter include healthcare needs of complex patients, difficulties in the doctor–patient relationship or in ward teamwork, medico-legal and ethical con-troversies, and the healthcare of care givers. The aim of this chapter is to provide practical indications on the most common clinical scenarios involving consulta-tion–liaison activities and basic skills in psychiatry.

Aim, historical development, and clinical settings

There is worldwide consensus on the use of the term 'consultation–liaison psychiatry' (the UK being an exception, using the term 'liaison psychiatry'). In the USA, this area of psychiatry was recognized formally as a subspecialty by the American Board of Med-ical Specialties in 2003, and is referred to by the name of psychosomatic medicine.[2] In Europe, similar acknowledgments were obtained in Switzerland, the Netherlands, and, though somewhat differently, in Germany.[3]

The development of CLP services was enabled by the integration of psychiatric de-partments in general hospitals (GH). CLP provides an opportunity to promote integra-tion of psychiatry into the other medical specialties.

Within the context of mere *consultation*, the psychiatrist is called ('upon demand') by colleagues of the somatic disciplines, to provide professional advice on diagnostics or for a particular treatment. The French term *liaison* refers to 'joining' or 'binding': in a *liaison* model, psychiatrists intermingle with other disciplines in joint patient care and are directly involved in the treatment of patients with psychiatric co-morbidity without exclusively operating at the request of the consultees.

Research has shown that patients with somatic illnesses, especially those suffering from chronic diseases, are at 1.5–2 times higher risk of developing a psychiatric co-morbidity in comparison with the rest of society.[4] Desan and colleagues[5] reported that over 50% of patients admitted to the GH had mental health needs, these being, most commonly, substance abuse (43%), mood/anxiety disorders (30%), psychotic disorders (13%), suicidal attempt/ideation (7%), and delirium/dementia (7%). Despite this, only about 3% of GH patients are referred to the psychiatrist,[6] with a European average of 1.4%.[7] Failure to recognize or address these needs may result in a prolonged length of hospital stay, increased healthcare costs, poorer outcomes (due to a higher number of diagnostic procedures, more complex drug regimens, more days off from work), and inappropriate admissions to accident and emergency departments.[8] Desan et al.[5] estimated an annual saving of up to $237,286 if these mental health needs are adequately addressed by a qualified CLP service.

Reasons for referral

Reasons for referral to psychiatry can be grouped into four main categories,[9] described in Table 29.1. While the first three reasons may be problematic and sometimes stem out of stigmatizing attitudes, the fourth situation is the most developed and favourable, being the result of a specific diagnostic reasoning or clinical protocol, and should be encouraged and reinforced by training activities.

The most common clinical reasons for referral to psychiatry are adjustment disorders and emotional disorders, including medically unexplained physical symptoms (the SAD triad: depression, anxiety, and somatization); behavioural disturbances; and delirium. Referrals for attempted suicide and risk of self-harm behaviours are less frequent. Finally, there may be specific reasons, within pre-agreed clinical protocols or research collaborations (e.g. bariatric surgery, interferon therapy, transplants), that mirror special activities of the local GH. Most psychiatric referrals come from medical

Table 29.1 Reasons for psychiatric referral

1. Generic, unspecified referral; one among all the other referrals of the diagnostic pathway

2. 'Magical' referral, at the end of a long diagnostic pathway which has not revealed the presence of a medical disease: psychiatric referral as *extrema ratio*

3. Referral for custody-control reasons, for 'difficult' patients (behavioural problems, not necessarily of psychiatric pertinence)

4. Specified referral, if the presence of a psychiatric disorder has been suspected by the ward physician, or when referral has screening purposes ('referral by contract', e.g. preliminary to organ transplantation or bariatric surgery)

Reproduced from Bonaviri G, Giordano PL, eds. Proceedings from the XL National Congress of the Italian Society of Psychiatry (Lo psichiatra e i suoi pazienti. Trasformazioni culturali in psichiatria) in Rigatelli M, Cavicchioli C. Ten suggestions for a CLP service in the general hospital (Dieci proposte per un servizio di consulenza psichiatrica in ospedale generale), p. 235–49, Copyright (1997).

wards (50–75%), while surgery accounts for another 15–20%. Referred patients are more often females and elderly. Outcomes of the psychiatric assessment are mostly diagnoses of affective and adjustment disorders, and organic psychoses, and psychotropic drugs are usually prescribed. Referral back is mostly to the GP, with admission to a psychiatric ward in around 10% of cases.[10]

The procedure of consultation

An important factor complicating the diagnosis of psychiatric co-morbidities in the GH setting is overlapping symptoms of somatic diseases. For example, fatigue caused by carcinosis can resemble a lack of motivation or drive caused by depression. Relationships vary: somatic illnesses may cause psychiatric symptoms (e.g. hypothyroidism causing depressive symptoms), while in other cases, somatic and psychiatric morbidity coexist without influencing each other too much. On the other hand, even subsyndromal psychiatric disorders can substantially influence the course of an illness.[11]

Additionally, physicians of other medical specialties are often unspecific and imprecise in their referral, leaving the CL psychiatrist with a wide array of questions to be answered within a limited amount of time and uncertainty as to whether the indication for a consultation arises in response to the needs of the patient or the treating team. Practical challenges also include a brief and unpredictable length of stay, and a lack of privacy. Yet, it is essential to establish a therapeutic alliance quickly and effectively.

Although the psychiatric consultation mainly relies on the clinical interview, the facts mentioned explain why CL interventions characteristically begin before meeting the patient. The first step consists of clarifying the reason for referral, identifying explicit and implicit reasons if necessary. Often, certain aspects of the problem can be solved at this early stage. For example, simple adjustments in the hospital ward setting may help to calm down geriatric patients in a state of agitation caused by numerous environmental changes. Early on in the consultation process, the CL psychiatrist should determine the time-span of the development of the psychopathological symptoms. Did the symptoms develop acutely or over a longer period of time? Information needs to be ascertained from interviewing the patient, the involved care givers, relatives, and physicians.

A well-structured 'assessment plan', along the following lines (see also Table 29.2), can serve as a 'road map' for the CL psychiatrist in the consultation process. During the process of exploration with the patient, obeying certain simple bedside manners (such as sitting down, smiling at the patient, shaking hands) can be simple but effective tools in establishing a more relaxed atmosphere and reducing interpersonal distance. Finding out the patient's most immediate concerns may help if the patient is preoccupied with an undisclosed fear or concern. Sometimes, doing something tangible for the patient, such as offering food or adjusting a pillow, can convey compassion and is much appreciated.

At the end of the consultation, the CL psychiatrist should integrate contributing psychosocial factors and formulate a diagnosis, as well as treatment and management recommendations including additional laboratory and radiological examinations, and psychological therapy as well as pharmacotherapy.

Table 29.2 Assessment plan for consultation (modified from Leentjens et al.[12])

Step	Activity
1	Obtaining presenting complaint and relevant history
2	Obtaining relevant past and family psychiatric history
3	Reviewing history and course of the current medical or surgical illness including treatment response and impact on functioning
4	Obtaining relevant past medical and surgical history
5	Assessing coping mechanisms and other psychological reactions to the medical or surgical condition
6	Assessing current medication, allergies, and substance use
7	Performing a mental status examination including cognitive examination and additional clinometric evaluation
8	Assessing relevant social considerations: is emotional support available?
9	Assessing decision-making capacity, if necessary

The why, what, and how of consultation–liaison psychiatry

The why of CLP

Box 29.1 summarizes some of the expected beneficial indirect effects of CLP activity, in addition to direct effects on morbidity, disability, and quality of life of patients and relatives. While the latter demonstrate the visible 'added value' of CLP activity, the outlined indirect effects should not be forgotten, especially as part of discussions with hospital administrations and healthcare planners regarding the advantages and disadvantages of establishing CLP services in a given hospital regional healthcare system.

Box 29.1 Why is CLP activity important, beyond direct patient care?

- Contributes to optimization of healthcare costs, via effects on length of hospital stay, number of admissions to emergency department, risk of readmission after discharge, number of diagnostics and consultations, and so on—all of which might be decreased [13]
- Relationship and integration of different areas of medicine, operationalization of biopsychosocial paradigm
- Fight to end stigma and neglect of medical health of the mentally ill

The what of CLP

The three specific clinical targets of CLP are summarized in Table 29.3 and are: medical–psychiatric co-morbidity, including coexisting psychiatric and non-psychiatric disorders affecting reciprocally; the once-called 'psychosomatic' disorders, including medically unexplained physical symptoms and functional disorders; and finally, liaison activities addressed to medical workers and teams.

To address these three targets, different models of liaison were conceived over time and adapted for adoption outside of the hospital, in primary care, and/or in the GH (Table 29.4). Some models are specific to the primary care clinical context (e.g. the 'shifted outpatient clinic' with a mental health professional/team periodically available at the primary care clinic for referral of selected cases), others are designed both for the GH and primary care (the traditional consultation–liaison model, or the more advanced integrated team model).

When performing CL activities, psychiatrists are often responsible for the appropriate causal attribution of either medical symptoms to underlying psychiatric conditions or psychiatric symptoms to underlying medical conditions. Both tasks may be tricky and demanding. Tables 29.6 and 29.7 list frequent clinically relevant syndromes, respectively. Medical symptoms (Table 29.5) are, by definition, the almost exclusive presentation of somatic symptom disorder (the new DSM-5 definition of the previous somatization disorder[14]) or functional neurological symptom disorder (the new DSM-5 definition of the previous conversion disorder[14]); otherwise, anxiety may very often express itself somatically (e.g. in panic attacks or in illness anxiety disorder). Internal medical conditions such as hypo-/hyperthyroidism or Addison's/Cushing's syndrome are well-known for their accompanying psychiatric symptomatology, which interestingly supports recent findings of a shared pathogenesis related to immunological dysfunctions (further examples are presented in Table 29.6).

Table 29.3 The three specific clinical targets of CLP

1. Medical–psychiatric co-morbidity	◆ Prevalently medical disorders presenting with psychiatric symptoms (e.g. delirium) or iatrogenic psychiatric symptoms (e.g. interferon, corticosteroids)
	◆ Medical disorders complicated by the onset or the pre-existence of a psychiatric disorder (e.g. depressive disorder in diabetes, or personality disorders affecting compliance in medically complex patients)
	◆ Prevalently psychiatric disorders presenting with medical symptoms or consequences (e.g. effects of suicidal attempts, eating disorders, substance-abuse related disorders)
2. 'Psychosomatic' disorders	A wide range of situations including medically unexplained physical symptoms (MUPS) and other *functional* disorders such as fibromyalgia, irritable bowel syndrome, chronic fatigue syndrome, etc.
3. Liaison activity addressed to other colleagues or teams	Conflicts in doctor–patient/relative relationship, medico-legal and ethical controversies (e.g. concerning incapacity or diminished responsibility, informed consent), integrated clinical procedures, etc.

Table 29.4 Different models of CLP provision

1. The 'community mental health team' model (for primary care)	◆ Aims at making multidisciplinary mental health treatment more widely available in the community
	◆ The team carries out a multidisciplinary approach to care in the primary care setting
	◆ Dedicated to address minor emotional disorders, such as mild anxiety or depressive disorders
	◆ The 'primary (level of) care' is differentiated from 'psychiatric secondary care' (the community mental health centre, addressing more complex/severe/specific psychiatric conditions)
2. The 'shifted outpatient clinic' (for primary care)	◆ The psychiatrist attends a certain primary care health centre (e.g. a GP's clinic) periodically, for first/occasional referrals or follow-up visits
	◆ May work independently of the GP
	◆ Based in primary care, yet has much in common with hospital outpatient services
	◆ Provides informal consultation–liaison service to the GPs and other primary care workers
3. The 'attached mental health professional' model (for primary care)	◆ Professionals other than psychiatrists (e.g. community psychiatric nurses, clinical psychologists, counsellors, social workers), employed by secondary care (e.g. hospitals) yet 'attached' to primary care services
	◆ Such professionals work with patients affected by minor anxiety or depressive disorders, or as consultants for GPs and other primary care workers
4. The 'consultation–liaison' model (for primary care and GH)	◆ Aims at reducing referrals for milder disorders
	◆ Encourages referrals of severe psychiatric disorders to the psychiatrist
	◆ Aims at enhancing and improving physicians' autonomous ability in detection and management of mental illness
	◆ Regular face-to-face contact between the psychiatrist and referring physicians, also to differentiate patients to be referred to secondary care from those to be treated by the primary care team
	◆ When referral is decided and takes place, feedback is provided to the primary care team

(*continued*)

Table 29.4 (continued) Different models of CLP provision

5. The 'integrated care' approach (for primary care and GH)	◆ Develops the 'consultation–liaison' model, moving from a multidisciplinary model to a transdisciplinary
	◆ Addresses physical and psychiatric multi-morbidity, by acknowledging that it is not sufficient to bring collaborating professionals together; rather, it is necessary to develop a theoretical framework of collaboration
	◆ Promotes integration of care, rather than integrated care by a single physician
	◆ Acknowledges complexity and helps other physicians to work with it

Source data from: *Br J Psychiatry*, 170, Gask L, Sibbald B, Creed F. Evaluating models of working at the interface between mental health services and primary care, p. 6–11, Copyright (1997) Royal College of Psychiatrists; *Aust N Z J Psychiatry*, 43, Smith GC. From consultation–liaison psychiatry to integrated care for multiple and complex needs, p. 1–12, Copyright (2009) SAGE Publications.

Table 29.5 Medical presentations of psychiatric disorders

Medical sign and symptoms	Disorder
◆ Presence of one or more somatic symptoms that are distressing or result in significant disruption of daily life	Somatic symptom disorder
◆ Presence of excessive thoughts, feelings, or behaviours related to the somatic symptoms or associated health concerns	
◆ The symptomatic state is persistent (more than 6 months)	
◆ Pain is the predominant somatic symptom that is distressing or results in significant disruption of daily life	Somatic symptom disorder with predominant pain ('Pain disorder' in the DSM-IV-TR)
◆ Presence of excessive thoughts, feelings, or behaviours related to pain or associated health concerns	
◆ The symptomatic state is persistent (more than 6 months)	
◆ Presence of one or more symptoms of altered voluntary motor or sensory function (weakness; paralysis; tremor; dystonic movement; myoclonus; gait disorder; swallowing; impaired speech such as dysphonia or slurred speech; seizures; anaesthesia or sensory loss; visual, olfactory, hearing disturbance or other special sensory symptoms; mixed symptoms)	Functional neurological symptom disorder (conversion disorder)
◆ Clinical findings provide clinical evidence of incompatibility between the symptom and recognized neurological or medical conditions	
◆ The symptom or deficit is not better explained by another medical or mental disorder	
◆ The symptom or deficit causes clinically significant distress or impairment in social, occupational, or other important areas of functioning or warrants medical evaluation	

(*continued*)

Table 29.5 (continued) Medical presentations of psychiatric disorders

Medical sign and symptoms	Disorder
◆ Preoccupation with having or acquiring a serious illness	Illness anxiety disorder
◆ Somatic symptoms are not present or, if present, are only mild in intensity; if another medical condition is present or there is a high risk for developing a medical condition, the preoccupation is clearly excessive	
◆ There is a high level of anxiety about health, and the individual is easily alarmed about personal health status	
◆ The individual performs excessive health-related behaviours or exhibits maladaptive avoidance (e.g. avoids doctors, check-up visits, and hospitals)	
◆ Illness preoccupation has been present for at least 6 months, but the specific illness that is feared may change over that period of time	
◆ The illness-related preoccupation is not better explained by another mental disorder	
◆ A medical symptom or condition (other than a mental disorder) is present	Psychological factors affecting other medical conditions
◆ Psychological or behavioural factors adversely affect the medical condition (e.g. determining poor adherence to the medications) and are not better explained by another mental disorder	
◆ Falsification of physical or psychological signs or symptoms, or induction of injury or disease, associated with identified deception	Factitious disorder (may be imposed on another, as well)
◆ The individual presents himself or herself to others as ill, impaired, or injured	
◆ The deceptive behaviour is evident even in the absence of obvious external rewards	
◆ The behaviour is not better explained by another mental disorder	

Source data from: American Psychiatric Association. *Diagnostic and statistical manual of mental disorders, fifth edition*. Copyright (2013) American Psychiatric Association.

Table 29.6 Psychiatric presentations of medical disorders

Psychiatric signs and symptoms	Disorder
Irritability, insomnia, psychosis, sense of sudden death	Hyperthyroidism
Psychomotor retardation, apathy, personality changes, paranoia, hallucinations, drowsiness, affective flattening	Hypothyroidism
Anxiety, confusion, agitation, tremors, restlessness, seizures	Hypoglycaemia
Anxiety, agitation, delirium, seizures	Hyperglycaemia

(continued)

Table 29.6 (continued) Psychiatric presentations of medical disorders

Psychiatric signs and symptoms	Disorder
Confusion, lethargy, stupor, seizure, coma, personality changes	Hyponatraemia
Depression, lethargy, psychosis, delirium	Addison's disease (adrenocortical insufficiency)
Depression, insomnia, mood lability, mania and euphoria, psychosis, delirium	Cushing's disease
Depression, paranoia, confusion	Hyperparathyroidism
Anxiety, agitation, confusion, depression, memory impairment	Hypoparathyroidism
Anxiety, anxious apprehension, panic attacks	Pheochromocytoma
Personality changes	Brain neoplasms
Mood changes, irritability, jocosity, memory impairment, aphasia, seizures, delirium, impaired judgement	Tumours affecting the frontal lobe of the brain
Aura, seizures, visual hallucinations	Tumours affecting the occipital lobe of the brain
Confusion, personality changes, memory impairment, seizures	Traumatic brain injury
Anxiety, euphoria, mania	Multiple sclerosis
Dissociation, confusion, psychosis, catatonia, aggressiveness, odd behaviour	Epilepsy
Cognitive impairment, disinhibition, depression, euphoria	Hepatic encephalopathy
Depression, agitation, visual hallucinations, paranoia	Acute intermittent porphyria
Personality changes, dementia, depression, mutacism, psychosis	HIV/AIDS
Depression, anhedonia, apathy, asthenia	Pancreatic neoplasms
Depression, psychosis, delirium, hallucination	Systemic lupus eryithematosus
Confusion, confabulation, language impairment, impaired concentration	B1 vitamin (thiamine) deficiency (beriberi)
Confusion, irritability, insomnia, memory impairment, depression, psychosis, dementia	B3 vitamin (niacinamide) deficiency (pellagra)
Apathy, irritability, memory impairment, seizures	B6 vitamin (pyridoxine) deficiency
Irritability, confusion, psychosis, dementia	B12 vitamin (cobalamin) deficiency
Agitation, paranoia, psychosis	Anti-NMDA encephalitis

Table adapted from Maurice Martin MD in Sadock BJ, Sadock VA. Kaplan and Sadock's *Pocket Handbook of Clinical Psychiatry*. Copyright (2010), with permission from Wolters Kluwer Health.

The how of CLP

Liaison psychiatry work requires a mix of skills including teamwork, partnership in working with other medical disciplines, skills of generic assessment of psychiatric problems, psychological management, knowledge of psychopharmacology, and a certain amount of clinical leadership. Diefenbacher and Strain[15] suggest that CL psychiatrists might even be forced to act less like physicians evaluating and treating specific patients, and to assume instead the role of 'case managers' (referring patients to psychiatric inpatient units and outpatient psychiatric follow-up), which suggests a move away from pure consultation to a liaison model. Kathol and colleagues[16] address a number of potential limitations of CLP services and provide suggestions for improvement (Table 29.7).

Regarding the interface between psychiatry and the somatic disciplines, 'soft skills' are a crucial element in the process of consultation. As previously stated, practical challenges to developing and maintaining a therapeutic relationship include a brief and unpredictable length of stay, a lack of privacy, and ambiguity as to whether the consultation arises in response to the needs of the inpatient, a family member, or the treating team. Hence, developing clear goals of intervention can be very difficult. Working in the role of a 'case manager' and an 'advocate' for the patient could mean that the CL psychiatrist has to insist on psychological aspects of care, if these are in danger of being disregarded. Understanding the global aspects of referral in the relationship between

Table 29.7 CLP services: main limitations and strategy for improvement

Main limitations	Suggestions for improvement
◆ Poor co-ordination with services provided by other mental health professionals such as psychiatric nurses and psychologists	◆ Develop proactive case finding
	◆ Adequate consultation team staffing to meet clinical demands
◆ Ineffective use of time	◆ Admission screening for the top 5% with 'red flags' for complexity
◆ Reactive involvement with patients, i.e. based on referral by non-psychiatric physicians	◆ Use of complexity assessment tools to quantify the level of complexity
◆ Referral of only a small percentage of patients admitted to the GH (0.5–3%)	◆ Implement preventive or active identification programmes such as delirium prevention programmes or screening for alcohol abuse
◆ Frequent inappropriate referral	
◆ Crisis-oriented (i.e. few preventive and/or active identification programmes are implemented, such as delirium prevention and proactive complex case finding)	◆ Improve communications among colleagues, (mental) healthcare professionals, and services
◆ Assessments performed late in hospitalization	◆ Regular follow-up throughout the hospital stay until symptom stabilization or maximum benefit is achieved
◆ Few follow-up visits	

physician, staff, and patients can be essential in the process of consultation. It is important to develop a feeling for aspects of the referral process which might not be overtly expressed by the consultee.

Table 29.8 offers some practical hints, including paying attention to the way we speak and write to colleagues, and investing time in developing integrated procedures, the

Table 29.8 Obstacles and indications for improving co-operation between co-workers

Obstacle	Action/solution
Stigma and prejudices	Organize dedicated seminars or round-table at local institutions
	Take some time at the end of the referral to explain to doctors and nurses who the patient is, and who the person is behind the patient
	Provide gentle reproach for stigmatizing attitudes of colleagues, to help increase self-awareness
	Be aware of your own stigmatizing attitudes
Language	Avoid too technical, abstract, or idiosyncratic expressions in favour of more user-friendly terms, but without sacrificing completeness and the need to convey the sense of complexity
Lack of/fear of basic clinical notions in reciprocal fields of competence	Keep updated, be curious, ask about things you are not familiar with (usually colleagues are happy to give you a little lecture!)
Lack of familiarity (with persons, procedures, etc.)	Let your colleagues know you; provide indications on how to find you (within the terms of your professional availability)
	Take some time to explain the appropriate procedures of referral to doctors *and* nurses
	Do not change procedures too often and clearly advertise any change
Excessive turnover of professionals	Establish a standardized procedure for transmission of information when colleagues move away and new others come
Previous negative experiences (during training and after)	Be aware that there might be a prejudice affecting your judgement, and give new people and new situations a chance
	Express your concerns as openly as possible, and make simple and clear suggestions to prevent bad things happening again
Pressure in clinical practice due to shortness of time and resources	Try and assume your colleagues' point of view, and ask them to do the same
	Be creative!
Fear of reciprocal manipulation (i.e. faking of severity to get urgent referrals)	Openly address your concern
	Do not manipulate yourself
	Take some time to 'educate' your colleagues about respecting you
Little time for face-to-face discussions on problems	Do not postpone discussions, as they nearly always prevent future waste of time

regular application of which may have long-term educational effects on the profession and professionalism. A CL psychiatrist should have skills in dealing with conflicts between physicians, which are a frequent obstacle to effective healthcare in many different clinical settings and occur almost exclusively at boundaries. Table 29.9 describes the three typical responses to conflict among colleagues that may arise in clinical practice. There are two possible reasons why negotiation is the least used strategy by physicians. Firstly, it may seem to require more time and energy by all the parties involved than avoidance or forceful imposition. Secondly, negotiation requires an explicit acknowledgement that there is a conflict.

Let us depict a common cause of conflict during the CLP activity: consultants are often asked to evaluate patients admitted to surgical or medical wards because of agitation or delirium. Behavioural impairments are experienced as difficult and disturbing by the ward personnel, so that the psychiatrist might be requested to move the patient to the psychiatric ward. In this case, conflict may originate from opposing views of the patient's problems. On the one side, the medical ward personnel might be scared or annoyed by the patient's (agitated) behaviour. On the other side, the psychiatrist might recognize such behaviour as being caused by a delirium requiring intensive medical intervention. In these cases, it is helpful that all involved parties meet face to face and can express their opinions and concerns. A first step in such discussion should be the recognition of points of consensus; for example, the fact that an agitated patient is, primarily, a suffering person, whose prompt recovery of well-being is a common goal for all clinicians. Then, the first point of divergence of opinion should be located. In our example, the somatic physician may believe that an agitated patient is a psychiatrist's concern; on the other hand, the psychiatrist may

Table 29.9 Responses to conflict among colleagues

Response	Definition, features, examples
Avoidance	◆ Simple neglect of different viewpoints and resulting tension, leading to refusal to address the conflict explicitly
	◆ As a consequence, both parties are not satisfied with each other's action, but just keep silent and let it go
Forceful imposition	◆ The more powerful of the two parties in conflict tries to force the other in their own direction
	◆ Decisions are imposed, sometimes with overt aggressive attitude: 'You will admit the patient to your ward without objection, and that's it!'
Negotiation	◆ Assertive and realistic addressing of the conflict
	◆ Willingness to consider each other's point of view
	◆ Co-operative attitude of search for compromise
	◆ 'I see your point, you see mine, let's work out how we can put them together for the sake of the patient'

believe that a patient whose agitation is due to a medical condition is a physician's concern.

A crucial step of negotiation is then agreeing on terms and definitions: conflict may sometimes arise simply because clinicians are using different words that mean the same thing. Negotiation implies 'respectfully disagreeing'—that is, overtly acknowledging differences of opinion and recognizing the conflict stemming from this discrepancy, without ceasing to respect each other.

Once a conflict has been recognized and the major points of agreement are emphasized, a plan should be generated in order to decide how to follow up the individual patient. This plan includes determining who is responsible for the case management and what contributions will be made by the other parties. Communication skills and emotional self-monitoring are also implied:

◆ Sarcasm, patronization, and condescension–that represent aggressive forms of the avoidance of discussion and conflict–should be avoided.

◆ Acknowledgment of one's feeling of annoyance or disapproval should be accepted rather than denied.

Experts in mental health have a responsibility towards colleagues from other branches of medicine, as 'living examples' and trainers of these skills.

The multiple roles and skills of the CL psychiatrist are summarized in Fig. 29.1.[12,17] The CL psychiatrist is expected to act both as a medical expert and also as a health advocate and communicator, as he or she contributes to the doctor–patient relationship. Teamwork, supervision, and leadership abilities are also valuable, to support a proactive clinical attitude.

Training in consultation–liaison psychiatry

Acquisition of CLP skills and competences is mandatory for postgraduate training in psychiatry, according to the European Union of Medical Specialists (UEMS). However, national fulfilment of this requirement varies throughout Europe. To begin the process of standardization, the European Association for Consultation–Liaison Psychiatry and Psychosomatics (EACLPP) conducted two surveys on CLP training across Europe and produced the 'European guidelines for training in consultation–liaison psychiatry and psychosomatics' (Box 29.2).[17]

Several scientific societies and academic and training institutions have been organizing and promoting interesting training initiatives dedicated to CLP during the past few years. A list of the more relevant materials is shown in Box 29.3.

Instruments and resources for clinical activity in CLP

Several online tools are available to assist the CL psychiatrist while consulting and prescribing medications. Table 29.10 provides a list of the most commonly used ones, with a short description of their more interesting features. Other online instruments and resources are listed in Box 29.4.

- Applies diagnostic and therapeutic skills to care for patients with somatic and psychiatric co-morbidity
- Effectively uses and recommends evidence-based guidelines and stays updated on newest developments in different fields
- Performs therapeutic interventions such as pharmacotherapy and brief psychotherapy

- Effectively and quickly able to form therapeutic alliance and effective professional relationship under a variety of clinical settings
- Communicates clinical findings and recommendations concisely

- Interacting with the consultee and relevant members of the health care team and primary physicians
- Educates a health care team in a way that enhances adherence to recommendations

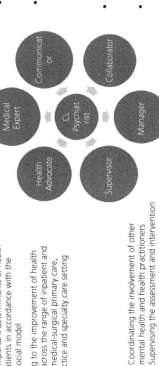

- Identifying important determinants of health affecting patients in accordance with the bio-psychosocial model
- Contributing to the improvement of health in patients across the range of inpatient and outpatient medical-surgical primary care, general practice and specialty care setting

- Coordinating the involvement of other mental health and health practitioners
- Supervising the assessment and intervention activity of the team members

- Utilizing resources effectively to balance the various aspects of care for patients with co-morbid or psychosomatic disorders

Fig. 29.1 Skills and competences of the CL psychiatrist.

Source data from: *Psychosomatics*, 52(1), Leentjens AF, Rundell JR, Wolcott DL, Guthrie E, Kathol R, Diefenbacher A, Psychosomatic Medicine and Consultation–Liaison Psychiatry: Scope of Practice, Processes, and Competencies for Psychiatrists or Psychosomatic Medicine Specialists: A Consensus Statement of the European Association of Consultation–Liaison Psychiatry and the Academy of Psychosomatic Medicine, p. 19–25, Copyright (2011) with permission from Elsevier; *J Psychosom Res*, 62(4), Söllner W, Creed F, and the European Association of Consultation–Liaison Psychiatry and Psychosomatics Workgroup on Training in Consultation–Liaison, European guidelines for training in consultation–liaison psychiatry and psychosomatics: report of the EACLPP Workgroup on Training in Consultation–Liaison Psychiatry and Psychosomatics, p. 501–9, Copyright (2007) with permission from Elsevier.

Box 29.2 European guidelines for training in consultation–liaison psychiatry and psychosomatics

♦ All residents in psychiatry or psychosomatics should be exposed to CL work as part of their clinical experience.

♦ A minimum of 6 months of full-time (or equivalent part-time) rotation to a CL department should take place on the second part of residency.

♦ Advanced training should last for at least 12 months.

♦ Supervision of trainees should be clearly defined and organized.

♦ Trainees should acquire knowledge and skills in the following:

   (a) assessment and management of psychiatric and psychosomatic disorders or situations (e.g. suicide/self-harm, somatization, chronic pain and psychiatric disorders, and abnormal illness behaviour in somatically ill patients);

   (b) crisis intervention and psychotherapy methods appropriate for medically ill patients;

   (c) psychopharmacology in physically ill patients;

   (d) communication with severely ill patients and dying patients, as well as with medical staff;

   (e) promotion of co-ordination of care for complex patients across several disciplines; and

   (f) organization of CL service in relation to GH and/or primary care.

♦ In addition, the workgroup elaborated recommendations on the form of training and on assessment of competency.

Reproduced from J Psychosom Res, 62, Söllner W, Creed F, and the European Association of Consultation-Liaison Psychiatry and Psychosomatics Workgroup on Training in Consultation-Liaison. European guidelines for training in consultation-liaison psychiatry and psychosomatics: report of the EACLPP Workgroup on Training in Consultation-Liaison Psychiatry and Psychosomatics.p. 501–9, Copyright (2007) with permission from Elsevier.

Box 29.3 Training initiatives for CLP

♦ http://www.apm.org/news/pdfs/KEH-EPA-course-2014.pdf

♦ http://estore.manchester.ac.uk/browse/product.asp?compid=1&modid=5&catid=216

♦ https://www.facebook.com/events/256016287856241/?ref=22

Table 29.10 Instruments and resources for clinical activity in CLP

Site	Developed by	Main features
Drug Interactions Explorer	University of Modena and Reggio Emilia (Italy)	Up to 30 selected drugs and active ingredients—including food, active ingredients of alternative medicines, herbs, and other commonly assumed substances—can be tested simultaneously
Drugs.com	Wolters Kluwer Health, American Society of Health-System Pharmacists, Cerner Multum and Thomson Reuters Micromedex	Includes links to the following: Harvard Health Topics A to Z, Harvard Health Decision Guides, a medical dictionary, an illustrated health encyclopaedia, a veterinary product database, and a section dedicated to FDA (Food and Drug Administration) drug alerts
WebMD	WebMD Health Professional Network	Provides medical information, support, and in-depth reference material about health and drugs; the WebMD editorial board is composed of a multidisciplinary staff that includes experts in journalism, content creation, community services, expert commentary, and medicine
RxList	WebMD Health Professional Network	Founded in 1995, it offers detailed and current pharmaceutical information on brand and generic drugs; content is continuously reviewed and updated following international scientific literature and other reliable sources (FDA, Cerner Multum, First Data Bank Inc.)
Medscape	WebMD Health Professional Network	Contains medical information and educational tools, delivered according to registration profile; includes a tool to check drug interactions
HIV Drug Interactions website	University of Liverpool	Specific for interactions with antiretroviral therapies
Healthline.com	Healthline Networks Inc.	Aims at delivering information in the field of health and medicine, educating and empowering users with relevant and responsible information, fostering better communication between doctors and patients; includes a section on drug interactions
Drug Interaction Tool	University of Maryland Medical Center	Free testing of different drug interactions

Box 29.4 Online instruments and resources to support the CL psychiatrist in drug prescription

- http://www.drug-interactions.eu
- http://www.drugs.com/
- http://www.webmd.com/
- http://www.rxlist.com/script/main/hp.asp
- http://reference.medscape.com/drug-interactionchecker
- http://www.hiv-druginteractions.org/Interactions.aspx
- http://www.healthline.com/druginteractions
- http://umm.edu/health/medical/drug-interaction-tool

Clinimetrics and communimetrics

In 1987, the term 'clinimetrics' was introduced by A. Feinstein to describe an approach to scale development different from the 'psychometric' one widely used in psychiatry, psychology, and mental health. This procedure privileges a more immediate approach and focuses on the use of measures in clinical practice (similar to that used in other branches of medicine, such as the Apgar score for newborns' health immediately after birth, or the New York Heart Association's functional classification system for heart failure).[18] While psychometric tools are based on homogeneous items selected through statistical methods (validity studies), clinimetric tools are derived from more heterogeneous items selected according to clinical criteria. Clinimetric tools have an independent face validity and are based upon more reliable information.

A further development was the use of clinimetric tools to improve communication (e.g. among colleagues of different backgrounds) and to directly translate clinical information into action steps (e.g. what should be done when the score of a certain test is above a clinically relevant threshold). This development is called 'communimetrics' and it is also designed to make thinking processes transparent.

An interesting example of a communimetric tool is the INTERMED, a screening instrument designed to predict complexity of care and acknowledged as the operationalization of the Engel biopsychosocial paradigm.[7,19] The INTERMED was developed in order to better assess, organize, and treat the biological, psychological, and social needs of patients. It allows for communication and comprehensive assessment that is sufficiently brief as to be clinically feasible and is readily translatable into specific interventions. As shown in Fig. 29.2, in the INTERMED, the risk factors are defined within a grid that includes four rows reflecting the biological, psychological, social, and healthcare systems. Each risk factor is assessed on four levels, using indicator colours similar to those of a traffic light. This grid includes a 'checklist' with operationalized interventions. The time perspective is reported in three columns: history, current State, and prognosis.

INTERMED - Rating Example

	PAST		CURRENT		PROGNOSIS
BIO-LOGICAL	Chronicity	③	Severity	⓪	②
	Complexity	①	Complexity	②	
PSYCHO-LOGICAL	Coping	①	Compliance	①	①
	Functioning	①	Symptoms	⓪	
SOCIAL	Integration	⓪	Stability	⓪	⓪
	Functioning	⓪	Network	⓪	
HEALTHCARE	Intensity	①	Organization	①	①
	Experiences	③	Referral	⓪	

③ SEVERE VULNERABILITY OR CARE NEED	① MILD VULNERABILITY OR CARE NEED
② MODERATE VULNERABILITY OR CARE NEED	⓪ NO VULNERABILITY OR CARE NEED

Fig. 29.2 INTERMED rating procedure.

Reproduced from *Med Clin N Am*, 90, Stiefel FC, Huyse FJ, Söllner W, Slaets JPJ, Lyons JS, Latour CHM, van der Wal N, de Jonge P. Operationalizing integrated care on a clinical level: the INTERMED project, p. 713–58, Copyright (2006) with permission from Elsevier.

The INTERMED is particularly useful for addressing complex patients, and possesses some interesting and useful features. First, the approach is based on a face-valid conceptual framework for identifying health risk factors by the operationalized biopsychosocial model of disease. Second, the approach is immediately interpretable through visualization. Third, it reinforces training approaches. However, the greatest potential for this decision-support approach is in the rapid communication of the patient's risk factors to the service delivery system. Another interesting characteristic of the INTERMED is that it can be used not only in the GH but also in outpatient settings, as a starting point to assess the needs of complex patients who require long-term case management.

In conclusion, clinimetric and communimetric tools represent good examples of how to convert knowledge derived from scientific research into clinical instruments that can assist everyday practice and improve delivery of care. This approach sounds particularly relevant in the field of CLP, considering the emphasis on communication, integration, and a proactive attitude typical of this area of medicine.[18]

Conclusions

To work on the interface between psychiatry and the rest of medicine is demanding, given the wide range of heterogeneous skills that are required. It is also one of the most stimulating areas of mental health and medicine, contributing to the improvement of knowledge on aetiology, diagnosis, treatment, prevention, and rehabilitation of both psychiatric and any other medical disorders.

CL psychiatrists may sometimes tend to suffer from 'omnipotence delusion', when they believe that medicine as a whole is psychosomatic. Though this may be true as a theoretical principle, more evidence is needed (mostly from research on translational pathways of disease) to convert it into practice for clinicians. For example, the evidence on the role of inflammation in the development of depression suggests new pharmacological strategies (e.g. augmentation of antidepressant therapy with non-steroidal anti-inflammatory drugs or omega-3 fatty acids); or the role of depression in the development of ischaemic heart disorders and metabolic syndrome may suggest the need to address depression at a very early stage, to impact on prognosis. In the future, CLP will probably have to work constantly 'on the boundaries', both of scientific–technical competences and of cultural backgrounds.

References

1 **Diefenbacher A, Burian R**. Liaison and consultation psychiatry. In: *International encyclopedia of social and behavioral sciences* (2nd edn) (ed. Wright J). Oxford: Elsevier; 2015.

2 **Angelino A, Lyketsos CG**. Training in psychosomatic medicine: a psychiatric subspecialty recognized in the United States by the American Board of Medical Specialties. *J Psychosom Res* 2011; **71**:431–2.

3 **Diefenbacher A**. Psychiatry and psychosomatic medicine in Germany: lessons to be learned? *Aust N Z J Psychiatry* 2005; **39**:782–94.

4 **Härter M, Baumeister H, Reuter K, et al**. Increased 12-month prevalence rates of mental disorders in patients with chronic somatic diseases. *Psychother Psychosom* 2007; **76**:354–60.

5 **Desan PH, Zimbrean PC, Weinstein AJ, Bozzo JE, Sledge WH**. Proactive psychiatric consultation services reduce length of stay for admissions to an inpatient medical team. *Psychosomatics* 2011; **52**:513–20.

6 **Rigatelli M, Ferrari S**. The Modena consultation–liaison psychiatry service, Italy. *Br J Psychiatry* 2004; **184**:268–9.

7 **Stiefel FC, Huyse FJ, Söllner W, et al**. Operationalizing integrated care on a clinical level: the INTERMED project. *Med Clin N Am* 2006; **90**:713–58.

8 **Diefenbacher, A**. Consultation and liaison psychiatry. In: *Contemporary psychiatry*. **Volume 1, Part 2: General psychiatry** (eds. Helmchen H, Henn F, Lauter H, Sartorius N). Berlin: Springer; 2000, pp. 253–67.

9 **Rigatelli M, Cavicchioli C**. Ten suggestions for a CLP service in the general hospital (Dieci proposte per un servizio di consulenza psichiatrica in ospedale generale). In: *Lo psichiatra e i suoi pazienti. Trasformazioni culturali in psichiatria. Proceedings from the XL National Congress of the Italian Society of Psychiatry, Napoli, 1997* (eds. Bonaviri G, Giordano PL). Napoli: Idelson; 1997, pp. 235–49 (in Italian).

10 **Ferrari S, Martire L, Rigatelli M**. The Psychiatric–Psychosomatic Consultation Service (PPCS) of Modena: eleven years of experience between clinical, training and research activities. *J Psychosom Res* 2012; **72**:479–80.

11 **Diefenbacher A, Burian R, Klesse C, Härter, M**. Konsiliar und liaisondienst für psychische erkrankungen. In: *Psychische erkrankungen klinik und therapie* (3rd edn) (eds. Berger M). Munich: Urban und Fischer; 2008 (in German).

12 **Leentjens AF, Rundell JR, Wolcott DL, Guthrie E, Kathol R, Diefenbacher A**. Psychosomatic medicine and consultation–liaison psychiatry: scope of practice, processes, and competencies for psychiatrists working in the field of CL psychiatry or psychosomatics. A consensus

statement of the European Association of Consultation–Liaison Psychiatry and Psychosomatics (EACLPP) and the Academy of Psychosomatic Medicine (APM). *J Psychosom Research* 2011(reprint); **70**:486–91.

13 **Hatcher SI, Gilmore K, Pinchen K**. A follow-up study of patients with medically unexplained symptoms referred to a liaison psychiatry service. *Int J Psychiatry Med* 2011; **41**:217–27.

14 **American Psychiatric Association**. *Diagnostic and statistical manual of mental disorders* (5th edn) (DSM-V). Arlington, VA: American Psychiatric Association; 2013.

15 **Diefenbacher A, Strain J**. Consultation–liaison psychiatry: stability and change over a ten-year-period. *Gen Hosp Psychiat* 2002; **24**:249–56.

16 **Kathol RG, Kunkel EJ, Weiner J, et al**. Psychiatrists for medically complex patients: bringing value at the physical health and mental health/substance-use disorder interface. *Psychosomatics* 2009; **50**:93–107.

17 **Söllner W, Creed F,** the European Association of Consultation–Liaison Psychiatry, Psychosomatics Workgroup on Training in Consultation–Liaison Psychiatry. European guidelines for training in consultation–liaison psychiatry and psychosomatics: report of the EACLPP Workgroup on Training in Consultation-Liaison Psychiatry and Psychosomatics. *J Psychosom Res* 2007; **62**:501–9.

18 **Engel GL**. The need for a new medical model: a challenge for biomedicine. *Science* 1977; **196**:129–36.

19 **Lyons JS**. *Communimetrics. A communication theory of measurement in human service setting*. New York: Springer Verlag; 2009.

Chapter 30

Presentation and treatment of mental disorders in migrants

Ilaria Tarricone, Iris Tatjana Graef-Calliess, Francesco Cazzola, Umut Altunoz, and Dinesh Bhugra

A new Europe

The needs in the mental healthcare system are necessarily diversified by global migration, particularly in Europe. Immigrants are such a heterogeneous group, and in working with them, it is crucial to take into account their country of emigration, their reasons for migration, their education, and their legal status.

Approximately over 200 million people move every year to find a better life through job opportunities, although the precise figure remains elusive. At the beginning of 2013, the EU population was 503 million, of which 20.4 million were third-country nationals (corresponding to 4% of the total population). Over 30 million people are defined as undocumented immigrants. The majority of immigrants who move to Central and Eastern Europe, or to Scandinavian countries, come from other European areas. Germany, Austria, and Finland are mostly an arriving point for migrants moving from Central and Eastern Europe. A high proportion of immigrants from outside the continent tend to move to Mediterranean countries, and to the UK and The Netherlands. Almost a third of UK's and Spain's immigrants come from outside Europe.[1] The total number of asylum applications in 2013 was 434,160, which represents a significant increase of around 100,000 applicants compared to the previous year. Thus, a new multicultural Europe is formed.

It may be hard for clinicians to relate to such a diversity of cultures, ethnicities, and reasons for migration, facing the challenge of understanding experiences of illness in migrants whose backgrounds are significantly different from theirs.[2] The way that symptoms of distress and illness present themselves is deeply related to culture, thus influencing the diagnostic process and treatment strategies in migrant populations. This may, in part, be due to differences in language, social background, religion, and moral values between the immigrant patients and the clinicians. Hence, mental healthcare is necessarily influenced in meeting the needs of people from different socio-cultural backgrounds.[2]

Introduction

In the last few decades, there has been a constant increase in the number of studies about the relationship between mental health and migration. The majority of these underline that, comparing migrants or ethnic minorities with natives or fellow coun-trymen without migratory experiences, the former show a higher prevalence of mental disorders.[3] Migrants' mental health is deeply affected by the travelling conditions and the social context in which they live in the receiving country. Mental health specialists must regularly contact such different cultural backgrounds. The wider determinants of the migrating patient's health are often different from those of the settled community, and a different approach by healthcare professionals is required. In order to effectively address the health needs of immigrants, it is essential to understand their background.

Definitions

Migration is defined as the process during which a person moves from one cultural setting to another, in order to settle for a longer period of time or permanently. The migration process can be characterized by a series of events, which are influenced by a number of factors, over a prolonged period of time, and these phases, in turn, are again influenced by other factors, such as social and individual ones.[4] A set of 'push and pull' factors permeate the reasons for migration, and could be found both at an individual and social level. Such factors determine the response in the individual, as well as in those who surround him or her.[5] In addition, migration implies the loss of the familiar: the language (especially colloquial and dialect), the attitudes, the val-ues, the social structures, and the support networks. Grieving for this loss could be accepted as a healthy and natural reaction of migration; otherwise, if the symptoms cause significant distress or impairment, and if they last for an extended period of time, psychiatric–psychotherapeutic intervention may become necessary.[2] As defined by Eisenbruch,[6] cultural bereavement is an experience resulting from the loss of social structures, cultural values, beliefs, and self-identity. The person tends to live in what he or she remembers, is visited by supernatural forces from the past while asleep or awake, and could experience feelings of guilt. Images of the past could be traumatic or, otherwise, intrude into the migrant's life, leaving the individual in a pool of anxieties, morbid thoughts, and anger.

The symptoms of cultural bereavement may be misdiagnosed due to problems with language and culture, and the use of Western diagnostic criteria in non-Western peo-ple.[2] Pre-migration factors and factors of influence during and after the migration pro-cess may play an important role as risk factors for mental disorders. Biological (age, gender), psychosocial, individual, and familial predispositions may also be taken into consideration. Migration factors include more than cultural bereavement and cultural shock, while post-migration factors include the discrepancy between expectations and achievements, and acceptance from the new nation.[2,4]

Mental health among immigrants

Rafnsson and Bhopal[7] reported that a major issue facing Europe is filling the current gap in the availability of high-quality data on health determinants, health status, and health service use among immigrant populations throughout the region. Decision making in public health greatly depends on the availability of relevant health informa-tion. Improving the availability of valid and comparable ethnic-minority health data should be regarded as a high priority.[7] A growing number of studies show that migrants have a higher risk of developing psychiatric disorders like depression, anxiety, suicidal behaviour, and psychosis.[5,8] Influencing factors, such as loneliness, homesickness, loss of status, language problems, resident permit status, unemployment, poverty, low education, poor living conditions, open racism, and dissonance between norms and values of the country of origin and the receiving country, play an important role. These influencing factors are identified as life events before, during, and after migration.[2]

Presentation of mental disorders in migrants

Migration and psychosis

In a meta-analysis by Cantor-Graae and Selten,[3] a moderate relative risk for schizophrenia of 2.7 (95% CI = 2.3–3.2) was found in first-generation migrants; the relative risk for schizophrenia was higher in the second generation, at 4.5 (95% CI = 1.5–13.1); and the greatest relative risk for schizophrenia was seen among immigrants from developing countries, at 3.3 (95% CI = 2.8–3.9), and 4.8 (95% CI = 3.7–6.2) for immigrants from countries with black people. Evidence of higher risk for psychosis was reported among Caribbean (Caribbean Black) immigrants in the UK;[9,10] among immigrants from Surinam, the Dutch Antilles, and Morocco in the Netherlands;[11] among immigrants from Australia, Africa, and Greenland in Denmark;[12] and among immigrants in Italy.[13,14]

The risk for mental illness was as high for second-generation immigrants as it was for non-immigrants in the study published by Cantor-Graae and Pedersen.[15] The authors reported that the increased risk found in second-generation immigrants cannot be explained by urbanization of birthplace or parental characteristics. Moreover, Bourque and colleagues[16] identified risk differences related to ethnic state and the host community: in the UK, black minorities showed higher risk, while in the Netherlands, the lighter and more recent North African migrants where at higher risk. Thus, it is very intriguing to understand which characteristics of each specific host society interact with each specific type of migrant and ethnic minority (first- or next-generation, economic migrants, political migrants, etc.) to increase the risk of psychoses.

Ethnic density has been reported to be an important factor in understanding the elevated rates of schizophrenia in some immigrant groups.[17] Bhugra and Becker,[18] however, postulated that cultural congruity, when people with similar cultural values live close to one another, may be more important in this respect. Further work is urgently needed to map cultural congruity and ethnic density with epidemiological data.[2]

To summarize, immigrants have a strongly increased risk for psychosis, which is associated with psychosocial stress factors such as social isolation, exclusion, and social defeat.[15,19,20] The most important factors of influence include discrimination and self-discrimination,[20–22] exposure to individual social adversities, and neighbourhood deprivation and social strain.[23] Ethnic density may be a protective factor and has been inversely linked to the prevalence of schizophrenia in migrant communities.[4]

Although various biological factors have been hypothesized in aetiology (such as intra-uterine infection in a population susceptible to local infections, relatively poor nutrition, use of cannabis and psychoactive substances, obstetric complications, and flu epidemics), the findings are not conclusive, except for the use of cannabis in vulnerable individuals. Thus, socio-cultural problems around identity, intergenerational differences, ambivalence towards both host and originating cultures, and dysfunctional acculturation, complicated by cumulative discrimination and racism (both overt and covert), may well prove to be significant factors in contributing to the stresses experienced by these groups, and need further exploration.[4]

Migration and affective disorders

Depression prevalence varies from 4.2% to 29.5% in different countries,[24] and the symptom presentation and prevalence[25] of depression are affected by cultural differences. The worldwide lifelong prevalence of depression is estimated to be 5.8% for men and 9.5% for women.[26] In a meta-analysis by Swinnen and Selten[27] regarding migration as a risk factor for affective disorders (including bipolar disorders), a slight increase of risk was found, but not for unipolar depressive disorder. In a cross-sectional study of a multi-ethnic working population, Sieberer et al.[28] found that first- and second-generation female migrants were more likely to suffer from depressiveness than non-migrant females. Thus, a history of migration was shown to be an independent risk factor for depression.

Possible triggers for depressive disorders among elder immigrants include disputes concerning remigration[19] or problems with acculturation, which may be particularly difficult towards the end of the lifespan and may contribute to cultural conflicts in the families. Poor social support in the new country may act as a precipitating factor.[4]

Depression was measured in a Survey of Health, Ageing, and Retirement in Europe (SHARE)—a cross-national, multidisciplinary, household-based panel survey using nationally representative probability samples of non-institutionalized populations aged 50 years and older (n = 28.517) from 11 European countries.[8] Effects of socio-demographic variables, physical co-morbidities, functional impairment, cognitive function, geographic region, and time lived in the current country of residence were assessed in a multivariate logistic regression analysis. The influence of migration status on the prevalence of depression was significantly greater in Northern and Western Europe compared to Southern Europe. A new study by Altunoz et al.[29] which compared Turkish immigrants with generalized anxiety disorder (GAD) in Germany with native Turkish patients with GAD, stated that higher depression severity in Turkish immigrants had an interaction with worry, GAD severity, and GAD-associated disability. In that study, only disability in social life was higher in immigrants with GAD independent of depression, which may suggest that a lack of social support also leads to higher depression rates in Turkish immigrants with GAD living in Germany.

Migration and dementia

The number of elderly immigrants is increasing in most European countries, but immigrant patients are underrepresented in dementia assessment and care facilities. The reasons can be found in different cultural perceptions of dementia and lack of knowledge about the available support among immigrants. Another important reason may be the difficult clinical assessment in immigrant patients with dementia. The interpretation of cognitive tests represents another major challenge.

Only a few studies on migrants with dementia are available. The Islington Study in London found prevalence of dementia among immigrants as 17.3%. The authors discussed increased cardiovascular co-morbidity as an explanation for the higher rates of dementia and its earlier onset among immigrants.[30] In Denmark, an increased frequency of dementia conditions (13.3%) compared to the expected prevalence of 7% in the Danish population was found, together with an increased frequency of Type 2 diabetes. The use of MMSE (mini mental state examination) as a guideline instrument of screening was shown to be applicable, with modifications, to persons who were illiterates and without any education, and to those first-generation immigrants who were only to a limited degree integrated as citizens.[31] In addition, the lack of medical healthcare in the country of origin, physically hard labour in the receiving society, a high risk of disintegration of social networks, and less or no utilization of a healthcare system could be factors which fasten the process of getting older. There is evidence that socioeconomic factors may initiate rapid development of dementia. The majority of immigrants are subjected to bad living conditions; therefore a higher prevalence of dementia among immigrants is expectable.

Migration and addictive disorders

The increased use of alcohol and various illicit substances has been linked to specific migrant populations.[4] There are a number of barriers to access for those migrants, including language difficulties, lack of knowledge about the public system of addiction treatment, mistrust towards government institutions, and fear of losing residence rights. However, access barriers can also result from a culturally different understanding of the causes and treatment of addictive behaviour.[3] All these findings suggest that information materials need to be adapted to the explanatory model used by each target group. Only by those means will it be possible to avoid misunderstandings and achieve greater effectiveness.[32] Due to cultural and social barriers, immigrants seldomly attend centres for information, counselling, and treatment of addictive disorders. In a study on cultural differences in the explanatory models of addictive behaviour among Turkish and German youths in Germany, relevant differences were found between the disorder concepts among the two groups.[32] Concerning substance abuse, German, but not Turkish youths, clearly differentiated between illegal drug abuse and alcohol or nicotine. Nearly half of all Turkish youths rejected central medical concepts such as 'physical dependence' or 'reduced control of substance intake' as completely inadequate to characterize problems of addictive behaviour.

Migration and eating disorders

Acculturation can produce elevated rates of eating disorders among migrants. In various studies, it has been reported that some migrant teenagers are more likely to develop eating disorders compared with native populations.[33] Eating disorders are known to be prevalent among girls and women in Western countries. In the United States, 90% of those who suffer from anorexia nervosa and bulimia nervosa are women. Research conducted in Israel shows results similar to those obtained in Western cultures. Since 1970, standards related to body ideals in the Western world have changed: the 'full', 'round' body image has been replaced by the extremely skinny 'ideal' body figure. Attitudes to eating may reflect cultural effects, with regards to eating disorders and the prevalence of obesity. It seems that the veteran immigrants have adopted Western cultural norms and eating patterns in a way that has erased the differences in tendency toward eating disorders between them and the Israeli-born women.

A few studies have investigated a cultural group's corporeal experiences in both its country of origin and host. Swami[34] evaluated the body image among 140 women in Harare, Zimbabwe, and an age-matched sample of 138 Zimbabwean migrants in Britain. Preliminary analyses showed that there were no significant differences in body mass index between the two groups. Further analyses showed that Zimbabwean women in Britain had significantly greater weight discrepancy and lower body appreciation than their counterparts in Zimbabwe. In addition, weight discrepancy and body appreciation among both samples were significantly associated with exposure to Western, but not Zimbabwean, media. These findings support the contention that transcultural migration may place individuals at risk for symptoms of negative body image.[34,35] Similar results are shown by a study comparing Polish migrants in Britain with native Poles in Poland.[36]

Migration and suicidality

Several studies reported a higher rate of suicide and suicide attempts among young migrant women. Several factors have been considered to explain this phenomenon including the tension arising from the difficulty of reconciling family expectations related to gender with the expectations of and experiences in the new community.[4] One of the central risk factors in this regard may be barriers to the healthcare system for immigrants. Insufficient knowledge about the structure of the healthcare system and lack of intercultural awareness by attending healthcare staff may be barriers to providing immigrant women in emotional crises with timely care. In comparison to young women of Turkish origin, the attempted rate of suicide among men of Turkish origin was lower. The Swiss WHO/EURO study,[37] which compared Turkish immigrants with Swiss natives, reported that women of Turkish origin had the highest rate of attempted suicides. The risk and precipitating factors for suicidality of immigrant women differ from the ones of immigrant men and native women.

Migration and special populations

Migration can affect mental health of special populations in several ways. Some risk factors for mental disorders related to migrant status are summarized in Table 30.1.

Table 30.1 Risk factors for mental disorders in migrant special populations

Special populations	Risk factors
Elderly	Dependent status
	Difficulty in developing new social network
Children	Separation from one or both parents
	Lonely migration
	Losses and reunion with families
	Trafficked children
Young	Acculturative stress
	Intergenerational differences
Refugees and asylum seekers	Experience of trauma and loss
	Forced migration
	Protracted asylum procedure
	Stay in detention
Women	Passive migration for family reunion
	Trafficked women
Undocumented/illegal migrants	Extremely precarious, health-threatening living conditions
	Extremely difficult access to care

Source data from: *Eur Psychiatry*, 29(2), Bhugra D, Gupta S, Schouler-Ocak M, Graeff-Calliess I, Deakin NA, Qureshi A, et al. EPA guidance on mental health care of migrants, p. 107–15, Copyright (2014) Elsevier

Treatment of mental disorders in migrants

Psychotherapy for immigrants

Studies on inpatient psychotherapy of immigrants stated a higher psychopathological burden at the beginning of the treatment, as well as lower efficacy of treatment at admission compared to native patients. Göbber et al.[38] identified the factor 'migration background' to be a negative predictor of therapeutic outcome. Several authors noted that immigrants tend to underuse mental health services and drop out from therapy prematurely. Important reasons for this are the lack of availability of modified mental health services and the inability of psychotherapists and counsellors to provide culturally sensitive psychotherapies for persons of different racial and ethnic backgrounds. The empirical evidence for the benefit of cultural adaptations in mental health interventions has been reviewed in two meta-analyses,[39] and four common methods of cultural adaptation have been summarized by Griner and Smith[37] (Box 30.1). The results of the meta-analytic review[39] indicate a moderate to strong benefit of culturally adapted interventions. It was found that interventions targeted at a specific cultural group were four times more effective than interventions provided to groups consisting

Box 30.1 The four methods of cultural adaptation

1 Cultural values of immigrant patients should be incorporated into therapy.

2 Immigrant patients can be matched with therapists of the same cultural or ethnic group.

3 Mental health interventions should be easily accessible and targeted to immigrant patients' circumstances.

4 Support resources available within immigrant patients' community, extended family members, tradition should be incorporated into therapy interventions.

Source data from: *Psychotherapy*, 43(4), Griner D, Smith TB. Culturally adapted mental health intervention: A meta-analytic review, p. 531–48. Copyright (2006) American Psychological Association

of patients from a variety of cultural backgrounds. Interventions conducted in patients' native languages were twice as effective as those conducted in English.

Further, the results of additional analyses indicated that the format of the intervention (individual therapy, group interventions) did not have any influence on the results.[39] In addition, the outcome of psychotherapy can be influenced fundamentally by the diverse concepts of illness and health, traditional values and beliefs, as well as by specific cultural factors. Reconciling two different cultures within the self is one of the most essential developmental tasks in the acculturative process.[40]

Psychotherapy in native languages cannot be realized everywhere because the number of qualified psychotherapists who speak a native language is insufficient. Therefore, the work with psychologically trained interpreters is of great importance and reduces the barrier to treatment with cross-cultural psychotherapy, and it decreases the treatment gap for traumatized immigrant patients.

Cultural competency

With the increased diversity of patients' multicultural backgrounds, there is the need for mental health professionals to recognize the coexistence of traditional approaches towards mental health care, with competent treatment exhibiting a willingness to forge a link between these and Western approaches to treatment.[41] According to Cross[42] and Kastrup,[41] cultural competence is not a static phenomenon but a developmental process moving along a continuum which includes:

1) cultural destructiveness

2) cultural incapacity

3) cultural blindness

4) cultural pre-competence

5) cultural competence, and

6) cultural proficiency.

To increase cultural competence of a healthcare system means to value diversity, to show sensitivity to cultural interactions, to facilitate incorporation and institutionalization of cultural knowledge, and to adjust service delivery to reflect understanding and awareness of diversity between and within cultures. Healthcare systems should make an effort to assess where they fall along the continuum.[41,42]

Cultural competence includes the ability to work with an interpreter. Professionals should be able to handle a clinical setting with an interpreter. Professional face-to-face interpretation is the most accurate method, but has many drawbacks, such as organizational requirements, training, and costs. Bilingual professionals with a command of the immigrant's language can fill gaps left by the scarcity of professional interpreters; however, their numbers are limited. Cultural mediators are useful if they can function as both health workers and interpreters, mediating between health professionals and service users.

According to Qureshi,[43] cultural competence represents a comprehensive response to the mental healthcare needs of immigrants. Cultural competence training involves the development of knowledge, skills, and attitudes that can improve the effectiveness of psychiatric–psychotherapeutic treatment. Cognitive cultural competence involves awareness of the various ways in which culture, immigration status, and race impact psychosocial development, psychopathology, and therapeutic transactions. Technical cultural competence requires proficiency in intercultural communication, the capacity to develop a therapeutic relationship with a culturally different patient, and the ability to adapt diagnosis and treatment in response to cultural differences[43,44] (see Box 30.2).

Cultural competence also means that individuals have to develop an understanding of the cultural knowledge, cultural sensitivity, cultural empathy (and appropriate

---

Box 30.2 Elements of cultural competency

1 Understand the concept of culture and how it can influence:
   - Human behaviour
   - Interpretations of that behaviour
   - Evaluations of that behaviour.

2 Demonstrate an openness/willingness to identify and explore one's own:
   - Cultural base (values, beliefs, and attitudes)
   - Emotions and thoughts generated by intercultural interactions.

3 Demonstrate an openness/willingness to explore the same things from the perspective of people from diverse cultures.

4 Demonstrate the ability to identify useful and culturally appropriate strategies for working with people from diverse cultural backgrounds.

Adapted from Schouler-Ocak et al.[10]

interactions), along with cultural insight, of both one's self and of the patient. Cultural competence is basically good clinical practice, where the clinician sees each patient in the context of the patient's cultural values and prejudices. Often, it is erroneously assumed that only ethnic minority patients have cultures. However, cultural competency is an ability to understand and be aware of cultural factors in all therapeutic interactions with all patients. These cultural factors include awareness of social and religious factors, attitudes, behaviours, models of illness, and possible beliefs about illness as held by the patients and their families and carers. Cultural knowledge, cultural skills, and cultural attitudes should be explored with the patients and their carers and families. Cultural competence should be considered at both the individual/clinical level as well as at the institutional level.

Cultural formulation

Cultural formulation is being increasingly advocated and has certainly major advantages. It allows both the patients and their families on the one side, and the clinicians on the other side, to engage in therapeutic interactions. The components of cultural formulation include cultural identity of the individual and their beliefs and values; how their distress and symptoms are seen in the cultural and environmental context and are reinforced by cultural factors; and how understanding between the patient and the clinician is shared, and whether shared therapeutic strategies are possible and can be developed along with the nature of the interaction.

Intercultural opening

One of the most fundamental barriers for immigrants in accessing health services in Europe is inadequate legal entitlement. Where such entitlements do exist, there need to be mechanisms for ensuring that they are known about and respected in practice.[45] Barriers preventing immigrants access to the healthcare system are often attributed to cultural differences and misunderstandings. However, 'culture' is a multifaceted term that is often (mis-)used as a putative, politically correct expression of 'ethnical differences', thus reifying social differences and neglecting discrimination. Nevertheless, immigrants and people suffering from mental health problems are among those subjects who experience the strongest barriers to accessing healthcare systems and the opening of mental healthcare institutions to immigrants remains a widely neglected topic.[1] A new approach is increasingly needed for dealing with barriers to social or healthcare systems and improving quality of treatment for immigrants, based on 'responsiveness to diversity'.[32,46,47] Healthcare systems need to address cultural issues in care, and health policy experts should understand how economic, political, and cultural processes influence each other to affect access, quality, adherence, and outcome.[48]

Mental healthcare in immigrants

Patients with an immigrant background often do not seek out mental health services to the same extent as native patients. In the case of Russian-Germans, the history of psychiatry in the former Soviet Union must be considered when examining the way that Russian-German immigrants view professional medical help, since it can contribute to their mistrust of medical and, in particular, psychiatric institutions. In former days, psychiatry in the Soviet Union was used as a political tool. Dissidents were often diagnosed with a mental disorder and treated for an unlimited period of time in psychiatric institutions with the aim of forcing them to revoke their opinions.

The European Psychiatric Association (EPA) guidance on mental healthcare of migrants underlines the need for cultural sensitivity and culturally competent treatment concepts for immigrant patients in *general* mental healthcare services.[4] However, for specific subgroups (e.g. refugees, asylum seekers, undocumented or traumatized immigrants), special services and cultural competent services may be helpful.[49,50] In general, the authors favour integrative concepts. The World Psychiatric Association (WPA) guidance[2] underlines a series of recommendations to policy makers, service providers, and clinicians, aimed at improving mental healthcare for immigrants, and the EPA guidance is in agreement with this (see Box 30.3).

Box 30.3 Summary of EPA guidance on mental healthcare of migrants

Service providers

- Providers should open their institutions to immigrants; intercultural opening is regular.
- Staff with immigrant background to be part of the multiprofessional teams.
- Cultural competence is a key issue for the staff and regular training is provided for them.
- Regular cross-cultural intervision/supervision is available.
- Culture-sensitive food, with regard to religious orientation, is offered.
- Cultural liaison is regularly provided.
- Prevention and awareness programmes for immigrants are covered.
- Information for immigrants (via pamphlets in their mother tongues) about the regional, community-based psychiatric, clinical, and outpatient care services should be improved.
- Institutions should have an official commissioner for issues relating to immigrants.

Policy makers

- Clear messages concerning equal treatment of immigrant and native patients; no discrimination of immigrant patients.

> **Box 30.3 Summary of EPA guidance on mental healthcare of migrants (continued)**
>
> ◆ Resources meeting the needs of all immigrants (asylum seekers, refugees, undocumented, traumatized, gender- and age-specific)–e.g. interpreter.
> ◆ Rights of immigrant patients should be also taken into consideration.
> ◆ Information for immigrants (via pamphlets in their mother tongues) on different diseases, treatment possibilities, psychotherapy and medication, websites in different languages; guide posts in different languages are available.
> ◆ More quantitative and qualitative research to better understand the interfaces (e.g. of gender, ethnicity, and immigration).
>
> Adapted from Bhugra et al.[4]

Therapists must be aware of several factors which can influence the therapeutic interaction (see Box 30.4). Such factors can include their own cultural heritage and whether they see themselves as mono-cultural, bi-cultural, or multicultural, and what this means; what type of communication style they have with each cultural group; and how these communications affect their therapeutic work. Perhaps more importantly, being able to recognize their abilities, strengths, and weaknesses which influence their 'worldview', and to know how this view differs from that of the patient, is an essential part of the therapeutic armamentarium.

Box 30.5 illustrates various assumptions that clinicians make in their dealings with patients.

Whether during psychotherapy or pharmacotherapy, it is important for therapists and clinicians to be aware of the impact that their assumptions may have on the patient and the therapeutic engagement.

Box 30.4 Therapist characteristics

◆ Aware of own likes, dislikes, beliefs, stereotypes
◆ Aware of own identity
◆ Ability to be neutral and open-minded
◆ Ability to learn about other cultures
◆ Awareness that there are differences
◆ Tendency to idealize one or other cultures
◆ Strengths and weaknesses of own/other cultures

Adapted from Schouler-Ocak et al.[10]

Box 30.5 Assumptions made by clinicians when dealing with patients

- Colour blindness: assume every ethnic minority patient is the same.
- Colour consciousness: all problems are due to ethnic minority status.
- Cultural transference: patient's feelings related to therapist's race.
- Cultural counter-transference: therapist's feelings related to patient's race.
- Cultural identification: ethnic minority therapists may over-identify.
- Identification with oppressor: ethnic minority therapists deny their status.

Adapted from Schouler-Ocak et al.[10]

Conclusions

Global migration and the increasing number of immigrants to Europe are a challenge to mental healthcare systems. There is growing evidence from recent years that there is greater emotional distress in migrants or even a higher prevalence of mental disorders when compared to natives or fellow countrymen without migratory experiences. Some migrant groups are at risk for higher rates of suicidality, affective disorders, addiction, and psychoses. This is why it is very important for clinicians and mental healthcare specialists to be aware of the wider determinants of the mental health of immigrants. Some of these may be identity conflicts, intergenerational differences, ambivalence towards both host and originating cultures, and dysfunctional acculturation, accompanied by cumulative discrimination or racism.

With increasing globalization, there is an urgent need to address problems with adequate diagnoses and treatment strategies for patients with a migration background. Mental health professionals should be trained in cultural competence and recognize:

a) the impact of cultural influence on symptom presentation;

b) culturally different attitudes towards the explanation of diseases;

c) the existence of traditional approaches towards mental healthcare.

If a healthcare system wants to increase its cultural competence, it needs to value diversity, be able to assess itself culturally, be aware of how cultures interact, incorporate and institutionalize cultural knowledge, and adjust service delivery in order to understand and be aware of diversity between and within cultures.

References

1 **Carta MG, Bernal M, Hardoy MC, Haro-Abad JM**. Migration and mental health in Europe (The State of the Mental Health in Europe Working Group: appendix 1). *Clin Pract Epidemiol Ment Health* 2005; **1**:13.

2 **Bhugra D, Gupta S, Bhui K, et al**. WPA guidance on mental health and mental health care in migrants. *World Psychiatry* 2011; **10**(1):2–10.

3 Cantor-Graae E, Selten J-P. Schizophrenia and migration: a meta-analysis and review. *Am J Psychiatry* 2005; **162**(1):12–24.

4 Bhugra D, Gupta S, Schouler-Ocak M, et al. EPA guidance on mental health care of migrants. *Eur Psychiatry* 2014; **29**(2):107–15.

5 Bhugra D. Migration and mental health. *Acta Psychiatr Scand* 2004; **109**(4):243–58.

6 Eisenbruch M. From post-traumatic stress disorder to cultural bereavement: diagnosis of Southeast Asian refugees. *Soc Sci Med* 1991; **33**(6):673–80.

7 Rafnsson SB, Bhopal RS. Migrant and ethnic health research: report on the European Public Health Association Conference 2007. *Public Health* 2008; **122**(5):532–4.

8 Aichberger M, Schouler-Ocak M, Mundt A, et al. Depression in middle-aged and older first generation migrants in Europe: results from the Survey of Health, Ageing and Retirement in Europe (SHARE). *Eur Psychiatry* 2010; **25**(8):468–75.

9 Sharpley MS, Hutchinson G, McKenzie K, Murray RM. Understanding the excess of psychosis among the African-Caribbean population in England. Review of current hypotheses. *Br J Psychiatry* 2001; **178**(40):s60–8.

10 Schouler-Ocak M, Graef-Calliess I T, Tarricone I, Qureshi A, Kastrup M C, Bhugra D. EPA guidance on cultural competence training. *Eur Psychiatry* 2015; **30**:431–40 DOI: 10.1016/j.eurpsy.2015.01.012

11 Fearon P, Kirkbride JB, Morgan C, Dazzan P, Morgan K, et al. Incidence of schizophrenia and other psychoses in ethnic minority groups: results from the MRC AESOP Study. *Psychol Med* 2006; **36**(11):1541–50.

12 Veling W, Selten JP, Veen N, Laan W, Blom JD, Hoek HW. Incidence of schizophrenia among ethnic minorities in the Netherlands: a four-year first-contact study. *Schizophr Res* 2006; **86**:189–93.

13 Cantor-Graae E, Pedersen CB, McNeil TF, Mortensen PB. Migration as a risk factor for schizophrenia: a Danish population-based cohort study. *Br J Psychiatry* 2003; **182**(2):117–22.

14 Tarricone I, Mimmi S, Paparelli A, et al. First-episode psychosis at the West Bologna Community Mental Health Centre: results of an 8-year prospective study. *Psychol Med* 2012; **42**(11):2255–64.

15 Lasalvia A, Bonetto C, Tosato S, et al. The PICOS-Veneto Group. First-contact incidence of psychosis in north-eastern Italy: influence of age, gender, immigration and socioeconomic deprivation. *Br J Psychiatry*, 2014;**205**:127–34. 2014.

16 Cantor-Graae E, Pedersen CB. Risk of schizophrenia in second-generation immigrants: a Danish population-based cohort study. *Psychol Med* 2007; **37**(4):485–94.

17 Bourque F, van der Ven E, Malla A. A meta-analysis of the risk for psychotic disorders among first- and second-generation immigrants. *Psychol Med* 2011; **41** (5):897–910.

18 Boydell J, van Os, J, McKenzie K. Incidence of schizophrenia in ethnic minorities in London: ecological study into interactions with environment. *BMJ* 2001; **323**(7325):1336.

19 Bhugra D, Becker M. Migration, cultural bereavement and cultural identity. *World Psychiatry* 2005; **4**:18–24.

20 Selten J-P, Cantor-Graae E. Hypothesis: social defeat is a risk factor for schizophrenia. **Br J Psychiatry Suppl.** 2007; **51**:s9–12.

21 Veling W, Hoek HW, Mackenbach JP. Perceived discrimination and the risk of schizophrenia in ethnic minorities. *Soc Psychiatry Psychiatr Epidemiol* 2008; **43**(12):953–9.

22 van Os J, Kenis G, Rutten BP. The environment and schizophrenia. *Nature* 2010; 11;468(7321):203–12.

23 **Veling W, Selten JP, Susser E, et al.** Discrimination and the incidence of psychotic disorders among ethnic minorities in The Netherlands. *Int J Epidemiol* 2007; **36**(4):761–8.

24 **Tarricone I, Stivanello E, Poggi F, et al.** Ethnic variation in the prevalence of depression and anxiety in primary care: a systematic review and meta-analysis. *Psychiatry Res* 2012; 28;**195**(3):91–106.

25 **Kirkbride JB, Boydell J, Ploubidis GB, et al.** Testing the association between the incidence of schizophrenia and social capital in an urban area. *Psychol Med* 2008; **38**(8):1083–94.

26 **Sartorius N, Ustün TB, Costa e Silva JA, et al.** An international study of psychological problems in primary care. Preliminary report from the World Health Organization Collaborative Project on 'Psychological Problems in General Health Care'. *Arch Gen Psychiatry* 1993; **50**(10):819–24.

27 **World Health Organization.** *World health report 2001: mental health—new understanding, new hope.* Geneva: World Health Organization; 2001.

28 **Swinnen SG, Selten J-P.** Mood disorders and migration meta-analysis. *Br J Psychiatry* 2007; **190**(1):6–10

29 **Altunoz U, Ozel-Kizil ET, Kokurcan A, Graef-Calliess IT.** P.4.b.022 Native Turkish patients and Turkish immigrants: a comparison in terms of clinical features of generalized anxiety disorder. *European Neuropsychopharmacology* October 2014, Vol.**24**:S599–S600, doi:10.1016/S0924-977X(14)70961–7.

30 **Sieberer M, Maksimovic S, Ersöz B, Machleidt W, Ziegenbein M, Calliess IT.** Depressive symptoms in first- and second-generation migrants: a cross-sectional study of a multi-ethnic working population. *Int J Soc Psychiatry* 2012; **58**(6):605–13.

31 **Pettit T, Livingston G, Manela M, Kitchen G, Katona C, Bowling A.** Validation and normative data of health status measures in older people: the Islington study. *Int J Geriatr Psychiatry* 2001; **16**(11):1061–70.

32 **Penka S, Krieg S, Hunner Ch, Heinz A.** Different explanatory models for addictive behavior in Turkish and German youths in Germany: significance for prevention and treatment. *Nervenarzt* 2003; **74**(7):581–6 (in German).

33 **Penka S, et al.** Explanatory models of addictive behaviour among native German, Russian-German, and Turkish youth. *Eur Psychiatry* 2008; **23**:36–42.

34 **Bhugra D, Bhui K.** Eating disorders in teenagers in East London: a survey. *Eur Eat Disord Rev* 2003; **11**(1):46–57.

35 **Swami V, Mada R, Tovée MJ.** Weight discrepancy and body appreciation of Zimbabwean women in Zimbabwe and Britain. *Body Image* 2012; **9**(4):559–62.

36 **Nasser M, Bhugra D.** Chow V. Concepts of body and self in minority groups. In: The Female Body in Mind. The Interface between the Female Body and Mental Health. Eds: Nasser M, Baistow K, Treasure J. New York: Taylor & Francis, 2007, p. 192–202.

37 **Göbber, J.,** Pfeiffer, W., Winkler, M., Kobelt, A., Petermann, F. Stationäre psychosomatische Rehabilitationsbehandlung von Patienten mit türkischem igrationshintergrund – Spezielle Herausforderungen und Ergebnisse der Behandlung. *Zeitschrift für Psychiatrie, Psychologie und Psychotherapie* 2010; **58**:181–187.

38 **Muheim F, Eichhorn M, Berger P, Czernin S, Stoppe G, Keck M, Riecher-Rössler A.** Suicide attempts in the county of Basel: results from the WHO/EURO Multicentre Study on Suicidal Behaviour. *Swiss Med Wkly* 2013 May 28; **143**:w13759.

39 **Taylor D, Szpakowska I, Swami V.** Weight discrepancy and body appreciation among women in Poland and Britain. *Body Image* 2013; **10**(4):628–31.

40 **Griner D, Smith TB**. Culturally adapted mental health intervention: a meta-analytic review. *Psychotherapy (Chic)* 2006; **43**(4):531–48.

41 **Calliess IT, Bauer S, Behrens K**. Culture dynamic model of bicultural identity. Intercultural psychotherapy with reference to the structure of the self. (Kulturdynamisches modell der bikulturellen identität. Interkulturelle psychotherapie unter berücksichtigung der struktur des selbst.) *Psychotherapeut* 2012; **57**:36–41.

42 **Kastrup M**. Staff competence in dealing with traditional approaches. *Eur Psychiatry* 2008; **23**(Suppl 1):59–68.

43 **Cross TL, Bazron BJ, Denis KW, Isacs MR**. Towards a culturally competent system of care: a monograph on effective services for minority children who are severely emotionally disturbed. Washington DC: CASSP Technical Centre; 1989.

44 **Qureshi A, Collazos F, Ramos M, et al**. Cultural competency training in psychiatry. *Eur Psychiatry* 2008; **23**:49–58.

45 **Braca M, Berardi D, Mencacci E, et al**. Understanding psychopathology in migrants: a mixed categorical-dimensional approach. *Int J Soc Psychiatry* 2014; **60**(3):243–53.

46 **Tarricone I, Stivanello E, Ferrari S, et al**. Migrant pathways to community mental health centres in Italy. *Int J Soc Psychiatry* 2012; **58**(5):505–11.

47 **Bischoff A, Chiarenza A, Loutan L**. 'Migrant-friendly hospitals': a European initiative in an age of increasing mobility. *World Hosp Health Serv* 2009; **45**(3):7–9.

48 **Rucci P, Piazza A, Perrone E, et al**. Disparities in mental health care provision to immigrants with severe mental illness in Italy. *Epidemiol Psychiatr Sci* 2014; **30**:1–11.

49 **Kleinman A**. Mental health in different groups of migrants and ethnic minorities in Europe and beyond. *Eur Psychiatry* 2012; **27**(Suppl 2):S81–2.

50 **Tarricone I, Braca M, Atti AR, et al**. Clinical features and pathway to care of migrants referring to the Bologna Transcultural Psychiatric Team. *Int J Cult Ment Health* 2009; **2**:1–15

Chapter 31

Management of mental disorders during pregnancy and the post-partum period

Zuzana Lattova, Olga Kazakova,
and Anita Riecher-Rössler

Introduction

For millennia, it has been argued that women express distress in different ways in comparison with men. Women suffer from double jeopardy in that they not only have higher rates of certain psychiatric disorders but also have problems in seeking help and are also expected to look after their families and commitments. There is little doubt that, often, men control political and economic levers, sometimes relegating women to second-class citizens. In addition, the patriarchal nature of societies can create further problems. Both biological and psychological differences are affected by social and cultural factors. Culture plays a major role in the development of our cognitive schemata and child-rearing patterns, thereby making it essential that we understand cultural and social patterns of behaviour. In addition, these behaviours affect attitudes towards women and the creation of gender roles and gender role expectations.

Women and psychiatry have had a rather tumultuous relationship in that, generally, male psychiatrists, at the behest of society, have controlled women's behaviour. Historically, for a number of reasons influenced by social norms, attitudes towards madness and women have varied dramatically. People with mental illness have been managed by priests and medical doctors, but there has always been the strong influence of social issues.

In this chapter, we aim to focus on specific peripartum illnesses. There is no doubt that women have an increased incidence of many psychiatric disorders and also happen to be carers in the family. We do not propose to discuss other psychiatric illnesses due to lack of space and since many textbooks are available. We also do not aim to cover historical phenomena regarding the development of attitudes to women and psychiatric disorders.

Post-partum illness

About 25–40% of mothers suffer from mood lability and mild depression during the first week after parturition (often called post-partum blues or post-partum dysphoria). About 10–15% suffer from a depressive disorder, and one or two of every thousand women present with psychosis during the infant's first year.[1-3] Patients with a history of bipolar disorder and schizophrenia are at higher risk of relapse in the post-partum months. Depression during pregnancy occurs as frequently as at any other given time in a woman's life.[4]

Psychiatric disorders in the puerperium have significant societal consequences. This topic brings up clinico-ethical questions of family planning with women who suffer from mental disorders, the care of them during pregnancy, interventions in the post-partum period, and child custody decisions. There is limited and often contradictory data about using psychotropic medication at this period and its outcomes for the fetus and child in case of breastfeeding.

In this chapter, we will focus on the most challenging psychiatric disorders in pregnancy and the post-partum period: post-partum psychosis and depression. Two sections are devoted to psychopharmacological treatment in pregnant and breastfeeding women.

Post-partum psychosis

Prevalence

The post-partum period has a much higher risk for psychosis than at any other time in a woman's life—up to 20 times higher in the first month after parturition.[5] One to two out of every thousand women present with post-partum psychosis (or puerperal psychosis, PP).[5-8]

Classification

Post-partum psychosis does not exist as a separate diagnostic category. According to the DSM-5 it can be classified under 'brief psychotic disorder with post-partum onset' (if onset is during pregnancy or within 4 weeks post-partum), code 298.8.[9] It is also possible to use a post-partum onset specifier for a mood or psychotic episode in patients with bipolar disorder, schizoaffective disorder, or major depressive disorder.[9,10]

The ICD-10 suggests coding mental disorders associated with the puerperium according to the presenting psychiatric disorder. That means using the usual classification number, while a second code (O99.3) indicates the association with the puerperium. Only in exceptional circumstances, ICD-10 also allows a special code, F53, to be used if there is 'insufficient' information to classify according to given classification criteria or if 'special additional features are noted'. [11,12]

Clinical features

The clinical picture of psychoses in the post-partum period does not usually differ significantly from that of psychoses occurring independently from parturition.[13] Symptom onset frequently occurs within the first 1–3 months after birth.[14] Onset and/or worsening of sleep disturbance may be the first symptoms of mental disorder, and this may lead to mood instability.[15] Symptoms of manic/mixed episodes are particularly common early on and usually precede the appearance of psychotic features.[16] Delusions may have post-partum-specific content; for example, ideas of grandiosity which are projected onto the child (e.g. the baby is believed to be Jesus).

Pathogenetic pathways and risk factors

There are several pathways to developing PP. Clinicians mainly see affective psychoses[17] but there are also some schizophrenic psychoses, and, more rarely, so-called atypical psychoses and organic psychoses.[13] The organic psychoses include post-eclamptic psychosis and psychosis due to obstetric complications (e.g. sepsis).[18] Antenatal care and antibiotics have almost eliminated most organic post-partum psychoses.

A previous diagnosis of a psychotic disorder is one of the strongest risk factors for PP. Further risk factors include a family history of a psychotic disorder. Other risk factors, such as unmarried status, giving birth for the first time, delivery complications, long duration of labour, night-time delivery, and prepartum hospitalization due to any mental disorder, have not been reported unequivocally.[16,19–23]

Screening

The Edinburgh Postnatal Depression Scale (EPDS)[24] and the Mood Disorder Questionnaire (MDQ)[25] can be used to screen for the first symptoms of depression and mania/hypomania. A mood diary can be useful in women with bipolar disorder.[10] The woman should be informed about the first symptoms of PP, if she is a high-risk patient, and so should her partner/significant other, if she agrees.

Management

As part of the pregnancy and birth plan, the risk of PP and the proposed management plan should be discussed in detail, and in advance, with women who are at risk of having post-partum psychosis and also with their partners and interested family members (see Table 31.1).[2,7,10,26]

Women with a high risk of post-partum psychosis should be offered prophylactic treatment. It is important to discuss, as early as possible, the increase of drug dosage right after delivery.

Table 31.1 Management of post-partum psychosis

Step 1	*Section 1.01 Close observation of the mother and the child after delivery*
	Particular attention needs to be paid to the monitoring of sleep pattern and normalization of sleep.
Step 2	*Section 1.02 Psychiatric hospitalization in case of (suspected) psychosis*
	Patients should be assessed for risk of self-harm or harm to others (particularly the infant), degree of insight, and functional capacity. Clinicians should be particularly vigilant in patients with rapid cycling, mixed features, or those who have delusions or command hallucinations involving their infant.
Step 3	*Section 1.03 Prescribing medication*
	The choice of treatment should be guided by past treatment response, degree of effectiveness, side-effects profile, patient preference, the acuity of illness, and breastfeeding status. Lithium, anticonvulsants, and neuroleptics may be prescribed as in an ordinary psychotic episode. Most psychotropic medications, including lithium, are excreted in breast milk and the risk to the neonate should be carefully considered.

(continued)

Table 31.1 (continued) Management of post-partum psychosis

	In recent studies oestrogen was considered as medication for PP, especially in patients with oestrogen deficiency.[27],[28] However, results of an open prospective study showed that oestrogen was not efficacious in the prevention of PP.[29] Oestrogen is not recommended for the management of PP in general psychiatry. [30] (For more information, see the section 'Psychotropic medication and breastfeeding'.)
Step 4	*Section 1.04 Advice to weigh up relative risks and benefits of breastfeeding* There are two main risks to be considered: secretion of the drug into breast milk with possible side-effects on the infant; interruption of mother's night sleep for breastfeeding. Possible solutions: careful selection of medication (see the section 'Psychotropic medication and breastfeeding'); milk expression during the day; or stopping breastfeeding.
Step 5	*Section 1.05 Risk assessment: considering the possibility of suicide and infanticide* Of 1000 women with post-partum psychosis, two complete suicide.[31] Among women hospitalized for post-partum psychosis, 9% had thoughts of harming the infant.[32]
Step 6	Psychoeducation, undertaken with partner/family
Step 7	Parenting training and supervision
Step 8	Planning maintenance treatment

Prognosis

Generally, prognosis is favourable. In a minority of women, the illness is characterized by a protracted course.[33] Women with bipolar disorder or schizoaffective disorder have a greater than 50% risk for another episode of post-partum psychosis.[34] This risk of relapse should be considered in planning future pregnancies.

Clinicians should remember that mental illness may affect mother–infant bonding. A significant proportion of mothers with psychotic disorders has parenting difficulties and may lose custody of their infant.[35] Untreated maternal mental disorder impacts on infant and childhood development, and is a risk factor for development of mental illness in the progeny.

Psychosis during pregnancy

For women with a history of psychosis, particularly psychosis in previous pregnancies, the risk of relapse during pregnancy increases mainly due to the (sometimes sudden) discontinuation of taking medication. Pregnancies of patients with psychosis are at an increased risk of obstetric complications, stillbirths, neonatal deaths, and psychiatric complications.[26],[36]

At the same time, women come into contact with many healthcare professionals who have numerous opportunities to help with the prevention and attenuation of these risks. Psychiatric services need to assist patients in engaging with primary care. Medications should be prescribed carefully with respect to consequences for the fetus, neonate, and the mother's health.[57] (For more information, see the section 'Psychotropic medication in pregnancy and breastfeeding'.)

Depression in pregnancy and the post-partum period

Epidemiology

In Europe, the incidence of depressive illness during pregnancy is around 10–15%, while post-partum depression occurs in around 10–22% of women.[37] A recent American study found that 40% of depressed mothers are depressed after birth and 34% during pregnancy; 26% had been depressed already before they became pregnant.[38]

Diagnosis and symptoms

The symptoms of depression in pregnancy in principle do not differ from depression at any other time, although some authors[39] report that women with post-partum major depression are less likely to report feeling sad, but often express feelings of guilt or worthlessness. They are typically much more anxious, with frequent preoccupation about their ability to parent their new child and the health of the infant. Obsessive thoughts to harm the child may be present. Furthermore, antenatal depression may go undiagnosed because of a focus on physical maternal and fetal well-being and the attribution of complaints to the physical and hormonal changes associated with pregnancy.[40,41]

Postnatal depression must be distinguished from the so-called 'baby blues' (see Table 31.2). Baby blues is a temporary emotional lability, usually during the first week after birth. It occurs in 40% of all new mothers. Baby blues lasts for several days and no treatment is needed.

Consequences

The most serious risk of untreated depression is suicide or, very rarely, even infanticide. Overall, suicide and attempted suicide during pregnancy and in the peripartum are rare. Nevertheless, suicide is the second most common cause of death associated with pregnancy and birth.[42]

Antenatal depression is linked with an elevated risk of premature birth, lower birth weight, and delayed intrauterine growth.[41,43] Depressed pregnant women often show inadequate weight gain, less frequent attendance at prenatal examinations, and increased substance abuse.[41]

Table 31.2 Distinguishing between baby blues and post-partum major depressive disorder

	Baby blues	**Major post-partum depression**
Prevalence	Up to 40%	Approximately 10%
Onset	3–5 days post-partum	Usually during the first month post-partum
Duration	<10 days	>2 weeks
Severity	Mild	Moderate to severe
Suicidality	Not present	May be present

Depression following birth may affect the mother's ability to care for the infant and may also impair maternal bonding. Depressed mothers show less verbal and visual communication toward their children. Children demonstrate more frequent breast-feeding and feeding problems, sleep problems, avoidance behaviours, and decreased affect regulation.[44] Maternal depression is a risk factor for cognitive, emotional, and socialization problems, as well as language problems, in later childhood.[45]

Treatment

The treatment of depression is based on psychoeducation, psychotherapy, and pharma-cotherapy. In post-partum depression, all evaluated psychotherapeutic methods were found to be effective and specific psychotherapies have been developed (e.g. see[46]). Es-pecially during pregnancy, all non-pharmacological treatment methods are preferred in order to avoid side-effects in the newborn. These include counselling for stress re-duction and sleep hygiene, relaxation therapy, involvement of the father, and some-times also social support.[41] Bright-light therapy has been successfully used in pregnant women with depression.[47] There is a lack of studies on the effects of psychotherapy in the treatment of depression during pregnancy, with the exception of a study on inter-personal therapy, which was shown to be effective.[48] Psychotropic treatment is used in more serious cases or where there is considerable risk. Selective serotonin reuptake in-hibitors (SSRIs), especially sertraline, are usually recommended as first-line treatment in breastfeeding.[57] (For more information, see the section 'Psychotropic medication and breastfeeding'.)

Psychotropic drugs in pregnancy

Approximately 3.5% of all pregnant women in the Western world use psychotropic drugs during pregnancy,[49] and the post-partum period is widely considered as a period of increased vulnerability to psychiatric disorders.

For every pregnancy, the baseline risk of a major congenital malformation is 1–3% of the population.[50] It is known that all psychotropic drugs pass the placenta.[51] The possible risks of psychotropic drug use during the first trimester of pregnancy include spontaneous abortion and malformations. In later pregnancy, risks of psychotropic medication might include pregnancy and perinatal complications such as low birth weight, prematurity, poor neonatal adaptation (feeding difficulties, irritability, tremor), and the possibility of long-term neurobehavioural effects (for a review, see [41,57]).

Data on the effects of psychotropic medication are limited and sometimes conflict-ing, especially as the effect of underlying depression is often neglected.[41] There is an in-creasing body of evidence-based information indicating that it may be more harmful to both the mother and her baby if she is not treated appropriately for a severe psychiatric disorder than when she is being treated with carefully selected medication.[41]

Pregnant women should be involved in the discussion about the risks and benefits of using pharmacological treatment (see Box 31.1).[41,52,57] Optimally, decision making should occur before pregnancy. If possible, drugs that are contraindicated during preg-nancy (most mood stabilizers, especially valproate) should be avoided in women of

---

Box 31.1 Use of psychotropic medication during pregnancy

- A single medication at a higher dose is favoured over multiple medications.
- Medications with fewer metabolites are preferred.
- Higher protein binding decreases placental passage.
- Changing medications increases the exposure to the baby.
- Dose increase is sometimes required in the third trimester due to increased blood volume; this changes rapidly post-partum and may require dose reduction.
- If a woman is being treated successfully with psychotropic medication before pregnancy, the same treatment should continue throughout pregnancy if there is no major risk of malformation.
- If pregnancy is planned and mental health is stable with a low risk of relapse, discontinuing psychotropic medication may be considered.
- Folic acid supplements are recommended for women on psychotropics, from preconception to at least the end of the first trimester.
- Specific ultrasound of the fetus should be performed in women on psychotropics, to exclude major malformations.

Source data from: *Adv Psychiatric Treatment*, 11, Kohen D. Psychotropic medication and breast feeding, p. 371–9, Copyright (2005) Royal College of Psychiatrists

---

childbearing age.[41] In cases where these drugs are prescribed, women should be carefully informed about their teratogenic potential.

Antidepressants

Selective serotonin reuptake inhibitors (SSRIs)

Although SSRIs are thought to be relatively safe, there are some reports of morphological teratogenicity.[53] However, specific patterns of congenital malformations have not been demonstrated with SSRIs across studies.[54] First-trimester paroxetine exposure seems to be associated with an increased prevalence of combined cardiac defects.[55] Generally, the slightly increased risk of malformations might also be connected to depression itself rather than to antidepressant medication.[41,56]

A possible increase of spontaneous abortions, earlier delivery, lower birth weight, and low APGAR scores have been noted in connection with use of SSRIs during pregnancy.[57] Some studies reported an increased risk of hypoglycaemia and hyperbilirubinaemia.[58]

Of all infants exposed to a SSRI *in utero*, around 30% develop symptoms of poor neonatal adaptation (PNA) such as hypotonia, hypothermia, respiratory depression, cyanosis, arrhythmias, and decreased sucking reflex. Some studies described an increased incidence of PNA after exposure to paroxetine and fluoxetine, compared to other SSRIs.[59]

There is conflicting evidence regarding an elevated risk of persistent pulmonary hypertension of the newborn (PPHN) after exposure to a SSRI. The absolute risk cannot be determined but is very small (less than 1%).[60]

Tricyclic antidepressants (TCAs)

Tricyclic antidepressants have been used extensively for several decades. There seems to be no increased risk of congenital malformations in first-trimester exposure to older TCAs.[57,61] Nulman et al.[62] found no increase of behavioural teratology or later behavioural problems in children born to mothers taking TCAs during pregnancy. Of all infants exposed to TCAs *in utero*, 20–50% develop PNA. Anticholinergic symptoms such as urine retention and constipation are extremely rare.[59]

Monoamine oxidase inhibitors (MAOIs)

There is little evidence of safety of MAOIs in pregnancy. There is a report of teratogenicity from an animal study.[63] Moreover, these drugs require the adoption of a low tyramine diet. MAOIs are therefore usually not recommended in pregnancy. Women on MAOIs should be switched to other antidepressants, ideally prior to pregnancy.

Other antidepressants

Venlafaxine, duloxetine, mirtazapine, trazodone, bupropion: There is a lack of studies on these antidepressants.[57] Prospective studies of mirtazapine,[64] trazodone and nefazadone,[65] as well as bupropion[66] revealed no increased risk of major malformations. There is one study of venlafaxine which suggests associations between periconceptional use of venlafaxine and some birth defects.[67] The risks of PNA are not known, except in relation to venlafaxine (where the risk seems comparable to the risk after exposure to a SSRI).[59]

Antipsychotics

Conventional antipsychotics

Conventional antipsychotics have been in use for half a century and have shown that generally there is no increased teratogenic risk with high-potency conventional antipsychotics. Low-potency antipsychotics seem to have a slightly increased risk of unspecific abnormalities.[68]

A meta-analysis of pregnancy and birth complications in women with schizophrenia found an increase in low birth weight, preterm birth, and perinatal infant death; however, the effect was small.[69] There is evidence that exposure to antipsychotics can lead to symptoms of PNA, but numbers on the incidence of PNA after exposure to antipsychotics are lacking. Extrapyramidal symptoms (increased muscle tone, tremors, agitation, dystonia, decreased sucking reflex, abnormal movements), jaundice, intestinal obstruction, unstable body temperature, respiratory distress, seizures, and transient neuro-developmental delay can also occur.[59,70]

Atypical antipsychotics

A prospective observational cohort comparing typical and atypical antipsychotics with a control group found that the malformation rate was about twofold higher among those on atypicals compared to the reference group. In the group exposed to atypicals, the most common major malformations were cardiovascular, and of the cardiac malformations, most were atrial or ventricular septal defects.[71]

Women receiving atypical antipsychotics, especially in polytherapy, experience more associated co-morbidities and instrumental deliveries. The exposed neonates were more likely to be born premature, were admitted more often to the neonatal intensive care unit, and presented with poor neonatal adaptation signs.[72]

Atypical antipsychotics are associated with weight gain in mothers, and induce maternal hyperglycaemia and impaired glucose tolerance.[73] There are conflicting data on birth weight after exposure to atypical antipsychotics: some studies found a significantly increased risk of low birth weight and infants small for their gestational age;[74] on the other hand, there are studies that found that neonates exposed to atypical antipsychotics were significantly more likely to be large for their gestational age compared with healthy controls;[75] and some studies did not find any differences.[76] Quetiapine appears to have a comparably safe profile during pregnancy, apart from metabolic syndrome.[57]

Mood stabilizers

Most mood stabilizers should be avoided during pregnancy; valproate, in particular, should *never* be given.[57] Quetiapine might be an alternative in some women.[57]

Lithium

Lithium is the most commonly prescribed mood stabilizer during pregnancy. First-trimester lithium exposure is associated with cardiovascular malformation, especially Ebstein's anomaly. The period of maximum risk is 2–6 weeks after conception. The absolute risk, however, is relatively small, reported at 0.05–0.1%.[77,78] A potential increase in the risk of neural tube defects should also be taken into consideration.[78]

Lithium exposure is associated with significantly more miscarriages and elective terminations of pregnancy.[79] The rate of preterm deliveries is higher in infants exposed to lithium.[79] After intrauterine exposure to lithium, the newborn might suffer from floppy infant syndrome. This syndrome is dose-related and consists of hypotonia, hypothermia, respiratory depression, cyanosis, arrhythmias, and decreased sucking reflex. Other described lithium-related symptoms are neonatal thyroid toxicity, nephrogenic diabetes insipidus, cardiovascular and renal dysfunctions, hyperbilirubinaemia, hepatotoxicity, and PPHN. These symptoms are generally self-limiting.[59]

In women on maintenance treatment, serum lithium levels should be monitored every 4 weeks throughout the pregnancy and weekly in the later half of pregnancy. Dosage should be adjusted to match the lower end of the therapeutic range. Renal excretion of lithium increases significantly during the third trimester and an increase of maternal dose is often necessary. Several days prior to delivery, the dosage should be gradually tapered to 60–70% of the original maintenance level. The full pre-pregnancy dose should be resumed immediately post-partum. High-resolution ultrasound and echocardiography of the fetus should be performed between the sixteenth and eighteenth week of gestation to identify possible abnormalities.

Valproic acid (VPA)

Valproic acid (VPA) is associated with a variety of congenital abnormalities. The types of birth defects most often reported in valproate exposure during pregnancy are neural tube defects, orofacial clefts, congenital heart defects, hypospadias, and skeletal abnormalities (polydactyly, craniosynostosis).[80] Morrow et al.[81] reported that for valproate monotherapy exposures, 1% of the pregnancy outcomes were neural tube defects, 1.5% orofacial clefts, 0.7% congenital heart defects, 0.9% hypospadias and/or genitourinary tract defects, 0.5% gastrointestinal tract defects, and 1.1% skeletal defects. A fetal valproate syndrome has been described, characterized by tall forehead with bifrontal narrowing, medial deficiency of eyebrows, infraorbital groove, trigonocephaly, flat nasal bridge, broad nasal root, anteverted nares, shallow philtrum, epicanthic folds, long upper lip with thin vermillion borders, thick lower lip, and small downturned mouth.[82]

The effect of valproate is dose-dependent; the risk of congenital malformations significantly increases at 600 mg/day, with the largest attributable risk observed at doses that exceeded 1000 mg/day. However, individual susceptibility is genetically determined and even very low daily dosages can be teratogenic in some highly sensitive individuals.[83]

Moreover, VPA is a behavioural teratogen. Prenatal exposure to VPA was associated with impaired cognitive function, a lower verbal intelligence quotient, poorer adaptive behaviour, and a higher rate of maladaptive behaviours.[84] Coagulopathies, hepatotoxicity, hypoglycaemia, and low birth weight are also described in association with VPA use in pregnancy.[68]

The use of VPA should be avoided in women of the fertile age group and stopped if pregnancy is planned or has already commenced.[41] Folate supplements should be taken and special ultrasound has to be performed to exclude malformations.

Carbamazepine

Carbamazepine is also associated with congenital abnormalities, although less so than VPA. Increased risk of spina bifida, craniofacial (especially orofacial cleft) and cardiovascular abnormalities, urogenital malformations, and growth retardation are documented.[68] On the other hand, some authors report that carbamazepine teratogenicity is relatively specific to spina bifida.[85] A 'fetal carbamazepine syndrome' has been described, characterized by hypertelorism with epicanthic folds, mongoloid slant of the palpebral apertures, short nose, long philtrum, and hypoplasia of the fingernails.[86]

Carbamazepine should be avoided during pregnancy. When already taken, folate supplements in the first months of gestation and the use of vitamin K during the last trimester are recommended, as well as special ultrasound.

Lamotrigine

Some evidence suggests that exposure to lamotrigine could increase the risk of orofacial clefts (especially cleft palate) in the offspring of women exposed to this drug in the first trimester of pregnancy.[87] If an antiepileptic is needed, lamotrigine can be given, with all precautions.

Sleeping medication

Benzodiazepines

Benzodiazepines during the first trimester are associated with a risk of oral cleft in newborns.[51] The evidence from meta-analyses is conflicting: the data from newer studies do not indicate an increased risk;[88] however, case-control studies suggest a twofold increased risk of oral cleft.[89]

Wikner et al.[90] found a higher than expected number of infants with pyloric stenosis or alimentary tract atresia (especially the small intestine) after benzodiazepine exposure. This was without association to any specific benzodiazepine or hypnotic benzodiazepine receptor agonist.

An increased risk for preterm birth and low birth weight was reported. Third-trimester use is associated with floppy infant syndrome. High-medication dosages (equivalent of diazepam 30 mg) and benzodiazepines with a long half-life appear to have the highest risk. Symptoms include hypotonia, hypothermia, respiratory depression, cyanosis, arrhythmias, and decreased sucking reflex. [59]

Barbiturates

Barbiturates should also be avoided as they are associated with malformations if given during the first trimester and with respiratory depression and withdrawal symptoms if given before delivery.[57]

Other sleeping medications

There are not enough safety data regarding other medications such as zolpidem, zopiclon, or zaleplon.[57] Safer alternatives for sedation might be quetiapine and, potentially, also amitriptyline (not in suicidal patients), diphenhydramine, or chlorpromazine.[57,70] Monotherapy should be achieved.

Psychotropic medication and breastfeeding

Breastfeeding carries numerous health advantages for the mother as well as for the baby. There is evidence for significant health-related, nutritional, immunological, developmental, psychological, social, economic, and environmental advantages.[91,92] On the other hand, with certain drugs, it can be safer to advise mothers against breastfeeding.[41,57]

Data on the safety of psychotropic medication in breastfeeding are mostly derived from case reports and small studies. A psychotropic drug has to pass several steps from intake by the mother to exert an effect on the baby. Most drugs are transferred into the milk by passive diffusion:[93]

1. Lower molecular weight and lipid solubility facilitate passage into breast milk.
2. The composition of milk, which changes with maturity, is one factor determining the drug's breast milk concentration.[94]
3. Breast milk has a lower pH than plasma. Therefore, many alkaline psychotropic drugs diffuse easily down a pH gradient.
4. Hindmilk has a higher lipid concentration and, therefore, a higher concentration of lipid-soluble drugs compared to foremilk.
5. Colostrum (produced only during the first days after birth) has a higher protein level and, therefore, higher concentration of protein-bound drugs.

For evaluation of the baby's exposure to a drug, a milk:plasma ratio is calculated from the concentration of the drug (or its metabolite) simultaneously measured in the mother's plasma and breast milk. A milk:plasma ratio greater than one suggests a high likelihood that the infant will be exposed to the drug.[95] The relative infant dose is the percentage of maternal plasma level received by the infant in a 24-hour period. For psychotropics, the arbitrary concentration in the infant's plasma of 10% of the established therapeutic maternal dose is used as the upper threshold, where the risk of side-effects is low and treatment is accepted as safe.[52]

The physiology of the newborn is immature, with a limited ability to metabolize drugs (hepatic and renal function immaturity, higher gastric pH, slower bowel motility, lower degree of plasma proteins). However, the capacity to metabolize drugs rapidly increases.[68] Preterm infants have a pronounced immaturity of all functions and should ideally not be exposed to psychotropic medication.[52]

Antidepressants

Tricyclic antidepressants (TCAs)

TCAs appear to be relatively safe during breastfeeding. The levels of the drugs ingested by an infant were found to be low. There are no adverse effects reported with amytriptyline, nortriptyline, imipramine, desipramine, dosulepine, and clomipramine.[52,96] Doxepine has a long-acting metabolite that may accumulate in infants. Respiratory depression in infants exposed to doxepine is an extremely rare complication.[97,98]

Selective serotonin reuptake inhibitors (SSRIs)

The excretion of a SSRI into breast milk ranges from low to undetectable levels. Citalopram has a high milk:plasma ratio; nevertheless, infant levels are still very low to undetectable.[99] According to Becker et al.,[91] sertraline and paroxetine should be considered first-line choices, whereas fluoxetine and citalopram should not. However, according to Riecher-Rössler and Heck,[57] paroxetine should not be established because of the teratogenic risk in potential further pregnancies.

No significant adverse effects on the infant have been reported with sertraline, fluvoxamine, and escitalopram. Fluoxetine has the active metabolite, norfluoxetine, with a very long half-life, which may accumulate in infants. There are several reports of adverse effects: irritability, excessive crying, colic, vomiting, and also a case of somnolence, hypotonia, and unresponsiveness.[91,100] Anyway, most reports show no adverse effects in the nursing infants but, rather, normal neurological development and normal weight gain.[101] Only very few cases of adverse effects with paroxetine have been reported and include hyponatraemia. However, causality was not clear because paroxetine levels were not determined in infant serum.[102] Citalopram may be associated with poor infant sleep,[103] hypotonia, colic, decreased feeding, and irritability.[104]

Other antidepressants

Experience on other antidepressants is limited, so they should not be first choice.[57]

Bupropion levels in infant serum were found to be low.[105] There is one case report of the development of seizures in a 6-month-old infant, which was possibly attributable to use of bupropion during breastfeeding.[106] **Venlafaxine** infant dose was variable and ranged up to 9.2%, which is relatively high but still below the 10% 'safe' level.[107]

Trazodone is excreted at the rate of 1% into breast milk: few cases of drowsiness and poor feeding have been reported.[52] The relative infant dose of mirtazapine (including the desmethyl metabolite) is 1.9%: no adverse effects in infants, including sedation or weight gain, were reported.[108]

Monoamine oxidase inhibitors (MAOIs)

There is a lack of studies on safety profiles of monoamine oxidase inhibitors during breastfeeding. Usual practice is discontinuation of this medication.

Antipsychotics

Conventional antipsychotics

Typical antipsychotics are excreted into breast milk usually at a rate less than 3% of maternal levels.[109] Haloperidol is excreted in relatively high amounts (two thirds of maternal serum levels) into breast milk.[110] There is one report of drowsiness and lethargy after chlorpromazine exposure.[111] Developmental delay at 12–18 months in babies exposed to chlorpromazine and haloperidol was described in one study.[110] On the other hand, most studies have shown no adverse effects. Levels of flupentixol and zuclopentixol in breast milk were low.[112] A potential relationship between the use of phenothiazines and the risk of sudden infant death syndrome is noted in the literature.[113]

Atypical antipsychotics

Risperidone,[114] quetiapine,[115] ziprasidone,[116] and sulpiride[117] infant serum levels were found in low to undetectable levels in exposed infants. No adverse effects were reported in monotherapy. Sulpiride is sometimes used as a galactagogue, to increase breast milk production. Olanzapine achieves very low infant plasma levels. Gentile[73] reported that olanzapine seems to be associated with an increased risk of inducing extrapyramidal reactions in breast-fed babies. Analyses of prospectively reported pregnancies, performed by the drug company, revealed that a total of 15.6% of the pregnancies reported an adverse event in the infant, the most common being somnolence (3.9%), irritability (2%), tremor (2%), and insomnia (2%).[118] Clozapine achieves relatively high concentrations in breast milk.[119] Among four infants who were breastfed by mothers taking clozapine, one infant experienced drowsiness and one infant experienced agranulocytosis possibly caused by clozapine, which resolved on stopping clozapine.[120] There is a case of a breastfed child of a mother taking clozapine with delayed speech development; fluent speech was not achieved until the age of 5 years.[121] The concentration of amisulpiride in breast milk is high and the relative infant dose was 10.7%, which is slightly above the usual 10% maximum recommendation.[122] No adverse effects on infants were reported. The reported levels of aripiprazole in breast milk were variable; authors estimated the infant dose from 0.7% to 8.3% of the maternal dosage.[123,124] No adverse side-effects in infants were reported.

Quetiapine seems relatively safe in pregnancy and breastfeeding. Furthermore, it does not reduce fertility in women who wish to get pregnant, as it does not induce hyperprolactinaemia. It is therefore an antipsychotic which allows pregnancy planning and therapy throughout the peripartum.[41,57]

Mood stabilizers

Lithium

Lithium level in breast milk is found to be at approximately 50% of maternal serum levels. Infant levels are variable, but also high. Furthermore, immature neonatal renal function increases the risk of toxicity. Transient laboratory abnormalities of elevated blood urea nitrogen, creatinine, and thyroid-stimulating hormone were observed in infants.[91] Cases of toxicity, including cyanosis, hypothermia, hypotonia, and electrocardiography (ECG) T-wave inversion are documented.[125] Opinions on the use of lithium while breastfeeding vary from absolute contraindication to prescribing on the mother's informed choice. However, if lithium is necessary, breastfeeding should not be recommended. If the mother insists on breastfeeding, the infant must be referred to a paediatrician for regular monitoring of lithium levels and blood urea nitrogen, creatinine, and thyroid-stimulating hormone.[93]

Carbamazepine

Carbamazepine and its active metabolite are found in breast milk in significant levels. Levels reported in infant plasma were variable, up to 65% of maternal levels. Transient hepatic toxicity, such as hyperbilirubinaemia and high concentrations of gamma-glutamyl-transferase, has been reported in neonates exposed to carbamazepine during breastfeeding.[126] Other documented side-effects include seizure-like activity, irritability, and poor feeding. Exposed infants should have serum levels monitored and liver function tests.[91]

Valproic acid (VPA)

The concentration of valproate in breast milk is up to 3% of maternal plasma levels.[127] There are no reports of major adverse events in children breastfed by mothers taking sodium valproate, apart from one adverse event of thrombocytopenia and anaemia. [128]

Other mood stabilizers

Lamotrigine is excreted in relatively high levels in breast milk; random infant serum levels are 30% of maternal levels.[91] There is concern about development of Stevens-Johnson syndrome. However, no cases have been reported. **Gabapentin** crosses into breast milk at nearly 100% of maternal concentrations and is therefore not recommended during breastfeeding.[129]

Sleeping medication

Benzodiazepines

Benzodiazepines have very low milk:plasma ratios; lower than other psychotropic medications, especially those with short half-lives.[109] Reported adverse effects include sedation, lethargy, and weight loss. There is a risk of accumulation of long-acting drugs in the infant's body; therefore, short-acting drugs are usually recommended. Exposed infants should be monitored for sedation and apnea. Avoid these drugs in prematurity.

Other hypnotics

Zaleplon and zopiclone achieve high concentrations in breast milk, and are therefore contraindicated during breastfeeding. Zolpidem might be compatible with breastfeeding (it is hydrophillic and rapidly excreted).[52] With other hypnotics, we do not have enough data with regard to breastfeeding, which is why they should be avoided.[57,129] If sedation during breastfeeding is needed, quetiapine or amitryptiline can be used (however, note the narrow therapeutic window of TCAs and do not use in suicidal patients).

References

1 O'Hara MW, Zekoski EM, Philipps LH, Wright EJ. Controlled prospective study of post-partum mood disorders: comparison of childbearing and nonchildbearing women. *J Abnorm Psych* 1990; **99**:3–15. DOI:10.1037/0021–843X.99.1.3

2 O'Hara MW. Post-partum 'blues,' depression, and psychosis: a review. *J Psychosom Obstet Gynaecol* 1987; **7**(3):205–27. DOI:10.3109/01674828709040280

3 Terp IM, Mortensen PB. Post-partum psychoses. Clinical diagnoses and relative risk of admission after parturition. *Br J Psychiatry* 1998; **172**:521–6. DOI:10.1192/bjp.172.6.521

4 Bennett HA, Einarson A, Taddio A, Koren G, Einarson TR. Prevalence of depression during pregnancy: systematic review. *Obstet Gynecol* 2004; **103**:698–709. DOI:10.1097/01.AOG.0000116689.75396.5f

5 Kendell RE, Chalmers JC, Platz C. Epidemiology of puerperal psychoses. *Br J Psychiatry* 1987; **150**:662–73.

6 Lusskin S. The epidemiology of postpartum depression. *Arch Womens Ment Health* 2001; **3**(Suppl 2):2, abstract S7.

7 Okano T, Nomura J, Kumar R, et al. An epidemiological and clinical investigation of postpartum psychiatric illness in Japanese mothers. *J Affect Disord* 1998; **48**(2–3):233–40.

8 Terp IM, Mortensen PB. Post-partum psychoses. Clinical diagnoses and relative risk of admission after parturition. *Br J Psychiatry* 1998; **172**:521–6.

9 American Psychiatric Association. *Diagnostic and statistical manual of mental disorders* (5th edn). Washington, DC: American Psychiatric Publishing; 2013 .DOI:10.1176/appi.books.9780890425596.744053

10 Sharma V. Treatment of postpartum psychosis: challenges and opportunities. *Curr Drug Saf* 2008; **3**(1):76–81.

11 Riecher-Rössler A. Prospects for the classification of mental disorders in women. *Eur Psychiatry* 2010; **25**(4):189–96. DOI:10.1016/j.eurpsy.2009.03.002

12 World Health Organization. *The ICD-10 classification of mental and behavioural disorders*. Geneva: World Health Organization; 1992. DOI:10.1002/1520–6505(2000)9:5 <201:AID-EVAN2>3.3.CO;2–P

13 Riecher-Rössler A, Rohde A. Diagnostic classification of perinatal mood disorders. In: *Perinatal stress, mood and anxiety disorders. From bench to bedside* (eds.Riecher-Rössler A, Steiner M). Basel: Karger; 2005, pp. 6–27.

14 Heron J, Robertson Blackmore E, McGuinness M, Craddock N, Jones I. No 'latent period' in the onset of bipolar affective puerperal psychosis. *Arch Womens Ment Health* 2007; **10**(2):79–81. DOI:10.1007/s00737–007–0174–z

15 Sharma V. Role of sleep loss in the causation of puerperal psychosis. *Med Hypotheses* 2003; **61**(4):477–81.

16 **Protheroe C**. Puerperal psychoses: a long term study 1927–61. *Br J Psychiatry* 1969; **115**(518):9–30.

17 **Chaudron LH, Pies RW**. The relationship between postpartum psychosis and bipolar disorder: a review. *J Clin Psychiatry* 2003; **64**(11):1284–92.

18 **Brockington I**. Diagnosis and management of post-partum disorders: a review. *World Psychiatry* 2004; **3**(2):89–95.

19 **Blackmore ER, Jones I, Doshi M, et al**. Obstetric variables associated with bipolar affective puerperal psychosis. *Br J Psychiatry* 2006; **188**:32–6. DOI:10.1192/bjp.188.1.32

20 **Harlow BL, Vitonis AF, Sparen P, Cnattingius S, Joffe H, Hultman CM**. Incidence of hospitalization for postpartum psychotic and bipolar episodes in women with and without prior prepregnancy or prenatal psychiatric hospitalizations. *Arch Gen Psychiatry* 2007; **64**(1):42–8. DOI:10.1001/archpsyc.64.1.42

21 **Platz C, Kendell RE**. A matched-control follow-up and family study of 'puerperal psychoses'. *Br J Psychiatry* 1988; **153**:90–4. DOI:10.1192/bjp.153.1.90

22 **Sharma V, Smith A, Khan M**. The relationship between duration of labour, time of delivery, and puerperal psychosis. *J Affect Disord* 2004; **83**(2–3):215–20. DOI:10.1016/j.jad.2004.04.014

23 **Whalley LJ, Roberts DF, Wentzel J, Wright AF**. Genetic factors in puerperal affective psychoses. *Acta Psychiatr Scand* 1982; **65**(3):180–93.

24 **Cox JL**. Postnatal depression: a comparison of African and Scottish women. *Soc Psychiatry* 1983; **18**(1):25–8.

25 **Hirschfeld RMA, Holzer C, Calabrese JR, et al**. Validity of the mood disorder questionnaire: a general population study. *Am J Psychiatry* 2003; **160**(1):178–80.

26 **Riecher-Rössler A**. Psychose in schwangerschaft und stillzeit. In: *Psychische erkrankungen in schwangerschaft und stillzeit* (ed. Riecher-Rössler A). Freiburg und Basel: Karger; 2012, pp. 34–42.

27 **Gregoire AJ, Kumar R, Everitt B, Henderson AF, Studd JW**. Transdermal oestrogen for treatment of severe postnatal depression. *Lancet* 1996; **347**(9006):930–3.

28 **Ahokas A, Aito M, Turiainen S**. Association between oestradiol and puerperal psychosis. *Acta Psychiatr Scand* 2000; **101**(2):167–9 (discussion 169–70).

29 **Kumar C, McIvor RJ, Davies T, et al**. Estrogen administration does not reduce the rate of recurrence of affective psychosis after childbirth. *J Clin Psychiatry* 2003; **64**(2):112–8. DOI:10.4088/JCP.v64n0202

30 **Sit D, Rothschild AJ, Wisner KL**. A review of postpartum psychosis. *J Womens Health (Larchmt)* 2006; **15**(4):352–68. DOI:10.1089/jwh.2006.15.352

31 **Weindling AM**. The confidential enquiry into maternal and child health (CEMACH). *Arch Dis Child* 2003; **88**(12):1034–7. DOI:10.1136/adc.88.12.1034

32 **Kumar R, Marks M, Platz C, Yoshida K**. Clinical survey of a psychiatric mother and baby unit: characteristics of 100 consecutive admissions. *J Affect Disord* 1995; **33**(1):11–22.

33 **Videbech P, Gouliaev G**. First admission with puerperal psychosis: 7–14 years of follow-up. *Acta Psychiatr Scand* 1995; **91**(3):167–73.

34 **Robertson E, Jones I, Haque S, Holder R, Craddock N**. Risk of puerperal and non-puerperal recurrence of illness following bipolar affective puerperal (post-partum) psychosis. *Br J Psychiatry* 2005; **186**:258–9. DOI:10.1192/bjp.186.3.258

35 **Seneviratne G**. Parenting assessment in a psychiatric mother and baby unit. *Br J Soc Work* 2003; **33**(4):535–55. DOI:10.1093/bjsw/33.4.535

36 Sacker A, Done DJ, Crow TJ. Obstetric complications in children born to parents with schizophrenia: a meta-analysis of case-control studies. *Psychol Med* 1996; **26**(2):279–87.

37 Altshuler LL, Cohen LS, Moline ML, et al. Treatment of depression in women: a summary of the expert consensus guidelines. *J Psychiatr Pract* 2001; **7**(3):185–208.

38 Wisner KL, Sit DK, McShea MC, et al. Onset timing, thoughts of self-harm, and diagnoses in postpartum women with screen positive depression findings. *JAMA Psychiatry* 2013; **70**:490–8.

39 Kammerer M, Marks MN, Pinard C, et al. Symptoms associated with the DSM-IV diagnosis of depression in pregnancy and post partum. *Arch Women Ment Health* 2009; **12**(3):135–41.

40 Bowen A, Muhajarine N. Antenatal depression. *Can Nurse* 2006; **102**(9):26–30.

41 Riecher-Rössler A. Depression in der peripartalzeit—diagnostik, therapie und prophylaxe. *Psych Up2date*; 2015.

42 Lindahl V, Pearson JL, Colpe L. Prevalence of suicidality during pregnancy and the postpartum. *Arch Women Ment Health* 2005; **8**:77–87.

43 Grote NK, Bridge JA, Gavin AR, Melville JL, Iyengar S, Katon WJ. A meta-analysis of depression during pregnancy and the risk of preterm birth, low birth weight, and intrauterine growth restriction. *Arch Gen Psychiatry* 2010; **67**:1012–24.

44 Field T. Postpartum depression effects on early interactions, parenting, and safety practices. *Infant Behav Develop* 2010; **33**:1–6.

45 Goodman SH, Rouse MH, Connell A, Broth MR, Hall CM, Heyward D. Maternal depression and child psychopathology: a meta-analytic review. *Clin Child Fam Psychol Rev* 2011; **14**:1–27.

46 Frisch U, Hofecker Fallahpour M, Stieglitz RD, Riecher-Rössler A. Group treatment for depression in mothers of young children: a controlled study. *Psychopathology* 2012; **46**:94–101.

47 Wirz-Justice A, Bader A, Frisch U, et al. A randomized, double-blind, placebo-controlled study of light therapy for antepartum depression. *J Clin Psychiatry* 2011; **72**:986–93.

48 Dennis CL, Hodnett ED. Psychosocial and psychological interventions for treating postpartum depression. *Cochrane Data Syst Rev* 2007; **4**:CD006116.

49 Munk-Olsen T, Laursen TM, Pedersen CB, Mors O, Mortensen PB. New parents and mental disorders: a population-based register study. *JAMA* 2006; **296**:2582–9.

50 McElhatton PR. General principles of drug use in pregnancy. *Pharm J* 2003; **270**:232–4.

51 Altshuler LL, Cohen L, Szuba MP, Burt VK, Gitlin M, Mintz J. Pharmacologic management of psychiatric illness during pregnancy: dilemmas and guidelines. *Am J Psychiatry* 1996; **153**(5):592–606.

52 Kohen D. Psychotropic medication and breast feeding. *Adv Psychiat Treat* 2005; **11**:371–9.

53 Myles N, Newall A, Ward H, Large M. Systematic meta-analysis of individual selective serotonin reuptake inhibitor medications and congenital malformation. *Austr N Z J Psychiatry* 2013; **47**(11):1002–12.

54 Byatt N, Deligiannidis KM, Freemann MP. Antidepressant use in pregnancy: a critical review focused on risks and controversies. *Acta Psychiatr Scand* 2013; **127**(2):94–114.

55 Wurst KE, Poole C, Ephross SA, Olsahn AF. First trimester paroxetine use and the prevalence of congenital, specifically cardiac, defects: a meta-analysis of epidemiological studies. *Birth Defects Res A Clin Mol Teratol* 2010; **88**:159–70.

56 **Jimenez-Solem E, Andersen JT, Petersen M, et al**. Exposure to selective serotonin reuptake inhibitors and the risk of congenital malformations: a nationwide cohort study. *BMJ Open* 2012; **2**(3):(iie001148).

57 **Riecher-Rössler A, Heck A**. Psychopharmakotherapie in schwangerschaft und stillzeit. In: *Psychische erkrankungen in schwangerschaft und stillzeit* (ed. Riecher-Rössler A). Freiburg und Basel: Karger; 2011, s. 69–89.

58 **Stewart DE**. Clinical practice. Depression during pregnancy. *N Engl J Med* 2011; **365**(17):1605–11.

59 **Kieviet M, Dolman AM, Honig A**. The use of psychotropic medication during pregnancy: how about the newborn? *Neuropsychiatr Dis Treat* 2013; **9**:1257–66.

60 **'t Jong GW, Einarson T, Koren G, Einarson A**. Antidepressant use in pregnancy and persistent pulmonary hypertension of the newborn (PPHN): a systematic review. *Reprod Toxicol* 2012; **34**(3):293–7.

61 **Ward RK, Zamorski MA**. Benefits and risks of psychiatric medications during pregnancy. *Am Fam Physician* 2002; **66**:629–36.

62 **Nulman I, Rovet J, Stewart DE, et al**. Child development following exposure to tricyclic antidepressants or fluoxetine throughout foetal life: a prospective controlled study. *Am J Psychiatry* 2002; **159**:1889–95.

63 **Poulson E, Robson J**. Effect of phenelzine and some related compounds in pregnancy. *J Endocrinol* 1964; **30**:205–15.

64 **Djulus J, Koren G, Einarson TR, et al**. Exposure to mirtazapine during pregnancy: a prospective, comparative study of birth outcomes. *J Clin Psychiatry* 2006; **67**:1280–4.

65 **Einarson A, Bonari L, Voyer-Lavignes S, et al**. A multicentre prospective controlled study to determine the safety of trazodone and nefazodone use during pregnancy. *Can J Psychiatry* 2003; **48**:106–10.

66 **Chun-Fai-Chan B, Koren G, Fayez I, et al**. Pregnancy outcome of women exposed to bupropion during pregnancy: a prospective comparative study. *Am J Obstet Gynaecol* 2005; **192**:932–6.

67 **Polen KN, Rasmussen SA, Riehle-Colarusso T, Reefhuis J**. National Birth Defects Prevention Study. Association between reported venlafaxine use in early pregnancy and birth defects; National Birth Defects Prevention Study, 1997–2007. *Birth Defects Res A Clin Mol Teratol* 2013; **97**(1):28–35.

68 **Menon SJ**. Psychotropic medication during pregnancy and lactation. *Arch Gynecol Obstet* 2008; **277**:1–13.

69 **Bennedsen BE**. Adverse pregnancy outcome in schizophrenic women: occurrence and risk factors. *Schizophr Res* 1998; **33**(1–2):1–26.

70 **Gentile S**. Antipsychotic therapy during early and late pregnancy. A systematic review. *Schizophr Bull* 2010; **36**:518–44.

71 **Habermann F, Fritzsche J, Fuhlbrück F, et al**. Atypical antipsychotic drugs and pregnancy outcome: a prospective, cohort study. *J Clin Psychopharmacol* 2013; **33**(4):453–62.

72 **Sadowski A, Todorow M, Yazdani Brojeni P, Koren G, Nulman I**. Pregnancy outcomes following maternal exposure to second-generation antipsychotics given with other psychotropic drugs: a cohort study. *BMJ Open* 2013; **13**:3(7); ii(e003062).

73 **Gentile S**. Infant safety with antipsychotic therapy in breast-feeding: a systematic review. *J Clin Psychiatry* 2008; **69**(4):666–73.

74 **Reis M, Källén B**. Maternal use of antipsychotics in early pregnancy and delivery outcome. *J Clin Psychopharmacol* 2008; **28**:279–88.

75 Newham JJ, Thomas SH, MacRitchie K, McElhatton PR, McAllister-Williams RH. Birth weight of infants after maternal exposure to typical and atypical antipsychotics: prospective comparison study. *Br J Psychiatry* 2008; **192**:333–7.

76 Lin H, Chen I, Chen Y, Lee HC, Wu FJ. Maternal schizophrenia and pregnancy outcome: does the use of antipsychotics make a difference? *Schizophr Res* 2010; **116**:55–60.

77 Cohen LS, Friedman JM, Jefferson JW, Johnson EM, Weiner ML. A re-evaluation of risk of in utero exposure to lithium. *JAMA* 1994; **271**:146–50.

78 Gentile S. Lithium in pregnancy: the need to treat, the duty to ensure safety. *Expert Opin Drug Saf* 2012; **11**(3):425–37.

79 Diav-Citrin O, Shechtman S, Tahover E, et al. Pregnancy outcome following in utero exposure to lithium: a prospective, comparative, observational study. *Am J Psychiatry* 2014; **171**(7):785–94. DOI:10.1176/appi.ajp.2014.12111402

80 Werler MM, Ahrens KA, Bosco JL, et al. Use of antiepileptic medications in pregnancy in relation to risks of birth defects. *Ann Epidemiol* 2011; **21**(11):842–50.

81 Morrow J, Russell A, Guthrie E, et al. Malformation risks of antiepileptic drugs in pregnancy: a prospective study from the UK Epilepsy and Pregnancy Register. *J Neurol Neurosurg Psychiatry* 2006; **77**:193–8.

82 Clayton-Smith J, Donnai D. Fetal valproate syndrome. *J Med Genet* 1995; **32**(9):724–7.

83 Diav-Citrin O, Shechtman S, Bar-Oz B, Cantrell D, Arnon J, Ornoy A. Pregnancy outcome after in utero exposure to valproate: evidence of dose relationship in teratogenic effect. *CNS Drugs* 2008; **22**:325–34.

84 Vinten J, Bromley RL, Taylor J, et al. The behavioral consequences of exposure to antiepileptic drugs in utero. *Epilepsy Behav* 2009; **14**(1):197–201.

85 Jentink J, Dolk H, Loane MA, et al. Intrauterine exposure to carbamazepine and specific congenital malformations: systematic review and case-control study. EUROCAT Antiepileptic Study Working Group. *BMJ* 2010; **341**:c6581.

86 Jones KL, Lacro RV, Johnson KA, Adams J. Pattern of malformations in the children of women treated with carbamazepine during pregnancy. *N Engl J Med* 1989; **320**(25):1661–6.

87 Holmes LB, Baldwin EJ, Smith CR, et al. Increased frequency of isolated cleft palate in infants exposed to lamotrigine during pregnancy. *Neurology* 2008; **70**:2152–8.

88 Bellantuono C, Tofani S, Di Sciascio G, Santone G. Benzodiazepine exposure in pregnancy and risk of major malformations: a critical overview. *Gen Hosp Psychiatry* 2013; **35**(1):3–8.

89 Enato E, Moretti M, Koren G. The fetal safety of benzodiazepines: an updated meta-analysis. *J Obstet Gynaecol Can* 2011; **33**(1):46–8.

90 Wikner BN, Stiller CO, Bergman U, Asker C, Källén B. Use of benzodiazepines and benzodiazepine receptor agonists during pregnancy: neonatal outcome and congenital malformations. *Pharmacoepidemiol Drug Saf* 2007; **16**(11):1203–10.

91 Becker MA, Mayor GF, Elisabeth JS. Psychotropic medications and breastfeeding. *Primary Psychiatry* 2009; **16**(3):42–51.

92 Lucas A, Morley R, Cole TJ, Lister G, Leeson-Payne C. Breast feeding and subsequent intelligence quotient in children born preterm. *Lancet* 1992; **339**:261–4.

93 Tripathi BM, Majumder P. Lactating mother and psychotropic drugs. *MSM* 2010; **8**:83–95. DOI: 10.4103/0973–1229.58821

94 Buist A, Norman TR, Dennerstein L. Breast-feeding and the use of psychotropic medication: a review. *J Affect Disord* 1990; **19**:197–206.

95 Suri RA, Altshuler LL, Burt VK, Hendrick VC. Managing psychiatric medications in the breast-feeding woman. *Meds Wom Health* 1998; **3**:1–10.

96 Eberhard-Gran M, Eskild A, Opjordsmoen S. Use of psychotropic medications in treating mood disorders during lactation. *CNS Drugs* 2006; **20**(3):187–8.

97 Frey OR, Scheidt P, von Brenndorff AI. Adverse effects in a newborn infant breast-fed by a mother treated with doxepin. *Ann Pharmacother* 1999; **33**(6):690–3.

98 Matheson I, Pande H, Alertsen AR. Respiratory depression caused by N-desmethyldoxepin in breast milk. *Lancet* 1985; **2**(8464):1124.

99 Rampono J, Kristensen JH, Hackett LP, Paech M, Kohan R, Ilett KF. Citalopram and demethylcitalopram in human milk; distribution, excretion and effects in breast fed infants. *Br J Clin Pharmacol* 2000; **50**(3):263–8.

100 Lester BM, Cucca J, Andreozzi L, Flanagan P, Oh W. Possible association between fluoxetine hydrochloride and colic in an infant. *J Am Acad Child Adolesc Psychiatry* 1993; **32**(6):1253–5.

101 Heikkinen T, Ekblad U, Palo P, Laine K. Pharmacokinetics of fluoxetine and norfluoxetine in pregnancy and lactation. *Clin Pharmacol Ther* 2003; **73**(4):330–7.

102 Abdul Aziz A, Agab WA, Kalis NN. Severe paroxetine induced hyponatremia in a breast fed infant. *J Bahrain Med Soc* 2004; **16**:195–8.

103 Schmidt K, Oleson OV, Jensen PN. Citalopram and breast-feeding: serum concentration and side effects in the infant. *Biol Psychiatry* 2000; **47**(2):164–5.

104 Lee A, Woo J, Ito S. Frequency of infant adverse events that are associated with citalopram use during breast-feeding. *Am J Obstet Gynecol* 2004; **190**(1):218–21.

105 Baab SW, Peindl KS, Wisner KL. Serum buproprion levels in two breastfeeding mother-infant pairs. *J Clin Psychiatry* 2002; **63**(10):910–11.

106 Chaudron LH, Schoenecker CJ. Buproprion and breastfeeding: a case of a possible infant seizure. *J Clin Psychiatry* 2004; **65**:881–2.

107 Ilett KF, Kristensen JH, Hackett LP, Paech M, Kohan R, Rampono J. Distribution of venlafaxine and its O-desmethyl metabolite in human milk and their effects in breastfed infants. *Br J Clin Pharmacol* 2002; **53**(1):17–22.

108 Kristensen JH, Ilett KF, Rampono J, Kohan R, Hackett LP. Transfer of the antidepressant mirtazapine into breast milk. *Br J Clin Pharmacol* 2007; **63**(3):322–7.

109 Moretti ME. Psychotropic drugs in lactation. *Can J Clin Pharmacol* 2009; **16**:49–57.

110 Yoshida K, Smith B, Craggs M, Kumar R. Neuroleptic drugs in breast-milk: a study of pharmacokinetics and of possible adverse effects in breast-fed infants. *Psychol Med* 1998; **28**(1):81–91.

111 Wiles DH, Orr MW, Kolakowska T. Chorpromazine levels in plasma and milk of nursing mothers. *Br J Clin Pharmacol* 1978; **5**(3):272–3.

112 Matheson I, Skjaeraasen J. Milk concentrations of flupenthixol, nortriptyline and zuclopenthixol and between-breast differences in two patients. *Eur J Clin Pharmacol* 1988; **35**(2):217–20.

113 Kahn A, Blum D. Phenothiazines and sudden infant death syndrome. *Pediatrics* 1982; **70**(1):75–8.

114 Ilett KF, Hackett LP, Kristensen JH, Vaddadi KS, Gardiner SJ, Begg EJ. Transfer of risperidone and 9-hydroxyrisperidone into human milk. *Ann Pharmacother* 2004; **38**(2):273–6.

115 Rampono J, Kristensen JH, Ilett KF, Hackett LP, Kohan R. Quetiapine and breast feeding. *Ann Pharmacother* 2007; **41**(4):711–4.

116 Schlotterbeck P, Saur R, Hiemke C, et al. Low concentration of ziprasidone in human milk: a case report. *Int J Neuropsychopharmacol* 2009; **12**:437–8.

117 Ylikorkala O, Kauppila A, Kivinen S, Viinikka L. Sulpiride improves inadequate lactation. *BMJ (Clin Res Ed)* 1982; **285**:249–51.

118 Brunner E, Falk DM, Jones M, Dey DK, Shatapathy CC. Olanzapine in pregnancy and breastfeeding: a review of data from global safety surveillance. *BMC Pharmacol Toxicol* 2013; **14**:38.

119 Barnas C, Bergant A, Hummer M, Saria A, Fleischhacker WW. Clozapine concentrations in maternal and fetal plasma, amniotic fluid, and breast milk. *Am J Psychiatry* 1994; **151**:945.

120 Dev VJ, Krupp P. Adverse event profile and safety of clozapine. *Rev Contemp Pharmacother* 1995; **6**:197–208.

121 Mendhekar DN. Possible delayed speech acquisition with clozapine therapy during pregnancy and lactation. *J Neuropsychiatry Clin Neurosci* 2007; **19**:196–7.

122 Teoh S, Ilett KF, Hackett LP, Kohan R. Estimation of rac-amisulpride transfer into milk and of infant dose via milk during its use in a lactating woman with bipolar disorder and schizophrenia. *Breastfeed Med* 2011; **6**(2):85–8.

123 Nordeng H, Gjerdalen G, Brede WR, Michelsen LS, Spigset O. Transfer of aripiprazole to breast milk: a case report. *J Clin Psychopharmacol* 2014; **34**:272–5.

124 Lutz UC, Hiemke C, Wiatr G, Farger G, Arand J, Wildgruber D. Aripiprazole in pregnancy and lactation a case report. *J Clin Psychopharmacol* 2010; **30**:204–5.

125 Chaudron LH, Jefferson JW. Mood stabilizers during breast-feeding: a review. *J Clin Psychiatry* 2000; **61**:79–90.

126 Merlob P, Mor M, Litin A. Transient hepatic dysfunction in an infant of an epileptic mother treated with carbamazepine during pregnancy and breast-feeding. *Ann Pharmacother* 1992; **26**:1563–5.

127 Nau H, Rating D, Koch S, Häuser I, Helge H. Valproic acid and its metabolite: placental transfer, neonatal pharmacokinetics, transfer via mother's milk and clinical status in neonates of epileptic mothers. *J Pharmac Exp Ther* 1981; **219**:768–77.

128 Stahl MM, Neiderud J, Vinge E. Thrombocytopenic purpura and anemia in a breast-fed infant whose mother was treated with valproic acid. *J Pediatr* 1997; **130**(6):1001–3.

129 Sivertz K, Kostaras X. The use of psychotropic medications in pregnancy and lactation. *BC Med J* 2005; **47**(3):135–8.

Chapter 32

Involuntary hospitalizations in psychiatry: what to do and what to avoid

Sarah B. Johnson, Corrado De Rosa, and Michael Musalek

Introduction

Patients must consent to the psychiatric care they receive, as with other medical treatments; however, there are specific circumstances in which treatments are compulsory and independent of the subject's will. Involuntary treatment in psychiatry has, since the advent of mental asylums and hospitals, been a controversial, but sometimes necessary, health procedure. It represents a crucial issue in mental health because of its impact upon the freedom of the subject involved. In several national mental health service systems, compulsory treatments are still frequent, and involuntary admission and treatment procedures vary widely by different countries. According to recent literature data, rates of involuntary hospital admission show a wide range, from 6–12.4 per 100,000 population in Portugal and Italy to 232.5 in Finland. Of course, such a degree of variation leads to speculation about the impact of specific features of the national mental health service organization and legislation.[1]

From a historical perspective, trends in involuntary hospitalization have evolved as increasing attention has been paid to the concept of patient rights. Working with patients who are admitted against their will can provide unique challenges to psychiatrists: it can be difficult to establish rapport, and an adversarial position may be taken by the patient because they feel as though their rights are being violated.

History

By the late 1700s, mental hospitals and asylums were beginning to be established in the United States and Europe. Both private and public hospitals existed and patients were typically retained on the basis of a doctor's judgement of need for treatment. There were essentially no procedures or laws in place to protect patient rights. Married women could be committed at the request of their husband, and children could be committed at the request of their parents. By the mid 1800s, courts were beginning to set standards and procedures to protect the rights of those committed. By the mid 1900s, increased attention was focused on patient's rights and liberties of the mentally ill. Commitment

Box 32.1 Legal basis for involuntary hospitalization

◆ *Patrens patriae*: refers to government's authority and responsibility to act for those who are unable to act for their own interests.

◆ *Police power*: refers to government's authority to act in the interest of maintaining order and public safety.

Source data from: Rosner R (ed), *Principles and Practice of Forensic Psychiatry*, 2nd edition, in Zerman et al., Hospitalization: voluntary and involuntary, Copyright (2003) Taylor and Francis.

criteria became more stringent, and more formalized procedures were developed with the intention of preventing unjust hospitalization against a patient's will.

Current state procedures on civil commitment are based on two legal doctrines: patrens patriae and police power (see Box 32.1). Key case law developments in the United States are summarized in Box 32.2.

In 1983, the American Psychiatric Association's Model Law on Civil Commitment[2] provided guidelines for emergency, involuntary hospitalization of persons exhibiting mental illness, and set time limits and procedures for extending hospitalization, if deemed necessary by the court. It also outlined other requirements including:

1 the individual must suffer from a severe mental disorder that is treatable;

2 hospitalization is the least restrictive treatment available;

Box 32.2 Case law development in the United States

◆ Lake v. Cameron (1966): 'least restrictive alternative' requirement for involuntary hospitalization

◆ The Lanterman-Petris-Short Act (1969): emphasized dangerousness

◆ Lessard v. Schmidt (1972): requirement for evidence of overt act of dangerousness within 30 days preceding admission

◆ Jackson v. Indiana (1972): placed limitations on involuntary hospitalization

◆ O'Connor v. Donaldson (1975): non-dangerous mentally ill could not be confined to a psychiatric hospital 'without more'

◆ Fasulo v. Arafeh (1977): need for continued hospitalization must be demonstrated by clear and convincing evidence; set standard for periodic review

◆ Parham v. J.R. (1979): required medical evaluation during commitment of minors

◆ Addington v. Texas (1979): set standard for 'clear and convincing evidence' requirement for civil commitment cases

Source data from: Rosner R (ed), *Principles and Practice of Forensic Psychiatry*, 2nd edition, in Zerman et al., Hospitalization: voluntary and involuntary, Copyright (2003) Taylor and Francis.

3   the person cannot consent to voluntary admission;

4   the person is incompetent to consent to treatment and without treatment the individual will be at risk of harm to self or others.

It has received wide review and criticisms, and is now reflected in many state commitment laws. Criteria for civil commitment have been substantially revised during the last decades in Europe, and similar reforms have paralleled those in the United States.[3]

From the 1950s and 1960s onwards, beside the changes in the mental health system and the achievement of the human rights movement, the focus shifted from a paternalistic approach to mental healthcare to the need to treat patients who were not able to take care of themselves. Alongside this development, the legal frameworks for the involuntary treatment of the mentally ill and the commitment laws have been reformed in many countries, with the aim of reducing the frequency of compulsory admissions. However, in several countries, reform of the commitment laws moved in the opposite way because of the need to protect society against the potential harmfulness of the mentally ill patients. This trend has emphasized the 'dangerousness criterion' as a mandatory prerequisite for compulsory admissions and contributed to the perception of mentally ill patients as being generally uncontrollable or dangerous persons, with extreme consequences for their stigmatization.[4,5]

Criteria for compulsory admission

Involuntary admissions in mental healthcare need to balance three different and often controversial interests:

1   the basic human rights of the persons concerned;

2   public safety;

3   the need for adequate treatment of the patients.

All the legislations are based on the assumption that individuals are not able to recognize their need for treatment because of the severe and acute symptoms of their illness. Compulsory admission leads to a conflict between a medical model and a civil liberties approach. The former emphasizes the need for treatment as a sufficient prerequisite for the involuntary treatment of a mentally ill patient; the latter approach accepts forced hospital admission only when a mentally ill person threatens to harm others or him/herself. In this case, 'dangerousness' is the only criterion justifying the involuntary treatment of someone.[6] However, some cultural movements refuse to consider dangerousness as a criterion for compulsory admission. In Italy, for example, the reason for involuntary treatment is no longer the dangerousness of the patient but the patient's need for care. From the law perspective, involuntary treatment must be provided if and when the 'mental condition of the person requires urgent treatment that the person does not accept'. The consequences are that:

1   non-acceptance of treatment by a mentally ill person is no longer an indication that he or she is socially dangerous;

2   the psychiatrist is no longer obliged to control and repress social dangerousness;

3   obliging mentally ill people to receive treatment is a way of protecting their rights not reducing them.

Experts nevertheless continue to debate other commitment criteria. One of the most discussed is the so-called 'Stone model', which stipulates several conditions for commitment:

1   a reliable diagnosis of a severe mental disorder

2   major distress of the patient

3   availability of an effective treatment

4   patient's incompetence to decide

5   reasonableness of applied treatment, which would be accepted by a competent person.[7,8]

These criteria provided the basis for the American Psychiatric Association's (APA) proposed model for civil commitment laws.[9] A patient's potential for harm to themself, either from suicidality or inability to care for themself, also meets the criteria for dangerousness.

Ethics

Involuntary admission should always be considered only as the last resort and should be applied only if all other possible specific strategies for the management of aggression or self-harm failed. The issue has been widely debated by critics, patient advocacy groups, patients, and family members of the mentally ill. Some argue that this type of treatment violates the fundamental patient rights of autonomy. On the other hand, physicians may also be criticized, or even face malpractice suits, if dangerous patients are released. Machlachlan and Mulder[10] outline key ethical principles that underlay involuntary hospitalization and can be used when making decisions in this area (Box 32.3).

Patient autonomy is often thought to be a key tenet of medical practice and informed consent. However, beneficence and social paternalism may take priority when dangerous patients must be hospitalized against their will. When patients become unable to make rational decisions due to psychosis or another mental defect, the principle of autonomy may not be applicable and beneficence becomes even more important. Social paternalism refers to interfering with a person's liberties in order to protect others or society as a whole. This is illustrated by using dangerousness as a criterion for involuntary hospitalization. This rationale for psychiatric hospitalization is used in cases where mental illness is the cause of the danger, and the illness can be expected to improve

---

Box 32.3 Ethical principles of involuntary hospitalization

◆ Autonomy

◆ Beneficence

◆ Social paternalism

◆ Medical paternalism

Box 32.4 Ethical aspects

- ◆ Make a quick and clear decision that is in the patient's interest. The whole procedure should have a limited time frame, avoiding overly long and stressful waits.

- ◆ Admit the patient to the closest hospital. If the patient asks, guarantee the presence, in the hospital, of their relatives.

- ◆ Hospitalize the patient after a psychiatrist's assessment, which should be carried out in the most comfortable conditions while ensuring the necessary level of safety.

- ◆ If at all possible, accommodate the admitted patient in a single room, in order to guarantee a safe and calm environment.

- ◆ Ensure the patient has regular contact with mental health professionals. These meetings should be held in an atmosphere of reciprocal respect and understanding.

- ◆ Communicate adequately to the patient about their clinical state. Inform them about their rights, diagnosis, prognosis, and treatment during each step of the procedure.

- ◆ Do not give information on the patient's clinical condition to other persons without the patient's consent.

with treatment, thus removing the danger. Individuals who do not suffer from mental illness and pose dangerousness may be more appropriately detained in jails. It can be difficult to predict dangerousness, and tips for assessing potentially dangerous patients will be presented later in this chapter. Medical paternalism refers to interfering with a patient's autonomy in order to provide benefit to him or her. This can apply in cases where patients are brought in for evaluation for mental deterioration and inability to care for themselves. Based on this principle, many areas also have procedures in place to enforce psychiatric medication if patients refuse treatment.

During involuntary hospital admissions, the patient's rights should be granted, and interventions provided should respect the principle of the 'less restrictive alternative' (Box 32.4).

Procedures

In the USA, there are different mechanisms for involuntary hospitalizations. The first is typically a certification by a physician or other mental health professional that serves as a holding order until more formal court proceedings can take place. It is typically time limited. A common setting for this type of procedure is the hospital emergency room. Patients are often brought for evaluation by the police or concerned family members, and a physician may detain the patient against his or her will if criteria for involuntary admission are met. The second mechanism typically involves filing a petition for commitment with the courts. The petition leads to a psychiatric evaluation and the court decides if the criteria for involuntary commitment are met, based on the evidence. These court-ordered commitments are typically of longer duration than emergency certifications. It is important for psychiatrists to familiarize themselves with national statutes and laws in their country regarding involuntary hospitalization.

Evaluation

Psychiatric evaluation

The evaluation of patients for involuntary hospitalization is one of the most daunting tasks for psychiatrists. Most physicians chose medicine as a career to 'help people' or for other altruistic reasons, and it is often difficult to establish therapeutic rapport or a working doctor–patient relationship with involuntary patients. Emergency rooms and inpatient units are the typical settings in which psychiatrists will encounter patients held on involuntary treatment orders.

It is important to conduct a thorough psychiatric and medical evaluation, and utilize collateral sources of information when patients are unable or unwilling to provide it on their own. Physicians should remain as objective as possible, reminding themselves that symptoms, and not diagnosis, tend to influence their judgements. It is crucial to proceed with a quick but complete evaluation to delineate the main factors leading to a treatment choice. Even though patients may become upset about the need for hospitalization, physicians must choose to better protect both the patient and the society. Table 32.1 outlines key components of a psychiatric evaluation for involuntary hospitalization.

Table 32.1 Components of psychiatric evaluation for involuntary admission

History of presentation	It includes how the patient arrived at the hospital (e.g. family, police), description of events in police or emergency medical report, and patient description of why he or she is at the hospital.
Past psychiatric history	It is important to determine the presence of an underlying psychiatric condition that may be the cause of dangerousness. It may be obtained from patients or records.
Medical history	It is important to recognize any medical conditions that may have contributed to the presentation of psychiatric symptoms and that should be treated during involuntary hospitalization.
Social history	Social stressors such as conflict with family, recent loss or divorce, legal problems, finances, and living situation may help assess for dangerousness and ability to care for self.
Substance use	Use of drugs or substances may contribute to or worsen psychiatric symptoms and increase risk for dangerousness. This may be obtained from the patient, collateral sources, or by conducting a drug screen test.

(continued)

Table 32.1 (continued) Components of psychiatric evaluation for involuntary admission

Violence history	A history of violence is an important predictor of future violence.
Mental status examination	Abnormalities on a mental status examination may indicate an active psychiatric condition that would benefit from treatment. Routinely investigate cognitive skills (memory, orientation), patient's thoughts and perceptions (delusions, hallucinations), thought processes (disorganization, incoherence, psychomotor retardation, or acceleration).
Risk of suicide	Socio-demographic and clinical factors, previous attempts, alcohol or substance use, loss of rational thinking, lack of social support, organized plans, sickness.
Assessment of patient's ability to give consent	Ability to take in appropriate information, ability to understand and listen, ability to reason, ability to express their decisions freely, ability to keep a decision over time.

Patients brought in for evaluation for involuntary admission may be challenging, in that they may feel as though their rights have been violated. They will often be uncooperative or even protest about being hospitalized and refuse treatment. When patients will not or cannot provide necessary information, hospital records and other sources of information may be helpful. Ambulance or police reports of the events leading to the patient being brought to the hospital may offer clues of violence potential. Family members and friends may also be able to provide valuable information. Patient privacy laws must be taken into consideration; however, many countries and areas have provisions that allow contact even without permission, in emergency situations.

Physical evaluation

Medical assessment must include a physical examination. Minimal requirements of physical examination should be level of consciousness, blood pressure, pulse, temperature, respiratory rate, and capillary blood glucose. Any sign of a significant abnormality should prompt a more thorough hospital investigation. If the patient has behavioural problems and refuses or protests, sedation may be indicated to facilitate the physical examination. The choice of drug should be guided by the patient's history and the situation. If the patient refuses to take the drug orally, the intramuscular route is the most common alternative.

Professionals involved in the procedure

Community psychiatrist

The physician who first visits the patient should collect all potentially useful information regarding the patient's situation from all available sources (relatives, friends, colleagues, social workers, police officers, other professionals). The first clinical examination should take place in a safe and quiet place, in the presence of preferably few persons, ideally with the participation of a nurse and possibly with a person whom the patient trusts. The physician should then issue a certificate on which the mental disturbances and other relevant elements causing the need for treatment should be clearly reported, including a statement that the necessary prerequisites are fulfilled.

After this preliminary clinical examination, the community psychiatrist can involve the medical professionals, defining clear tasks for each of them. The patient can be moved to a first aid station if there is a need for a general medical check or if it is necessary to ascertain the presence of any alcohol or drug intoxication which may have contributed to the development of psychiatric symptoms. Information on patients' socio-demographic and clinical characteristics must be transferred to the hospital team before his or her admission.

Hospital team

At the patient's arrival, a full mental status examination should be performed by the ward psychiatrist. The ward psychiatrist, after a careful examination of the patient, has the responsibility for the final decision on their involuntary hospital admission. Moreover, information about the patient's hospital admission must be provided by the psychiatrist, as soon as possible, to the relevant authorities. Nurses and other medical professionals must prepare the room and the bed before the patient's arrival; if the physician agrees, they can take part in the clinical evaluation. They must check the patient's personal belongings and guarantee direct daily contact with him or her, displaying calm and supportive communicative behaviours at all times. Moreover, they must inform the patient about the ward's rules and report on the patient's physical monitoring in appropriate records.

Police

Upon a documented request from the physician, and only when all alternatives have been considered, the police can be requested to conduct the patient's examination and/or to take the patient to the hospital for involuntary admission. Police officers should inform the patient clearly about the procedures and his or her rights; they must avoid aggressive physical and verbal behaviours toward the patient. All the applied coercive measures should be recorded in a specific file, including reasons for these and a clear description on how they have been performed. This file should always be at the judge's disposal.

Judges

The judge, before making any decision about the patient's admission, must collect information from all reliable sources (including the mental health community team, relatives, police officers), enquiring about the patient's clinical situation from the ward physician directly. In cases where orders that led to an involuntary hospitalization were not carried out within 48 hours, the circumstances under which the orders were issued should be re-examined. As explicitly required in local legislations, the hearing should ideally take place in a comfortable and safe room located in the ward.

During the hearing, the judge should involve the ward physician in order to supplement his or her information with clinical details. The judge's decision should be based on information obtained from all persons participating in the involuntary admission procedure.

Working with involuntary patients in inpatient settings

Working with involuntary patients can pose unique challenges because of the nature of the treatment relationship. It can be more difficult to establish therapeutic rapport because the patient does not necessarily see the need for, or desire, psychiatric treatment. Patients involuntarily hospitalized may also have potential for violence, or may not be willing to co-operate with evaluation or provide personal historical information. Evidence-based principles and specific guidelines for working with involuntary patients are limited; however, respecting patients' rights and adhering to institutional policies regarding involuntary hospitalization are good practices.

Patients who have been involuntarily hospitalized due to potential for harm to others may be at increased risk of violence. During their initial assessment, violence potential should be considered. If a patient is agitated, the following measures may be used:[11]

◆ Remove the patient to a safe environment.

◆ Remove any objects that could be used as weapons.

◆ Express sympathetic concerns about the patient and their complaints.

◆ Respond in a confident and supportive manner.

◆ Ask the patient what can be done to address their complaints.

If these measures do not de-escalate the situation, physical restraint or medication may be required to maintain safety.

Involuntarily hospitalized patients may not be able or willing to make treatment decisions and participate with evaluation. Family members or healthcare proxies may be able to supply details about the patient's history and may also help to guide treatment by providing information about the patient's preferences. Patient privacy must be respected and privacy laws should be followed.[12]

To build rapport with involuntarily hospitalized patients, physicians should provide reassurance that they respect the patient's rights and follow institutional policies and procedures regarding involuntary commitment. Although specific statutes differ, most provide some type of representation for the patient, and reassurance of this may encourage the doctor–patient relationship. Patients should be provided with copies of legal documents, as permitted by the enforced policy.

Conclusions

Understanding procedures for involuntary hospitalization and respecting patients' rights through all phases of the evaluation and treatment increase a physician's ability to work with this patient population. Although working with involuntary patients is a common challenge for psychiatrists, hospitalization in this situation ensures the safety of the patient and of society as a whole.

References

1 Fiorillo A, Giacco D, De Rosa C, et al. Patient characteristics and symptoms associated with perceived coercion during hospital treatment. *Acta Psychiatr Scand* 2012; **125**:460–7.

2 Stromberg C, Stone A. A model state law on civil commitment of the mentally ill. *Harv J Legis* 1983; **20**:275–396.

3 Applebaum P. A theory of ethics for forensic psychiatry. *J Am Acad Psychiatry Law* 1997; **25**:233–47.

4 Angermeyer M, Matschinger H. Violent attacks on public figures by persons suffering from psychiatric disorders. Their effect on the social distance towards the mentally ill. *Eur Arch Psychiatry Clin Neurosci* 1995; **245**:159–64.

5 Phelan J, Link B. The growing belief that people with mental illnesses are violent: the role of the dangerousness criterion for civil commitment. *Soc Psychiatry Psychiatr Epidemiol* 1998; **33**(Suppl 1):S7–12.

6 Chodoff P. Involuntary hospitalization of the mentally ill as a moral issue. *Am J Psychiatry* 1984; **141**:384–9.

7 Stone A. Comment: Is dangerousness an issue for physicians in emergency commitment? *Am J Psych* 1975; **132**:829–31.

8 Hoge SK, Sachs G, Appelbaum PS, Greer A, Gordon C. Limitations on psychiatrists' discretionary civil commitment authority by the Stone and dangerousness criteria. *Arch Gen Psychiatry* 1988; **45**:764–9.

9 American Psychiatric Association. Guidelines for legislation of the psychiatric hospitalization of adults. *Am J Psychiatry* 1983; **140**:672–9.

10 Machlachlan A, Mulder R. Criteria for involuntary hospitalization. *Austr N Z J Psychiatry* 1998; **33**:729–33.

11 Doebbeling C. *Behavioral emergencies. The Merck manual for healthcare professionals.* Merck Manuals: Online Medical Library; 2012. Available at: http://www.merckmanuals.com/professional/psychiatric-disorders/approach-to-the-patient-with-mental-symptoms/behavioral-emergencies.

12 Byatt N, Pinals D, Arikan R. Involuntary hospitalization of medical patients who lack decisional capacity: an unresolved issue. *Psychosomatics* 2006; **47**:443–8.

Chapter 33

Sexual variation and mental health

Gurvinder Kalra, Antonio Ventriglio,
Christian Foerster, and Dinesh Bhugra

Case study

James and John, both aged 32, are referred to a sex clinic as they are having relationship problems. They have been together for five years and both are committed to their relationship. James is 'out' at work and to his family, whereas very few friends know about John. As far as John's family is concerned, he and James share the flat. This has caused a lot of tension in their relationship and John is beginning to feel insecure about it. Occasionally, this has caused erectile dysfunction in James and it is affecting their relationship. They have been referred to the psychiatrist for treatment and investigation of the erectile dysfunction and for help with dealing with the stress within the relationship.

Introduction

Sexuality is an innate and crucial part of our personal identity. Sexuality defines us not only as individuals but also as social beings, helping us to connect with others in different ways and at varying levels of intimacy. Individuals can be affected by their sexual attraction to others and also by their abilities to sexually satisfy themselves and others. Sexuality is part of the reproductive ability and is also meant for pleasure. As sexuality forms such an important part of who we are, it is inevitable that any variation in it may also affect our identities equally.

Sexual variation or diversity is sexual behaviour that varies from the usual and commonly understood 'hetero'-sexual behaviour. Historically, due to social mores and attitudes, sexual variation has often been reduced to a symptom of psychopathology, with expectations for treatment. However, with an increasing understanding of different aspects of sexuality, it is now generally accepted that these variations are not always to be seen as pathological. In this chapter, we look at what sexual variation is and how it relates to mental health. We do not propose to cover every sexual variation but to present some examples of the more common ones.

What is sexual variation?

Sexual variation, or diversity, is defined as any sexual orientation, identity, or behaviour that lies outside what is defined as so-called 'normal' heterosexual penetrative intercourse. It is worth remembering that such a variation can be seen as a statistical variation or 'abnormality', or a variation defined by the society or the culture. There are various aspects of sexual functioning that we need to bear in mind. Sexual orientation refers to a person's preference for a sexual and emotional relationship with another person of a particular sex[1] and can be heterosexual, homosexual, bisexual, or asexual (no sexual attraction to any sexes). Sexual identity is self-ascribed and refers to what the person labels (identifies) themself as—gay (including lesbian), straight, or bisexual. Sexual behaviour refers to the actual behavioural component of one's sexual relations, indicating the gender of the person one has sexual relations with: again, it can be heterosexual, homosexual, or bisexual.

It is important to note that these three components of one's sexuality may or may not be congruent with each other, and it is a matter of personal choice as to how one identifies (or does not identify) oneself. These personal choices are very strongly influenced by social and cultural mores. The sexual act has three components including fantasy and arousal, the act itself, and the availability of a sexual partner. It is possible that a heterosexual male with heterosexual fantasies may not have the option of having heterosexual sex, perhaps because he is in prison or some other all-male environment. His sexual orientation may remain heterosexual, as well as his fantasies, but the actual sexual act may be same-sex. Thus, there can be sexual fluidity in many individuals.

There is every possibility though that sexual identity may be more closely related to sexual behaviour than sexual orientation. Thus, an individual who has homosexual orientation and engages in homosexual sexual relations (behaviour) may identify him/herself as homosexual, but this is a very simplistic possibility. There are many individuals who may have homosexual orientation but engage in heterosexual relations due to social and cultural pressures, and may hence identify themselves as heterosexual or, very rarely, as bisexual. However, it is crucial that clinicians are aware of how individuals see themselves—as heterosexual or homosexual—and sexual behaviour must be separated from identity and orientation.

Individuals have multiple identities related to gender, religion, and culture, and similarly may have private and public identities which are moulded according to external and internal pressures. Self-perceived and self-identified gender identity can also play a role in determining how an individual feels, behaves, and is expected to behave. Gender identity has very strong social components to it. Thus, a person's intrinsic sense of being male, female, or an alternative gender (boygirl, girlboy, transgender, genderqueer, eunuch, agender) starts to play a major role in identity development.

Sexual variation and mental health

There is an expanse of literature that points to a higher rate of mental health problems including psychosocial distress, leading to negative mental health outcomes, in individuals with sexually variant orientation, behaviour, and identity.[2] A meta-analysis by King et al.[3] pointed towards a one and a half times higher risk of depression and anxiety disorders over a period of 12 months or a lifetime in the lesbian, gay, and bisexual (LGB) population. The rates of substance use, such as cigarette smoking and alcohol consumption (including risky single-occasion drinking, RSOD), were also shown to be much higher in lesbian, gay, bisexual, and transgender (LGBT) populations.[4]

These associations have been found to be more marked for males than females.[5] It is not very clear whether this is due to genuine differences or because questions may have been wrongly framed. It is also possible that females have higher rates of certain psychiatric disorders and yet may be less willing to seek help for themselves as they are also much more likely to be carers—the double jeopardy situation. These hypotheses deserve population studies to be confirmed. Furthermore, we know that cultures not only have specific gender roles assigned but also have different gender role expectations, and this discrepancy may further contribute to increased alienation leading to higher rates of mental disorders. In addition, cultures have been described as sex-positive and sex-negative:[6] sex-positive cultures have a strong emphasis on sexual activity as a means for pleasure; whereas in sex-negative cultures, sexual activity is about procreation and propagation of the family name. Thus, attitudes to alternative sexuality and alternative sexual activity will vary dramatically.

In addition, it is also possible that socio-economic and educational status will play a role in self-identification of gender, gender role, and emotional distress which may or may not be linked with gender role. Francoeur and Noonan[7] present the data from 60 countries on various sexual habits of populations. They note that sexual variations appear across all countries, though the actual figures may vary slightly. This variation may be ascribed to differences in methods of data collection.

In an interesting series of studies, it has been demonstrated that policies applicable to same-sex relationships do affect rates of mental disorders in the group. In a survey of 34,653 participants (of whom 577 were identified as LGBT), Hatzenbuehler et al.[8] reported that where there were no policies in place providing protection to LGBT individuals, the rates of any mood disorder in this population were twice those of the heterosexual sample (20.4% compared to 10.2%), as were those of anxiety disorder (30.1% in comparison with 16.1%). Alcohol use was almost two and a half times more common, and drug disorders, five times more common, in LGBT individuals in comparison with heterosexual participants. Psychiatric co-morbidity among LGBT individuals was three and a half times higher. Interestingly, for those who lived where there were no protective policies, rates of every psychiatric disorder were nearly double, suggesting that political steps are needed to reduce the incidence of such disorders.

The same group[9] also found that, after the legalization of same-sex marriage, there was a significant decrease in the number of mental healthcare visits made by sexual-minority men, as well as a reduction in the number of their hospital visits related to physical ill health, in comparison with the 12 months prior to legalization. This seems again to suggest that social factors play an important role in the mental health of sexual-minority individuals. In a study of 31,852 high-school students (including 1413 LGBT students), the same group[10] found that living in a geographical area with a religious climate that was supportive of homosexuality resulted in lower rates of alcohol abuse and, interestingly, fewer sexual partners. Once again, this study illustrates that social factors affect LGBT individuals perhaps more disproportionately.

Results from a longitudinal study of the health of Australian women showed that 38% of same-sex attracted female respondents aged 22–27 years had experienced depression, compared to only 19% of heterosexual female respondents. They had also experienced higher levels of anxiety (17.1% versus 7.9%).[11] In the same study, sexually variant women were more likely to have tried to harm or kill themselves in the previous six months. Higher rates of self-harm and suicidal thoughts have been linked to violence and harassment in same-sex attracted individuals,[12] confirming findings from other parts of the world. Sexually variant women were also significantly more likely to report cigarette smoking,[13] risky alcohol use (7% compared to 3.9%), marijuana use (58.2% versus 21.5%), use of other illicit drugs (40.7% versus 10.2%), and injecting drug use (10.8% versus 1.2%).[14] In a population-based telephone survey in Los Angeles,[2] depressed women who identified themselves as lesbians were more likely to be using an antidepressant medication and reported significantly more days of poor mental health compared to heterosexual women. These studies indicate that further work is needed to develop this area of research, especially with validated questions being asked.

Not entirely surprisingly, these mental health disparities are not only found in adults but also in adolescents and young adults, with sexual-minority youth (less than 18 years old) reporting significantly higher suicidality and depression symptoms.[15] An interesting longitudinal study followed up a birth cohort of 1265 children born in Christchurch (New Zealand) over a 21-year period.[16] At 21 years of age, 1007 sample members were questioned about their sexual orientation, with 28 subjects (2.8%) being classified as of gay, lesbian, or bisexual orientation. Data was gathered on a range of psychiatric disorders, including suicidal ideation and suicidal attempts, over the period from age 14 years to 21 years. Although the numbers are small, it was observed that LGB young people were at increased risk of major depression, generalized anxiety disorder, conduct disorder, nicotine dependence, other substance abuse and dependence, multiple disorders, suicidal ideation, and suicidal attempts. More recent studies show that these disparities persist over time, and in fact increase in relation to substance use, as the sexually variant youth transitions into adulthood.[17,18,19] The finding that sexually variant youth report higher substance use compared to heterosexual youth is confirmed by findings from other countries. However, it is important to emphasize that more data are needed from low- and middle-income countries and from countries where homosexual behaviour is proscribed.

It should not come as a surprise that those with sexual variation do not just have mental health issues but also physical health issues, with LGB individuals reporting significantly higher odds of experiencing physical health problems.[20] It has been observed that these individuals have a greater likelihood than the general population of having anonymous sex with multiple partners,[21] which puts them at a greater risk for sexually transmitted infections[22] such as HIV/AIDS.[23] It can be hypothesized that the reasons for this increase include early sexual debut during adolescence, unprotected sexual intercourse with multiple sexual partners, and engagement in illicit substance use.[24] It is also extremely likely that these poor health behaviours and negative physical and mental health outcomes are associated with poor access to healthcare for sexual-variant individuals.[25] For a number of reasons, including the illegal nature of such behaviours in many countries, individuals either resist or delay seeking healthcare from mainstream healthcare providers,[26] contributing to the chronic nature of some of the conditions.

Minority stress hypothesis

Meyer[27] has described an interesting and useful explanatory framework known as the 'minority stress model' that can be used to describe and understand the relationship between mental health and sexual variation. The minority stress theory posits that the stigma, discrimination, and prejudice that sexually variant individuals experience give rise to minority status, stress, and, eventually, mental health problems by adding an extra burden over and above the everyday life stressors that they experience (see Fig. 33.1).

Sexually variant individuals have to deal with a number of phase-of-life issues that are unique to this population. Phase-of-life issues are major changes that happen at certain periods in our life cycle or development and that can have a dramatic impact upon us. Some of these phase-of-life issues are starting school, graduating, starting a new job, discovering one's sexuality, relationships, marriage, having children, retiring, and death of a loved one. Sexually variant individuals may have additional difficulties during these phase-of-life times, including challenges relating to 'coming out', as illustrated in Box 33.1.

Individuals with a higher level of internalized homo-negativity (i.e. negative attitudes towards homosexuality which will be influenced by societal attitudes and discrimination) and those that more often encounter negative reactions from other people on their sexual variance report more mental health problems.[28] Thus, a series of social processes that centre on homophobic and transphobic attitudes expose the sexually variant individuals to serious personal stresses, increasing their likelihood of suicidal behaviour and the overall negative quality of their lives in terms of mental health.

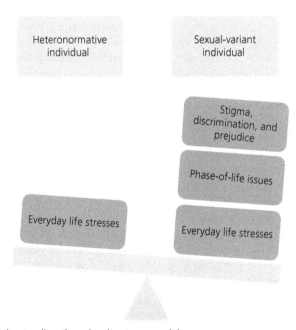

Fig. 33.1 Understanding the minority stress model.

Box 33.1 Phase-of-life issues in sexual variance

- Childhood sexual and gender-variant behaviour
- 'Coming out'
- Dealing with family and socio-cultural pressures
- Discrimination and prejudice (including educational institute and workplace-based issues)
- Violence and sexual abuse
- Romantic relationships
- Issues in old age
- End-of-life issues

Cultural issues

As mentioned previously, one of the major issues is how societies view the purpose of sexual behaviour. By legitimizing negativity towards sexual variation, societies add to discrimination. There is little doubt that sexual variation has existed across generations and across cultures, though rates may vary. Ford and Beach[29] found that homosexuality was rare or absent in 29 of the 79 cultures that they surveyed. Homosexuality was very rare in the Siriono, although they did not prohibit homosexual relationships. Similarly, it was noted to be very rare among Orthodox Jews.[30,31] It would be interesting, however, to see how these figures compare with more recent times.

Three models of homosexuality— the Greek model, the Melanesian model, and the Western model—have been described[32] as coexisting today. Ancient Greek culture allowed an older married man to have sexual relations with a younger boy by acting as a mentor to him and training him into manhood. Thus, in the Greek model, a boy starts out as exclusively homosexual (in his relationship with a bisexual mentor) but then later on goes on to become bisexual himself. Interestingly, apart from this sanctioned homosexuality, any homosexual relation between adults were discouraged in ancient Greek culture.[32] The Melanesian model existed in the islands of Papua New Guinea, wherein a man passed through three stages in his sexual life: passive exclusive homosexuality, active exclusive homosexuality, and exclusive adult heterosexuality. This culture required adolescent boys to engage in fellatio with younger boys from the age of about seven years until puberty. This was considered a form of social obligation and duty. They were expected to perform this throughout their adolescence until they reached marriageable age, when they had to stop all homosexual activity and marry, becoming exclusively heterosexual. Any man who still wanted to engage in homosexual activity with either other men of his age or of a younger age was considered aberrant or deviant.[32] The Western model is different from the Greek and the Melanesian models and is basically characterized by homosexual relations between adults.[32] These relationships also reflect prevalent social mores and norms, as well as social expectations and attitudes towards sexual activity.

Transgender and gender-variant individuals have also existed since ancient times and in different cultures; for example, the *hijras* in India,[33] *kathoeys* in Thailand,[34] Xanith in Oman,[35] gallae in the Roman Empire,[36] the mahu of Polynesia,[37] and the two-spirit person in native North America.[38] Much has been written on the tolerability towards transgender and gender-variant individuals in different cultures, but a more pertinent and common underlying theme in almost all the cultures is that of marginalization, which can happen in a different manner compared to gay and lesbian individuals. Inevitably, this often leads to a poor quality of life and poor mental health outcomes among gender-variant people. The interaction between cultures and sexual variance is quite complex, with more tolerant countries (such as the Netherlands) having a higher rate of suicidal risk in sexually variant individuals compared to heterosexual individuals.[39]

The psychiatrist's role when assessing mental health in sexually variant individuals

It is highly likely that individuals who experience being different in their sexual lives will consult mental health professionals at some point, either to have the conflict resolved or as part of other psychiatric problems. Thus, the professionals need to be equipped with the necessary skills and knowledge to help them. When it comes to helping individuals in 'alternate consultations', a psychiatrist plays multiple roles, which are illustrated in Table 33.1.

It is clear that human sexuality has a large number of variances which affect sexual and social functioning. It is important that psychiatrists recognize and deal with their own prejudices before seeing patients whose sexual proclivities they may find difficult to accept. Furthermore, it is critical that at all levels of medical training, some training in cultural competence and cultural awareness is made available. Such approaches are about good clinical practice and the humane nature of medicine, rather than anything else. It is also critical that patients whose lifestyles are at variance with that of the psychiatrist are made to feel comfortable and able to open up in clinical settings which, at the best of times, can be scary places. It is also part of a doctor's role to advocate for their patients, and this may, in some countries, lead to legal issues. Under those conditions, legal rules have to be obeyed. However, by working with advocacy organizations, regulators, and policy makers, it should be possible to help and support patients at a broader level. Nevertheless, the main aim of the psychiatric consultation has to be to maximize a person's overall psychological well-being, quality of life, and self-fulfilment. A brief overview of the different roles of a psychiatrist is provided in Table 33.1.

Table 33.1 Roles of a psychiatrist in alternate consultations

◆ Assessor	◆ Referrer	◆ Supporter
◆ Diagnostician	◆ Psychotherapist	◆ Counsellor
◆ Educator	◆ Advocate	◆ Healer

Assessment and diagnosis

The first step in the assessment of issues related to sexual variation and mental health is that the psychiatrist needs to be comfortable with their own personal views and prejudices, so that they feel at ease in asking the right questions about sexual orientation, sexuality, and sexual behaviours. Only then can they make the patient feel relaxed enough about opening up. Psychiatrists' communication skills will be extremely important in such settings. Patients may not open up immediately, and different patients will use different strategies to do so, choosing words that they feel comfortable with. It is important that clinicians use clear terms when discussing sexuality and are not afraid to ask the patient about specific terms they may be using.

It is vital to obtain a clear and comprehensive history. There must be accounts and details of childhood and early life experiences in terms of gender/sexual orientation, behaviour, and identity. As in other cases, absolute patient confidentiality within the local legal framework is vital. Clinicians must not pathologize sexual variation in individuals since it is an important part of their core identity. This acknowledgement can be made by maintaining a respectful and non-judgemental attitude, providing empathic validation to their experiences. Clinicians must also refrain from labelling different experiences of the patient with diagnoses and pathology which may further make the individual feel discriminated against. It is important that clinicians are sensitive to non-verbal cues that suggest discomfort in the patient, probably using normalization techniques to diffuse some of this discomfort.

Although ICD and DSM are the major diagnostic classification systems used across different services, it is useful to know that not all experiences of individuals, especially those with sexual variation, can be put into these codes of disorders. Therefore, it may be safer and perhaps more acceptable to call them phase-of-life issues (see Box 33.1), rather than giving diagnostic labels which may prove to be inaccurate and unhelpful. Perhaps the best option is to ask the patients themselves to define who they are and how they perceive their identity. Being non-judgemental and patient-centric will help elicit honest and relevant responses and information.

Clinicians must also pay particular attention to the specifics of the language that they use when talking with sexually variant individuals (Box 33.2) and avoid using any terms that reflect their own discomfort as embedded in heterosexist assumptions and stereotypes. The use of careful and sensitive language conveys very clearly to the patient that the clinician is comfortable in exploring intimate issues, and this can make it easier for the patient to open up. It has been shown that being open about one's sexual orientation may be related to better mental health outcomes, most particularly among sexual-minority women.[28]

During the clinical interview, it is important that the psychiatrist is aware of their own personal feelings and attitudes towards the patient, particularly in response to sexuality and sexual practices which may seem particularly shocking (e.g. anonymous sex, various fetishes).

Box 33.2 Using appropriate language in alternate consultations

Do NOT ask (inappropriate language)

- Are you married or single?
- Do you have a girlfriend/boyfriend? (addressing a male/female)
- How many girls/boys have you dated in the past? (addressing a boy/girl)
- How many children do you have?
- Are you the 'top' or the 'bottom' partner?
- What is your sexual preference? (since the word 'preference' indicates a conscious choice)

Appropriate language

- Ask: Are you in a relationship?
- Ask: Are you dating anybody currently?
- Use blank for gender instead of writing 'male/ female/ others'

'Coming out' issues

An important phase-of-life issue in sexually variant individuals is the process of 'coming out', which involves self-disclosure of one's sexual and/or gender identity to others at different levels of intimacy. This phase-of-life issue has been widely studied by a number of scholars and researchers. Cass[40] proposed a clear and comprehensive model, shown in Table 33.2.

The Cass model does not take specific socio-cultural factors into account and assumes the process to be a straightforward one, with a linear nature. In reality though, individuals may take many sidesteps in the process of revealing their sexuality to different people at different times. It has been suggested that those who do not go through each of the described stages in order may not be considered as well-adjusted gay individuals.[41] However, it is important that individuals reach a certain level of contentment before moving on to tell others. Thus, each stage can be a plateau as well as a step. It is entirely possible that the Cass model reflects attitudes prevalent in the 1970s and needs modifications. Further development comes from Coleman,[42] who proposed an additional model for the coming out process, especially among homosexual males and lesbians, which focuses on romantic attachments too. This model comprises five stages:

1) pre-coming out (no awareness of same-sex feelings but often a slight awareness of feeling different from others);

2) coming out (selective coming out to individuals in one's life and contact with other sexually variant individuals);

3) exploration of one's sexual identity (usually with increased contact with other sexually variant individuals);

Table 33.2 Coming out stages

Age (years)	Stage	Common questions and cognitions facing the individual	Needs of the client
0–13			
13–18	Identity confusion	First awareness of thoughts, feelings, attractions, and behaviours as homosexual, leading to confusion ('fog'), turmoil, and often denial of these feelings.	'Who am I?' 'Am I different?'	May explore internal positive and negative judgements; may need to know about the spectrum of sexual behaviour; may need permission and encouragement to explore sexuality as a normal experience.
	Identity comparison	Begin to come out of the 'fog' and start accepting 'I might be homosexual'. Although accept identity, it inhibits behaviour. Compartmentalize their sexuality—accept LG definition of behaviour but maintain 'heterosexual identity'.	'It's only temporary.' 'I'm just in love with this man/woman and it will end with this.' 'May be I am gay.' 'What are gay people like?' 'I'm alone... am I?'	May need information about sexuality, identity, LGBT community resources; may need to talk with someone.
15–21	Identity tolerance	Realize 'they are not the only one'. Seek out other lesbian and gay people to combat feelings of isolation. Task is to decrease social isolation. May try out various 'stereotypical roles' with more self-tolerance towards these roles.	'Where are other gay people like me?'	Need to be supported in exploring own feelings of shame derived from heterosexism and internalized homophobia; need support in finding positive LGBT resources.

(continued)

Table 33.2 (continued) Coming out stages

Age (years)	Stage	Common questions and cognitions facing the individual	Needs of the client
	Identity acceptance	Start accepting (vs. tolerance from earlier stage) and attaching a positive connotation to their identity.	Need exploration of grief and loss of heterosexual life expectation and of any internalized homophobia; need to know about where, when, and to whom to disclose.
		May start coming out to selective people and attempt to bring congruence between public and private views of self-image.	'I am gay.' 'Am I okay?' 'I can come out to some people.'
		Continued contact with lesbian and gay culture and decreased contact with heterosexual community.	
18+	Identity pride	Feel pride in self-identity and immerse oneself in the lesbian and gay culture, often acquiring all gay friends and social connections.	'I am proud to be gay.' 'I don't and won't pass for straight.' 'I want people to know who I am.'
			Need to explore issues of heterosexism and receive support for exploring anger issues or other existential issues.
		Deep rage towards 'majority culture' and 'heterosexist viewpoints' leading to confrontation with heterosexist ideologies.	
18+	Identity synthesis	Gay/lesbian identity integrated with other aspects of life.	'I'm an OK person who happens to be gay.'
		Sexual identity becomes only one aspect of self, rather than the entire identity.	Common issues may need to be addressed as per the individual.
		Recognize supportive heterosexual others and is more at peace with self.	

Reproduced from *J Homosex*, 4(3), Cass VC. Homosexual identity formation: a theoretical model, p. 219–35, Copyright (1979) Taylor and Francis

Box 33.3 Exploring coming out issues

- Do you want to come out?
- On a scale of 1–10 (1 = not at all important; 10 = very important), how important is it for you to come out?
- Why do you want to come out?
- What do you think will happen if you do not come out at all?
- What are the practical implications of you coming out: abandonment by family, homelessness, unemployment, social outcast, losing relationships including marriage (non-heterosexual), victimization, marginalization?
- Who do you want to come out to? Why do you think coming out to these individuals is fine?
- Who can you look to for support following any negative outcomes in your coming out process?

Source data from: *Indian J Homosex*, 54(3), Kalra, G. Breaking the ice: IJP on homosexuality, p. 299–300, Copyright (2012) Indian Psychiatric Society

4) first relationship (with or without physical and emotional attraction; most of these relationships may not last for a long time);

5) integration of public and private identities into one's self-image (more stable relationships are usually established in this stage and are more likely to be based on mutual trust and honesty, with a higher likelihood for success).

In clinical settings, it is important to understand and explore the main issues related to the actual process of coming out. Some examples are provided in Box 33.3.[43] The psychiatrist has an obligation to help the individual explore the various implications, including personal guilt and social shame, that coming out will have on his or her life and on those around them. Inevitably, this will depend on the socio-cultural context and will vary between different countries and even within the same country.

As in other clinical assessments (but perhaps more relevant in assessing individuals with sexual variation), it is helpful for the clinician to understand what social support is available to the individual in order to determine what else may be needed to avoid alienation and social isolation. Alternate sexuality has different meanings and impact across genders too; therefore, this needs to be considered carefully. The impact of perceived and real stigma and discrimination in various areas of the patient's life will also affect their therapeutic engagement and alliance, and must be explored.

Management-related issues

Clinical management of patients with sexual variation must take into account additional factors such as stigma, discrimination, and prejudice, as well as the psychiatrist's own attitude and prejudices. Thus, clinical engagement and the therapeutic alliance can be quite complex given the range of sexual and gender issues that patients bring to the consultation.

The main resource for managing issues related to sexual variation remains psychotherapy, although some problems may also be treated with pharmacological agents.

Psychotherapies/psychoeducation

A major part of the management of patients with sexual variations is education and providing information and support about diversity in sexuality and gender identities, expressions, and experiences. The clinician needs to talk about sexual variation, given that silence may reinforce stigma and taboo surrounding the issue. Psychotherapy with patients will be dictated by their clinical needs but would most commonly involve supportive psychotherapy, providing them with a holding environment wherein they can feel safe enough to talk about their concerns.

It is crucial to conceptualize sex, gender, and sexuality as a multidimensional construct rather than a rigid entity which seeks to fit every individual into predefined pigeon holes. An example that may be used is that of a ball of clay, which is easy to mould but continues to remain clay, even as it changes shape.

Using gay- and gender-affirmative therapy means sticking to the assumptions that LGBT identities are normal and part of a spectrum, and that changing a patient's sexual and/or gender identity is not the goal of treatment. Such affirmative therapy embraces and encourages a positive view of LGBT identities and addresses the negative influences that homophobia, transphobia, and heterosexism have on the lives of such patients.

To be a gay-affirmative therapist, it is crucial that he or she examines any negative attitudes and prejudices towards sexual variation that they themselves may have, and explore how these are reflected to the patient during therapy sessions. They may also want to reflect on their ideas and beliefs about gender binaries. Promoting oneself as a gay-affirmative therapist would require creating a LGBT-friendly clinical setting with reading material, information on resources, and also the use of affirmative language (without using heteronormative assumptions) on all paperwork. Gay-affirmative therapists may also challenge heterosexist attitudes in heterosexual patients and thus act as advocates towards more gay-affirming practices. There have been instances, for example, where therapists have introduced religious learnings into therapeutic sessions to indicate to the patient that such variant behaviours are pathological, sinful, and may hence warrant treatment,[44] without realizing that religion can induce shame and guilt in the patient and increase their distress.

One of the common and first major issues that a clinician has to confront is that sexual variations are not pathologies. Curative therapies have no role to play. If the patient is feeling uncomfortable about their sexual identity and is looking for a cure, they have to be dissuaded. Legal issues may make things difficult but the clinician must look at the scientific evidence and practice accordingly. It is critical that clinicians explore the underlying reasons for sexual variation in an empathic manner. It is also important not to pathologize some of a patient's phase-of-life issues. For example, patients may be quite distressed during the coming out phase of their lives and have a very delicate and vulnerable sense of self and self-image. They may also appear quite impulsive, often persuading the clinician to diagnose them with borderline personality disorder and treat them accordingly. There is a high likelihood of borderline personality individuals having engaged in same-sex behaviour but this does not necessarily translate into self-labelling as gay or lesbian.[45] Sexual orientation must be clearly differentiated from sexual behaviour.

When a patient presents with any concern, it helps if the therapist discusses with him or her, the various implications, in terms of their life, of the particular issue and of approaching it in different ways. For instance, the clinician can provide a safe holding space in the therapy room and can collaboratively explore options of which family members the patient can come out to by calculating the relative risks given the patient's life story. This would thus involve not only the patient but also their family and significant others. Often families, friends, and others may have to participate in therapy and may need psychoeducation, as parental and family support remains an important correlate of health-related outcome in patients' lives[46] in many cultures.

Some patients (especially transitioning gender-variant individuals) may request workplace- related support that may require the clinician to write accompanying letters of endorsement. The clinician must take into account the socio-cultural context of such approaches and decisions, but often assisting the individual to move from a socio-centric identity construct to an ego-centric identity construct helps. This would involve gentle but repeated questioning of the socio-centric inclinations in the patient—the way they worry too much about 'others' in society, and the way this worrying attitude restricts them from living their life to its full potential. In doing this, the therapist needs to be careful not to encourage patients who are questioning their identity to come out prematurely or to simply reassure them by saying 'it is okay to be gay'. The best role would be that of a facilitator, helping their patients to resolve their complex issues in their own time instead of pushing them to a premature resolution.

Sexually variant individuals may present with the same clinical problems that heterosexuals do, including depression, anxiety disorders, substance use issues, relationship issues, and work-related issues.[47] Many of these issues may sometimes have no relevance to a patient's sexual orientation or identity, but as the clinician starts working with these patients, such matters may begin to become increasingly relevant and may need to be addressed. One can successfully use various therapies, such as cognitive behavioural models, with sexually variant patients.[48] Often, lesbian and gay couples may enter therapy to deal with issues specific to sexually variant individuals. However, they may also present with issues such as faulty communication patterns or conflict negotiation strategies.[49] In working with gay and lesbian couples, it must be remembered that the couple may be at different stages of coming out, so that must be part of the therapy process. It can happen that the partner who is already out can put pressure on the one who may not be ready to take this step, thus creating tensions which will need to be addressed before therapy can move forward. It is worthwhile to also note that the usual expectations in heterosexual relationships (such as monogamy, pooled finances, dividing household roles along gender lines, moving together for each other's career advancement, caring for one another's families in old age, mutual inheritance) may not necessarily apply in same-sex couples unless discussed by the partners.[49] With legalization of same-sex marriage and adoption rights of gay couples, the differential patterns are changing, but for some therapists, these changes may well prove difficult to accept.

Appropriate referrals form an important part of management plans for transgender individuals and would include referrals to specialists in this area, endocrinologists and surgeons, various support groups, and non-governmental organizations. Often meeting others dealing with the same issues (who can share experiences and provide personalized, non-professional support) helps to alleviate many of the associated negative emotions. Such social networks act as a buffer against the negative impact of minority stress.[50]

Pharmacotherapies

The role of psychopharmacology is limited to the presence of any psychiatric illness, but it has to be considered only after ruling out the reactive response to phase-of-life issues. It is more helpful to consider alternative, non-pharmacological approaches to alleviating the stress due to these issues. However, it is important to note that pharmacotherapy may be a more effective short-term treatment for dysthymia in this population, whereas in the long term, psychotherapy or combination treatment may be more helpful.[51] While treating with psychotropic agents, the clinician will need to also take into consideration if the patient is receiving treatment for any co-morbid infections and diseases (such as HIV/AIDS), to avoid any drug–drug interactions. The choice of medication will differ depending on the individual, but it is advisable to choose an agent with the least sexual side-effects.

Pharmacotherapy for psychiatric illnesses in transgender individuals may also need to be tailored after taking into consideration if they are on any hormonal treatment or have already begun to transition. This is both important and sensible, given that hormonal treatment has a positive effect on a transgender individual's mental health, with a reduction in both psychiatric distress and functional impairment.[52]

Conclusions

Sexual variation is both a challenge and an opportunity to recognize the nature of human diversity and human nature. There is no doubt that sexual activity plays a major role in 'being' human and also for propagation of the species. Sexual activity (meant as a pleasurable activity) and objects of attraction (person one is attracted to) are important factors to recognize in all history taking and management, no matter what psychiatric or physical condition is being treated. It is absolutely vital that clinicians are aware of their own prejudices and discriminatory attitudes, and of feelings and factors which may be influencing these. Good clinical practice demands that a patient's needs and values are paramount, rather than those of the clinician. It is to the advantage of the profession to take the lead and educate society at large about sexual variation and its implications for both physical and mental health.

References

1 **Weiten W**. Motivation and emotion. In: *Psychology: themes and variations* (3rd edn.) (ed. Weiten W). Pacific Grove, California: Brooks/Cole Publishing Company; 1995, pp. 375–415.
2 **Diamant AL, Wold C**. Sexual orientation and variation in physical and mental health status among women. *J Womens Health (Larchmt)* 2003; **12**(1):41–9.
3 **King M, Semlyen J, Tai SS, et al**. A systematic review of mental disorder, suicide, and deliberate self harm in lesbian, gay and bisexual people. *BMC Psychiatry* 2008; **8**:70.

4 Hagger-Johnson G, Taibjee R, Semlyen J, et al. Sexual orientation identity in relation to smoking history and alcohol use at age 18/19: cross-sectional associations from the Longitudinal Study of Young People in England (LSYPE). *BMC Open* 2013; **3**(8):e002810.

5 Fergusson DM, Horwood LJ, Ridder EM, Beautrais AL. Sexual orientation and mental health in a birth cohort of young adults. *Psychol Med* 2005; **35**(7):971–81.

6 Bullough V. *Sexual variance in society and history*. Chicago: University of Chicago Press; 1976.

7 Francoeur RT, Noonan RJ. *The continuum complete encyclopedia of sexuality*. New York: Continuum International Publishing Group; 2004.

8 Hatzenbuehler ML, Keyes KM, Hasin D. State-level policies and psychiatric morbidity in lesbian, gay and bisexual populations. *Am J Public Health* 2009; **99**:2275–81.

9 Hatzenbuehler ML, O'Cleingh C, Grasso C, Meyer K, Safren S, Bradford J. Effect of same sex marriage laws on health care use and expenditures in sexual minority men: a quasi-natural experiment. *Am J Public Health* 2012; **102**:285–91.

10 Hatzenbuehler ML, Pachanks JE, Wolff J. Religious climate and health risk behaviors in sexual minority youths: a population based study. *Am J Public Health* 2012; **102**:657–63.

11 McNair R, Kavanagh A, Agius P, Tong B. The mental health status of young adult and mid-life non-heterosexual Australian women. *Aust N Z J Public Health* 2004; **29**(3):265–71.

12 Hillier L, Turner A, Mitchell A. *Writing themselves in again: the 2nd national report on the sexual health and wellbeing of same-sex attracted young people in Australia. Australian Research Centre in Sex, Health and Society (ARCSHS)*. Melbourne: La Trobe University; 2005.

13 Hughes TL, Jacobson KM. Sexual orientation and women's smoking. *Curr Womens Health Rep* 2003; **3**(3):254–61.

14 Hillier L, de Visser RO, Kavanagh A, McNair R. The drug-use patterns of heterosexual and non-heterosexual women: data from the Women's Health Australia Study. In: *Out in the Antipodes: Australian and New Zealand perspectives on gay and lesbian issues in psychology* (eds. Riggs DW, Walker GA). Bentley, WA: Brightfire Press; 2004.

15 Marshal MP, Dietz LJ, Friedman MS, et al. Suicidality and depression disparities between sexual minority and heterosexual youth: a meta-analytic review. *J Adolesc Health* 2011; **49**(2):115–23.

16 Fergusson DM, Horwood L, Beautrais AL. Is sexual orientation related to mental health problems and suicidality in young people? *Arch Gen Psychiatry* 1999; **56**(10):876–80.

17 Marshal MP, Dermody SS, Cheong J, et al. Trajectories of depressive symptoms and suicidality among heterosexual and sexual minority youth. *J Youth Adolesc* 2013; **42**(8):1243–56.

18 Needham BL. Sexual attraction and trajectories of mental health and substance use during the transition from adolescence to adulthood. *J Youth Adolesc* 2012; **41**(2):179–90.

19 Marshal MP, Friedman MS, Stall R, Thompson AL. Individual trajectories of substance use in lesbian, gay and bisexual youth and heterosexual youth. *Addiction* 2009; **104**(6):974–81.

20 Frost DM, Lehavot K, Meyer IH. Minority stress and physical health among sexual minority individuals. *J Behav Med* 2015;**38**:1–8.

21 Bimbi DS, Nanin JE, Parsons JT, Vicioso KJ, Missildine W, Frost D. Assessing gay and bisexual men's outcome expectancies for sexual risk under the influence of alcohol and drugs. *Subst Use Misuse* 2006; **41**:643–52.

22 Halkitis PN, Zade DD, Shrem M, Marmor M. Beliefs about HIV non-infection and risky sexual behavior among MSM. *AIDS Educ Prev* 2004; **16**:448–58.

23 Halkitis PN, Green KA, Mourgues P. Longitudinal investigation of methamphetamine use among gay and bisexual men in New York City: findings from project bumps. *J Urban Health* 2005; **82**:18–25.

24 Rosario M, Meyer-Bahlburg HF, Hunter J, Gwadz M. Sexual risk behaviors of gay, lesbian and bisexual youths in New York City: prevalence and correlates. *AIDS Educ Prev* 1999; **11**(6):476–96.

25 Diamant AL, Wold C, Spritzer K, Gelberg L. Health behaviors, health status, and access to and use of health care: a population-based study of lesbian, bisexual, and heterosexual women. *Arch Fam Med* 2000; **9**(10):1043–51.

26 McNair R, Anderson S, Mitchell A. Addressing health inequalities in Victorian lesbian, gay, bisexual and transgender communities. *Health Promot J Austr* 2001; **11**(1):32–9.

27 Meyer IH. Prejudice, social stress, and mental health in lesbian, gay and bisexual populations: conceptual issues and research evidence. *Psychol Bull* 2003; **129**:674–97.

28 Kuyper L, Fokkema T. Minority stress and mental health among Dutch LGBs: examination of differences between sex and sexual orientation. *J Couns Psychol* 2011; **58**(2):222–33.

29 Ford CS, Beach FA. *Patterns of sexual behaviour*. London: Eyre and Spottiswoode; 1952.

30 Kinsey AC, Pomeroy WB, Martin CE. *Sexual behavior in the human male*. Philadelphia: W.B. Saunders; 1948.

31 Prager D. Judaism, homosexuality and civilization. *Ultimate Issues* 1990; **6**(2):24.

32 Blackwood E. *The many faces of homosexuality: anthropological approaches to homosexual behavior*. New York: Routledge; 1986.

33 Nanda S. Hijras: an alternative sex and gender role in India. In: *Third sex, third gender: essays from anthropology and social history* (ed. Herdt G). New York: Zone Books; 1994, pp. 373–418.

34 Brummelhuis H. Transformations of transgender. *J Gay Lesbian Soc Serv* 1999; **9**(2–3):121–39.

35 Shapiro J. Transsexualism: reflections on the persistence of gender and the mutability of sex. In: *Same sex cultures and sexuality: an anthropological reader* (ed. Robertson J). Malden, MA: Blackwell Publishing; 2005.

36 Roscoe W. *Priests of the goddess: gender transgression in the ancient world. The 109th annual meeting of the American Historical Association*. San Fransisco, CA: American Historical Association; 1994.

37 Besnier, N. Polynesian gender liminality through time and space. In: *Third sex, third gender: essays from anthropology and social history* (ed. Herdt G). New York: Zone Books; 1994, pp. 285–328.

38 Roscoe W. (ed.) *Living the spirit: a gay American Indian anthology*. New York: St. Martin's Press; 1988.

39 de Graaf R, Sandfort TG, ten Have M. Suicidality and sexual orientation: differences between men and women in a general population-based sample from the Netherlands. *Arch Sex Behav* 2006; **35**(3):253–62.

40 Cass VC. Homosexual identity formation: a theoretical model. *J Homosex* 1979; **4**(3):219–35.

41 Kaufman J, Johnson C. Stigmatized individuals and the process of identity. *Sociol Q* 2004; **45**(4):807–33.

42 Coleman E. Developmental stages of the coming-out process. *J Homosex* 1982; **7**(2–3):31–43.

43 **Kalra G**. Breaking the ice: IJP on homosexuality. *Ind J Psychiatry* 2012; **54**(3):299–300.

44 **Kalra G**. A psychiatrist's role in 'coming out' process: context and controversies post-377. *Ind J Psychiatry* 2012; **54**:69–72.

45 **Reich DB, Zanarini MC**. Sexual orientation and relationship choice in borderline personality disorder over ten years of prospective follow-up. *J Pers Disord* 2008; **22**:564–72.

46 **Needham BL, Austin EL**. Sexual orientation, parental support, and health during the transition to young adulthood. *J Youth Adolesc* 2010; **39**(10):1189–98.

47 **Hart TA, Heimberg RG**. Presenting problems among treatment-seeking gay, lesbian, and bisexual youth. *J Clin Psychol* 2001; **57**(5):615–27.

48 **Safren SA, Rogers T**. Cognitive-behavioral therapy with gay, lesbian, and bisexual clients. *J Clin Psychol* 2001; **57**(5):629–43.

49 **Green RJ, Mitchell V**. Gay and lesbian couples in therapy: minority stress, relational ambiguity and families of choice. In: *Clinical handbook of couple therapy* (ed. Gurman AS). New York: Guilford Press; 2008, pp. 662–80.

50 **Kuyper L, Fokkema T**. Loneliness among older lesbian, gay, and bisexual adults: the role of minority stress. *Arch Sex Behav* 2010; **39**(5):1171–80.

51 **Levounis P, Drescher J, Barber ME**. *The LGBT casebook*. Virginia: American Psychiatric Publishing; 2012.

52 **Colizzi M, Costa R, Todarello O**. Transsexual patients' psychiatric comorbidity and positive effect of cross-sex hormonal treatment on mental health: results from a longitudinal study. *Psychoneuroendocrinology* 2014; **39**:65–73.

Chapter 34

Translational neuroimaging

Felipe Picon, Umberto Volpe, Philipp Sterzer, and Andreas Heinz

Case study

Felix has just completed his psychiatric training. He is the best achieving doctor of his 2055 graduation class. Worldwide efforts to understand how the brain works have thrived and now many of these neuroscientific findings are used daily to help ease and cure the myriad of psychiatric disorders. Felix has been trained on how to interview psychiatric patients, to understand their suffering, and to diagnose and treat them; however, as a modern-day core competence, he has also been trained on how to apply neuroimaging techniques as a tool to better differentiate diagnosis, choose between different treatments, and make predictions on the outcomes of the interventions made. Felix is about to decide if he should complete his PhD in neuroradiology, in order to have a better chance of been hired in his hometown psychiatric hospital.

Introduction

The futuristic picture described in the case study is something that many psychiatrists long for. It would be the ultimate translation of neuroscientific discoveries into real psychiatric applications.[2] The availability of objective measures of brain functioning and the deep understanding of the neurobiological underpinnings of mental disorders would be of great help in everyday psychiatric practice. This would be the best outcome of the efforts being made by many neuroscientists around the world. The various modalities of neuroimaging would, then, be an essential part of the diagnostic and prognostic process, providing either actual images for clinical classification or different data, depending on the technique used, to help in defining the prognosis or to predict the response to a certain treatment.

It is with this hopeful state of mind that this chapter has been written. Its goal is to foster interest in neuroimaging among future psychiatrists and also to highlight the nomenclature and details of the technology already available.

History of neuroimaging

The history of neuroimaging, a field comprising methods that image or map the structure and function of the brain, is intertwined with the history of neurosciences and neuroradiology. In the sixteenth century, Vesalius performed neuroanatomical studies and considered that thoughts and feelings were stored in the cerebral ventricles.[3]

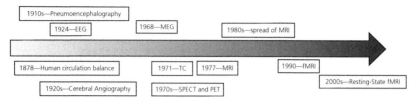

Fig. 34.1 Timeline of the evolution of neuroimaging techniques.

Interestingly, centuries later, in 1976, the first modern psychiatric neuroimaging study using computerized tomography with schizophrenic patients also studied the ventricular volumes.[4] In 1878, Mosso described the 'human circulation balance' and introduced the important idea of blood flow variations during mental activities, which still remains a key concept for functional neuroimaging.[1,5] In the 1910s, Dandy produced the first image of the brain in a painful procedure called pneumoencephalography in which air injected into the ventricles was the contrast to form the X-ray image of the brain. The evolution of neuroimaging continued in the 1920s when Moniz introduced cerebral angiography, making X-ray images of blood vessels by injecting contrast (a process we are familiar with today).[6] In 1924, Berger recorded the first human electroencephalogram (EEG),[7] allowing the first recordings of event-related potentials later on. In 1968, Cohen demonstrated alternating magnetic fields outside the human scalp, thus initiating magnetoencephalography (MEG).[6,8]

The evolution of the usage of X-rays to acquire images of the brain came a few decades later, in 1971, when the efforts of many scientists created computerized tomography (CT). It was not long after that the developments of radioactive compounds were put together with CT and, as a consequence, single-positron emission computerized tomography (SPECT) and positron emission tomography (PET) were added to the list of neuroimaging techniques. At the same time, magnetic resonance imaging (MRI) was also being developed, with the first clinical MRI image being produced in 1977.

The following years were filled with the improvement of all modalities and the spread of MRI into clinical settings. In 1990, Ogawa introduced the concept of the blood–oxygen level dependent (BOLD) contrast and created the functional MRI (fMRI).[9] Following this, there has been an exponential growth of published papers using fMRI.[10] Since 2001, a different functional technique, known as 'resting state' functional connectivity, has received considerable attention. This technique enables the measurement of functional connectivity among different brain regions, without the use of any cognitive task in the scanner. It is therefore stated that the person is 'resting', although we know that the brain is actually restless.[11]

Fig. 34.1 presents a summary timeline of key developments in neuroimaging over recent decades.

Current neuroimaging modalities

Nowadays, clinical neuroimaging is mainly the domain of neurologists, neuroradiologists (for diagnostic purposes), as well as psychiatrists (when trying to rule out a neurological aetiology for psychiatric symptoms). This aspect of neuroimaging is not covered within this chapter. Instead, we provide an overview of the specificities of the main structural and functional modalities.

Traditionally, neuroimaging modalities are categorized as either structural or functional. Current structural approaches are provided mainly by structural magnetic resonance imaging (sMRI) and diffusion tensor imaging (DTI) which focuses on the structural connectivity. Functional neuroimaging is currently represented by SPECT, PET, EEG, MEG, near infrared spectroscopic (NIRS) imaging, fMRI, and magnetic resonance spectroscopy (MRS). Table 34.1 provides a brief description of these various techniques and Table 34.2 compares the main functional modalities in terms of their strengths and limitations. The most recent technical developments in this field include 'voxel-wise correction' and 'biological parametric mapping' (which correct for brain volume differences between patients and controls).[12]

Table 34.1 Neuroimaging modalities

Neuroimaging modality	Brief description
Structural magnetic resonance imaging (sMRI) (See Figures in Table 34.3)	Evolving from CT, sMRI studies began looking at ROI (regions of interest); this approach provides information on one brain structure of interest at a time. sMRI is based on the T1 contrast of MR images, elucidating peculiarities and differences in the volume of brain regions in each psychiatric disorder compared to control subjects. For further details, also see Table 34.2.
Diffusion tensor imaging (DTI) (see Fig. 34.2 in colour plate section)	DTI uses the restriction of movement of water molecules within the myelin sheath to determine the morphology of axonal bundles in the white matter (tractography) and to calculate its anisotropy (as reported in most of the studies, the fractional anisotropy—FA). DTI provides information on the structural connectivity between brain regions.[13]
Single-positron emission computerized tomography (SPECT) (see Fig. 34.3 in colour plate section)	A single photon-emitting radiopharmaceutical (contrast) is injected into the bloodstream of the patient who is then placed in the SPECT scanner. The device captures the single photon emission, thus generating a brain image with greater intensity where the radiopharmaceutical has more activity. For example, if the contrast is linked to a dopamine transporter molecule, it is possible to map where this transporter protein is available in the brain.[14]
Positron emission tomography (PET) (see Fig. 34.4 in colour plate section)	PET uses the same principle as SPECT, but the PET radiopharmaceutical contrasts emit positrons, have a shorter half-life (the cyclotron has to be placed near the scanner), and a better spatial resolution. Hence, PET provides images with greater resolution than with SPECT. PET uses radionuclides such as ^{15}O, ^{13}N, ^{11}C, and ^{18}F, with half-lives of $^{15}O = 2$ min, $^{13}N = 10$ min, $^{11}C = 20$ min, and $^{18}F = 110$ min. Each with a specific decay, they are thus used in different ways, depending on the focus of the study.[15]

(continued)

Table 34.1 (continued) Neuroimaging modalities

Neuroimaging modality	Brief description
Electroencephalography (EEG) (see Fig. 34.5 in colour plate section)	The electrodes placed on the scalp of the subject measure the voltage oscillations of the flow of ionic currents from brain cortical neurons; the recorded bioelectrical measure provides a topographical and momentary expression of the brain activity.[16]
Magnetoencephalography (MEG) (see Fig. 34.6 in colour plate section)	MEG captures the electromagnetic fields produced by brain electrical currents, by using highly sensitive magnetometers; it provides electromagnetic measures of brain functioning.[8,17]
Near infrared spectroscopic imaging (NIRSI) (see Fig. 34.7 in colour plate section)	Transmitters and detectors of near infrared light are placed on the head of the subject to detect differences in transmission and absorption of the infrared light reflected on the haemoglobin. Therefore, NIRSI can measure the cortical changes in blood flow, which indicate neuronal activity.[18] It has a relatively low spatial resolution and only covers the cortex, but has the advantages of being easily moved to more naturalistic environments (outside a research facility or hospital) and is non-invasive.
Functional magnetic resonance imaging (fMRI) (see Fig. 34.8 in colour plate section)	FMRI studies brain activity by detecting changes in blood flow related to brain function. It uses a contrast called BOLD (blood oxygenated level dependent), which utilizes the distortion of the electromagnetic field in the MRI scanner to show where the oxygenated blood ceases to be oxygenated, thus revealing where substantial brain function occurs.[9]
Magnetic resonance spectroscopy (MRS) (See Fig. 34.9 in colour plate section)	MRS shows the concentration of, for example, N-acetyl aspartate (NAA), choline (Cho), creatine (Cr), lipids, lactate (Lac), myo-inositol (mI), glutamate (Glu), and glutamine (Gln) in a selected brain area. Each metabolite has its specific characteristic as a marker of a particular neuronal activity.[19] MRS gives a metabolic measure of brain function.

Table 34.2 Strengths and limitations of the main functional neuroimaging modalities

Neuroimaging modality	Temporal resolution	Spatial resolution	Invasiveness
SPECT	> 60 seconds	6–8 mm	Yes (uses radiotracers)
PET	45 seconds	4 mm	Yes (uses radiotracers)
MEG	1 millisecond	5 mm	Non-invasive
fMRI	2–5 seconds	1–1.15 mm	Non-invasive

Table 34.3 Voxel- and surface-based morphometric sMRI techniques

Technique	Description
Voxel-based morphometry (VBM) (See Fig. 34.10 in colour plate section)	VBM allows the study of regional differences in brain structure. It compares the brains of groups of individuals at the level of each voxel (tridimensional pixel), usually measuring 1mm.[20] VBM was first developed as an analytical element of the Statistical Parametric Mapping (SPM) software package.[21]
Surface-based morphometry (SBM) (See Fig. 34.11 in colour plate section)	SBM uses surfaces to set limits/boundaries in structural brain images to measure distances between brain regions. One such boundary lies between grey and white matter, while another one is set between the outer border of the grey matter to the cerebrospinal fluid (CSF) space. Thus, the technique allows estimation of the thickness of the cerebral cortex. In addition, SBM allows measurement of the gyral curvature, depth, area, and volume of various brain regions.[22] The best known software that uses this method is Freesurfer.[23]

Brain images acquired with MRI can be processed with different software, thus providing different data outputs. Among the methods used for structural images, two approaches most commonly referred to in the literature are voxel-based morphometry (VBM) and surface-based morphometry (SBM), also used for measuring the cortical thickness. The details of each approach are given in Table 34.3. Other relevant software used in neuroimaging pre-processing and analysis is presented in Table 34.4.

Functional MRI is traditionally known for showing which brain areas are activated during a specific task, executed by the subject while inside the scanner, with the BOLD signal increasing and diminishing according to the neuronal activity. This approach is also known as task-based fMRI. In addition to investigating functional specialization in terms of increases and decreases of the BOLD signal in specific brain regions, fMRI can also be used to examine functional integration—that is, task-related interactions between brain regions in terms of functional connectivity.[27] A straightforward way to measure functional connectivity is to assess how the BOLD signal time course in one brain region co-varies with the signal in other regions as a function of task[28] or of between-subject factors such as genotype[29] or psychopathology.[30] In contrast to such correlative approaches, other methods, such as Granger causality[31] or dynamic causal modelling (DCM),[32] aim at inferring causal interactions between brain regions from fMRI signal time courses. For example, DCM for fMRI has been used to show reduced

Table 34.4 Neuroimaging software

Software	Institution of origin	Main characteristics
Statistical Parametric Mapping (SPM)	University College London, UK	SPM is a free software package designed to carry out statistical parametric mapping of functional and structural brain images (fMRI and PET).[21]
		Available at: http://fil.ion.ucl.ac.uk/spm
Functional Magnetic Resonance Imaging of the Brain Software Library (FSL)	Oxford University, UK	FSL is a free software library of image analysis and statistical tools for functional, structural, and diffusion MRI brain imaging data[24]
		Available at: http://www.fmrib.ox.ac.uk/fsl
Analysis of Functional NeuroImages (AFNI)	National Institute of Mental Health (NIMH), Bethesda, MD, USA	AFNI is an open-source agglomeration of programs for processing and displaying functional MRI data.[25]
		Available at: http://afni.nimh.nih.gov/afni
FreeSurfer	MGH/HST Athinoula A. Martinos Center for Biomedical Imaging, Charleston, MA, USA	FreeSurfer is free software for analysing MR structural, functional, and diffusion images. Its most known feature is the measurement of the cerebral cortical thickness.[23]
		Available at: http://www.freesurfer.net
BioImage Suite	Yale University, New Haven, CT, USA	BioImage Suite is free software for the analysis of neuro, cardiac, and abdominal images.
		Available at: http://www.bioimagesuite.org
MRIcron	University of South Carolina, Columbia, SC, USA	MRIcron is a free software program used to view and convert the DICOM image format (original format of the images acquired by the scanner) into the NIfTI[26] format (the image format mostly used in the MRIcron software).
		Available at: http://www.nitrc.org/projects/mricron

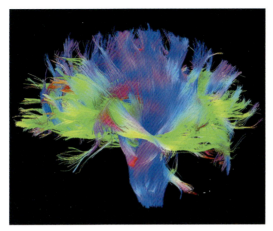

Fig. 34.2 Diffusion tensor imaging (DTI). Tractography image showing the morphology of axonal bundles in the white matter. Blue represents tracts going in the rostral–caudal direction; red, latero–lateral direction; and green, antero–posterior direction. Other colours are a mixture of those directions.

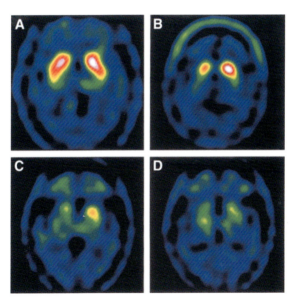

Fig. 34.3 Single-positron emission computerized tomography (SPECT). SPECT images of four subjects showing the decreasing binding of 99mTc-TRODAT-1 in bilateral putamen comparing a healthy subject (A) with three others with different stages of Parkinson's disease.

Reproduced from *J Nucl Med*, 45(3), Weng Y-H, Yen T-C, Chen M-C, Kao P-F, Tzen K-Y, Chen R-S, et al., Sensitivity and specificity of 99mTc-TRODAT-1 SPECT imaging in differentiating patients with idiopathic Parkinson's disease from healthy subjects, p. 393–401, Copyright (2004), with permission from The Society of Nuclear Medicine and Molecular Imaging.

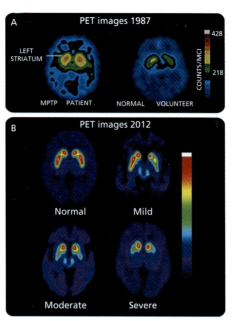

Fig. 34.4 Positron emission tomography (PET). Comparison of (A) 18F-spiperone (a D2-like antagonist) PET image from 1987 and (B) a 18F-FPCIT PET image from 2012, showing the increased resolution and definition between the caudate nuclei and putamen in B compared to A.

Reproduced from *Neurology*, 80(10), Portnow LH, Vaillancourt DE, Okun MS, The history of cerebral PET scanning: from physiology to cutting-edge technology, p. 952–6, Copyright (2013), with permission from Wolters Kluwer Health.

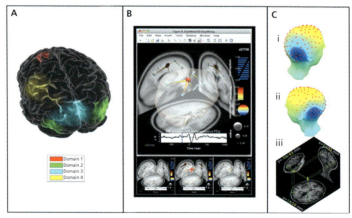

Fig. 34.5 Electroencephalography (EEG). Examples of EEG source imaging: (A) source decomposition of EEG data; (B) EEG-based brain connectivity analysis and visualization; (C) (i) and (ii) showing the scalp projections (green = 0, yellow = positive, blue = negative), and (iii) location of the equivalent current dipole in the subject MRI-based head model.

Reproduced from *Am J Med Genet*, 165(2), McLoughlin G, Makeig S, Tsuang MT, In search of biomarkers in psychiatry: EEG-based measures of brain function, p. 111–21, Copyright (2013), with permission from John Wiley & Sons Ltd.

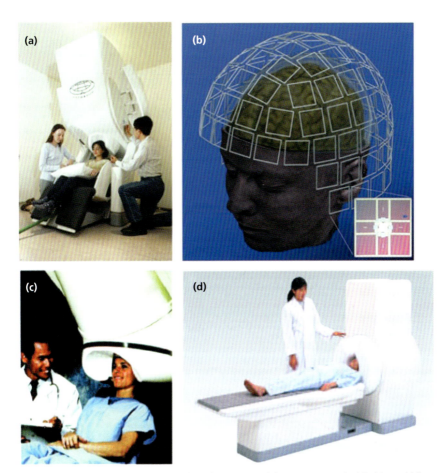

Fig. 34.6 Magnetoencephalography (MEG). Commercial MEG systems in (a), (c), and (d); (b) shows the placement of each magnetometer over the scalp.

Reproduced from Hansen P, Kringelbach M, Salmelin R, *MEG: An Introduction to Methods*, Copyright (2010), with permission from Oxford University Press, USA.

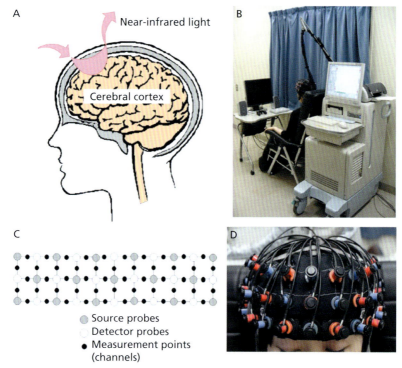

A — Near-infrared light / Cerebral cortex

B

C
○ Source probes
○ Detector probes
● Measurement points (channels)

D

Fig. 34.7 Near infrared spectroscopic (NIRS) imaging. (A) Illustration showing the near infrared light being emitted from a source probe onto the human scalp, passing and being scattered through the brain tissue, which will be detected by a detector probe; (B) shows commercial NIRS equipment; (C) shows the disposition of the source probes, detector probes, and measurement points (channels); and (D) shows the NIRS helmet in place over the scalp of the subject.

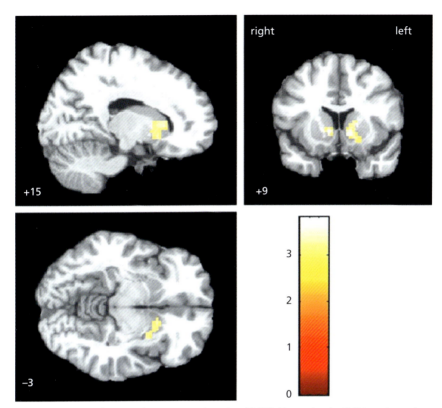

Fig. 34.8 Functional magnetic resonance imaging (fMRI). Example of a fMRI study results display showing the areas of increased activation for 17 euthymic bipolar patients relative to healthy comparison subjects submitted to emotional and non-emotional tasks.

Reproduced from *Am J Psychiatry*, 164(4), Wessa M, Houenou J, Paillère-Martinot M-L, Berthoz S, Artiges E, Leboyer M, et al., Fronto-striatal overactivation in euthymic bipolar patients during an emotional go/nogo task, p. 638–46, Copyright (2007), reproduced with permission from *American Journal of Psychiatry*.

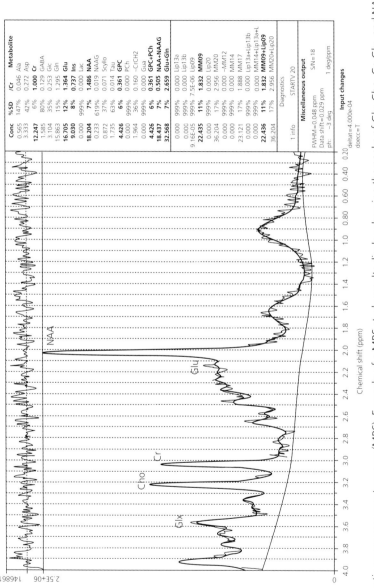

Fig. 34.9 Magnetic resonance spectroscopy (MRS). Example of a MRS study results display showing the peaks of Glx, Cho, Cr, Glu, and NAA from a previously selected area of the brain.

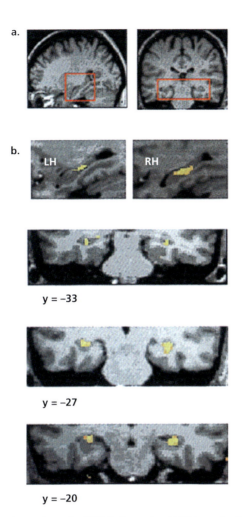

a.

b.

LH   RH

y = −33

y = −27

y = −20

Fig. 34.10 Voxel-based morphometry (VBM). Example of VBM results display: (a) shows a sagittal section of an MRI scan with the hippocampus indicated by the red box; (b) shows the group results superimposed on an MRI image.

Reproduced from *Proc Natl Acad Sci USA*, 97(8), Maguire EA, Gadian DG, Johnsrude IS, Good CD, Ashburner J, Frackowiak RS, et al., Navigation-related structural change in the hippocampi of taxi drivers, p. 4398–403, Copyright (2000), reproduced with permission from National Academy of Sciences, USA.

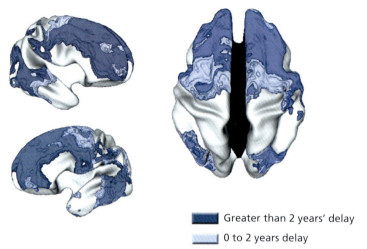

■ Greater than 2 years' delay

▨ 0 to 2 years delay

Fig. 34.11 Surface-based morphometry (SBM). Example of SBM study results display. This image shows the regions where the ADHD group had delayed cortical maturation.

Reproduced from *Proc Natl Acad Sci USA*, 104(49), Shaw P, Eckstrand K, Lerch JP, Greenstein D, Clasen L., Attention-deficit/hyperactivity disorder is characterized by a delay in cortical maturation, p. 4398–403, Copyright (2007), reproduced with permission from National Academy of Sciences, USA.

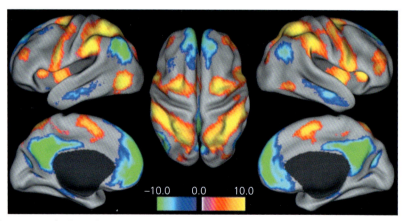

Fig. 34.12 Default mode network (DMN) regions (in green-blue) shown anticorrelated with regions involved in attention and working memory (in yellow-red).

interactions between frontal and parietal regions during a working memory task in patients with schizophrenia.[33]

In addition to task-based fMRI, functional connectivity between different brain areas can also be assessed in resting-state fMRI (RS-fMRI), in which the subject is not required to attend to any task; instead, the subject lies still inside the scanner, with the eyes closed or opened and fixed on a specific point. In RS-fMRI, the BOLD signal oscillations of the whole brain are interpreted as meaning that wherever the signal is synchronically rising or diminishing, these areas are 'communicating' with each other. This fMRI technique is gaining ground within the neuroimaging scientific community. For further details on this technique, see Table 34.5

RS-fMRI has aroused much interest in the field of cognitive neuroscience since the first studies in the early 2000s.[35] The technique explores the intrinsic activity of the brain, not necessarily related to any motor or sensorial event, and became best known by the study of the so-called 'default mode network' (DMN).[36] RS-fMRI also reveals the functional status of other basic brain networks, such as the auditory system, visual system, sensorimotor system, 'salience' network, 'executive control' network, and the 'dorsal attention' network.[11] The exploration of the activity of all these networks can be obtained during any task performance. Possibly this is one of the most relevant reasons why this technique recently blossomed within the psychiatric research community. Furthermore, RS-fMRI allows the study of patients of different ages and with various mental disorders and levels of cognitive functioning, with no need to train the patient with regards to a specific task. This flexibility of application is very useful for psychiatric research, and this method has already been used to analyse aberrations, disruptions, and modifications of functional connectivity involved in several mental disorders: bipolar disorder,[37–39] major depression,[40–42] schizophrenia,[43–45] attention deficit hyperactivity disorder (ADHD),[46–48] panic disorder,[49–51] social anxiety disorder,[52–56]

Table 34.5 Task-based fMRI and resting-state fMRI

fMRI approach	Description
Task-based fMRI	This is the traditional fMRI approach that uses blood flow fluctuations, through the BOLD signal, to generate images of brain activity while the subject is performing a specific task. Task-based fMRI can be analysed using different neuroimaging software, such as SPM,[34] AFNI,[25] and FSL.[24] Several different neuropsychological tests have been used (flanker test, go/no go test, etc.) and the field is always trying to develop new tasks in order to answer different questions or to reach more accurate responses inside the scanner.
Resting-state fMRI (RS-fMRI)	RS-fMRI shows which regions are 'communicating' with each other, making it possible to elucidate functional networks during rest and their potential alterations in mental disorders. It reveals the functional connectivity without the need to execute any neuropsychological task while inside the scanner—hence, the word 'resting' in its name.[35] RS-fMRI can be analysed using the same neuroimaging software as task-based fMRI, although the way to interpret the findings is different.

post-traumatic stress disorder (PTSD),[57,58] generalized anxiety disorder (GAD),[59,60] obsessive compulsive disorder (OCD),[61,62] autism,[63,64] borderline personality disorder,[65,66] anorexia,[67–69] bulimia,[70,71] alcohol dependence,[72,73] cocaine addiction,[74–78] cannabis addiction,[79,80] heroin addiction,[81–83] internet gaming addiction,[84,85] pathological gambling,[86,87] among others.

The DMN consists of a set of brain regions, including cortical midline structures such as the ventromedial prefrontal cortex and the posterior cingulate gyrus, and areas of the lateral parietal cortex and superior temporal gyrus bilaterally, which are more activated when one is thinking about the future, remembering the past, or day-dreaming.[88] The DMN was discovered during the study of moments of 'rest' that occurred during task-based functional studies (moments in which the subject was not performing the cognitive task). Ever since Raichle coined the term 'default mode network' in 2001,[36] exploration of this network has been non-stop. Many of the aforementioned psychiatric studies assess the disruption and alteration of the DMN. Its function has already been described in other mammals as well,[89–91] and its reliability[92] and consistency[93–95] strengthens its translational use to psychiatry as a possible future biomarker (See Fig. 34.12 in colour plate section)

The quest for neuroimaging biomarkers for psychiatric disorders

A biomarker, as defined by the Biomarkers Definitions Working Group, is a 'characteristic that is objectively measured and evaluated as an indicator of normal biological processes, pathogenic processes, or pharmacologic responses to a therapeutic intervention'.[97] Considering that the techniques of neuroimaging map the function and status of the living human brain, it is plausible to consider that they are the most appropriate techniques to generate biomarkers of psychiatric disorders. Neuroimaging biomarkers of psychiatric disorders would improve considerably the routine of psychiatrists. They would provide objective measures of brain function for the purpose of differential diagnosis, classification, staging, prediction of course of the disorder, and prediction of response to treatment.[98] As a prognostic biomarker, a specific set of neuroimaging features could predict future occurrence of a disorder in healthy childhood samples, for instance. With this foreseeability, prevention of future negative psychiatric outcomes would be highly and accurately enhanced. Unfortunately, as we know, this goal has not yet been reliably reached. Even so, this quest for a useful neuroimaging biomarker in psychiatry already counts with many studies that apply structural and functional modalities.

Structural MRI scans of individuals with ADHD, schizophrenia, Tourette's syndrome, bipolar disorder, and at familial risk for major depression were discriminated from the sMRI scans of healthy subjects through the use of a statistical algorithm that analyses the differences in all images, differentiating one group from the other only by the features of the images.[99] In another study, grey matter density was calculated from sMR images of 36 patients with recent-onset psychosis and 36 matched controls, and a pattern classification analysis was applied. The method was able to classify both groups with 86.1% accuracy.[100] A similar approach, using support vector machine classification (a machine-learning approach to BOLD signal patterns of task-based fMRI), analysed the functional brain images of adolescents with ADHD and controls. The pattern of brain activation correctly classified up to 90% of patients (sensibility) and 63% of controls (specificity), achieving an overall classification accuracy of 77%.[101] Another study, using the same approach, but with a different task, also showed a pattern of brain activation that correctly classified up to 80% of patients (sensitivity) and 70% of controls (specificity), achieving an overall classification accuracy of 75%.[102] Using RS-fMRI of 98 ADHD patients and 141 healthy controls, another group was able to demonstrate 76.15% accuracy, and sensitivity of 63.27% and specificity of 85.11% in the discrimination of both groups with the use of a support vector machine classifier.[103] The approach can be used to elucidate gene × gene effects on brain structure.[104]

Besides the use of sMRI and fMRI signals, functional NIRS data can also differentiate patients with schizophrenia from healthy controls. Hahn and colleagues[105] enrolled 40 patients with schizophrenia and 40 controls who undertook a working memory task while wearing the fNIRS helmet. The method was able to classify the different groups with 76% accuracy. However, these promising findings need to be replicated in independent samples in order to achieve external validity and to eventually become a useful biomarker.

In the attempt to use neuroimaging as a biomarker of prediction of treatment outcome, Wrase et al.[106] observed that amygdala volume reductions predict relapse in alcohol-dependent subjects. McGrath and colleagues[107] used glucose PET scans of 38 patients prior to randomization to treatment for depression with either escitalopram (10–20 mg/d) or 16 sessions of cognitive behaviour therapy. They found that insula hypometabolism was associated with remission to cognitive behaviour therapy and poor response to escitalopram, while insula hypermetabolism was associated with remission to escitalopram and poor response to cognitive therapy. Another study enrolled 24 patients suffering from depression and compared them with 51 healthy controls, with the use of PET with a serotonin-binding radiotracer. They found that elevated serotonin binding in raphe nuclei was associated with subsequent remission with the use of escitalopram.[108] DTI was also applied to 18 subjects with depression prior to 8 weeks' treatment with a selective serotonin reuptake inhibitor (SSRI). Average fractional anisotropy (FA) in the tracts to the right amygdala was significantly lower in non-remitters than remitters. These results suggest that the integrity and/or the number of white matter fibres terminating in the right amygdala may be compromised in SSRI non-remitters.[109]

The aforementioned are just some examples of different ways to address the quest for an objective measure of brain function in psychiatric disorders using neuroimaging techniques. Each modality has its strengths and weaknesses related to how it acquires the biological signals of the brain. One possible explanation for why no reliable biomarker is yet available is the lack of neurochemical specificity in any particular disorder when referring to neurotransmitters and the use of SPECT and PET, for instance.[98] The absence of a gold standard of functional activity in fMRI is also a major challenge to be overcome. Moreover, several clinically diagnosed disorders share common neurobiological dysfunctions (e.g. during reward anticipation).[110] Besides that, the wide variety of software used and the lack of a gold standard of statistical analysis are also sources of concern. This diversity makes it difficult to compile data and, therefore, affects an overall analysis.

Another important aspect that hampers the extrapolation of neuroimaging findings on psychiatric disorders is sample sizes. As there are many studies with small sample sizes, some findings cannot be extrapolated to the general population, making this a future challenge for all young psychiatrists who venture in this field of research.[111] As already shown, the application of pattern-based analysis (e.g. using machine-learning techniques) is a promising way to predict the course of psychiatric diseases. Perhaps the most important translational use for a neuroimaging biomarker would be to differentiate between psychiatric disorders, not between cases and controls, since that can be easily done clinically without any scans. As an example, the differentiation of whether a child presenting distractibility has ADHD or bipolar disorder is of extreme importance, because the treatment is totally different from one situation to the other. Even more important would be to predict the onset of psychosis before it happened, hopefully preventing its onset with early treatment.

Conclusions

Despite all the progress in neuroimaging techniques in the last 30 years, there are still several questions left unanswered. One of the most fundamental questions for neuroscientists—how does the brain function?—is still awaiting a clinically meaningful answer. This exemplifies one caveat of fMRI: that there is no gold standard for brain activation or deactivation. Recent discoveries shown through brain images usually make sensational headlines in lay journals and magazines, but, for the most part, these results only enlighten the research path of the specific disorder studied. This relates to the issue of external validity of neuroimaging studies.

Some initiatives are already in place to manage some of the limitations described here. Regarding the sample size of neuroimaging studies, some international collaborations are in progress, with the open sharing of online, large samples of structural and functional neuroimaging data.[112] Initiatives with a specific focus on children at risk for the development of psychopathology,[113] ADHD,[114] autism,[63] and addiction,[115] and large community-based samples to study psychiatric disorder through the life span[116] with multi-modality neuroimaging are already in progress. Many groups from different parts of the world are collaborating to investigate, through neuroimaging, the human connectome,[117] and substantial public funding and support have been added to the worldwide effort to understand how the brain functions, in the quest to eliminate brain dysfunctions.[118,119] Hopefully, in the years to come, the results from these initiatives will help us to better understand the brain and lead us to solve some of the difficulties in finding a neuroimaging biomarker for psychiatric disorders.

The scope of the methods presented here shows the numerous possibilities and increasing opportunities for the early career psychiatrist interested in psychiatric neuroimaging research. For those not inclined to research, it is our hope that this brief review will provide the background to future discoveries of psychiatric neuroimaging.

Translational neuroimaging is still in its infancy, but if the exponential growth of possibilities seen in the last decade continues, the futuristic picture described at the beginning of the chapter will inevitably become reality.

References

1 **Holmes OW**. *The autocrat of the breakfast-table*. Boston: Phillips, Sampson, Co.: 1858. 1858.

2 **Machado-Vieira R**. Tracking the impact of translational research in psychiatry: state of the art and perspectives. *J Transl Med* 2012; **10**:175.

3 **Vesalius A**. *De humani corporis fabrica libri septem*. 1543.

4 **Johnstone EC, Crow TJ, Frith CD, Husband J, Kreel L**. Cerebral ventricular size and cognitive impairment in chronic schizophrenia. *Lancet* 1976; **2**(7992):924–6.

5 **Sandrone S, Bacigaluppi M, Galloni MR, Martino G**. Angelo mosso (1846–910). *J Neurol* 2012; **259**(11):2513–4.

6 **Alper MGM**. Three pioneers in the early history of neuroradiology: the Snyder lecture. *Doc Ophthalmol* 1999; **98**(1):29–49.

7 **Haas LF**. Hans Berger (1873–1941), Richard Caton (1842–926), and electroencephalography. *J Neurol Neurosurg Psychiatr* 2003; **74**(1):9.

8 **Cohen D**. Magnetoencephalography: evidence of magnetic fields produced by alpha-rhythm currents. *Science* 1968; **161**(3843):784–6.

9 **Ogawa S, Lee TM, Kay AR, Tank DW**. Brain magnetic resonance imaging with contrast dependent on blood oxygenation. *Proc Natl Acad Sci USA* 1990; **87**(24):9868–72.

10 **Bandettini P**. Functional MRI today. *Int J Psychophysiol* 2007; **63**(2):138–45.

11 **Raichle ME**. The restless brain. *Brain Connect* 2011; **1**(1):3–12.

12 **Beck A, Wustenberg T, Genauck A, et al**. Effect of brain structure, brain function, and brain connectivity on relapse in alcohol-dependent patients. *Arch Gen Psychiatry* 2012; **69**(8):842–52.

13 **Tournier J-D, Mori S, Leemans A**. Diffusion tensor imaging and beyond. *Magn Reson Med* 2011; **65**(6):1532–56.

14 **Holman BL, Devous MD**. Functional brain SPECT: the emergence of a powerful clinical method. *J Nucl Med* 1992; **33**(10):1888–904.

15 **Raichle ME**. A brief history of human brain mapping. *Trends Neurosci* 2009; **32**(2):118–26.

16 **da Silva FL**. EEG and MEG: relevance to neuroscience. *Neuron* 2013; **80**(5):1112–28.

17 **Hansen P, Kringelbach M, Salmelin R (eds)**. *MEG: an introduction to methods* (1st edn). New York: Oxford University Press; 2010, p. 1.

18 **Owen-Reece H, Smith M, Elwell CE, Goldstone JC**. Near infrared spectroscopy. *Br J Anaesth* 1999; **82**(3):418–26.

19 **Gujar SK, Maheshwari S, Björkman-Burtscher I, Sundgren PC**. Magnetic resonance spectroscopy. *J Neuroophthalmol* 2005; **25**(3):217–26.

20 **Ashburner J, Friston KJ**. Voxel-based morphometry—the methods. *NeuroImage* 2000; **11**(6):805–21.

21 **Ashburner J**. SPM: a history. *NeuroImage* 2012; **62**(2):791–800.

22 **Fischl B, van der Kouwe A, Destrieux C, et al**. Automatically parcellating the human cerebral cortex. *Cereb Cortex* 2004; **14**(1):11–22.

23 **Fischl B**. FreeSurfer. *NeuroImage* 2012; **62**:774–81.:1–15.

24 Jenkinson M, Beckmann CF, Behrens TEJ, Woolrich MW, Smith SM. FSL. *NeuroImage* 2012; **62**(2):782–90.

25 Cox RW. AFNI: software for analysis and visualization of functional magnetic resonance neuroimages. *Comput Biomed Res* 1996; **29**(3):162–73.

26 Larobina M, Murino L. Medical image file formats. *J Digit Imaging* 2014; **27**(2):200–6.

27 Stephan KE. On the role of general system theory for functional neuroimaging. *J Anat* 2004; **205**(6):443–70.

28 Friston KJ, Buechel C, Fink GR, Morris J, Rolls E, Dolan RJ. Psychophysiological and modulatory interactions in neuroimaging. *NeuroImage* 1997; **6**(3):218–29.

29 Heinz A, Braus DF, Smolka MN, et al. Amygdala-prefrontal coupling depends on a genetic variation of the serotonin transporter. *Nat Neurosci* 2005; **8**(1):20–1.

30 Schmack K, Gòmez-Carrillo de Castro A, Rothkirch M, et al. Delusions and the role of beliefs in perceptual inference. *J Neurosci* 2013; **33**(34):13701–12.

31 Roebroeck A, Formisano E, Goebel R. Mapping directed influence over the brain using Granger causality and fMRI. *NeuroImage* 2005; **25**(1):230–42.

32 Friston KJ, Harrison L, Penny W. Dynamic causal modelling. *NeuroImage* 2003; **19**(4):1273–302.

33 Deserno L, Sterzer P, Wustenberg T, Heinz A, Schlagenhauf F. Reduced prefrontal-parietal effective connectivity and working memory deficits in schizophrenia. *J Neurosci* 2012; **32**(1):12–20.

34 Ashburner J. SPM: a history. *NeuroImage* 2012, 15;**62**:791–800.

35 Raichle ME, Snyder AZ. A default mode of brain function: a brief history of an evolving idea. *NeuroImage* 2007; **37**(4):1083–90 (discussion 1097–9).

36 Raichle ME, MacLeod AM, Snyder AZ, Powers WJ, Gusnard DA, Shulman GL. A default mode of brain function. *Proc Natl Acad Sci USA* 2001; **98**(2):676–82.

37 Favre P, Baciu M, Pichat C, Bougerol T, Polosan M. fMRI evidence for abnormal resting-state functional connectivity in euthymic bipolar patients. *J Affect Disord* 2014; **165**:182–9.

38 Teng S, Lu C-F, Wang P-S, et al. Altered resting-state functional connectivity of striatal-thalamic circuit in bipolar disorder. *PLoS ONE* 2014; **9**(5):e96422.

39 Vargas C, Lopez-Jaramillo C, Vieta E. A systematic literature review of resting state network—functional MRI in bipolar disorder. *J Affect Disord* 2013; **150**(3):727–35.

40 Kerestes R, Davey CG, Stephanou K, Whittle S, Harrison BJ. Functional brain imaging studies of youth depression: a systematic review. *Neuroimage Clin* 2013; 4:209–31.

41 Schilbach L, Müller VI, Hoffstaedter F, et al. Meta-analytically informed network analysis of resting state FMRI reveals hyperconnectivity in an introspective socio-affective network in depression. *PLoS ONE* 2014; **9**(4):e94973.

42 Ramasubbu R, Konduru N, Cortese F, Bray S, Gaxiola-Valdez I, Goodyear B. Reduced intrinsic connectivity of amygdala in adults with major depressive disorder. *Front Psychiatry* 2014; **5**:17.

43 Cocchi L, Harding IH, Lord A, Pantelis C, Yücel M, Zalesky A. Disruption of structure-function coupling in the schizophrenia connectome. *Neuroimage Clin* 2014; 4:779–87.

44 Tomasi D, Volkow ND. Mapping small-world properties through development in the human brain: disruption in schizophrenia. *PLoS ONE* 2014; **9**(4):e96176.

45 Yang GJ, Murray JD, Repovs G, et al. Altered global brain signal in schizophrenia. *Proc Natl Acad Sci USA* 2014; **111**(20):7438–43.

46 Castellanos FX, Margulies DS, Kelly C, et al. Cingulate-precuneus interactions: a new locus of dysfunction in adult attention-deficit/hyperactivity disorder. *Biol Psychiatry* 2008; **63**(3):332–7.

47 Posner J, Park C, Wang Z. Connecting the dots: a review of resting connectivity MRI studies in attention-deficit/hyperactivity disorder. *Neuropsychol Rev* 2014; **24**:3–15.

48 Cortese S, Kelly C, Chabernaud C, et al. Toward systems neuroscience of ADHD: a meta-analysis of 55 fMRI studies. *Am J Psychiatry* 2012; **169**(10):1038–55.

49 Pannekoek JN, Veer IM, van Tol M-J, et al. Aberrant limbic and salience network resting-state functional connectivity in panic disorder without comorbidity. *J Affect Disord* 2013; **145**(1):29–35.

50 Lai C-H, Wu Y-T. Decreased regional homogeneity in lingual gyrus, increased regional homogeneity in cuneus and correlations with panic symptom severity of first-episode, medication-naïve and late-onset panic disorder patients. *Psychiatry Res* 2013; **211**(2):127–31.

51 Shin Y-W, Dzemidzic M, Jo HJ, et al. Increased resting-state functional connectivity between the anterior cingulate cortex and the precuneus in panic disorder: resting-state connectivity in panic disorder. *J Affect Disord* 2013; **150**(3):1091–5.

52 Arnold Anteraper S, Triantafyllou C, Sawyer AT, Hofmann SG, Gabrieli JD, Whitfield-Gabrieli S. Hyper-connectivity of subcortical resting-state networks in social anxiety disorder. *Brain Connect* 2014; **4**(2):81–90.

53 Dodhia S, Hosanagar A, Fitzgerald DA, et al. Modulation of resting-state amygdala-frontal functional connectivity by oxytocin in generalized social anxiety disorder. *Neuropsychopharmacology* 2014; **39**:2061–9.

54 Liu F, Guo W, Fouche J-P, et al. Multivariate classification of social anxiety disorder using whole brain functional connectivity. *Brain Struct Func* 2013; **220**:101–15.

55 Pannekoek JN, Veer IM, van Tol M-J, et al. Resting-state functional connectivity abnormalities in limbic and salience networks in social anxiety disorder without comorbidity. *Eur Neuropsychopharmacol* 2013; **23**(3):186–95.

56 Hahn A, Stein P, Windischberger C, et al. Reduced resting-state functional connectivity between amygdala and orbitofrontal cortex in social anxiety disorder. *NeuroImage* 2011; **56**(3):881–9.

57 Chen AC, Etkin A. Hippocampal network connectivity and activation differentiates post-traumatic stress disorder from generalized anxiety disorder. *Neuropsychopharmacology* 2013; **38**(10):1889–98.

58 Brown VM, LaBar KS, Haswell CC, et al. Altered resting-state functional connectivity of basolateral and centromedial amygdala complexes in posttraumatic stress disorder. *Neuropsychopharmacology* 2014; **39**(2):351–9.

59 Roy AK, Fudge JL, Kelly C, et al. Intrinsic functional connectivity of amygdala-based networks in adolescent generalized anxiety disorder. *J Am Acad Child Adolesc Psychiatry* 2013; **52**(3):290–2.

60 Andreescu C, Sheu LK, Tudorascu D, Walker S, Aizenstein H. The ages of anxiety–differences across the lifespan in the default mode network functional connectivity in generalized anxiety disorder. *Int J Geriatr Psychiatry* 2014; **29**(7):704–12.

61 Stern ER, Fitzgerald KD, Welsh RC, Abelson JL, Taylor SF. Resting-state functional connectivity between fronto-parietal and default mode networks in obsessive-compulsive disorder. *PLoS ONE* 2012; **7**(5):e36356.

62 Posner J, Marsh R, Maia TV, Peterson BS, Gruber A, Simpson HB. Reduced functional connectivity within the limbic cortico-striato-thalamo-cortical loop in unmedicated adults with obsessive-compulsive disorder. *Hum Brain Mapp* 2013; **35**(6):2852–60.

63 Di Martino A, Yan C-G, Li Q, et al. The autism brain imaging data exchange: towards a large-scale evaluation of the intrinsic brain architecture in autism. *Mol Psychiatry* 2014; **19**(6):659–67.

64 Washington SD, Gordon EM, Brar J, et al. Dysmaturation of the default mode network in autism. *Hum Brain Mapp* 2014; **35**(4):1284–96.

65 Wolf RC, Sambataro F, Vasic N, et al. Aberrant connectivity of resting-state networks in borderline personality disorder. *J Psychiatry Neurosci* 2011; **36**(6):402–11.

66 Doll A, Sorg C, Manoliu A, et al. Shifted intrinsic connectivity of central executive and salience network in borderline personality disorder. *Front Hum Neurosci* 2013; **7**:727.

67 Cowdrey FA, Filippini N, Park RJ, Smith SM, McCabe C. Increased resting state functional connectivity in the default mode network in recovered anorexia nervosa. *Hum Brain Mapp* 2014; **35**(2):483–91.

68 Favaro A, Clementi M, Manara R, et al. Catechol-O-methyltransferase genotype modifies executive functioning and prefrontal functional connectivity in women with anorexia nervosa. *J Psychiatry Neurosci* 2013; **38**(4):241–8.

69 Favaro A, Santonastaso P, Manara R, et al. Disruption of visuospatial and somatosensory functional connectivity in anorexia nervosa. *Biol Psychiatry* 2012; **72**(10):864–70.

70 Amianto F, D'Agata F, Lavagnino L, et al. Intrinsic connectivity networks within cerebellum and beyond in eating disorders. *Cerebellum* 2013; **12**(5):623–31.

71 Lee S, Ran Kim K, Ku J, Lee J-H, Namkoong K, Jung Y-C. Resting-state synchrony between anterior cingulate cortex and precuneus relates to body shape concern in anorexia nervosa and bulimia nervosa. *Psychiatry Res* 2014; **221**(1):43–8.

72 Müller-Oehring EM, Jung Y-C, Pfefferbaum A, Sullivan EV, Schulte T. The resting brain of alcoholics. *Cereb Cortex* 2014. [Epub ahead of print]

73 Spagnolli F, Cerini R, Cardobi N, et al. Brain modifications after acute alcohol consumption analyzed by resting state fMRI. *Magn Reson Imaging* 2013; **31**(8):1325–30.

74 Ding X, Lee S-W. Cocaine addiction related reproducible brain regions of abnormal default-mode network functional connectivity: a group ICA study with different model orders. *Neurosci Lett* 2013; 548:110–4.

75 Konova AB, Moeller SJ, Tomasi D, Volkow ND, Goldstein RZ. Effects of methylphenidate on resting-state functional connectivity of the mesocorticolimbic dopamine pathways in cocaine addiction. *JAMA Psychiatry* 2013; **70**(8):857–68.

76 Wisner KM, Patzelt EH, Lim KO, MacDonald AW. An intrinsic connectivity network approach to insula-derived dysfunctions among cocaine users. *Am J Drug Alcohol Abuse* 2013; **39**(6):403–13.

77 Cisler JM, Elton A, Kennedy AP, et al. Altered functional connectivity of the insular cortex across prefrontal networks in cocaine addiction. *Psychiatry Res* 2013, 30;**213**:39–46

78 Kelly C, Zuo X-N, Gotimer K, et al. Reduced interhemispheric resting state functional connectivity in cocaine addiction. *Biol Psychiatry* 2011; **69**(7):684–92.

79 Pujol J, Blanco-Hinojo L, Batalla A, et al. Functional connectivity alterations in brain networks relevant to self-awareness in chronic cannabis users. *J Psychiatr Res* 2014; **51**:68–78.

80 Orr C, Morioka R, Behan B, et al. Altered resting-state connectivity in adolescent cannabis users. *Am J Drug Alcohol Abuse* 2013; **39**(6):372–81.

81 Qiu Y-W, Han L-J, Lv X-F, et al. Regional homogeneity changes in heroin-dependent in-
    dividuals: resting-state functional MR imaging study. *Radiology* 2011; **261**(2):551–9.

82 Wang Y, Zhu J, Li Q, et al. Altered fronto-striatal and fronto-cerebellar circuits in heroin-
    dependent individuals: a resting-state FMRI study. *PLoS ONE* 2013; **8**(3):e58098.

83 Jiang G, Wen X, Qiu Y, et al. Disrupted topological organization in whole-brain func-
    tional networks of heroin-dependent individuals: a resting-state FMRI study. *PLoS ONE*
    2013; **8**(12):e82715.

84 Ding W-N, Sun J-H, Sun Y-W, et al. Altered default network resting-state functional con-
    nectivity in adolescents with internet gaming addiction. *PLoS ONE* 2013; **8**(3):e59902.

85 Dong G, Huang J, Du X. Alterations in regional homogeneity of resting-state brain activity
    in internet gaming addicts. *Behav Brain Func* 2012; **8**(1):41.

86 Koehler S, Ovadia-Caro S, van der Meer E, et al. Increased functional connectivity between
    prefrontal cortex and reward system in pathological gambling. *PLoS ONE* 2013; **8**(12):e84565.

87 Tschernegg M, Crone JS, Eigenberger T, et al. Abnormalities of functional brain networks
    in pathological gambling: a graph-theoretical approach. *Front Hum Neurosci* 2013; **7**:625.

88 Buckner RL, Andrews-Hanna JR, Schacter DL. The brain's default network: anatomy,
    function, and relevance to disease. *Ann N Y Acad Sci* 2008; 1124:1–38.

89 Mantini D, Gerits A, Nelissen K, et al. Default mode of brain function in monkeys. *J Neu-
    rosci* 2011; **31**(36):12954–62.

90 Upadhyay J, Baker SJ, Chandran P, et al. Default-mode-like network activation in awake
    rodents. *PLoS ONE* 2011; **6**(11):e27839.

91 Lu H, Zou Q, Gu H, Raichle ME, Stein EA, Yang Y. Rat brains also have a default mode
    network. *Proc Natl Acad Sci USA* 2012; **109**(10):3979–84.

92 Zuo X-N, Di Martino A, Kelly C, et al. The oscillating brain: complex and reliable. *Neuro-
    Image* 2010; **49**(2):1432–45.

93 Harrison BJ, Pujol J, López-Solà M, et al. Consistency and functional specialization in the
    default mode brain network. *Proc Natl Acad Sci USA* 2008; **105**(28):9781–6.

94 Long X-Y, Zuo X-N, Kiviniemi V, et al. Default mode network as revealed with multiple
    methods for resting-state functional MRI analysis. *J Neurosci Meth* 2008; **171**(2):349–55.

95 Damoiseaux JS, Rombouts SARB, Barkhof F, et al. Consistent resting-state networks
    across healthy subjects. *Proc Natl Acad Sci USA* 2006; **103**(37):13848–53.

96 Fox MD, Snyder AZ, Vincent JL, Corbetta M, van Essen DC, Raichle ME. The human
    brain is intrinsically organized into dynamic, anticorrelated functional networks. *Proc Natl
    Acad Sci USA* 2005; **102**(27):9673–8.

97 Biomarkers Definitions Working Group. Biomarkers and surrogate endpoints: preferred
    definitions and conceptual framework. *Clin Pharmacol Ther* 2001; **69**(3): 89–95.

98 Linden DEJ. The challenges and promise of neuroimaging in psychiatry. *Neuron* 2012;
    73(1):8–22.

99 Bansal R, Staib LH, Laine AF, et al. Anatomical brain images alone can accurately diag-
    nose chronic neuropsychiatric illnesses. *PLoS ONE* 2012; **7**(12):e50698.

100 Sun D, van Erp TGM, Thompson PM, et al. Elucidating a magnetic resonance imaging-
    based neuroanatomic biomarker for psychosis: classification analysis using probabilistic
    brain atlas and machine learning algorithms. *Biol Psychiatry* 2009; **66**(11):1055–60.

101 Hart H, Chantiluke K, Cubillo AI, et al. Pattern classification of response inhibition in
    ADHD: toward the development of neurobiological markers for ADHD. *Hum Brain Mapp*
    2014; **35**(7):3083–94.

102 **Hart H, Marquand AF, Smith A, et al**. Predictive neurofunctional markers of attention-deficit/hyperactivity disorder based on pattern classification of temporal processing. *J Am Acad Child Adolesc Psychiatry* 2014; **53**(5):569–78.

103 **Cheng W, Ji X, Zhang J, Feng J**. Individual classification of ADHD patients by integrating multiscale neuroimaging markers and advanced pattern recognition techniques. *Front Syst Neurosci* 2012; **6**:58.

104 **Puls I, Mohr J, Wrase J, et al**. Synergistic effects of the dopaminergic and glutamatergic system on hippocampal volume in alcohol-dependent patients. *Biolog Psychol* 2008; **79**(1):126–36.

105 **Hahn T, Marquand AF, Plichta MM, et al**. A novel approach to probabilistic biomarker-based classification using functional near-infrared spectroscopy. *Hum Brain Mapp* 2013; **34**(5):1102–14.

106 **Wrase J, Makris N, Braus DF, et al**. Amygdala volume associated with alcohol abuse relapse and craving. *Am J Psychiatry* 2008; **165**(9):1179–84.

107 **McGrath CL, Kelley ME, Holtzheimer PE, et al**. Toward a neuroimaging treatment selection biomarker for major depressive disorder. *JAMA Psychiatry* 2013; **70**(8):821–9.

108 **Miller JM, Hesselgrave N, Ogden RT, et al**. Brain serotonin 1A receptor binding as a predictor of treatment outcome in major depressive disorder. *Biol Psychiatry* 2013; **74**(10):760–7.

109 **Delorenzo C, Delaparte L, Thapa-Chhetry B, Miller JM, Mann JJ, Parsey RV**. Prediction of selective serotonin reuptake inhibitor response using diffusion-weighted MRI. *Front Psychiatry* 2013; **4**:5.

110 **Hägele C, Schlagenhauf F, Rapp M, et al**. Dimensional psychiatry: reward dysfunction and depressive mood across psychiatric disorders. *Psychopharmacology (Berl)* 2015; **232**:331–41.

111 **Button KS, Ioannidis JPA, Mokrysz C, et al**. Power failure: why small sample size undermines the reliability of neuroscience. *Nat Rev Neurosci* 2013; **14**(5):365–76.

112 **Biswal BB, Mennes M, Zuo X-N, et al**. Toward discovery science of human brain function. *Proc Natl Acad Sci USA* 2010; **107**(10):4734–9.

113 **Salum GA, Sergeant J, Sonuga-Barke E, et al**. Specificity of basic information processing and inhibitory control in attention deficit hyperactivity disorder. *Psychol Med* 2013; **8**:1–15.

114 **HD-200 Consortium**. The ADHD-200 Consortium: a model to advance the translational potential of neuroimaging in clinical neuroscience. *Front Syst Neurosci* 2012; **6**:62.

115 **Schumann G, Loth E, Banaschewski T, et al**. The IMAGEN study: reinforcement-related behaviour in normal brain function and psychopathology. *Mol Psychiatry* 2010; **15**(12):1128–39.

116 **Nooner KB, Colcombe SJ, Tobe RH, et al**. The NKI-Rockland sample: a model for accelerating the pace of discovery science in psychiatry. *Front Neurosci* 2012; **6**:152.

117 **Craddock RC, Jbabdi S, Yan C-G, et al**. Imaging human connectomes at the macroscale. *Nat Meth* 2013; **10**-:524–39.

118 **Hampton T**. European-led project strives to simulate the human brain. *JAMA* 2014; **311**:1598–600.; 1598–600.

119 **Underwood E**. Neuroscience. BRAIN project meets physics. *Science* 2014; **30**:954–5.

Chapter 35

Psychotherapy in practice

Ana Moscoso, Jordan Sibeoni,
Nikolina Jovanovic, and Fritz Hohagen

Case study

Karen, a woman in her thirties, enters Marco's office. She is tall, dressed in a black coat and purple hat, very pale, and appears confused and frightened. She has asked for an appointment because she is depressed, having trouble coping with work and family, and wants antidepressant medication—at least that is what she has said to the nurse. The interview reveals that she has been suffering from depressive mood, lack of energy, and insomnia for a few months. It all started after her father died, but she remembers having mood changes in her early twenties, too. The father was abusive to her mother and did not dedicate much attention to Karen or her younger sister. At the end of the interview, she says she desperately needs help, but not medication—'I just want to talk with someone, you know . . . I need to talk with someone; I don't want to feel like this anymore . . . Can you help me?'

Marco is a young psychiatrist who just finished his training last year. The training was mainly biologically oriented, so he is very skilled in psychopharmacology. He did attend a few psychotherapy workshops, but feels insecure about using what he learned in clinical practice. During the interview, he manages to convert patient's symptoms into potential neurobiological abnormalities and has a very clear idea what medication to prescribe. However, now that the patient says she does not want medication, and only wants to talk, he is not sure what to do. Have you ever felt like Marco? How would you treat a patient like Karen?

Introduction

Psychotherapies are treatments performed through psychological means, based on specific techniques which stem from different theoretical models. Conducted either with an individual or in a group situation, they are all operate through an inter-human relationship that implies a 'changing process'.

If we consider a patient as a biopsychosocial unit, psychiatry needs to address all the disciplines that might enhance the knowledge and treatment of mental disease. From biology to anthropology, from psychology through sociology, psychiatric semiology needs to associate and integrate itself with the approach of the psychic functioning of the subject.

The 'changing process', the result of an effective psychotherapy, can be perceived subjectively, but might also be assessed with certain tools (quantitative and/or qualitative) and may even be seen through the modification of brain activity.[1] Therefore, psychotherapy might be turning a new page, as neuroimaging and specialized electroencephalograms help to define the neurophysiological basis of psychotherapeutic change.[2] These findings highlight how psychotherapy can be both a *psychological* and a *neurobiological* treatment.

Whether or not you find it relevant to become a psychotherapist (Table 35.1), psychiatrists will often find themselves placed in a psychotherapeutic position. However, being a psychotherapist does not just happen, and no one should be practicing psychotherapy without proper training.

Table 35.1 To train or not to train in psychotherapy?

'I'm not sure I need psychotherapy training at all. I am very skilled in psychopharmacology and if someone really needs psychotherapy, I can always make an appointment with a psychotherapist.'	Many colleagues work that way—one psychiatrist is focused on pharmacological treatment, and the other on psychotherapy. If that option makes you feel most comfortable, by all means continue to work like that.
	Not every psychiatrist should be a psychotherapist, but at least some basic psychotherapeutic training will be useful for you and your clinical practice, as it will improve your communication skills, understanding of non-verbal communication, as well as understanding of psychopathology.
'Not to forget the most important point—there is very little evidence that psychotherapy works! I am interested in evidence-based treatments.'	We agree that many studies in this field have significant methodological problems. The field urgently needs to develop more appropriate methodology to be able to grasp subtle changes that occur during the psychotherapeutic processes—most probably, a combined qualitative and quantitative approach, together with the use of novel technologies. However, at the same time, there are well-designed studies that point out that patients exposed to psychotherapy do get better, and when treatment combines biological and psychosocial methods, this is even more beneficial for them. Besides, many drug trials have severe methodological problems, too.
'It's time consuming! Training usually takes years to complete. Come on, who has that much time in life?'	This is true! It can take up to 4–5 years to complete the training. However, acquiring expertise does take time; it is as simple as that. We all agree that *ars longa, vita brevis est* . . . but if you want to take care of your patients in the best possible way, at least some talking therapy will come in very handy. The key point here is to plan your life, as well as your career, wisely. Probably the best time to do this training would be when you are a medical trainee, as that is when you are likely to have the least obligations in your private life.

(continued)

Table 35.1 (continued) To train or not to train in psychotherapy?

'It costs money! Did you know that my colleague calculated that the whole psychotherapy training costs the same value as one brand new BMW? I can't afford that, not with the mortgage, a second baby on the way…'	Again, you are right! Bills need to be paid, that is reality. However, try to look at this as investment in your future, because that is what it is basically. As stated previously, plan your career, choosing the timing wisely, and talk with your colleagues to see how are they dealing with this issue. Many training programmes give discounts and even loans for students.
	Another important point: studies suggest that in many European countries, patients prefer psychotherapy to drug treatment.[3] Besides, approximately half of our patients are suffering from disorders which also need to be treated through psychotherapy (BPD, OCD, anxiety, depression, etc.). Thus, psychiatrists will lose half of their patients to other professional groups if they are not well trained in psychotherapy.
'There are so many psychotherapy schools. How do I know which one to choose?'	Take your time! As we have just discussed, the training is costly and time-consuming, and you want to choose the school that is closest to your understanding of the world, and fits best with your personality and approach to patients. Worst case scenario would be that after three years you realize that you should have gone for, say, CBT instead of systemic therapy. To avoid that, get familiar with schools in your country— visit their open days, seminars, workshops; talk with other trainees. Do not be afraid to ask questions and discuss all you want before choosing what is best for you. This might take 6–12 months, or even longer.

How to practice psychotherapy

Psychotherapy is an art, but psychotherapies are techniques. Young psychiatrists train in psychotherapy very often at their own initiative and expense, to gain theoretical and technical expertise. Yet, once in practice, they will often perceive a gap. They will find, hidden in the gap, their own intimate and affective contribution to the psychotherapeutic practice, since good psychotherapy requires the therapist 'to prescribe himself'.[4] This 'personal prescription' and the patient–therapist match can be ultimately more important than the technique itself.[5]

Becoming a psychotherapist is, before anything else, a story of solitude and singularity. Not necessarily the therapist's singularity but the singularity of the interaction, of the asymmetric encounter between two persons, which is, definitely, what makes it beautiful.

The therapeutic part of any psychiatric consultation

The idea that psychiatric observation could be entirely scientific, neutral, reproducible, impartial, objective, and complete seems to be utopistic.[6]

The expression of a symptom is a reflection of a singular and individual experience and, at the same time, a reflection of a relationship which involves the psychiatrist. Therefore, the psychiatric encounter is decidedly subjective—moreover, *intersubjective*. Intersubjectivity should be present in every medical encounter, regardless of the specialty, but is often of increased importance in psychiatry where, most of the time, assessment relies on the interview itself. In psychiatry, the specific technical interview, validated by experience and clinical efficiency, should create a safe surrounding in which the patient feels comfortable to reveal their own narrative. Here again, the psychiatrist uses his own presence (his attitude, his awareness) as a part of a process that is simultaneously diagnostic and therapeutic. It is the therapeutic contact that allows the gathering of relevant information and assessment of psychopathology. It is within the intersubjective space that the patient can explore their feelings and thoughts.

Not only is the psychotherapeutic perspective essential throughout the interview, but it is also important to be aware that without a therapeutic alliance, the patient will less likely to take the prescribed treatment and the chances of improvement will also be lower.[7]

Non-specific determinants of psychotherapy

Throughout the years, some authors have tried to grasp what is common to every therapy. Psychotherapy integration grew out of increasing dissatisfaction with the continuous creation of new schools of therapy.[8]

Box 35.1 summarizes some of the *core processes* occurring within a psychotherapeutic setting. Every school will carry out these core processes differently, but the aim should still be the same.

There are also *non-specific factors* in all kinds of psychotherapy (Fig. 35.1). These present themselves in the patient, the therapist, and in the working alliance. The act of psychotherapy implies a relationship between one person (or a group) who suffers

---

Box 35.1 The core processes of psychotherapy

1 Engagement (or establishing and maintaining a therapeutic alliance)

2 Activating the patient's observing self

3 Searching for maladaptive patterns of functioning

4 Initiating and then maintaining change in those patterns

5 Saying good-bye

Source data from: Gabbard GO, *Textbook of Psychotherapeutic Treatments*, in Beitman BD, Chapter 26, Theory and Practice of Psychotherapy Integration, Copyright (2009), American Psychiatric Publishing.

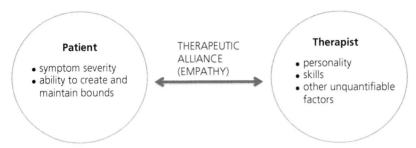

Fig. 35.1 Key non-specific factors in every psychotherapy treatment.

Source data from: Gabbard GO, *Textbook of Psychotherapeutic Treatments*, in Beitman BD, Chapter 26, Theory and Practice of Psychotherapy Integration, Copyright (2009), American Psychiatric Publishing.

and another person (or another group) invested with the role of psychotherapist. This therapeutic relationship hinges on the humane and ethical features of the therapist and the patient's ability to create an alliance.

On the patient's side, there is a reason for being in therapy, an ability to create and maintain bonds, and a motivation and expectations regarding the therapy. On the psychotherapist's side stand their personality, warmth, tolerance, ability to listen, and especially their empathy, along with other unquantifiable factors. All psychotherapy is based on the phenomenon of empathy, as defined as the ability of being in the place of the other, of representing the other, both emotionally and cognitively.[9] The dynamics of empathy rely on the interactions between therapist and patient; on the ability of the therapist to reflect (questioning his own representations and practice) and to recognize the otherness of the patient.

Why do some psychiatrists relate to psychotherapy more than others?

What makes a psychiatrist feel enthusiastic about psychotherapy? And within the field of psychotherapy, what makes him choose particular models? Several reasons can be given. Notable among them is the degree of exposure to psychotherapy and different kinds of psychotherapy, particularly during training, and also the psychiatrist's personality or propensity for the field itself.

'Believing' in psychotherapy implies the rejection of Cartesian dualism in which mind and brain are artificially separated from each other. Psychotherapy must work by changing the brain, and the mind is the activity of the brain.[10]

In order to become a psychotherapist, the psychiatrist needs to be willing to detach himself from what is clinical and theoretical a priori, and to apprehend the situation through the bias of his feelings, his sensations, his intuition, himself. The psychiatrist needs to constantly reflect on and question his own subjectivity. Therefore, he needs *to observe, to observe himself*, and, at a *meta* level, *to observe himself while observing*.

The psychiatrist also needs to continuously review his relationship with psychopathology, acknowledging that his psychiatric knowledge is 'formed/deformed by his history, his parents, his educators, his mentors, his personal experiences, his curiosity, his capacity for judgement and critique, his ability to question what he has or hasn't learned'.[11]

The psychiatrist who wants to become a psychotherapist cannot, unlike in many other fields, function within a role 'that excludes the connoisseur from his own knowledge'.[12] We do not propose here to embrace subjectivism; rather, to place psychiatry in a permanent dialogue between the objective knowledge and the subjective reflection.

Supervision in psychotherapy

The psychiatrist-psychotherapist should benefit from individual supervision, thought of as an asymmetrical relationship that co-builds and is based on empathy and recognition of otherness. It is also important to meet and form supervisory groups, to elaborate on and confront perspectives.

Models and theory applied to practice

To date, there are numerous psychotherapeutic strategies used across the world. In this section, we aim to present well-established theories and techniques currently used in mental health, through a short description of each and with reference to the clinical example from the beginning of the chapter. As the chapter title suggests, the idea is to describe psychotherapy in practice, and not necessarily to discuss, exhaustively, every model. Therefore, with the help of our clinical case study example, Karen, we will illustrate how therapists from different schools would treat this patient.

It is important to bear in mind that, despite their empirical use, not every technique has been equally evidence-base tested. For instance, cognitive and behavioural therapy is by far better evidence-base tested than all the other therapies. On the other hand, one should remember that what works in research, what has been 'tested', does not necessarily work in community settings.

Theoretical models (the main roots)

Cognitive behavioural therapy (CBT)

CBT stands for a range of psychotherapies focusing on human behavioural, cognitive, emotional, and social development and human functioning. CBT is now an established approach as it has proved its efficacy in a wide range of conditions such as anxiety and depressive disorders,[13] psychotic disorders, and other diagnostic groups. It can be applied individually and in group settings.

The therapeutic work can progress both during sessions and outside them. Between sessions, the patient might have some assignments (or homework) to do, in order to test and challenge the dysfunctional beliefs and behaviour. A CBT therapist tends to be directive: he/she instructs and coaches, so that his/her patients can learn how to identify dysfunctional and negative thoughts from healthy ones.

Usually, the therapist sets a therapeutic programme during the first interview to decide the main goals and the number of sessions required to achieve them (usually between 10 and 20). During sessions, several CBT techniques can be used, as stated in Table 35.2.

Table 35.2 CBT techniques

Cognitive theory[14,15]	Enables the exploration of mental processes such as thinking, knowing, remembering, judging, and problem solving—gathered under the umbrella of 'cognition'.
	Psychopathological symptoms are seen as the consequence of distortions in cognitive processes, which produce cognitive patterns of malfunctioning (such as selective abstraction, arbitrary inference, or overgeneralization). The aim of cognitive therapy is to correct these cognitive distortions.
Behaviourism[16]	Its main assumption is that human behaviour is learned and influenced by the environment, which selects the adaptive behaviours. Thus, behavioural responses are conditioned, especially during the learning process.
'Third wave' psychotherapies[17] Dialectical behaviour therapy[18]	The focus of the therapy goes beyond just cognition and behaviour.
Metacognitive therapy[19] Mindfulness-based cognitive therapy (MBCT)[20,21] Acceptance and commitment therapy[22]	They are more integrative, and take into account interpersonal, environmental, and emotional factors.

Case study (continued)

In CBT, depression can be understood as the result of depressive cognitions. While focusing on the *cognitive modification of thoughts and emotions*, you can help Karen to learn how to identify pessimistic verbalization and how to counter her depressive thoughts/cognitions in order to have a more rational, than emotional, representation of reality. She will learn how to question herself by saying 'How can I think differently in this particular situation?' She will then identify her cognitive patterns/distortions. Each cognitive pattern will then be treated separately, before being finally integrated together, in order to exit these patterns.

You might also apply *behavioural interventions* which focus on reinforcing more adaptive responses such as habituation or exposure (real or imaginary); operant conditioning (positive or negative reinforcement to increase or inhibit behaviour) can be used. If you want to address Karen's difficulties of performance (at work and at home with the family), a progressive reattribution of tasks that promotes the recovery of activity can be also included.

Psychodynamic and psychoanalytical therapies

Since the conceptualization of psychoanalysis by Freud, many authors have added their own concepts and techniques. Nowadays, there is no homogeneity in the field of psychoanalysis, neither in its practice, nor in its theory.

The main assumption of psychoanalysis is the existence of the unconscious (i.e. mental activity taking place outside of the conscious sphere of the mind). The unconscious would be made from sexual instincts that have been repressed in order to solve a psychic conflict between these instincts and reality. When repression fails, what has been repressed returns into consciousness in the shape of dreams, lapses, missteps, and psychopathological symptoms. Psychoanalysis aims to make the patient discover the link between their symptoms and past experience.

Three core elements are to be considered in psychodynamic practice: active listening, free association of ideas, and interpretation. Free association of ideas by the patient provides access to the underlying thoughts behind fantasies. Listening to the patient, respecting the silences and the unspoken, allows transference (the projection of the patient's unconscious desires to the analyst). The interpretation of this transference, and also of the therapist's counter-transference (therapist's own reaction to the patient's projections) is the very core of psychoanalytic treatment.

It is common to make a distinction between the standard psychoanalytical cure and psychodynamic individual psychotherapy (PIP). The psychoanalytical cure is based on a framework made of rules decided jointly by the therapist and the patient. Basically, the patient lies on a couch, with the therapist sitting behind him or her. Sessions are regular (often several per week) and the location, duration, and timings are fixed. Usually, the cure takes place over several years. This form of psychoanalytical treatment is indicated in the case of neurosis. PIP is based on psychoanalytic concepts but therapists and patients are face to face, duration of the treatment is shorter, and indications are broader, including personality disorders.

Case study (continued)

If treating Karen through psychoanalysis, you will certainly address her in a less directive and more global fashion. Your treatment will most probably be intense (at least one session per week) and over a long period (months, possibly years). You will be non-directive, and you will take interest in her past experiences, conscious and unconscious.

In the case of Karen, her depression could be linked to the loss (of the love)[23] of an object (actual or ancient) and the mourning process that goes with that loss.[24] This object might be between conscious and unconscious. During the session, the loss of the object will be re-enacted within the relationship between the psychotherapist and Karen. Additionally, growing up in a dysfunctional family with an abusive and neglectful father counts as a traumatic experience that might be reflected in Karen's perception of trust, reliability on other people, and intimate relations. This is also something that could be resolved through a positive emotional experience with a therapist (so-called 'corrective emotional experience').

Karen will be more suited for PIP, as are most psychiatric (non-neurotic) patients. Later in her treatment, Karen might benefit from psychodynamic group therapy.

Mentalization-based therapy

Mentalization-based therapy (MBT) has been developed by Peter Fonagy and Anthony Bateman, and has roots in psychodynamic psychotherapy. The process of mentalizing is a preconscious, imaginative mental activity, which consists of giving a sense to our subjective mental state and to who we are within the context of personal and social interactions. MBT is also intuitive and emotional, and highlights the importance of the therapist rather than the technique.

According to Bateman and Fonagy,[25] focusing on mentalization provides an appropriate domain for therapeutic intervention in many disorders, such as borderline personality disorders (BPD), in which disturbance of mentalizing could have contributed to its development. Indeed, those suffering BPD have shown a fragile mentalizing and reflective capacity, especially in the context of attachment relationships. BPD perfectly suits this technique, and most studies and papers about MBT focus on the treatment of individuals with BPD. However, recent developments have included its use in other situations such as depression, post-traumatic stress disorder (PTSD), eating disorders,[26] and in family therapy and adolescence.[27]

Steps towards progressive mentalization are displayed in Table 35.3.

Table 35.3 Steps towards progressive mentalization

Step 1: Explore the patient's subjective experience	The therapist must consider that it is impossible to know what the patient has in mind, regarding the opacity of mental state, and that it is better not to make assumptions about the patient's feelings. Instead, it is better to actively question the patient, exploring his/her subjective experience in order to elicit all perspectives and points of view.
Step 2: Work within the attachment framework	The therapist has to work within the attachment framework since any one-to-one psychotherapy will activate the attachment system.
Step 3: Adapt according to the mentalizing capacity of the patient	In adapting, the therapist will move from less complex interventions (when the patient has high emotional intensity and low mentalizing), to much more complex interventions (when the patient has moderate–low emotional intensity and high mentalizing). In this process, the therapist may move backwards and forwards between interventions, according to the moment and the patient's state of mind (e.g. emotional arousal, intensity of attachment, need to avoid a perceived threat).
Step 4: Maintain mentalizing and reinstate it in both the therapist and the patient	This is the ultimate task for the therapist.

Source data from: Gabbard GO, *Textbook of Psychotherapeutic Treatments*, in Bateman A, Fonagy P, Allen, JG, Chapter 28, Theory and Practice of Mentalization-Based Therapy, Copyright (2009), American Psychiatric Publishing.

Case study (Continued)

Within MBT, you might start to acknowledge, with Karen, how depression impairs her ability to mentalize. Indeed, the lack of energy to live and think leads to a lack of initiative to mentalize. As depression is very often associated with self-absorption and social isolation, Karen's other mental states will also be impaired. This distorted mentalizing contributes to a vicious cycle of depression.[28] With Karen, you might then pursue the process of getting free from 'being locked into the reality of one view' by generating multiple perspectives. This process develops by engaging the patient in a real dialogue, and not by leading Karen to pre-established conclusions. In other words, she will be able to move from the psychic equivalence mode (mind = world) to the mentalizing mode (mind represents the world in many different ways). In order to achieve it, the therapist's goals are: 'to promote (1) mentalizing about oneself, (2) mentalizing about others and (3) mentalizing of relationships'.[29] Within MBT, you will also explore the relationship Karen had with her father throughout the years. This might open a door to her attachment framework, which is very probably a key determinant to the development of her depressive state.

Family therapy

Appearing in the USA in the 1950s, family psychotherapy (whether treating individuals/children, their parents, or families) focuses on the relational context, addresses patterns of interaction and meaning, and aims to facilitate personal and interpersonal resources within a system (i.e. a functional unit).

In a chain of influence, every action is also a reaction; interactions within the system are treated as having circular dynamics rather than linear causality.

Historically, we can distinguish two main theoretical models: *psychoanalytic family therapy*, focused on the present and transgenerational family history as well as on the psychic apparatus of the group; and *systemic family therapy*, initially conceptualized from communication theory (Palo Alto School) and general systems theory, and later enriched by new theoretical–practical approaches (Whitaker's symbolic–experiential approach, structural family therapy from Minuchin, contextual therapy from Boszormenyi-Nagy, strategic model of Jay Haley, etc.). In practice, there are many applications and indications, and the approach can change from one team to the other.

Sessions that are performed in active co-therapy, with direct supervision that allows a supervisor to observe the session and intervene if needed, are becoming increasingly popular. Very often, sessions are also recorded to allow supervision work between sessions.

Case study (continued)

In family therapy, the whole family is invited to the session (in the case of Karen, her husband and children are invited to the session) and their interactions become the scope of therapy. Despite the children's age, the observation of the interactions between parents and children can give us important information, and they are usually welcome to the sessions. However, if the couple's problems are significant, we might think about excluding the children from couple therapy, just as one would close the bedroom door.[30]

During the first sessions, it might be useful to *map the family system*, and this can be achieved by using genograms and timelines. A *genogram* will help in tracking the family system (the ones who live together but also significant others). A *timeline*[31] will allow the identification of nodal events and important stressors (very often associated with developmental transitions such as the beginning of a family and children going to school, and other unrelated ones such as unemployment and racism). A timeline will also help to detect repetitive patterns of behaviour, covert linkage, and unresolved conflict and losses, particularly when similar developmental challenges are confronted. The therapist will help the family to make meaning of their crisis and to regain a positive outlook,[32] which will contribute to problem resolution.

It is important to bear in mind that, in Karen's case, the family therapist should be addressing her individual problems through the scope of the whole family. The latter is not to be considered as source to the pathology, but as a partner in delivering the treatment, since Karen's symptoms might display a function on family communication or homoeostatis.

Psychotherapy with specific populations

Psychotherapy with babies

Psychotherapy in early stages is of extreme importance, given the limitations of psychopharmacology. The scope is generally the interaction between the primary caregiver (usually the mother, but also the father, together or alone) and the baby.

Child–parent psychotherapy is a relationship-based treatment for infants, toddlers, and pre-schoolers who are experiencing mental health problems or who are at risk for such disturbances due to parental mental illness, maladaptive parenting practices, discordant parent–child temperament styles, and/or adverse life experiences.[33] The practice has psychoanalytic origins, in the work of Anna Freud and Melanie Klein, with later eminent inputs from Bolwby's theory of attachment and Margaret Mahler and Selma Feinberg's observation of babies, among other relevant authors.

This work enables a better adjustment in the parent–child dyad, in turn helping to solve sleeping problems, eating disorders, or excessive crying. The early recognition and treatment of autism is also within the scope of infant psychotherapy.

Later developments of these techniques, such as the approach proposed by Greenspan,[34] strengthen the importance of cognitive and affective development through interactive play. This technique is often used in the evaluation and detection of autism spectrum disorders.

Early childhood family-based therapy and MBT are also practiced, to a lesser extent.

Psychotherapy with children

Working with children implies that the therapist must alter the developmental stage of the children in question (which is not necessarily the chronological age), replacing behaviours and other patterns typical of earlier development with more mature adaptive capacities.[35] In others words, the therapist aims to help children to return to the path of normal development.[36]

It is important to bear in mind that younger children respond better to more frequent sessions.[37] Parent coaching and their implication in the treatment is important, but this also depends on the technique being used. Common techniques are psychodynamic play therapy (the first one to be created), CBT applied for children, and family therapy. All child psychotherapies aim to reduce risk and enhance developmental processes that constitute resilience. As important as the work with the individual child is, the home emotional environment will necessarily also need to be addressed.

Psychotherapy with adolescents

Remembering that psychotherapy with adolescents is also developmentally based, the need for individual assessment and follow-up is increasingly important.

From the first psychoanalytic techniques, to CBT and systemic models, or the more recent adaptations of interpersonal therapy (IPT-A) and MBT-A, the range of therapies that can be applied to adolescents is quickly being developed.

Adolescence is a time of transition that implies the maturation of psychical, cognitive, emotional, and social abilities, enabling the individual to reach adulthood. However, asynchronies in development across these domains are very frequent and almost expectable. Therapists might enable transition in moments of crisis (how to adapt to change) or emergent psychopathology.

Despite the increasing experience of autonomy during adolescence (individually and culturally determined), engaging with parents and family in the treatment is usually required, and the working alliance needs to address both. Group therapy with peers is also a very popular strategy during this phase of development.

Psychotherapy in old age

Despite the early doubts of using psychotherapy to treat people in old age, research in the field has been impressively developed. Beliefs that this population group were less able to change (and for a shorter time), are now being put aside, given the overwhelming evidence of an increasingly ageing society and of the specific needs of this group.

Beforehand, it is important to remember how ageing can be a source of prejudice and discriminatory practice,[38] leading practitioners to work on a denial basis (e.g. 'you look much younger than you are' is commonly heard in health facilities). It is also important to bear in mind intersubjectivity when addressing this age group (e.g. they are not homogeneous, they are not necessarily cognitive impaired).

Conditions such as depression have been addressed extensively, by using tools such as CBT and psychodynamic and interpersonal therapies. Reminiscence therapy (a counselling tool, usually group-based, that is often used to enable the elderly to gain perspective on their lives) and life review therapy (a more in-depth tool that might enable the reworking of past conflicts) were specially designed for this age group. Family therapy is not often used, developed, or researched, except in situations where families are confronted with cognitively impaired elders.[38]

Psychotherapy with migrants and culture-based therapies

Since Kraepelin[39] and his travels to Java Island in 1904, many authors have tried to address the link between culture and psychiatry. The question of culture has been tackled in psychotherapeutic settings for quite some time now, and it is becoming more important every day, given the increased flow of migration as a result of globalization.

Culture can be defined as 'a set of meanings, behavioural norms, values, everyday practices and beliefs used by members of a given group in society as a way of conceptualizing their view of the world and their interactions with the environment'.[40]

Table 35.4 Different culture-based therapies

Intracultural therapy	Patient and therapist share the same cultural background.
Intercultural or cross-cultural therapy	Patient and therapist are not from the same culture but the therapist has an anthropological knowledge of the patient's culture.
	This model is in line with cross-cultural research and leads to the acknowledgement of specific psychotherapeutic issues for particular cultural or ethnic groups, and also to the creation of specific psychotherapeutic settings.
Transcultural therapy	Patient and the therapist are not from the same culture but the therapist is aware of the importance of culture for mankind.
	Ethnopsychiatry is inscribed in this model.

Source data from: Devereux G, *Essais d'ethnopsychiatrie generale*, Copyright (1983), Gallimard.

According to Georges Devereux,[41] there are three possibilities when considering the cultural backgrounds of therapist and patient: intracultural therapy; intercultural or cross-cultural therapy; and transcultural or *meta*-cultural therapy, as explained in Table 35.4.

The model of ethnopsychiatry (or ethnopsychoanalysis), conceptualized by Devereux, belongs to the last category. Ethnopsychiatry relies on the principles of psychic universality (that psychic functioning is what defines being human and that every human being and every cultural or psychic production have then the same value) and of cultural encoding (that every man moves towards the universal through the particularities of his culture). The 'complementary method' prescribes that anthropology and psychoanalysis should not be used simultaneously to treat migrants and to explore the patient's discourse on both a cultural and individual level. A transcultural therapist will analyse both individual and cultural counter-transference.

Based on this theoretical framework, some specific care devices have been created for first- and second-generation migrants.[42] The classic setting is of group therapy, with one lead therapist surrounded by a number of co-therapists from several cultural and linguistic backgrounds. An interpreter is present, who can translate back and forth between the patient's native language and the language of the new country.

Status of the psychiatric psychotherapist and training issues across Europe

Whether or not psychotherapy becomes part of psychiatry is clearly an issue of ongoing debate across Europe, and relates to epistemological conflicts between the different paradigms found in psychiatry and to the broad diversity of psychotherapies.

Recognized institutions such as the European Union of Medical Specialties (UEMS) Section of Psychiatry[43] and Child and Adolescent Psychiatry,[44] acknowledge the need of psychotherapy as a treatment tool in psychiatry and the importance of it being taught during training. As UEMS recently stated:

> It is crucial for psychiatry that the scope of psychotherapy is well defined and that all psychiatrists are qualified to use psychotherapeutic interventions in everyday treatment of psychiatric patients. The psychiatrist should therefore be familiar with the effective factors common to all psychotherapies and the way of assessing, defining the treatment plan, the setting and evaluation. Any type of psychotherapeutic training—independent of theoretical school—should put emphasis on the above mentioned.
>
> Reproduced from European Union of Medical Specialists.
> Report of the UEMS Section of Psychiatry, Copyright (2004) UEMS

However, the way psychotherapy is carried out across Europe is clearly heterogeneous, despite ongoing efforts at standardization. A survey conducted by the UEMS Section of Psychiatry in 2004 revealed many differences across European countries; for example, in its recognition as a core professional aspect, in its use as a therapeutic tool, in professional renumeration.[43] Heterogeneity is also perceived by early career psychiatrists who, nevertheless, do not seem dissatisfied, in general, with the training they receive in psychotherapy and feel confident to use it in their daily work. [45]

Some specific concerns from trainees regarding psychotherapy were highlighted by Nawka and relate to three specific areas: concerns about clinical opportunities, concerns about funding and availability of psychotherapy courses, and finally, concerns regarding personal psychotherapy (considered important but only encouraged and financially supported in a few European countries).[46]

Training in psychotherapy remains a crucial cornerstone for psychiatric training. The European Federation of Psychiatric Trainees (EFPT) have also endorsed the importance of a working knowledge of psychotherapy as an integral part of being a psychiatrist.[47] A statement from the Board of Psychiatry of UEMS[43] recommended training in the theory of psychotherapy that lasts at least 120 hours, with supervision (preferably individual and group) provided on a regular basis for at least 100 hours. The recommendations of the Child and Adolescent Psychiatry Section of UEMS mentioned the need of an academic base for psychotherapeutic work with children, adolescents, and their families, as well as the need for training in specific models such as psychoanalytic/psychodynamic individual psychotherapy, cognitive behavioural psychotherapy, or family psychotherapy.[44] Despite these recommendations, several European countries fail to include any form of psychotherapeutic training in their curricula.[48]

Conclusion

In conclusion, psychotherapeutic treatments are alive and well in psychiatry and will remain so in the future. However, the field desperately needs more focused research and development of appropriate methodology that will be able to detect subtle changes that occur during the psychotherapeutic process. We agree with UEMS and fully support their view that it is crucial, for psychiatry, that the scope of psychotherapy is well defined and that all psychiatrists are qualified to use psychotherapeutic interventions in everyday treatment of psychiatric patients. We can only hope that trainees and young psychiatrists are aware of this and will search for opportunities to train in psychotherapy.

References

1 Barsaglini A, Sartori G, Benetti S, Pettersson-Yeo W, Mechelli A. The effects of psychotherapy on brain function: a systematic and critical review. *Prog Neurobiol* 2014; **114**:1–14.

2 Beitman BD, Viamontes GI, Soth AM, et al. Toward a neural circuitry of engagement, self-awareness, and pattern search. *Psychiatr Ann* 2006; **36**:272–82.

3 McHugh RK, et al. Patient preference for psychological vs pharmacologic treatment of psychiatric disorders: a meta-analytic review. *J Clin Psychiatry* 2013; **74**(6):595–602.

4 Balint M. The crisis of medical practice. *Am J Psychoanal* 2002; **62**(1):7–15.

5 Blow AJ, et al. Is who delivers the treatment more important than the treatment itself? The role of the therapist in common factors. *J Marital Fam Ther* 2007; **33**(3):298–317.

6 Lempérière T, et al. *Psychiatrie de l'adulte* (2nd edn). Paris: Elsevier Masson; 2006.

7 Krupnick JL, et al. The role of the therapeutic alliance in psychotherapy and pharmacotherapy outcome: findings in the National Institute of Mental Health Treatment of Depression Collaborative Research Program. *J Consult Clin Psychol* 1996; **64**:532–9.

8 Prochaska JO, Norcross JC. *Systems of psychotherapy: a trans-theoretical analysis*. New York: Thompson Books/Cole; 2007.

9 Beitman BD. Theory and Practice of Psychotherapy Integration. In: Textbook of Psychotherapeutic Treatments. (ed. Gabbard GO). American Psychiatric Publishing; 2009.

10 Gabbard GO. Preface. In: *Textbook of psychotherapeutic treatments* (ed. Gabbard GO). American Psychiatric Publishing; 2009.

11 Bogaert E. Le diagnostique et une écriture. *Sud/Nord* 2009; **24**:1–43.

12 Morin E. La connaissance de la connaissance. La methode 3. Paris: Seuil; 1986.

13 Hofmann S, et al. The efficacy of cognitive behavioural therapy: a review of meta-analyses. *Cogn Ther Res* 2012; **36**:427–40.

14 Beck A, et al. *Cognitive therapy of depression*. New York: Guilford Press; 1979.

15 Beck J. *Cognitive behaviour therapy: basics and beyond* (2nd edn). New York: Guilford; 2011.

16 Skinner BF. The operational analysis of psychological terms. *Behav Brain Sci* 1984; **7**(4):547–81.

17 Beck AT. Comparing CBT with third wave therapies. *Cogn Ther Today* 2012; **17**:1–2, 6.

18 Linehan MM. *Cognitive behavioural training for borderline personality disorder*. New York: Guilford Press; 1993.

19 Wells A. *Metacognitive therapy for anxiety and depression*. New York: Guilford Press; 2009.

20 Sipe WE, Eisendrath SJ. Mindfulness-based cognitive therapy: theory and practice. *Can J Psychiatry* 2012; **57**(2);63–9.

21 Segal ZV, Williams JMG, Teasdale JD. *Mindfulness-based cognitive therapy for depression: a new approach to preventing relapse*. New York: Guilford Press; 2002.

22 Hayes SC, Strosahl KD, Wilson KG. *Acceptance and commitment therapy: an experiential approach to behavior change*. New York: Guilford Press; 1999.

23 **Coimbra de Matos A**. *A depressão: episódios de um percurso em busca do seu sentido* (3rd edn). Lisboa: Climepsi Editores; 2007.

24 **Freud S**. Trauer und melancholie. *Intern Zeitschrift Psychoanalyse* 1917; **4**(6):288–301.

25 **Bateman A, Fonagy P**. *Mentalization-based treatment for borderline personality disorder: a practical guide*. Oxford, UK: Oxford University Press; 2006.

26 **Skardelud F**. Eating one's words. Part III: mentalisation-based psychotherapy for anorexia nervosa-an outline for a treatment and training manual. *Eur Eat Disord Rev* 2007; **15**:323–39.

27 **Fearon P et al**. Short-term mentalization and relational therapy (SMART): an integrative family therapy for children and adolescents. In: *Handbook of mentalization-based treatment* (eds. Allen JG, Fonagy P). Chichester, UK: Wiley; 2006, pp. 201–22.

28 **Tobias G**. et al. Enhancing mentalizing through psycho-education. In: *Handbook of mentalization-based treatment* (eds. Allen JG, Fonagy P). Chichester, UK: Wiley; 2006, pp. 249–269.

29 **Bateman A, Fonagy P, Allen, JG**. Chapter 28. Theory and practice of mentalization-based therapy. In: *Textbook of psychotherapeutic treatments* (ed. Gabbard GO). American Psychiatric Publishing; 2009.

30 **Rolland JS, Walsh F**. Chapter 18. Family systems theory and practice. In: *Textbook of psychotherapeutic treatments* (ed. Gabbard GO). American Psychiatric Publishing; 2009.

31 **Haley J**. *Problem-solving therapy*. San Francisco, CA: Jossey-Bass; 1976.

32 **Griffith J, Griffith ME**. *Encountering the sacred in psychotherapy: how to talk with people about their spiritual lives*. New York: Guilford Press; 2002.

33 **Lieberman A, Van Horn P**. Child-parent psychotherapy: a developmental approach to mental health treatment in infancy and early childhood. In: *Handbook of infant mental health* (3rd edn) (ed. Zeanah CH). New York: Guilford Press, 2009, p. 439–449.

34 The Greenspan Floortime Approach. Homepage at: http://www.stanleygreenspan.com/

35 **Target M**, et al. Psychosocial therapies with children. In: *Oxford textbook of psychotherapy* (ed. Gabbard GO, Beck JS, Holmes J). Oxford: Oxford University Press; 2005, p. 341.

36 **Freud A**. *Normality and pathology in childhood: assessments of development*. Madison, CT: International Universities Press; 1965.

37 **Target M, Fonagy P**. The efficacy of psychoanalysis for children with emotional disorders. *JAACAP* 1994; **33**:361–71.

38 **Cook JM, et al**. (2005). Psychotherapy with older adults. In: *Oxford textbook of psychotherapy* (ed. Gabbard GO, Beck JS, Holmes J). Oxford: Oxford University Press; 2005, p. 381.

39 **Hufschmitt L**. Kraepelin à Java. *Synapse* 1992; **86**:69–75.

40 **Alarcon RD, Ruiz P**. Theory and practice of cultural psychiatry in the United States and abroad. *Rev Psychiatry* 1995; **14**:599–626.

41 **Devereux G**. *Essais d'ethnopsychiatrie generale*. Paris: Gallimard; 1983.

42 **Moro MR**. *Psychopathologie transculturelle des enfants et des adolescents*. Paris: Dunod; 2000.

43 **UEMS**. *Psychotherapy: report of the UEMS Section for Psychiatry*. Edinburgh; 2004. Available at: http://uemspsychiatry.org/wp-content/uploads/2013/09/2004Apr-Psychotherapy.pdf

44 **Tsiantis J, Piha J, Deboutte D**. *Guidelines on psychotherapy*. UEMS Section-Board on Child and Adolescent Psychiatry/Psychotherapy (CAPP)/Working Group on Psychotherapy; 2009. Available at: http://www.uemscap.eu/training

45 **Fiorillo A**. Training and practice of psychotherapy in Europe: results of a survey. *World Psychiatry* 2011; **10**(3): 238.

46 **Nawka A, et al**. Mental health reforms in Europe: challenges of postgraduate psychiatric training in Europe: a trainee perspective. *Psychiatr Serv* 2010; **61**(9):862–4.

47 EFPT Psychotherapy Working Group. Homepage at: http://www.efpt.eu/page.php/ Psychotherapy

48 **Kuzman MR, et al**. Psychiatry training in Europe: views from the trenches. Med Teach2012; **34**(10):e708–7017.

Index